1. Amsler's Grid

The chart on the opposite page is patterned after the grid devised by Professor Marc Amsler. It can provide for the rapid detection of small irregularities in the central 20° of the field of vision. The chart is composed of a grid of lines containing a central white fixation spot. The squares on the grid are 5 mm in size and subtend a visual angle of 1° at 30 cm viewing distance.

The chart is to be viewed in modest light monocularly at a distance of 28-30 cm utilizing the correct refraction for this distance. Viewing should be accomplished without previous ophthalmoscopy and without instillation of any drugs affecting pupillary size or accommodation.

A series of questions should be asked while the patient is viewing the central white spot.

1) Is the center spot visible? The absence of the spot may indicate the presence of a central scotoma.

2) While viewing the center white spot can you see all four sides? The inability to perceive these areas may indicate the presence of an arcuate scotoma of glaucoma encroaching upon the central area or a centrocecal scotoma.

3) Do you see the entire grid intact? Are there any defects? If an area of the grid is not visible, then a paracentral scotoma is present.

4) Are the horizontal and vertical lines straight and parallel? If not, then metamorphopsia is present. The parallel lines may "bend" inwards giving rise to micropsia or "bend" outwards giving rise to macropsia.

5) Do you see any blur or distortion in the grid? Any movement? A color aberration? These changes may be present prior to the appearance of a definite scotoma.

Complete your drug reference library with these 5 essential volumes!

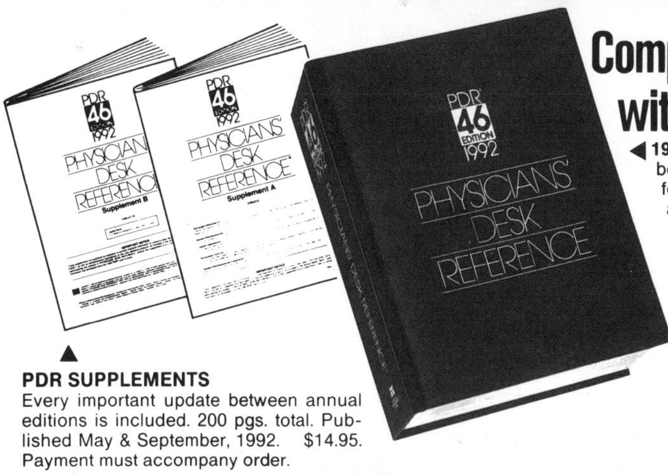

PDR SUPPLEMENTS
Every important update between annual editions is included. 200 pgs. total. Published May & September, 1992. $14.95. Payment must accompany order.

1992 PHYSICIANS' DESK REFERENCE® Scores of new drugs have been added making previous volumes obsolete. Features include four complete indices • full-color, actual-size photographs • fast, accurate look-ups of all FDA-required information • use-in-pregnancy ratings • and much more. 2,500 pgs. Published December, 1991. $54.95.

1992 PDR FOR NONPRESCRIPTION DRUGS®
Vital information on OTC drug products: ingredients, indications, drug interactions, dosage, administration, and more. Four complete indices, full-color photo section. 800 pgs. Published February, 1992. $35.95.

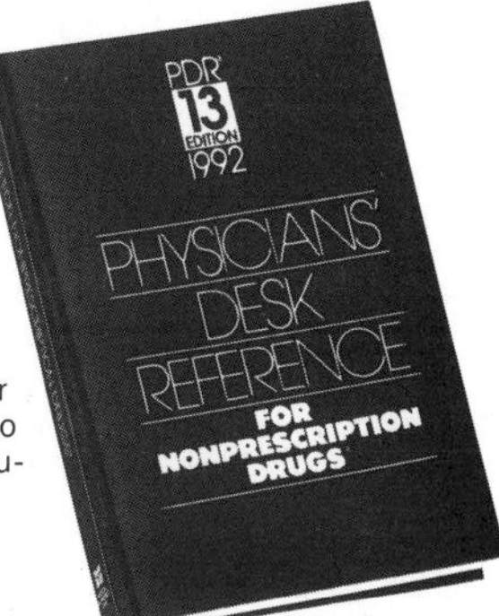

1992 PDR FOR OPHTHALMOLOGY®
Complete directory of drug and product information relating to Optometry and Ophthalmology: specialized instrumentation, equipment, lenses, product photographs, color grids for rapid product and drug identification, color-blind test. 400 pgs. Published October, 1991. $39.95.

1992 PDR DRUG INTERACTIONS & SIDE EFFECTS INDEX®
The perfect companion volume to make your PDR a more powerful reference tool than ever before! Includes food interactions. 1220 pgs. Published January, 1992 $36.95.

1992 PDR INDICATIONS INDEX™
Gives full range of drugs specifically indicated for precise clinical situations. Double-check prescriptions, identify alternatives. Flexible binding 4" x 7". 350 pgs. Published January, 1992. $20.95.

DETACH ALONG DOTTED LINE AND MAIL.

USE THIS CARD TO ORDER PDR PRINT AND ELECTRONIC PRODUCTS

Send ____	copies of 1992 Physician's Desk Reference®	092031	$54.95 each
Send ____	copies of 1992 PDR for Ophthalmology®	092023	$39.95 each
Send	copies of 1992 PDR Supplements A	092080	
____	and B	092098	$14.95 set
Send ____	copies of 1992 PDR Drug Interactions and Side Effects Index®	092049	$36.95 each
Send ____	copies of 1992 PDR Indications Index™	092056	$20.95 each
Send ____	copies of 1992 PDR for Nonprescription Drugs®	092064	$35.95 each

☐ SAVE TIME AND MONEY EVERY YEAR AS A SUBSCRIBER.
Check here to enter a standing order for future editions of the publications ordered. Next year we'll confirm your order, and you are guaranteed to receive the lowest price available.

☐ Pocket PDR® .... $249.00 each

PDR® on CD-ROM (CD-ROM drive required)

☐ PDR on CD-ROM containing all 5 PDR volumes and The Merck Manual .... $895.00 each

☐ PDR on CD-ROM containing all 5 PDR volumes .... $595.00 each

Check Format: ☐ 360K 5¼" diskettes ☐ 720K 3½" diskettes

☐ PDR Drug Interactions and Side Effects Diskettes™ .... $219.00 each

Check Format: ☐ 360K 5¼" diskettes ☐ 720K 3½" diskettes

For fastest service call toll free
1-800-232-7379,
or **FAX YOUR ORDER:**
201-573-4956

(Do not mail a confirmation order in addition to this fax.)

CHECK METHOD OF PAYMENT:

☐ Payment enclosed (shipping and handling are free).

☐ Check ☐ VISA ☐ MasterCard

Account # ____ Exp. Date Mo. ____ Yr. ____

Signature ____

☐ Bill me later. Add $3.95 shipping and handling per unit.
Residents of NJ, IL, IA, CA, VA, and KY please add sales tax.
Orders shipped in USA only.

Purchase of reference materials for professional use may be tax deductible.

Name ____

Institution ____

Address ____

City ____ St. ____ Zip ____

Occupation ____

512954

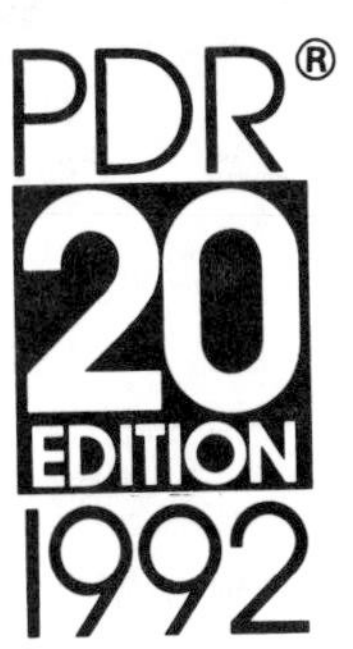

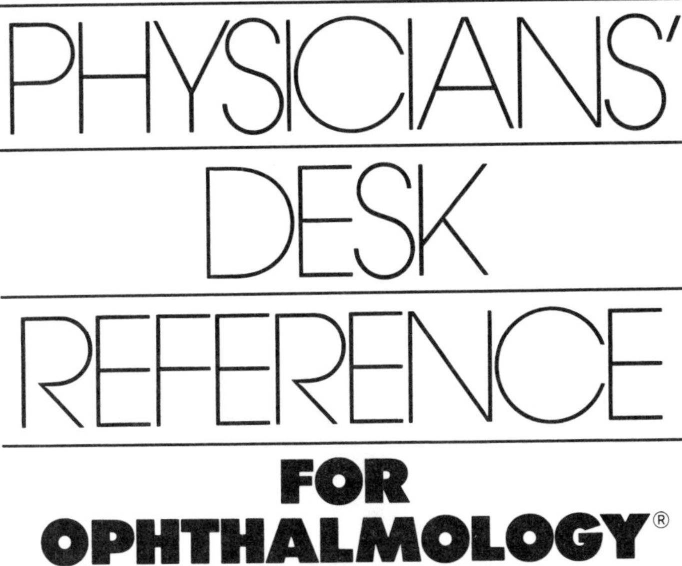

FOR OPHTHALMOLOGY®

Editorial Consultants

JOSEPH B. WALSH, M.D.
Professor and Chairman
Department of Ophthalmology
New York Medical College
New York Eye and Ear Infirmary

ARTHUR GOLD, M.D.
Associate Professor
Department of Ophthalmology
Albert Einstein College of Medicine
Montefiore Medical Center

HOWARD CHARLES, M.D.
Assistant Professor of Ophthalmology
Albert Einstein College of Medicine
Montefiore Medical Center

Director of Production: MARJORIE A. DUFFY

Assistant Director of Production: CARRIE WILLIAMS

Manager of Production Services: ELIZABETH H. CARUSO

Index Editor: ADELE L. DOWD

Production Coordinator: ELIZABETH A. KARST

Art Associate: JOAN K. AKERLIND

Product Manager: JOHN A. MALCZYNSKI

National Sales Manager: CHARLIE J. MEITNER

Account Managers: CHAD E. ALCORN
MICHAEL S. SARAJIAN
JOANNE C. TERZIDES

Commercial Sales Manager: ROBIN B. BARTLETT

Database Manager: MUKESH MEHTA, R.Ph.

Fulfillment Manager: KERRY MACKERELL

Officers of Medical Economics Data, a division of Medical Economics Inc.: President and Chief Executive Officer: Norman R. Snesil; Senior Vice President and Chief financial Officer: Joseph T. Deithorn; Senior Vice President of Business Development: Stephen J. Sorkenn; Vice President, Sales and Marketing: Thomas F. Rice; Vice President of Circulation: Scott J. Rockman; Vice President of Operations: Mark L. Weinstein; Vice President, Information Services: Edward J. Zecchini.

ISBN 1-56363-002-8

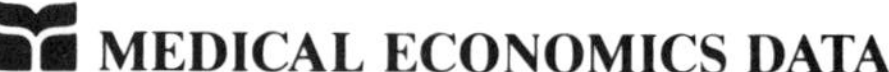
MEDICAL ECONOMICS DATA

Foreword to the Twentieth Edition

PHYSICIANS' DESK REFERENCE For OPHTHALMOLOGY®is published by Medical Economics Data with the cooperation of the manufacturers whose products are described in the Product Information Section. This reference provides physicians in the field of ophthalmology with information on pharmaceutical products, lenses and equipment used primarily in this specialty.

PDR For Ophthalmology®also contains a special editorial section prepared to provide basic information for the practicing ophthalmologist. Editorial has been prepared by Joseph B. Walsh, M.D. of New York Medical College, New York Eye and Ear Infirmary, Arthur Gold, M.D. and Howard Charles, M.D. of the Albert Einstein College of Medicine in New York, with a chapter on Ocular Toxicology by F.T. Fraunfelder, M.D. The editorial section presented in this edition represents their opinions and is not necessarily endorsed by Medical Economics Data.

The twentieth edition of Physicians' Desk Reference For Ophthalmology contains an updated Product Identification Section. This section is included to help you identify products by displaying actual size color reproductions of drug products—tablets and capsules—used in the practice of ophthalmology. Some products such as eye drops, ointments and solutions have been reduced in size to fit available space.

As an adjunct to this section there is a Color Vision Screening Chart which can be used to test patients for color blindness.

Under the Federal Food, Drug & Cosmetic (FD&C) Act, a drug approved for marketing may be labeled, promoted, and advertised by the manufacturer only for those uses for which the drug's safety and effectiveness have been established. The Code of Federal Regulations 201.100(d)(1) pertaining to labeling for prescription products require that for PDR For Ophthalmology content, "indications, effects, dosages, routes, methods, and frequency and duration of administration and any relevant warnings, hazards, contraindications, side effects, and precautions" must be the "*same in language and emphasis*" as the approved labeling for the products. FDA regards the words "*same in language and emphasis*" as requiring VERBATIM use of the approved labeling providing such information.

PDR For Ophthalmology includes a section for manufacturers of specialized instrumentation, equipment, lenses, lens care products and sutures. Participating companies have described or listed categories of products manufactured and the locations of their sales and service offices.

The function of the publisher is the compilation, organization, and distribution of this information. Each product description has been prepared by the manufacturer, and edited and approved by the manufacturer's medical department, medical director, and/or medical consultant. In organizing and presenting the material in Physicians' Desk Reference For Ophthalmology, the publisher does not warrant or guarantee any of the products described herein or perform any independent analysis in connection with any of the product information contained herein. Physicians' Desk Reference For Ophthalmology does not assume, and expressly disclaims, any obligation to obtain and include information other than that provided to it by the manufacturer. In making this material available it should be understood that the publisher is not advocating the use of any product described herein. Additional information on any product may be obtained through the manufacturer.

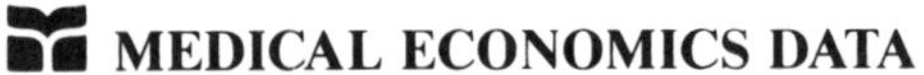
MEDICAL ECONOMICS DATA

Contents

Section 1

Indices ..... Page I
1. Manufacturers' Index I
2. Product Name Index V
3. Product Category Index IX
4. Active Ingredients Index XV
5. Instrumentation, Lenses, and Sutures Index XXI

Section 2

Pharmaceuticals in Ophthalmology ..... Page 1
1. Mydriatics and Cycloplegics 2
2. Miotics 3
3. Antimicrobial Therapy 3
4. Ocular Anti-Inflammatory Therapy 9
5. Anesthetic Agents 10
6. Agents for the Treatment of Glaucoma 11
7. Medications for the Dry Eye 12
8. Ocular Decongestants 13
9. Ophthalmic Irrigating Solutions 14
10. Hyperosmolar Agents 14
11. Diagnostic Agents 15
12. Other Agents 16
13. Ocular Toxicology 17

Section 3

Suture Materials ..... Page 20

Section 4

Ophthalmic Lenses ..... Page 22
1. Absorptive and Tinted Lenses 22
2. Multifocal Lenses 23
3. Non-Visible Segment Lenses 24
4. Fresnel Lenses and Prisms 26
5. Soft Contact Lenses 27
6. Rigid Gas Permeable 37
7. Aphakia 40
   Aphakic Extended Wear Hydrogels 41
   Intraocular Lenses 42
8. Relative Magnification, Lens Effectivity,
   Index of Refraction, Conversion Tables 43

Section 5

Vision Standards and Low Vision .... Page 47
1. Vision Standards 47
2. Low Vision 50

Section 6

Evaluation of Permanent Visual Impairment .... Page 52
1. Criteria and Methods for Evaluation 53
Central Visual Acuity 53
Visual Fields 54
Abnormal Ocular Motility and Binocular Diplopia 56

Section 7

Product Identification Section .... Page 101
Color Vision Screening Chart 106

Section 8

Pharmaceutical Product Information .... Page 201

Products are listed alphabetically by manufacturer. The information concerning the products described in this section has been prepared by the manufacturer, and edited and approved by the medical department, medical director or medical counsel of each manufacturer.

Section 9

Lenses and Lens Care .... Page 317
Part 1: Contact Lenses (Hard and Soft) 317
Part 2: Intraocular Lenses 323
Part 3: Lens Care Products 325
Part 4: Spectacle Lenses and Products 349

Section 10

Instrumentation, Equipment, Sutures .... Page 351
Part 1. Specialized Instruments and Equipment 351
Part 2. Sutures 359

Amsler's Grid .... Inside Front Cover
Near Vision Chart .... Inside Back Cover

SECTION 1

The Indices

The Indices are divided into six parts:

Part I—Manufacturers' Index; names, addresses and telephone numbers of participating advertisers.

Part 2—Product Name Index; products are listed alphabetically.

Part 3—Product Category Index: lists products by indications.

Part 4—Active Ingredients Index; lists products alphabetically by generic name.

Part 5—Instrumentation, Equipment, Lenses and Sutures.

Part 1 – Manufacturers' Index

PAGE

AKORN, INC. 103, 201
100 Akorn Drive
Abita Springs, LA 70420

Address inquiries to:
David H. Turner (800) 535-7155
Vice President (504) 893-9300
In LA (800) 344-2291

Manufacturing Facility:
1340 N. Jefferson Street
Anaheim, CA 92807
(714) 579-7545

ALCON LABORATORIES, INC. 210
and its affiliates
CORPORATE HEADQUARTERS
6201 South Freeway
Fort Worth, TX 76134

Address inquiries to:
Sales Service (817) 293-0450

ALCON SURGICAL, INC. 230, 323, 351, 359
6201 South Freeway
Fort Worth, TX 76134

Address inquiries to:
Marketing Dept. (817) 293-0450
(800) TO-ALCON
(800) 862-5266

ALLERGAN HUMPHREY 352
2992 Alvarado Street
San Leandro, CA 94577

Address inquiries to:
(Toll Free) (800) 227-1508
(Toll Free in CA) (800) 826-6566
Telex 470714
FAX (415) 483-8025

ALLERGAN MEDICAL OPTICS 236
9701 Jeronimo Road
Irvine, CA 92718

ALLERGAN OPTICAL 325
A Division of Allergan, Inc.
2525 Dupont Drive
P.O. Box 19534
Irvine, CA 92713-9534

Address inquiries to:
Medical Director (714) 752-4500

ALLERGAN PHARMACEUTICALS 238
A Division of Allergan Inc.
2525 Dupont Drive
P.O. Box 19534
Irvine, CA 92713-9534

Address inquiries to:
Product/Medical Information
Outside CA (800) 433-8871
CA (714) 752-4500
Customer Service/Order Entry
Outside CA (800) 854-7149
CA (714) 752-4500

ALZA CORPORATION 256
950 Page Mill Road
P.O. Box 10950
Palo Alto, CA 94303-0802

Address ordering inquiries to:
Customer Service
(800) 227-9953

Address Medical/Technical Inquiries to:
Marianne Peschon (800) 634-8977

PAGE

AYERST LABORATORIES 258
As a result of a merger of Wyeth Laboratories and Ayerst Laboratories, all prescription products formerly of both companies are products of Wyeth-Ayerst Laboratories. All nonprescription products formerly of Ayerst are products of Whitehall Laboratories.

BAUSCH & LOMB INCORPORATED, CONTACT LENS DIVISION 317
1400 North Goodman Street
Rochester, NY 14692

Address inquiries to:
Customer Service
US (800) 828-9030
NY State (800) 462-1720

BAUSCH & LOMB PERSONAL PRODUCTS DIVISION 258
1400 North Goodman Street
Rochester, NY 14692-0450

BAUSCH & LOMB PHARMACEUTICALS DIVISION 103, 259
8500 Hidden River Parkway
Tampa, FL 33637

Address inquiries to:
Customer Service Department
(800) 227-1427
(813) 975-5000

BURROUGHS WELLCOME CO. 263
3030 Cornwallis Road
Research Triangle Park, NC 27709
(800) 722-9292

For Medical or Drug Information:
Contact Drug Information Department
Business hours only (8:15 AM to 4:15 PM EST) (800) 443-6763
For 24-hour Medical Emergency Information, call (800) 443-6763

For Sales Information:
Contact Sales Distribution Department

Address Other Inquiries To:
Public Affairs Department

CANON U.S.A., INC. 354
One Canon Plaza
Lake Success, NY 11042

Address inquiries to:
Mr. Richard Weiss
(516) 488-6700

CIBA VISION CORPORATION 343
2910 Amwiler Court
Atlanta GA 30360

Address inquiries to:
Customer Service Department
(800) 241-5999
Consultation Services
(800) 241-7468

CIBA VISION OPHTHALMICS 103, 268
2910 Amwiler Court
Atlanta, GA 30360

COOPERVISION, INC. 269
3495 Winton Place
Rochester, NY 14623

Address inquiries to:
Kristine Banister (716) 272-3749

EAGLE VISION, INC. 269
6263 Poplar Avenue, Suite 650
Memphis, TN 38119 U.S.A.

Address inquiries to:
Customer Service Department
Nationwide (800) 222-7584
Local (901) 682-9400
FAX (901) 761-5736

PAGE

FISONS CORPORATION 103, 270
P.O. Box 1710
Rochester, NY 14603

Address inquiries to:
Professional Services Department
(716) 475-9000

HEALTH MAINTENANCE PROGRAMS, INC. 270
7 Westchester Plaza
Elmsford, NY 10523

Address inquiries to:
Joel Ross (800) 362-8673
(914) 592-3155

IOLAB CORPORATION 323
a Johnson & Johnson Company
500 Iolab Drive,
Claremont, CA 91711

Address inquiries to:
Marketing Services
(800) 423-1871
CA only (800) 352-1891
See also SITE MICROSURGICAL SYSTEMS, INC. and IOLAB PHARMACEUTICAL

IOLAB CORPORATION PHARMACEUTICAL DIVISION 103, 271
a Johnson & Johnson Company
500 Iolab Drive
Claremont, CA 91711

Address inquiries to:
(714) 624-2020

KABI PHARMACIA OPHTHALMICS INC. 279
605 East Huntington Drive
Monrovia, CA 91017

Address inquiries to:
Customer Service (800) 423-4866

LA HAYE LABORATORIES, INC. 280
2205 152nd Street
Redmond, WA 98052

Address inquiries to:
Joyce Bales (206) 644-2020

LACRIMEDICS, INC. 281
9008 Newby Street
Rosemead, CA 91770

Address inquiries to:
Customer Service
7:00 AM to 6:00 PM (PST)
US (800) 367-8327
FAX (714) 357-9889

LEDERLE LABORATORIES 282
Division of American Cyanamid Co.
Business Center Drive
One Cyanamid Plaza
Wayne, NJ 07470

Address medical/pharmacy inquiries on marketed products only to:
Professional Services Department
LEDERLE LABORATORIES
Pearl River, NY 10965
During business hours (8 AM to 4:30 PM EST)
(914) 735-2815

All other inquiries and after hours emergencies
(914) 732-5000
LEDERLE PARENTERALS, INC.
Carolina, Puerto Rico 00630

Inquiries on ordering/billing should be directed to Distribution Centers

ATLANTA
Contact EASTERN (Philadelphia) Distribution Center

CHICAGO
Bulk Address
1100 E. Business Center Drive
Mt. Prospect, IL 60056
Mail Address
P.O. Box 7614
Mt. Prospect, IL 60056-7614
(800) 533-3753
(312) 827-8871

DALLAS
Bulk Address
7611 Carpenter Freeway
Dallas, TX 75247
Mail Address
P.O. Box 655731
Dallas, TX 75265
(800) 533-3753
(214) 631-2130

LOS ANGELES
Bulk Address
2300 S. Eastern Avenue
Los Angeles, CA 90040
Mail Address
T.A. Box 2202
Los Angeles, CA 90051
(800) 533-3753
(213) 726-1016

EASTERN (Philadelphia)
Bulk Address
202 Precision Drive
Horsham, PA 19044
Mail Address
P.O. Box 993
Horsham, PA 19044
(800) 533-3753
(215) 672-5400
See STORZ OPHTHALMICS, INC.

MARCO EQUIPMENT, INC. 355
11825 Central Parkway
P.O. Box 16938
Jacksonville, FL 32245-6938
Toll Free Number US (800) 874-5274
(904) 642-9330
TELEX: 756172
FAX (904) 642-9338
Address inquiries to:
Brad Santora (904) 642-9330

MARCO TECHNOLOGIES 356
11825 Central Parkway
P.O. Box 16938
Jacksonville, FL 32245-6938
Toll Free Number US (800) 874-5274
(904) 642-9330
TELEX: 756172
FAX (904) 642-9338
Address inquiries to:
Robert Kalapp (904) 642-9330

MERCK SHARP & DOHME 103, 282
Division of Merck & Co., Inc.
West Point, PA 19486
(215) 661-5000
For Product Information:
Write: Professional Information
West Point, PA 19486-9989
Call: (215) 661-7300
Business hours only
8:30 AM to 4:45 PM (EST)
Address other inquiries to:
Professional Services Department
West Point, PA 19486-9989
Branch Offices:
Arlington, TX 76011
925-111th Street (817) 640-5657
Atlanta Area: see Norcross, GA
Baltimore Area: see Columbia, MD
Boston Area: see Needham Heights, MA
Chicago Area: see Oak Brook, IL
Columbia, MD 21045
9199 Red Branch Rd.
(301) 730-8240
Columbus, OH 43228
4242 Janitrol Road (614) 276-5308
Dallas/Fort Worth Area: see Arlington, TX
Denver, CO 80216
4900 Jackson Street (303) 355-1602
Kansas City Area: see Overland Park, KS
Kenner, LA 70062
1431 E. Airline Hwy. (504) 464-0111
Los Angeles, CA 90040
6409 E. Gayhart St. (213) 723-9661
Memphis, TN 38106
1980 Latham Street (901) 948-8501
Minneapolis, MN 55441
12955 State Hwy. 55
(612) 559-4445
Needham Heights, MA 02194
40 A Street (617) 444-5510
New Orleans Area: see Kenner, LA
New York Area: see Somerset, NJ
Norcross, GA 30071
2825 Northwoods Parkway
(404) 662-7200
Oak Brook, IL 60522
2010 Swift Drive (708) 574-2160
Overland Park, KS 66215
9001 Quivira Rd. (913) 888-1110
Portland, OR 97211
717 N.E. Lombard St.
(503) 285-2582
Somerset, NJ 08873
300 Franklin Square Drive
(908) 805-0300

OCUMED, INC. 297
119 Harrison Avenue
Roseland NJ 07068
Address inquiries to:
Alfred R. Caggia (201) 226-2330

OPTICAL RADIATION CORPORATION 325
1300 Optical Drive
Azusa, CA 91702
Address inquiries to:
(818) 969-3344
(800) 423-1887
FAX (818) 812-0283

PARKE-DAVIS 104, 298
Division of Warner-Lambert Company
201 Tabor Road
Morris Plains, NJ 07950
(201) 540-2000
Address inquiries to:
During working hours:
Product Information (800) 223-0432
NJ & HI (201) 540-2117
Medical Information (201) 540-3950
After hours or on weekends:
(201) 540-2000
Regional Sales Offices
Atlanta, GA 30328
5901 Peachtree Dunwoody Road
(404) 396-4080
Baltimore (Cockeysville), MD 21030
311 International Circle
(301) 584-7810
Chicago (Schaumburg), IL 60173
1750 East Golf Road
(708) 240-1740
Cincinnati, OH 45242
4445 Lake Forest Drive
(513) 563-6658
Dallas, TX 75234
12200 Ford Road (214) 484-5566
San Francisco (San Ramon), CA 94583
4000 Executive Parkway
(415) 867-1109
Los Angeles (Irvine), CA 92715
18201 Von Karman Avenue
(714) 852-0905
New York (Paramus, NJ) 07652
Paramus Plaza IV
12 Route 17 North (201) 368-0733
St. Louis, MO 63105
101 South Hanley Road
(314) 863-7706

PFIZER CONSUMER HEALTH CARE DIVISION 104, 303
Division of Pfizer Incorporated
235 East 42nd Street
New York, NY 10017 (212) 573-3131

POLYMER TECHNOLOGY CORPORATION 104, 348
100 Research Drive
Wilmington, MA 01887
Address Inquiries To:
Customer Affairs (800) 333-4730

ROCHE LABORATORIES 105, 304
a division of Hoffmann-La Roche Inc.
Nutley, NJ 07110
For Medical Information:
Write:
Professional Services Department
For: Medical Emergency Information
(24-hour service)
Product Information
Reporting Adverse Events
(800) 526-6367
Branch Warehouse
Belvidere, NJ 07823-0200
200 Roche Drive
(201) 475-5337

RODENSTOCK USA INC. LENS DIVISION 349
69 Kenosia Avenue
Danbury, CT 06813-3333
Address inquiries to:
Marketing Department (800) 458-0620
In CT (203) 748-4311
Canada (800) 387-7750

ROSS LABORATORIES 105, 304
Columbus, Ohio 43216
Division of Abbott Laboratories, USA

SCHERING CORPORATION 305
Address inquiries to:
Professional Services Department
Galloping Hill Road
Kenilworth, NJ 07033
9:00 AM to 5:00 PM EST:
(800) 526-4099
After regular hours and on weekends:
(201) 298-4000

SITE MICROSURGICAL SYSTEMS, INC. 357
Division of IOLAB CORPORATION
a Johnson & Johnson company
135 Gilbralter Road
Horsham, PA 19044-0963
Address inquiries to:
Carol A. Edwards, R.N.
M. Kelly Rodrigues 800-445-SITE

STORZ OPHTHALMICS, INC. 105, 307
3365 Tree Court Industrial Blvd.
St. Louis, MO 63122-6694

TOPCON INSTRUMENT CORPORATION OF AMERICA 357
65 West Century Road
Paramus, NJ 07652-9990
Address inquiries to:
Medical Instrument Division
(201) 261-9450

VISTAKON JOHNSON & JOHNSON VISION PRODUCTS, INC. 321
4500 Salisbury Road
Jacksonville, FL 32216
Address inquiries to:
Philip Fitzsimmons (904) 443-1066
FAX (904) 443-1252

VOLK OPTICAL **358**
7893 Enterprise Drive
Mentor, OH 44060

Address inquiries to:
Toll Free (800) 345-VOLK
(216) 942-6161

WALKER PHARMACAL COMPANY **313**
4200 Laclede Avenue
St. Louis, MO 63108

Address inquiries to:
Customer Service Dept.
(314) 533-9600
P.O. Box 8080
St. Louis, MO 63156

WYETH-AYERST LABORATORIES **105, 314**
Div. of American Home Products Corp.
Post Office Box 8299
Philadelphia, PA 19101

Address inquiries to:
Professional Service

For General Information call:
(215) 688-4400

Part II — Product Name Index

A

A.C.S. Alcon Closure System (Alcon Surgical) p 359
ACP-6R and ACP-6S Chart Projectors (Topcon Instrument) p 357
AKWA Tears Ointment (Akorn) p 208
AKWA Tears Solution (Akorn) p 208
AMO Vitrax Solution (Allergan Medical Optics) p 236
AMVISC (IOLAB) p 324
AMVISC Plus (IOLAB) p 323
AODISC Disinfection/Neutralization System (CIBA Vision Corp.) p 343
AOSEPT Disinfection/Neutralization Solution (CIBA Vision Corp.) p 343
AOSEPT Disinfection/Neutralization System (CIBA Vision Corp.) p 343
Achromycin Ophthalmic Ointment 1% (Storz Ophthalmics) p 307
◆**Achromycin Ophthalmic Suspension 1%** (Storz Ophthalmics) p 105, 308
Acuvue Contact Lenses (Vistakon) p 321
Adsorbonac 2% and 5% (Alcon Laboratories) p 210
Adsorbotear (Alcon Laboratories) p 210
Akarpine Ophthalmic Solution (Akorn) p 201
AK-Chlor Sterile Ophthalmic Ointment & Solution (Akorn) p 201
AK-Cide Sterile Ophthalmic Ointment & Suspension (Akorn) p 202
AK-Con (Akorn) p 202
AK-Con-A (Akorn) p 203
AK-Dex 0.05% Ointment (Akorn) p 203
AK-Dex 0.1% Solution (Akorn) p 203
AK-Dilate Solution 2.5% and 10% (Akorn) p 203
AK-Fluor Injection 10% and 25% (Akorn) p 204
AK-Mycin Ointment (Akorn) p 204
AK-NaCl 5% Ointment & Solution (Akorn) p 204
AK-Pentolate (Akorn) p 204
AK-Poly-Bac Ointment (Akorn) p 205
◆**AK-Pred** (Akorn) p 103, 205
AK-Spore H.C. Ointment (Akorn) p 206
AK-Spore H. C. Suspension (Akorn) p 206
AK-Spore Ointment (Akorn) p 205
AK-Spore Solution (Akorn) p 205
◆**AK-Sulf** (Akorn) p 103, 207
AK-Taine (Akorn) p 207
AK-Trol Ointment & Suspension (Akorn) p 207
Albalon Solution with Liquifilm (Allergan Pharmaceuticals) p 238
Albalon-A Liquifilm (Allergan Pharmaceuticals) p 238
Alcaine (Alcon Laboratories) p 210
Alcon A-OK Ophthalmic Knife (Alcon Surgical) p 351
Alcon Intraocular Lenses (Alcon Surgical) p 323
Allergan Enzymatic Contact Lens Cleaner (Allergan Optical) p 327
Allergan Eyewash (Allergan Pharmaceuticals) p 238
Allergan Hydrocare Cleaning and Disinfecting Solution (Allergan Optical) p 325
Allergan Hydrocare Preserved Saline Solution (Allergan Optical) p 326
Allergan Sorbi-Care Saline Solution (Allergan Optical) p 327
Allergy Drops (Bausch & Lomb Personal) p 258
Argyrol S.S. 10% (IOLAB Pharmaceuticals) p 271
Argyrol S.S. 20% Dropperettes (IOLAB Pharmaceuticals) p 271
Aspherical Lenses - Topcon (Topcon Instrument) p 357
ASSIST-O.R. Suture Pack (Alcon Surgical) p 359
Atropine Sulfate Ophthalmic Ointment, Sterile (Bausch & Lomb Pharmaceuticals) p 259
Atropine Sulfate Ophthalmic Solution, Sterile (Bausch & Lomb Pharmaceuticals) p 259
Atropine Sulfate Sterile Ophthalmic Solution and S.O.P. Sterile Ophthalmic Ointment (Allergan Pharmaceuticals) p 239
Atropisol Dropperettes ½%, 1% and 2% (IOLAB Pharmaceuticals) p 271
Auroemycin Ophthalmic Ointment 1.0% (Storz Ophthalmics) p 308
Autoref Keratometer RK-2 (Canon) (Canon U.S.A.) p 355

B

◆**BIO-COR 12, 24, and 72 Collagen Corneal Shield** (Bausch & Lomb Pharmaceuticals) p 103, 260
BSS (15 mL & 30 mL) Sterile Irrigation Solution (Alcon Surgical) p 230
BSS (250 mL) Sterile Irrigation Solution (Alcon Surgical) p 231
BSS (500 mL) Sterile Irrigation Solution (Alcon Surgical) p 231
BSS and BSS PLUS Irrigation Administration Set (Alcon Surgical) p 351
BSS PLUS (500 mL) Sterile Irrigation Solution (Alcon Surgical) p 231
Bacitracin Ophthalmic Ointment-Sterile (Bausch & Lomb Pharmaceuticals) p 259
Bacitracin Zinc and Polymyxin B Sulfate Ophthalmic Ointment, Sterile (Bausch & Lomb Pharmaceuticals) p 259
Balanced Salt Solution (Allergan Pharmaceuticals) p 239
Balanced Salt Solution (Bausch & Lomb Pharmaceuticals) p 259
Basol-S Sterile Surgical Solution (Ocumed) p 297
Bausch & Lomb Medalist Tinted Contact Lenses (Bausch & Lomb Contact Lens) p 317
Bausch & Lomb NaturalTint Hydrophilic Contact Lenses (Bausch & Lomb Contact Lens) p 317
Bausch & Lomb P.A.1 Bifocal Hydrophilic Contact Lenses (Bausch & Lomb Contact Lens) p 317
Bausch & Lomb Soflens Hydrophilic Contact Lenses (Bausch & Lomb Contact Lens) p 317
Betagan Liquifilm (Allergan Pharmaceuticals) p 239
Betagan Liquifilm with C Cap Compliance Cap (Allergan Pharmaceuticals) p 239
Betoptic Sterile Ophthalmic Solution (Alcon Laboratories) p 211
Betoptic S Sterile Ophthalmic Suspension (Alcon Laboratories) p 212
Bladesaver Foam Blade Protector (Alcon Surgical) p 351
Bleph-10 Ophthalmic Solution with Liquifilm (Allergan Pharmaceuticals) p 241
Bleph-10 Ophthalmic Ointment (Allergan Pharmaceuticals) p 241
Blephamide Liquifilm (Allergan Pharmaceuticals) p 242
Blephamide S.O.P. (Allergan Pharmaceuticals) p 242
Blink-N-Clean Contact Lens Solution (Allergan Optical) p 328
◆**Boston Advance Cleaner** (Polymer Technology) p 104, 348
Boston Advance Conditioning Solution (Polymer Technology) p 348
Boston Advance Rewetting Drops (Polymer Technology) p 348

C

CF-60UV Fundus Camera (Canon) (Canon U.S.A.) p 354
CIBA Vision Saline Solution (CIBA Vision Corp.) p 344
CL-2000 Lensmeter (Topcon Instrument) p 358
CP-600 Automatic Chart Projector (Marco Equipment) p 355
CP-5D Chart Projector (Topcon Instrument) p 357
CT-20 Computerized Tonometer (Topcon Instrument) p 357
CV-1000 and CV-2000 Computerized Vision Testers (Topcon Instrument) p 357
Canon Autorefractometer R-22 (Canon U.S.A.) p 354
Canon CR4-45NM Dual Non-Mydriatic Retinal Camera (Canon U.S.A.) p 354
Canon KU-1 IOL Estimator (Canon U.S.A.) p 354
Catarase 1:5000 (IOLAB Pharmaceuticals) p 271
Cellufresh Lubricant Ophthalmic Solution (Allergan Pharmaceuticals) p 243
Celluvisc Lubricant Ophthalmic Solution (Allergan Pharmaceuticals) p 243
Cetamide Ointment (Alcon Laboratories) p 220
Cetapred Ointment (Alcon Laboratories) p 220
◆**Chibroxin Sterile Ophthalmic Solution** (Merck Sharp & Dohme) p 103, 282
Chloramphenicol Ophthalmic Ointment, Sterile (Bausch & Lomb Pharmaceuticals) p 259
Chloramphenicol Ophthalmic Solution, Sterile (Bausch & Lomb Pharmaceuticals) p 259
◆**Chloromycetin Hydrocortisone Ophthalmic** (Parke-Davis) p 104, 298
◆**Chloromycetin Ophthalmic Ointment, 1%** (Parke-Davis) p 104, 299
◆**Chloromycetin Ophthalmic Solution** (Parke-Davis) p 104, 300
Chloroptic S.O.P. (Allergan Pharmaceuticals) p 243
Chloroptic Sterile Ophthalmic Solution (Allergan Pharmaceuticals) p 243
Ciloxan Sterile Ophthalmic Solution (Alcon Laboratories) p 214
Clean-N-Soak Hard Contact Lens Cleaning & Soaking Solution (Allergan Optical) p 328
Clean-N-Soakit Hard Contact Lens Storage Case (Allergan Optical) p 328
Clean-N-Stow Hard Contact Lens Storage Case (Allergan Optical) p 328
◆**Clear Eyes ACR** (Ross) p 105, 305
Clear Eyes Lubricating Eye Redness Reliever (Ross) p 304
Color Bar Schirmer Tear Test (Eagle Vision) p 269
Collagen Implants (Intracanalicular) for Lacrimal Efficiency Test (Lacrimedics) p 281
◆**Collyrium for Fresh Eyes** (Wyeth-Ayerst) p 105, 314
◆**Collyrium Fresh** (Wyeth-Ayerst) p 105, 314
Colormatic Hard Resin Spectacle Lenses (Rodenstock) p 349
Cortisporin Ophthalmic Ointment Sterile (Burroughs Wellcome) p 263
Cortisporin Ophthalmic Suspension Sterile (Burroughs Wellcome) p 264
Cosmolit Bifo 28 Spectacle Lenses (Rodenstock) p 349
Cosmolit Single Vision Spectacle Lenses (Rodenstock) p 349
Cryophake (Alcon Surgical) p 351
Cyclogyl (Alcon Laboratories) p 215
Cyclomydril (Alcon Laboratories) p 216

D

Dacriose (IOLAB Pharmaceuticals) p 271
◆**Daranide Tablets** (Merck Sharp & Dohme) p 103, 284

◆**Decadron Phosphate Sterile Ophthalmic Ointment** (Merck Sharp & Dohme) p 103, 285
◆**Decadron Phosphate Sterile Ophthalmic Solution** (Merck Sharp & Dohme) p 103, 285
Dexacidin Ointment (IOLAB Pharmaceuticals) p 272
Dexacidin Suspension (IOLAB Pharmaceuticals) p 272
Dexamethasone Sodium Phosphate Injection, USP (IOLAB Pharmaceuticals) p 271
Dexamethasone Sodium Phosphate Ophthalmic Ointment, Sterile (Bausch & Lomb Pharmaceuticals) p 259
Dexamethasone Sodium Phosphate Ophthalmic Solution, Sterile (Bausch & Lomb Pharmaceuticals) p 259
Dexamethasone Sodium Phosphate Ophthalmic Solution, USP (IOLAB Pharmaceuticals) p 271
Dexasporin Ointment (Bausch & Lomb Pharmaceuticals) p 259
Dexasporin Suspension (Bausch & Lomb Pharmaceuticals) p 259
Diamox Parenteral (Storz Ophthalmics) p 308
◆**Diamox Sequels (Sustained Release)** (Storz Ophthalmics) p 105, 310
◆**Diamox Tablets** (Storz Ophthalmics) p 105, 308
Dropperettes (1mL) (IOLAB Pharmaceuticals) p 271
Dry Eyes Solution (Bausch & Lomb Pharmaceuticals) p 259
Dry Eye Therapy (Bausch & Lomb Personal) p 258
Duolube Eye Ointment (Bausch & Lomb Personal) p 258
Duratears Naturale (Alcon Laboratories) p 216

E

E-Pilo-1, E-Pilo-2, E-Pilo-3, E-Pilo-4, E-Pilo-6 (IOLAB Pharmaceuticals) p 271
EV Lid-Cleanser Kit II (Eagle Vision) p 269
EV Monocanalicular Stent (Eagle Vision) p 269
EV Rose Bengal (Eagle Vision) p 269
EZVUE Violet Haptic Lenses (IOLAB) p 323
Eagle Vision-Freeman Punctum Plug (Eagle Vision) p 269
EasyClean/GP Daily Cleaner (Allergan Optical) p 328
⅛% Econopred & 1% Econopred Plus (Alcon Laboratories) p 217
Enuclene (Alcon Surgical) p 232
Epifrin (Allergan Pharmaceuticals) p 244
Epinephrine 1:1000 Dropperettes (IOLAB Pharmaceuticals) p 271
Erythromycin Ophthalmic Ointment, Sterile (Bausch & Lomb Pharmaceuticals) p 259
Eserine Sulfate Ophthalmic Ointment 0.25% (IOLAB Pharmaceuticals) p 271
Esterman Binocular/Monocular Tests (Allergan Humphrey) p 352
Excalibur Spatulated Needles (Alcon Surgical) p 359
Extenzyme Protein Cleaner (Allergan Optical) p 329
Eye Drops (Bausch & Lomb Pharmaceuticals) p 259
Eye-Pak Ophthalmic Drapes (Alcon Surgical) p 351
Eye Wash (Bausch & Lomb Personal) p 258
Eye Wash (Bausch & Lomb Pharmaceuticals) p 259
Eye-Stream (Alcon Laboratories) p 217
Eye-Zine Sterile Eye Drops (Ocumed) p 297
EYEscrub Eyelid Cleanser (CooperVision) p 269

F

FML Forte Liquifilm (Allergan Pharmaceuticals) p 245
FML Liquifilm (Allergan Pharmaceuticals) p 244
FML S.O.P. (Allergan Pharmaceuticals) p 245
FML-S Sterile Ophthalmic Suspension (Allergan Pharmaceuticals) p 246
◆**Floropryl Sterile Ophthalmic Ointment** (Merck Sharp & Dohme) p 103, 286
Fluoracaine (Akorn) p 208
Fluorescein Sodium 2% Dropperettes (IOLAB Pharmaceuticals) p 271
Fluorescite Injection (Alcon Laboratories) p 217
Fluorescite Syringe (Alcon Laboratories) p 217
Fluorets Ophthalmic Strips (Akorn) p 208
◆**Fluor-I-Strip** (Wyeth-Ayerst) p 105, 314
◆**Fluor-I-Strip A.T.** (Wyeth-Ayerst) p 105, 314
Fluor-Op Ophthalmic Suspension (IOLAB Pharmaceuticals) p 272
Funduscein 10% and Funduscein 25% (IOLAB Pharmaceuticals) p 271

G

◆**Gantrisin Ophthalmic Ointment/Solution** (Roche) p 105, 304
Garamycin Ophthalmic Ointment—Sterile (Schering) p 305
Garamycin Ophthalmic Solution—Sterile (Schering) p 305
Genoptic Liquifilm Sterile Ophthalmic Solution (Allergan Pharmaceuticals) p 247
Genoptic S.O.P. Sterile Ophthalmic Ointment (Allergan Pharmaceuticals) p 247
Gentacidin Ointment (IOLAB Pharmaceuticals) p 273
Gentacidin Solution (IOLAB Pharmaceuticals) p 273
Gentak Ointment & Solution (Akorn) p 208
Gentamicin Ointment (Bausch & Lomb Pharmaceuticals) p 259
Gentamicin Solution (Bausch & Lomb Pharmaceuticals) p 259
Gentamicin Sulfate Injection, USP (IOLAB Pharmaceuticals) p 271
Glaucon (Alcon Laboratories) p 218
Gonak Ophthalmic Demulcent Solution (Akorn) p 209
Gonioscopic Prism Solution (Alcon Laboratories) p 218
Goniosol Ophthalmic Solution (IOLAB Pharmaceuticals) p 271

H

HMS Liquifilm (Allergan Pharmaceuticals) p 247
Healon (Kabi Pharmacia Ophthalmics) p 279
Healon Yellow (Kabi Pharmacia Ophthalmics) p 280
Herplex Liquifilm (Allergan Pharmaceuticals) p 248
Herrick Lacrimal Plug (Lacrimedics) p 281
Homatropine Hydrobromide 2% and 5% Dropperettes (IOLAB Pharmaceuticals) p 271
Homatropine Hydrobromide Ophthalmic Solution 2% and 5% (IOLAB Pharmaceuticals) p 271
◆**Humorsol Ophthalmic Solution** (Merck Sharp & Dohme) p 103, 287
Humphrey A/B/ Scan System (Allergan Humphrey) p 352
Humphrey Auto Keratometer (Allergan Humphrey) p 352
Humphrey Automatic Refractors Models 580, 585 and 590 (Allergan Humphrey) p 352
Humphrey Field Analyzer (Allergan Humphrey) p 352
Humphrey Lens Analyzer Model 306 (Allergan Humphrey) p 353
Humphrey Lens Analyzer Model 330 (Allergan Humphrey) p 353
Humphrey Lens Analyzer Model 340 (Allergan Humphrey) p 353
Humphrey STATPAC Single Test Analysis (Allergan Humphrey) p 352
Humphrey Ultrasonic Biometer (Allergan Humphrey) p 354
Humphrey Ultrasonic Pachometer (Allergan Humphrey) p 353
HypoTears Lubricating Eye Drops (IOLAB Pharmaceuticals) p 273
HypoTears Ointment (IOLAB Pharmaceuticals) p 273
HypoTears PF Preservative-Free Lubricating Eye Drops (IOLAB Pharmaceuticals) p 273

I

ICAPS Plus (La Haye) p 280
ID-5 & ID-10 Binocular Indirect (Topcon Instrument) p 357
I-Knife Microsurgical Knives (Alcon Surgical) p 351
I-Knife II Microsurgical Knives (Alcon Surgical) p 351
IMAGEnet Digital Imaging Systems 512 and 1024 (Topcon Instrument) p 357
IOLAB Intraocular Lenses (IOLAB) p 323
IS-100 Ophthalmic Stand (Topcon Instrument) p 357
Inflamase Forte 1% (IOLAB Pharmaceuticals) p 274
Inflamase Mild ⅛% (IOLAB Pharmaceuticals) p 274
Intracanalicular Collagen Implants-Temporary (Eagle Vision) p 269
Iocare Balanced Salt Solution 15 ml (IOLAB Pharmaceuticals) p 271
Iocare Balanced Salt Solution 500 ml (IOLAB Pharmaceuticals) p 271
IOLAB Microsurgical Equipment (IOLAB) p 323
IOLAB Viscoelastics (IOLAB) p 323
IOPIDINE (Alcon Surgical) p 232
Iri-Sol Sterile Isotonic Buffered Solution (Ocumed) p 297
Irrigation & Aspiration Sets (Alcon Surgical) p 351
ISMOTIC (Alcon Surgical) p 233
Isopto Atropine (Alcon Laboratories) p 218
Isopto Carbachol (Alcon Laboratories) p 219
Isopto Carpine (Alcon Laboratories) p 219
Isopto Cetamide Solution (Alcon Laboratories) p 220
Isopto Cetapred Suspension (Alcon Laboratories) p 220
Isopto Homatropine (Alcon Laboratories) p 221
Isopto Hyoscine (Alcon Laboratories) p 222

K

KR-3000 Auto Refractometer (Topcon Instrument) p 357
Keratometer I (Marco Equipment) p 355

L

LC-65 Daily Contact Lens Cleaner (Allergan Optical) p 330
LM-820 Automatic Lensmeter (Marco Equipment) p 355
LM-P5 Lensmeter (Topcon Instrument) p 358
Lacril Lubricant Ophthalmic Solution (Allergan Pharmaceuticals) p 248
Lacri-Lube NP Lubricant Ophthalmic Ointment (Allergan Pharmaceuticals) p 249
Lacri-Lube S.O.P. Sterile Ophthalmic Ointment (Allergan Pharmaceuticals) p 249

◆**Lacrisert** (Merck Sharp & Dohme) p 104, 289
Lactoplate (Eagle Vision) p 269
Lens Clear Soft Lens Cleaner (Allergan Optical) p 331
Lens Fresh Lubricating & Rewetting Drops (Allergan Optical) p 331
Lens Plus Daily Cleaner (Allergan Optical) p 332
Lens Plus Oxysept Disinfection System (Allergan Optical) p 332
Lens Plus Oxysept 1 Disinfecting Solution (Allergan Optical) p 335
Lens Plus Oxysept 2 Rinse & Neutralizer (Allergan Optical) p 334
Lens Plus Rewetting Drops (Allergan Optical) p 336
Lens Plus Sterile Saline Solution (Preservative Free) (Allergan Optical) p 336
Lensept Disinfection Solution (CIBA Vision Corp.) p 345
Lensept Disinfection System (CIBA Vision Corp.) p 345
Lensept Neutralizer & Rinsing/Storage Solution (CIBA Vision Corp.) p 345
LensKeeper Contact Lens Carrying Case (Allergan Optical) p 337
Lensrins Preserved Saline Solution (Allergan Optical) p 337
Lens-Wet Lubricating & Rewetting Solution (Allergan Optical) p 338
Liquifilm Forte Lubricant Ophthalmic Solution (Allergan Pharmaceuticals) p 249
Liquifilm Tears Lubricant Ophthalmic Solution (Allergan Pharmaceuticals) p 249
Liquifilm Wetting Solution (Allergan Optical) p 338
LubriTears Ointment (Bausch & Lomb Pharmaceuticals) p 259

M

MT-336 Automatic Perimeter (Marco Technologies) p 356
Marco AR-1000 and AR-1600 Automatic Refractors (Marco Technologies) p 356
Marco AR-1200 Automatic Refractor (Marco Technologies) p 356
Marco ARK-2000 Automated Refractor/Keratometer (Marco Technologies) p 356
Marco Bio-Scan Ultrasonic A-Scan (Marco Technologies) p 356
Marco Chairs and Stands (Marco Equipment) p 355
Marco International Chair and Stand (Marco Equipment) p 355
Marco Laseron Yag Laser (Marco Technologies) p 356
Marco Lensmeters (Marco Equipment) p 355
Marco Projection Perimeter (Marco Equipment) p 356
Marco Radiusgauge (Marco Equipment) p 356
Marco Slit Lamps IIB, III, IV, V, and V-G (Marco Equipment) p 356
Marco Slit Lamps G-II and G-XX (Marco Equipment) p 356
Marco Standard Chart Projector (Marco Equipment) p 356
Marco Surgiscope 2 (Marco Equipment) p 355
Marco TRS-1200 Total Refraction System (Marco Technologies) p 357
Marco Trial Sets and Frames (Marco Equipment) p 356
MarcoTilt Chair (Marco Equipment) p 356
Maxidex Sterile Ophthalmic Ointment (Alcon Laboratories) p 222
Maxidex Sterile Ophthalmic Suspension (Alcon Laboratories) p 223
Maxitrol Ophthalmic Ointment/Suspension (Alcon Laboratories) p 223
Metimyd Ophthalmic Ointment—Sterile (Schering) p 306
Metimyd Ophthalmic Suspension—Sterile (Schering) p 306
LubriTears Solution (Bausch & Lomb Pharmaceuticals) p 259
Microsponge Teardrop (Alcon Surgical) p 352
◆**Miochol with Iocare Steri-Tags, Miochol System Pak and Miochol System Pak Plus** (IOLAB Pharmaceuticals) p 103, 274
MIOSTAT (Alcon Surgical) p 233
MiraFlow Extra-Strength Cleaner (CIBA Vision Corp.) p 346
Moist Eye Moisture Panels for the Eye (Eagle Vision) p 269
Moisture Drops (Bausch & Lomb Personal) p 258
Murine Eye Lubricant (Ross) p 305
Murine Plus Lubricating Eye Redness Reliever (Ross) p 305
◆**Muro 128 Sodium Chloride Ophthalmic Ointment** (Bausch & Lomb Pharmaceuticals) p 103, 260
◆**Muro 128 Solution 2% and 5%** (Bausch & Lomb Pharmaceuticals) p 103, 260
Murocel (Bausch & Lomb Pharmaceuticals) p 259
Murocoll-2 Sterile Ophthalmic Solution (Bausch & Lomb Pharmaceuticals) p 261
Mydfrin 2.5% (Alcon Laboratories) p 224
Mydriacyl (Alcon Laboratories) p 225

N

Naphcon (Alcon Laboratories) p 226
Naphcon Forte (Alcon Laboratories) p 226
Naphcon-A Ophthalmic Solution (Alcon Laboratories) p 226
Natacyn (Alcon Laboratories) p 227
Neo-Dexair Ophthalmic Solution (Bausch & Lomb Pharmaceuticals) p 259
◆**NeoDecadron Sterile Ophthalmic Ointment** (Merck Sharp & Dohme) p 104, 290
◆**NeoDecadron Sterile Ophthalmic Solution** (Merck Sharp & Dohme) p 104, 291
Neomycin and Polymyxin B Sulfates and Gramicidin Ophthalmic Solution (IOLAB Pharmaceuticals) p 271
Neomycin and Polymyxin B Sulfates and Hydrocortisone Ophthalmic Suspension (IOLAB Pharmaceuticals) p 271
Neomycin Sulfate-Dexamethasone Sodium Phosphate Ophthalmic Solution, USP (IOLAB Pharmaceuticals) p 271
Neosporin Ophthalmic Ointment Sterile (Burroughs Wellcome) p 265
Neosporin Ophthalmic Solution Sterile (Burroughs Wellcome) p 266
◆**Neptazane Tablets** (Storz Ophthalmics) p 105, 311

O

OC-10M, OC-20T & OC-30A Automated Ophthalmic Chairs (Topcon Instrument) p 357
OM 2000 Operation Microscope (Marco Equipment) p 355
OM-4 Ophthalmometer (Topcon Instrument) p 358
OMS-60, OMS-70 and OMS-600 Operation Microscopes (Topcon Instrument) p 358
OU-180 Ophthalmic Chair & Stand (Topcon Instrument) p 357
◆**Occucoat** (Storz Ophthalmics) p 105, 312
Ocu-Caine Sterile Ophthalmic Solution (Ocumed) p 297
Ocu-Carpine Sterile Ophthalmic Solution (Ocumed) p 297
Ocu-Chlor Sterile Ophthalmic Solution (Ocumed) p 297
Ocu-Chlor Sterile Ophthalmic Ointment (Ocumed) p 297
OcuClear Eye Drops (Schering) p 306
Ocu-Cort Sterile Ophthalmic Ointment (Ocumed) p 297
Ocu-Dex Sterile Ophthalmic Ointment (Ocumed) p 297
Ocu-Dex Sterile Ophthalmic Solution (Ocumed) p 297
Ocufen (Allergan Medical Optics) p 237
Ocu-Lone-C Sterile Ophthalmic Ointment (Ocumed) p 297
Ocu-Lone-C Sterile Ophthalmic Suspension (Ocumed) p 297
Ocu-Lube Sterile Ophthalmic Ointment (Ocumed) p 297
Ocu-Mycin Sterile Ophthalmic Ointment (Ocumed) p 297
Ocu-Mycin Sterile Ophthalmic Solution (Ocumed) p 297
Ocu-Pentolate Sterile Ophthalmic Solution (Ocumed) p 297
Ocu-Phrin Sterile Eye Drops (Ocumed) p 297
Ocu-Phrin Sterile Ophthalmic Solution (Ocumed) p 297
Ocu-Pred Forte Sterile Ophthalmic Solution (Ocumed) p 297
Ocu-Pred Sterile Ophthalmic Solution (Ocumed) p 297
Ocu-Pred-A Sterile Ophthalmic Suspension (Ocumed) p 297
Ocusert Pilo-20 and Pilo-40 Ocular Therapeutic Systems (Alza) p 256
Ocu-Sol Sterile Antiseptic Wetting & Lubricating Solution (Ocumed) p 297
Ocu-Spor-B Sterile Ophthalmic Ointment (Ocumed) p 297
Ocu-Spor-G Sterile Ophthalmic Solution (Ocumed) p 297
Ocu-Sul-10 Sterile Ophthalmic Ointment (Ocumed) p 297
Ocu-Sul-10, -15, -30 Sterile Ophthalmic Solution (Ocumed) p 297
Ocu-Tears Sterile Ophthalmic Solution (Ocumed) p 297
Ocutricin HC Ointment (Bausch & Lomb Pharmaceuticals) p 259
Ocutricin HC Suspension (Bausch & Lomb Pharmaceuticals) p 259
Ocutricin Ointment (Bausch & Lomb Pharmaceuticals) p 259
Ocutricin Solution (Bausch & Lomb Pharmaceuticals) p 259
Ocu-Trol Sterile Ophthalmic Ointment (Ocumed) p 297
Ocu-Trol Sterile Ophthalmic Suspension (Ocumed) p 297
Ocu-Tropic Sterile Ophthalmic Solution (Ocumed) p 297
Ocu-Tropine Sterile Ophthalmic Ointment (Ocumed) p 297
Ocu-Tropine Sterile Ophthalmic Solution (Ocumed) p 297
Ocuvite Vitamin and Mineral Supplement (Storz Ophthalmics) p 312
Ocu-Zoline Sterile Ophthalmic Solution (Ocumed) p 297
Opcon Ophthalmic Solution (Bausch & Lomb Pharmaceuticals) p 259
Opcon-A Ophthalmic Solution (Bausch & Lomb Pharmaceuticals) p 262
◆**Ophthalgan** (Wyeth-Ayerst) p 105, 315
Ophthalmic Nutrients (Health Maintenance) p 270
Ophthetic (Allergan Pharmaceuticals) p 249
◆**Ophthochlor Ophthalmic Solution** (Parke-Davis) p 104, 300
◆**Ophthocort** (Parke-Davis) p 104, 301
Optemp (Alcon Surgical) p 352
◆**Opticrom 4% Ophthalmic Solution** (Fisons) p 103, 270
◆**OptiPranolol Sterile Ophthalmic Solution** (Bausch & Lomb Pharmaceuticals) p 103, 261
Orcolon (Optical Radiation) p 325
OSMOGLYN (Alcon Surgical) p 234
OxyCup Lens Case (Allergan Optical) p 339
OxyTab Cup (Allergan Optical) p 332

P

PR-1000 Auto Refractometer (Topcon Instrument) p 357
PAIR-PAK II Suture Pack (Alcon Surgical) p 359
Pentolair Solution (Bausch & Lomb Pharmaceuticals) p 259
Petrolatum Ointment (Bausch & Lomb Pharmaceuticals) p 259
Phacoemulsification Kits (Alcon Surgical) p 352
Phenylephrine HCl 10% (Rfg.) Dropperettes (IOLAB Pharmaceuticals) p 271
Phenylephrine Hydrochloride Ophthalmic Solution 2.5%, Sterile (Bausch & Lomb Pharmaceuticals) p 259
Phenylephrine Hydrochloride 2.5% Ophthalmic Solution, USP (IOLAB Pharmaceuticals) p 271
◆**Phospholine Iodide** (Wyeth-Ayerst) p 105, 315
Photocolor Hard Resin Spectacle Lenses (Rodenstock) p 349
Pilagan Liquifilm Sterile Ophthalmic Solution (Allergan Pharmaceuticals) p 250
Pilagan Liquifilm Sterile Ophthalmic Solution with C Cap Compliance Cap (Allergan Pharmaceuticals) p 250
◆**Pilocar** (IOLAB Pharmaceuticals) p 103, 275
◆**Pilocar Dropperettes 1%, 2% and 4%** (IOLAB Pharmaceuticals) p 103, 271
◆**Pilocar Twin Pack** (IOLAB Pharmaceuticals) p 103, 275
Pilopine HS Gel (Alcon Laboratories) p 227
Pilostat Sterile Ophthalmic Solution 0.5%, 1%, 2%, 3%, 4%, 5%, 6% (Bausch & Lomb Pharmaceuticals) p 263
Polymacon Hydrophilic Contact Lenses (Bausch & Lomb Contact Lens) p 317
Poly-Pred Liquifilm (Allergan Pharmaceuticals) p 250
Polysporin Ophthalmic Ointment Sterile (Burroughs Wellcome) p 266
Polytrim Ophthalmic Solution Sterile (Allergan Pharmaceuticals) p 251
Pred Forte (Allergan Pharmaceuticals) p 252
Pred Mild (Allergan Pharmaceuticals) p 254
Pred-G Liquifilm Sterile Ophthalmic Suspension (Allergan Pharmaceuticals) p 252
Pred-G S.O.P. Sterile Ophthalmic Ointment (Allergan Pharmaceuticals) p 253
Prednisolone Sodium Phosphate Ophthalmic Solution, Sterile (Bausch & Lomb Pharmaceuticals) p 259
Prefrin Liquifilm Vasoconstrictor and Lubricant Eye Drops (Allergan Pharmaceuticals) p 254
Prefrin-A (Allergan Pharmaceuticals) p 255
Profenal Sterile Ophthalmic Solution (Alcon Surgical) p 234
ProFree/GP Weekly Enzymatic Cleaner (Allergan Optical) p 339
Progressiv R Spectacle Lenses (Rodenstock) p 349
Progressiv S Spectacle Lenses (Rodenstock) p 349
Proparacaine Hydrochloride Ophthalmic Solution, Sterile (Bausch & Lomb Pharmaceuticals) p 259
Proparacaine Hydrochloride and Fluorescein Sodium Ophthalmic Soluton, Sterile (Bausch & Lomb Pharmaceuticals) p 259
Propine with C Cap Compliance Cap (Allergan Pharmaceuticals) p 255

R

RM-A2000 & RM-A2300 Refractometers (Topcon Instrument) p 357
Refresh Lubricant Ophthalmic Solution (Allergan Pharmaceuticals) p 256
Refresh P.M. Lubricant Ophthalmic Ointment (Allergan Pharmaceuticals) p 256
Relief Vasoconstrictor and Lubricant Eye Drops (Allergan Pharmaceuticals) p 256
Resolve/GP Daily Cleaner (Allergan Optical) p 339
Rēv-Eyes Ophthalmic Eyedrops 0.5% (Storz Ophthalmics) p 312
Rose Bengal 1% (Akorn) p 209

S

SITE-TXR Microsurgical System (SITE) p 357
SLIMFIT Ovoid Optic Lenses (IOLAB) p 323
Sno Strips Tear Flow Test Strips (Akorn) p 209
Soakare Hard Contact Lens Soaking Solution (Allergan Optical) p 340
Sodium Sulamyd Ophthalmic Ointment 10%-Sterile (Schering) p 307
Sodium Sulamyd Ophthalmic Solution 10%-Sterile (Schering) p 307
Sodium Sulamyd Ophthalmic Solution 30%-Sterile (Schering) p 307
SoftWear Sterile Saline Solution for Sensitive Eyes (CIBA Vision Corp.) p 347
Solitaire Small Incision Closure Needles (Alcon Surgical) p 359
STERI-UNITS (Alcon Surgical) p 235
Style Keeper Contact Lens Carrying Case (Allergan Optical) p 340
Succus Cineraria Maritima (SCM-Walker) (Walker Pharmacal) p 313
Sulf-10 Dropperettes 10% (IOLAB Pharmaceuticals) p 271
Sulf-10 Ophthalmic Solution 10% (IOLAB Pharmaceuticals) p 271
Sulfacetamide Sodium Ophthalmic Ointment 10%, Sterile (Bausch & Lomb Pharmaceuticals) p 259
Sulfacetamide Sodium Ophthalmic Solution, 10%, 15% and 30%, Sterile (Bausch & Lomb Pharmaceuticals) p 259
Sulphrin Ointment (Bausch & Lomb Pharmaceuticals) p 259
Sulphrin Suspension (Bausch & Lomb Pharmaceuticals) p 259
Sulpred Suspension (Bausch & Lomb Pharmaceuticals) p 259
SureVue Contact Lenses (Vistakon) p 322

T

Tearisol Ophthalmic Solution (IOLAB Pharmaceuticals) p 271
Tears Naturale II Lubricant Eye Drops (Alcon Laboratories) p 228
Tears Naturale Free (Alcon Laboratories) p 228
Tears Plus Lubricant Ophthalmic Solution (Allergan Pharmaceuticals) p 256
Tears Renewed Ointment (Akorn) p 209
Tears Renewed Solution (Akorn) p 209
Tetracaine HCl Dropperettes ½% (IOLAB Pharmaceuticals) p 271
Tetracaine Hydrochloride Ophthalmic Solution, Sterile (Bausch & Lomb Pharmaceuticals) p 259
◆**Timoptic in Ocudose** (Merck Sharp & Dohme) p 104, 294
◆**Timoptic Sterile Ophthalmic Solution** (Merck Sharp & Dohme) p 104, 292
TobraDex Ophthalmic Suspension and Ointment (Alcon Laboratories) p 228
Tobrex Ophthalmic Ointment and Solution (Alcon Laboratories) p 229
Topcon Retinal Cameras (Topcon Instrument) p 358
Topcon Slit Lamps (Topcon Instrument) p 358
Topcon Trial Lens Set and Frame (Topcon Instrument) p 358
Total All-In-One Hard Contact Lens Solution (Allergan Optical) p 340
Tropicacyl (Akorn) p 209
Tropicamide Ophthalmic Solution, Sterile (Bausch & Lomb Pharmaceuticals) p 259

U

Ultrazyme Enzymatic Cleaner (Allergan Optical) p 340

V

VT-10 Vision Tester (Topcon Instrument) p 358
VT-D5 Vision Tester (Topcon Instrument) p 358
VT-SE Vision Tester (Topcon Instrument) p 358
Vasocidin Ointment (IOLAB Pharmaceuticals) p 275
Vasocidin Ophthalmic Solution (IOLAB Pharmaceuticals) p 276
Vasocon Regular (IOLAB Pharmaceuticals) p 271
Vasocon-A (IOLAB Pharmaceuticals) p 278
Vasosulf (IOLAB Pharmaceuticals) p 279
◆**Vira-A Ophthalmic Ointment, 3%** (Parke-Davis) p 104, 302
Viroptic Ophthalmic Solution, 1% Sterile (Burroughs Wellcome) p 267
Viscoat Sterile Viscoelastic Ophthalmic (Alcon Surgical) p 235
◆**Visine A.C. Eye Drops** (Pfizer Consumer) p 104, 303
◆**Visine EXTRA Eye Drops** (Pfizer Consumer) p 104, 303
◆**Visine Eye Drops** (Pfizer Consumer) p 104, 303
◆**Visine L.R. Eye Drope** (Pfizer Consumer) p 104, 303
Volk 60D, 78D and 90D Double Aspheric Lenses (Volk Optical) p 358
Volk Area Centralis Fundus Laser Lenses (Volk Optical) p 358
Volk Double Aspheric Lenses (Volk Optical) p 358
Volk QuadrAspheric Fundus Laser Lenses (Volk Optical) p 358
Volk TransEquator Fundus Laser Lenses (Volk Optical) p 358
◆**Voltaren Ophthalmic Sterile Ophthalmic Solution** (CIBA Vision Ophthalmics) p 103, 268

W

Wet-N-Soak Wetting and Soaking Solution (Allergan Optical) p 342
Wet-N-Soak Plus Wetting and Soaking Solution (Allergan Optical) p 342

Z

Zincfrin (Alcon Laboratories) p 230
Zolyse (Alcon Surgical) p 236

Part 3— Product Category Index

A

ALLERGY RELIEF PRODUCTS, OPHTHALMIC
Allergy Drops (Bausch & Lomb Personal) p 258
Clear Eyes ACR (Ross) p 105, 305
Naphcon-A Ophthalmic Solution (Alcon Laboratories) p 226
Opticrom 4% Ophthalmic Solution (Fisons) p 103, 270

ALPHA ADRENERGIC AGONIST
IOPIDINE (Alcon Surgical) p 232

ANESTHETICS
TOPICAL/OPHTHALMIC
AK-Taine (Akorn) p 207
Alcaine (Alcon Laboratories) p 210
Ocu-Caine Sterile Ophthalmic Solution (Ocumed) p 297
Ophthetic (Allergan Pharmaceuticals) p 249
Proparacaine Hydrochloride Ophthalmic Solution, Sterile (Bausch & Lomb Pharmaceuticals) p 259
Tetracaine HCl Dropperettes ½% (IOLAB Pharmaceuticals) p 271
Tetracaine Hydrochloride Ophthalmic Solution, Sterile (Bausch & Lomb Pharmaceuticals) p 259

ANTIBACTERIALS (see under ANTIBIOTICS & ANTISEPTICS)

ANTIBIOTICS
VIRAL AGENTS (see under VIRAL AGENTS)

ANTIBIOTICS (TOPICAL/OPHTHALMIC)
ANTIBACTERIALS
Chibroxin Sterile Ophthalmic Solution (Merck Sharp & Dohme) p 103, 282
Ciloxan Sterile Ophthalmic Solution (Alcon Laboratories) p 214
ANTIBIOTICS & COMBINATIONS
Achromycin Ophthalmic Ointment 1% (Storz Ophthalmics) p 307
Achromycin Ophthalmic Suspension 1% (Storz Ophthalmics) p 105, 308
AK-Chlor Sterile Ophthalmic Ointment & Solution (Akorn) p 201
AK-Mycin Ointment (Akorn) p 204
AK-Poly-Bac Ointment (Akorn) p 205
AK-Spore Ointment (Akorn) p 205
AK-Spore Solution (Akorn) p 205
Auroemycin Ophthalmic Ointment 1.0% (Storz Ophthalmics) p 308
Bacitracin Ophthalmic Ointment-Sterile (Bausch & Lomb Pharmaceuticals) p 259
Bacitracin Zinc and Polymyxin B Sulfate Ophthalmic Ointment, Sterile (Bausch & Lomb Pharmaceuticals) p 259
Chibroxin Sterile Ophthalmic Solution (Merck Sharp & Dohme) p 103, 282
Chloramphenicol Ophthalmic Ointment, Sterile (Bausch & Lomb Pharmaceuticals) p 259
Chloramphenicol Ophthalmic Solution, Sterile (Bausch & Lomb Pharmaceuticals) p 259
Chloromycetin Ophthalmic Ointment, 1% (Parke-Davis) p 104, 299
Chloromycetin Ophthalmic Solution (Parke-Davis) p 104, 300
Chloroptic S.O.P. (Allergan Pharmaceuticals) p 243
Chloroptic Sterile Ophthalmic Solution (Allergan Pharmaceuticals) p 243
Ciloxan Sterile Ophthalmic Solution (Alcon Laboratories) p 214
Cortisporin Ophthalmic Ointment Sterile (Burroughs Wellcome) p 263
Cortisporin Ophthalmic Suspension Sterile (Burroughs Wellcome) p 264
Erythromycin Ophthalmic Ointment, Sterile (Bausch & Lomb Pharmaceuticals) p 259
Garamycin Ophthalmic Ointment—Sterile (Schering) p 305
Garamycin Ophthalmic Solution—Sterile (Schering) p 305
Genoptic Liquifilm Sterile Ophthalmic Solution (Allergan Pharmaceuticals) p 247
Genoptic S.O.P. Sterile Ophthalmic Ointment (Allergan Pharmaceuticals) p 247
Gentacidin Ointment (IOLAB Pharmaceuticals) p 273
Gentacidin Solution (IOLAB Pharmaceuticals) p 273
Gentak Ointment & Solution (Akorn) p 208
Gentamicin Ointment (Bausch & Lomb Pharmaceuticals) p 259
Gentamicin Solution (Bausch & Lomb Pharmaceuticals) p 259
Neosporin Ophthalmic Ointment Sterile (Burroughs Wellcome) p 265
Neosporin Ophthalmic Solution Sterile (Burroughs Wellcome) p 266
Ocu-Chlor Sterile Ophthalmic Solution (Ocumed) p 297
Ocu-Chlor Sterile Ophthalmic Ointment (Ocumed) p 297
Ocu-Mycin Sterile Ophthalmic Ointment (Ocumed) p 297
Ocu-Mycin Sterile Ophthalmic Solution (Ocumed) p 297
Ocu-Spor-B Sterile Ophthalmic Ointment (Ocumed) p 297
Ocu-Spor-G Sterile Ophthalmic Solution (Ocumed) p 297
Ocutricin HC Ointment (Bausch & Lomb Pharmaceuticals) p 259
Ocutricin HC Suspension (Bausch & Lomb Pharmaceuticals) p 259
Ocutricin Ointment (Bausch & Lomb Pharmaceuticals) p 259
Ocutricin Solution (Bausch & Lomb Pharmaceuticals) p 259
Ophthochlor Ophthalmic Solution (Parke-Davis) p 104, 300
Polysporin Ophthalmic Ointment Sterile (Burroughs Wellcome) p 266
Polytrim Ophthalmic Solution Sterile (Allergan Pharmaceuticals) p 251
TobraDex Ophthalmic Suspension and Ointment (Alcon Laboratories) p 228
Tobrex Ophthalmic Ointment and Solution (Alcon Laboratories) p 229

ANTIFUNGAL
Natacyn (Alcon Laboratories) p 227

CORTICOSTEROIDS & COMBINATIONS
AK-Cide Sterile Ophthalmic Ointment & Suspension (Akorn) p 202
AK-Spore H.C. Ointment (Akorn) p 206
AK-Spore H. C. Suspension (Akorn) p 206
AK-Trol Ointment & Suspension (Akorn) p 207
Blephamide Liquifilm (Allergan Pharmaceuticals) p 242
Blephamide S.O.P. (Allergan Pharmaceuticals) p 242
Cetapred Ointment (Alcon Laboratories) p 220
Chloromycetin Hydrocortisone Ophthalmic (Parke-Davis) p 104, 298
Cortisporin Ophthalmic Ointment Sterile (Burroughs Wellcome) p 263
Cortisporin Ophthalmic Suspension Sterile (Burroughs Wellcome) p 264
Decadron Phosphate Sterile Ophthalmic Ointment (Merck Sharp & Dohme) p 103, 285
Decadron Phosphate Sterile Ophthalmic Solution (Merck Sharp & Dohme) p 103, 285
Dexacidin Ointment (IOLAB Pharmaceuticals) p 272
Dexacidin Suspension (IOLAB Pharmaceuticals) p 272
Dexamethasone Sodium Phosphate Ophthalmic Ointment, Sterile (Bausch & Lomb Pharmaceuticals) p 259
Dexamethasone Sodium Phosphate Ophthalmic Solution, Sterile (Bausch & Lomb Pharmaceuticals) p 259
Dexasporin Ointment (Bausch & Lomb Pharmaceuticals) p 259
Dexasporin Suspension (Bausch & Lomb Pharmaceuticals) p 259
FML-S Sterile Ophthalmic Suspension (Allergan Pharmaceuticals) p 246
Isopto Cetapred Suspension (Alcon Laboratories) p 220
Maxitrol Ophthalmic Ointment/Suspension (Alcon Laboratories) p 223
Metimyd Ophthalmic Ointment—Sterile (Schering) p 306
Metimyd Ophthalmic Suspension—Sterile (Schering) p 306
Neo-Dexair Ophthalmic Solution (Bausch & Lomb Pharmaceuticals) p 259
NeoDecadron Sterile Ophthalmic Ointment (Merck Sharp & Dohme) p 104, 290
NeoDecadron Sterile Ophthalmic Solution (Merck Sharp & Dohme) p 104, 291
Ocu-Cort Sterile Ophthalmic Ointment (Ocumed) p 297
Ocu-Dex Sterile Ophthalmic Ointment (Ocumed) p 297
Ocu-Dex Sterile Ophthalmic Solution (Ocumed) p 297
Ocu-Lone-C Sterile Ophthalmic Ointment (Ocumed) p 297
Ocu-Lone-C Sterile Ophthalmic Suspension (Ocumed) p 297
Ocu-Pred Forte Sterile Ophthalmic Solution (Ocumed) p 297
Ocu-Pred Sterile Ophthalmic Solution (Ocumed) p 297
Ocu-Pred-A Sterile Ophthalmic Suspension (Ocumed) p 297
Ocu-Trol Sterile Ophthalmic Ointment (Ocumed) p 297
Ocu-Trol Sterile Ophthalmic Suspension (Ocumed) p 297
Ophthocort (Parke-Davis) p 104, 301
Poly-Pred Liquifilm (Allergan Pharmaceuticals) p 250
Pred-G Liquifilm Sterile Ophthalmic Suspension (Allergan Pharmaceuticals) p 252
Pred-G S.O.P. Sterile Ophthalmic Ointment (Allergan Pharmaceuticals) p 253
Prednisolone Sodium Phosphate Ophthalmic Solution, Sterile (Bausch & Lomb Pharmaceuticals) p 259
Sulphrin Ointment (Bausch & Lomb Pharmaceuticals) p 259
TobraDex Ophthalmic Suspension and Ointment (Alcon Laboratories) p 228
Vasocidin Ointment (IOLAB Pharmaceuticals) p 275
Vasocidin Ophthalmic Solution (IOLAB Pharmaceuticals) p 276

SULFONAMIDES & COMBINATIONS
AK-Cide Sterile Ophthalmic Ointment & Suspension (Akorn) p 202
AK-Sulf (Akorn) p 103, 207
Bleph-10 Ophthalmic Solution with Liquifilm (Allergan Pharmaceuticals) p 241
Bleph-10 Ophthalmic Ointment (Allergan Pharmaceuticals) p 241

Blephamide Liquifilm (Allergan Pharmaceuticals) p 242
Blephamide S.O.P. (Allergan Pharmaceuticals) p 242
Cetamide Ointment (Alcon Laboratories) p 220
Gantrisin Ophthalmic Ointment/Solution (Roche) p 105, 304
Isopto Cetamide Solution (Alcon Laboratories) p 220
Ocu-Sul-10 Sterile Ophthalmic Ointment (Ocumed) p 297
Ocu-Sul-10, -15, -30 Sterile Ophthalmic Solution (Ocumed) p 297
Sodium Sulamyd Ophthalmic Ointment 10%-Sterile (Schering) p 307
Sodium Sulamyd Ophthalmic Solution 10%-Sterile (Schering) p 307
Sodium Sulamyd Ophthalmic Solution 30%-Sterile (Schering) p 307
Sulf-10 Dropperettes 10% (IOLAB Pharmaceuticals) p 271
Sulf-10 Ophthalmic Solution 10% (IOLAB Pharmaceuticals) p 271
Sulpred Suspension (Bausch & Lomb Pharmaceuticals) p 259
Vasosulf (IOLAB Pharmaceuticals) p 279

ANTIGLAUCOMATOUS AGENTS

BETA ADRENERGIC BLOCKING AGENT (TOPICAL)
Betagan Liquifilm (Allergan Pharmaceuticals) p 239
Betagan Liquifilm with C Cap Compliance Cap (Allergan Pharmaceuticals) p 239
Betoptic Sterile Ophthalmic Solution (Alcon Laboratories) p 211
Betoptic S Sterile Ophthalmic Suspension (Alcon Laboratories) p 212
OptiPranolol Sterile Ophthalmic Solution (Bausch & Lomb Pharmaceuticals) p 103, 261
Timoptic in Ocudose (Merck Sharp & Dohme) p 104, 294
Timoptic Sterile Ophthalmic Solution (Merck Sharp & Dohme) p 104, 292

CARBONIC ANHYDRASE INHIBITORS
Daranide Tablets (Merck Sharp & Dohme) p 103, 284
Diamox Parenteral (Storz Ophthalmics) p 308
Diamox Sequels (Sustained Release) (Storz Ophthalmics) p 105, 310
Diamox Tablets (Storz Ophthalmics) p 105, 308
Neptazane Tablets (Storz Ophthalmics) p 105, 311

EPINEPHRINE PREPARATIONS
E-Pilo-1, E-Pilo-2, E-Pilo-3, E-Pilo-4, E-Pilo-6 (IOLAB Pharmaceuticals) p 271
Epifrin (Allergan Pharmaceuticals) p 244
Epinephrine 1:1000 Dropperettes (IOLAB Pharmaceuticals) p 271
Glaucon (Alcon Laboratories) p 218
Propine with C Cap Compliance Cap (Allergan Pharmaceuticals) p 255

HYPEROSMOTIC AGENT
ISMOTIC (Alcon Surgical) p 233
OSMOGLYN (Alcon Surgical) p 234

MIOTIC (DIRECT ACTING)

PARASYMPATHOMIMETICS
Akarpine Ophthalmic Solution (Akorn) p 201
E-Pilo-1, E-Pilo-2, E-Pilo-3, E-Pilo-4, E-Pilo-6 (IOLAB Pharmaceuticals) p 271
Isopto Carbachol (Alcon Laboratories) p 219
Isopto Carpine (Alcon Laboratories) p 219
Ocu-Carpine Sterile Ophthalmic Solution (Ocumed) p 297
Ocusert Pilo-20 and Pilo-40 Ocular Therapeutic Systems (Alza) p 256
Pilagan Liquifilm Sterile Ophthalmic Solution (Allergan Pharmaceuticals) p 250
Pilagan Liquifilm Sterile Ophthalmic Solution with C Cap Compliance Cap (Allergan Pharmaceuticals) p 250
Pilocar (IOLAB Pharmaceuticals) p 103, 275
Pilocar Dropperettes 1%, 2% and 4% (IOLAB Pharmaceuticals) p 103, 271
Pilocar Twin Pack (IOLAB Pharmaceuticals) p 103, 275
Pilopine HS Gel (Alcon Laboratories) p 227
Pilostat Sterile Ophthalmic Solution 0.5%, 1%, 2%, 3%, 4%, 5%, 6% (Bausch & Lomb Pharmaceuticals) p 263

MIOTIC (INDIRECT ACTING)

CHOLINESTERASE INHIBITOR
Floropryl Sterile Ophthalmic Ointment (Merck Sharp & Dohme) p 103, 286
Humorsol Ophthalmic Solution (Merck Sharp & Dohme) p 103, 287
Phospholine Iodide (Wyeth-Ayerst) p 105, 315

ANTIHISTAMINES
AK-Con-A (Akorn) p 203
Albalon-A Liquifilm (Allergan Pharmaceuticals) p 238
Opcon-A Ophthalmic Solution (Bausch & Lomb Pharmaceuticals) p 262
Prefrin-A (Allergan Pharmaceuticals) p 255
Vasocon-A (IOLAB Pharmaceuticals) p 278

ANTI-INFLAMMATORY AGENTS

NON-STEROIDALS
Voltaren Ophthalmic Sterile Ophthalmic Solution (CIBA Vision Ophthalmics) p 103, 268

ANTIOXIDANTS
ICAPS Plus (La Haye) p 280
Ophthalmic Nutrients (Health Maintenance) p 270

ANTIVIRAL AGENTS (see under VIRAL AGENTS)

ARTIFICIAL EYE CLEANSER/LUBRICANT
Enuclene (Alcon Surgical) p 232

ARTIFICIAL TEARS PREPARATIONS
Adsorbotear (Alcon Laboratories) p 210
Celluvisc Lubricant Ophthalmic Solution (Allergan Pharmaceuticals) p 243
Dry Eye Therapy (Bausch & Lomb Personal) p 258
HypoTears Lubricating Eye Drops (IOLAB Pharmaceuticals) p 273
HypoTears PF Preservative-Free Lubricating Eye Drops (IOLAB Pharmaceuticals) p 273
Lacril Lubricant Ophthalmic Solution (Allergan Pharmaceuticals) p 248
Liquifilm Forte Lubricant Ophthalmic Solution (Allergan Pharmaceuticals) p 249
Liquifilm Tears Lubricant Ophthalmic Solution (Allergan Pharmaceuticals) p 249
LubriTears Ointment (Bausch & Lomb Pharmaceuticals) p 259
LubriTears Solution (Bausch & Lomb Pharmaceuticals) p 259
Moisture Drops (Bausch & Lomb Personal) p 258
Murocel (Bausch & Lomb Pharmaceuticals) p 259
Prefrin Liquifilm Vasoconstrictor and Lubricant Eye Drops (Allergan Pharmaceuticals) p 254
Refresh Lubricant Ophthalmic Solution (Allergan Pharmaceuticals) p 256
Relief Vasoconstrictor and Lubricant Eye Drops (Allergan Pharmaceuticals) p 256
Tearisol Ophthalmic Solution (IOLAB Pharmaceuticals) p 271
Tears Naturale II Lubricant Eye Drops (Alcon Laboratories) p 228
Tears Naturale Free (Alcon Laboratories) p 228
Tears Plus Lubricant Ophthalmic Solution (Allergan Pharmaceuticals) p 256
Tears Renewed Solution (Akorn) p 209

C

COLLAGEN IMPLANTS
Collagen Implants (Intracanalicular) for Lacrimal Efficiency Test (Lacrimedics) p 281

COLLAGEN SHIELD
BIO-COR 12, 24, and 72 Collagen Corneal Shield (Bausch & Lomb Pharmaceuticals) p 103, 260

COMPLIANCE AIDS
Betagan Liquifilm with C Cap Compliance Cap (Allergan Pharmaceuticals) p 239
Pilagan Liquifilm Sterile Ophthalmic Solution with C Cap Compliance Cap (Allergan Pharmaceuticals) p 250
Propine with C Cap Compliance Cap (Allergan Pharmaceuticals) p 255

CONTACT LENS APPLIANCES & ACCESSORIES

STORING SYSTEMS
Clean-N-Soakit Hard Contact Lens Storage Case (Allergan Optical) p 328
Clean-N-Stow Hard Contact Lens Storage Case (Allergan Optical) p 328
Lens Plus Oxysept Disinfection System (Allergan Optical) p 332
Lensept Disinfection System (CIBA Vision Corp.) p 345
LensKeeper Contact Lens Carrying Case (Allergan Optical) p 337
OxyCup Lens Case (Allergan Optical) p 339
OxyTab Cup (Allergan Optical) p 332
Style Keeper Contact Lens Carrying Case (Allergan Optical) p 340

CONTACT LENS (SOFT LENS)

DAILY WEAR, VISION CORRECTION
Acuvue Contact Lenses (Vistakon) p 321
Bausch & Lomb NaturalTint Hydrophilic Contact Lenses (Bausch & Lomb Contact Lens) p 317
Bausch & Lomb P.A.1 Bifocal Hydrophilic Contact Lenses (Bausch & Lomb Contact Lens) p 317
Bausch & Lomb Soflens Hydrophilic Contact Lenses (Bausch & Lomb Contact Lens) p 317
Polymacon Hydrophilic Contact Lenses (Bausch & Lomb Contact Lens) p 317
SureVue Contact Lenses (Vistakon) p 322

EXTENDED WEAR, VISION CORRECTION
Acuvue Contact Lenses (Vistakon) p 321
Bausch & Lomb Medalist Tinted Contact Lenses (Bausch & Lomb Contact Lens) p 317
Bausch & Lomb NaturalTint Hydrophilic Contact Lenses (Bausch & Lomb Contact Lens) p 317

Bausch & Lomb Soflens Hydrophilic Contact Lenses (Bausch & Lomb Contact Lens) p 317
Polymacon Hydrophilic Contact Lenses (Bausch & Lomb Contact Lens) p 317

CONTACT LENS—HARD LENS CARE PRODUCTS

CLEANING SOLUTION
Blink-N-Clean Contact Lens Solution (Allergan Optical) p 328
Clean-N-Soak Hard Contact Lens Cleaning & Soaking Solution (Allergan Optical) p 328
EasyClean/GP Daily Cleaner (Allergan Optical) p 328
LC-65 Daily Contact Lens Cleaner (Allergan Optical) p 330
MiraFlow Extra-Strength Cleaner (CIBA Vision Corp.) p 346
Resolve/GP Daily Cleaner (Allergan Optical) p 339

GENERAL PURPOSE
Total All-In-One Hard Contact Lens Solution (Allergan Optical) p 340

REWETTING AND LUBRICATING
Blink-N-Clean Contact Lens Solution (Allergan Optical) p 328
Lens Fresh Lubricating & Rewetting Drops (Allergan Optical) p 331
Lens-Wet Lubricating & Rewetting Solution (Allergan Optical) p 338
Ocu-Sol Sterile Antiseptic Wetting & Lubricating Solution (Ocumed) p 297

SOAKING
Clean-N-Soak Hard Contact Lens Cleaning & Soaking Solution (Allergan Optical) p 328
Ocu-Sol Sterile Antiseptic Wetting & Lubricating Solution (Ocumed) p 297
Soakare Hard Contact Lens Soaking Solution (Allergan Optical) p 340
Wet-N-Soak Wetting and Soaking Solution (Allergan Optical) p 342
Wet-N-Soak Plus Wetting and Soaking Solution (Allergan Optical) p 342

WETTING
Liquifilm Wetting Solution (Allergan Optical) p 338
Ocu-Sol Sterile Antiseptic Wetting & Lubricating Solution (Ocumed) p 297
Wet-N-Soak Wetting and Soaking Solution (Allergan Optical) p 342
Wet-N-Soak Plus Wetting and Soaking Solution (Allergan Optical) p 342

CONTACT LENS—RIGID GAS PERMEABLE LENS CARE PRODUCTS

CLEANERS
Boston Advance Cleaner (Polymer Technology) p 104, 348
EasyClean/GP Daily Cleaner (Allergan Optical) p 328
LC-65 Daily Contact Lens Cleaner (Allergan Optical) p 330
ProFree/GP Weekly Enzymatic Cleaner (Allergan Optical) p 339
Resolve/GP Daily Cleaner (Allergan Optical) p 339

DISINFECTION
Boston Advance Conditioning Solution (Polymer Technology) p 348

PROTEIN REMOVERS
Boston Advance Cleaner (Polymer Technology) p 104, 348

REWETTING & LUBRICATING
Boston Advance Rewetting Drops (Polymer Technology) p 348

SOAKING
Boston Advance Conditioning Solution (Polymer Technology) p 348
Wet-N-Soak Wetting and Soaking Solution (Allergan Optical) p 342
Wet-N-Soak Plus Wetting and Soaking Solution (Allergan Optical) p 342

WETTING
Wet-N-Soak Wetting and Soaking Solution (Allergan Optical) p 342
Wet-N-Soak Plus Wetting and Soaking Solution (Allergan Optical) p 342

CONTACT LENS—SOFT LENS CARE PRODUCTS

CLEANERS
Allergan Enzymatic Contact Lens Cleaner (Allergan Optical) p 327
Allergan Hydrocare Cleaning and Disinfecting Solution (Allergan Optical) p 325
Extenzyme Protein Cleaner (Allergan Optical) p 329
LC-65 Daily Contact Lens Cleaner (Allergan Optical) p 330
Lens Clear Soft Lens Cleaner (Allergan Optical) p 331
Lens Plus Daily Cleaner (Allergan Optical) p 332
MiraFlow Extra-Strength Cleaner (CIBA Vision Corp.) p 346
Ultrazyme Enzymatic Cleaner (Allergan Optical) p 340

NEUTRALIZERS
Lens Plus Oxysept 2 Rinse & Neutralizer (Allergan Optical) p 334
Lensept Disinfection System (CIBA Vision Corp.) p 345
Lensept Neutralizer & Rinsing/Storage Solution (CIBA Vision Corp.) p 345

PROTEIN REMOVERS
Allergan Enzymatic Contact Lens Cleaner (Allergan Optical) p 327
Extenzyme Protein Cleaner (Allergan Optical) p 329
Ultrazyme Enzymatic Cleaner (Allergan Optical) p 340

REWETTING & LUBRICATING
Lens Fresh Lubricating & Rewetting Drops (Allergan Optical) p 331
Lens Plus Rewetting Drops (Allergan Optical) p 336
Lens-Wet Lubricating & Rewetting Solution (Allergan Optical) p 338

RINSING (COLD)
Allergan Hydrocare Preserved Saline Solution (Allergan Optical) p 326
Allergan Sorbi-Care Saline Solution (Allergan Optical) p 327
Lens Plus Oxysept Disinfection System (Allergan Optical) p 332
Lens Plus Oxysept 2 Rinse & Neutralizer (Allergan Optical) p 334
Lens Plus Sterile Saline Solution (Preservative Free) (Allergan Optical) p 336
Lensept Disinfection System (CIBA Vision Corp.) p 345
Lensept Neutralizer & Rinsing/Storage Solution (CIBA Vision Corp.) p 345
Lensrins Preserved Saline Solution (Allergan Optical) p 337
SoftWear Sterile Saline Solution for Sensitive Eyes (CIBA Vision Corp.) p 347

RINSING (HEAT)
Allergan Hydrocare Preserved Saline Solution (Allergan Optical) p 326
Allergan Sorbi-Care Saline Solution (Allergan Optical) p 327
CIBA Vision Saline Solution (CIBA Vision Corp.) p 344
Lens Plus Sterile Saline Solution (Preservative Free) (Allergan Optical) p 336
Lensrins Preserved Saline Solution (Allergan Optical) p 337
SoftWear Sterile Saline Solution for Sensitive Eyes (CIBA Vision Corp.) p 347

STORAGE & DISINFECTION (COLD)
AODISC Disinfection/Neutralization System (CIBA Vision Corp.) p 343
AOSEPT Disinfection/Neutralization Solution (CIBA Vision Corp.) p 343
AOSEPT Disinfection/Neutralization System (CIBA Vision Corp.) p 343
Allergan Hydrocare Cleaning and Disinfecting Solution (Allergan Optical) p 325
Lens Plus Oxysept Disinfection System (Allergan Optical) p 332
Lens Plus Oxysept 1 Disinfecting Solution (Allergan Optical) p 335
Lensept Disinfection Solution (CIBA Vision Corp.) p 345
Lensept Disinfection System (CIBA Vision Corp.) p 345
Lensept Neutralizer & Rinsing/Storage Solution (CIBA Vision Corp.) p 345
SoftWear Sterile Saline Solution for Sensitive Eyes (CIBA Vision Corp.) p 347

STORAGE & DISINFECTION (HEAT)
Allergan Hydrocare Preserved Saline Solution (Allergan Optical) p 326
Allergan Sorbi-Care Saline Solution (Allergan Optical) p 327
Lens Plus Sterile Saline Solution (Preservative Free) (Allergan Optical) p 336
Lensrins Preserved Saline Solution (Allergan Optical) p 337
SoftWear Sterile Saline Solution for Sensitive Eyes (CIBA Vision Corp.) p 347

CORTICOSTEROIDS & COMBINATIONS, OPHTHALMIC
AK-Dex 0.05% Ointment (Akorn) p 203
AK-Dex 0.1% Solution (Akorn) p 203
AK-Pred (Akorn) p 103, 205
Blephamide Liquifilm (Allergan Pharmaceuticals) p 242
Blephamide S.O.P. (Allergan Pharmaceuticals) p 242
⅛% Econopred & 1% Econopred Plus (Alcon Laboratories) p 217
FML Forte Liquifilm (Allergan Pharmaceuticals) p 245
FML Liquifilm (Allergan Pharmaceuticals) p 244
FML S.O.P. (Allergan Pharmaceuticals) p 245
FML-S Sterile Ophthalmic Suspension (Allergan Pharmaceuticals) p 246
Fluor-Op Ophthalmic Suspension (IOLAB Pharmaceuticals) p 272
HMS Liquifilm (Allergan Pharmaceuticals) p 247
Inflamase Forte 1% (IOLAB Pharmaceuticals) p 274
Inflamase Mild ⅛% (IOLAB Pharmaceuticals) p 274
Maxidex Sterile Ophthalmic Ointment (Alcon Laboratories) p 222
Maxidex Sterile Ophthalmic Suspension (Alcon Laboratories) p 223
Poly-Pred Liquifilm (Allergan Pharmaceuticals) p 250
Pred Forte (Allergan Pharmaceuticals) p 252
Pred Mild (Allergan Pharmaceuticals) p 254
Pred-G Liquifilm Sterile Ophthalmic Suspension (Allergan Pharmaceuticals) p 252

Pred-G S.O.P. Sterile Ophthalmic Ointment (Allergan Pharmaceuticals) p 253
Sulfacetamide Sodium Ophthalmic Ointment 10%, Sterile (Bausch & Lomb Pharmaceuticals) p 259
Sulfacetamide Sodium Ophthalmic Solution, 10%, 15% and 30%, Sterile (Bausch & Lomb Pharmaceuticals) p 259
Sulphrin Suspension (Bausch & Lomb Pharmaceuticals) p 259

D

DECONGESTANTS, OPHTHALMIC

DECONGESTANT COMBINATIONS
AK-Con-A (Akorn) p 203
Albalon-A Liquifilm (Allergan Pharmaceuticals) p 238
Naphcon-A Ophthalmic Solution (Alcon Laboratories) p 226
Opcon-A Ophthalmic Solution (Bausch & Lomb Pharmaceuticals) p 262
Prefrin-A (Allergan Pharmaceuticals) p 255
Vasosulf (IOLAB Pharmaceuticals) p 279
Visine EXTRA Eye Drops (Pfizer Consumer) p 104, 303

DECONGESTANT/ASTRINGENT COMBINATIONS
Clear Eyes ACR (Ross) p 105, 305
Visine A.C. Eye Drops (Pfizer Consumer) p 104, 303

DECONGESTANTS
AK-Con (Akorn) p 202
Albalon Solution with Liquifilm (Allergan Pharmaceuticals) p 238
Clear Eyes Lubricating Eye Redness Reliever (Ross) p 304
Collyrium Fresh (Wyeth-Ayerst) p 105, 314
Eye Drops (Bausch & Lomb Pharmaceuticals) p 259
Eye-Zine Sterile Eye Drops (Ocumed) p 297
Murine Plus Lubricating Eye Redness Reliever (Ross) p 305
OcuClear Eye Drops (Schering) p 306
Ocu-Phrin Sterile Eye Drops (Ocumed) p 297
Ocu-Phrin Sterile Ophthalmic Solution (Ocumed) p 297
Ocu-Zoline Sterile Ophthalmic Solution (Ocumed) p 297
Phenylephrine HCl 10% (Rfg.) Dropperettes (IOLAB Pharmaceuticals) p 271
Phenylephrine Hydrochloride Ophthalmic Solution 2.5%, Sterile (Bausch & Lomb Pharmaceuticals) p 259
Prefrin Liquifilm Vasoconstrictor and Lubricant Eye Drops (Allergan Pharmaceuticals) p 254
Relief Vasoconstrictor and Lubricant Eye Drops (Allergan Pharmaceuticals) p 256
Vasocon Regular (IOLAB Pharmaceuticals) p 271
Visine Eye Drops (Pfizer Consumer) p 104, 303
Visine L.R. Eye Drope (Pfizer Consumer) p 104, 303

VASOCONSTRICTOR/ASTRINGENT COMBINATIONS
Zincfrin (Alcon Laboratories) p 230

DEMULCENT
Celluvisc Lubricant Ophthalmic Solution (Allergan Pharmaceuticals) p 243
Clear Eyes ACR (Ross) p 105, 305
Clear Eyes Lubricating Eye Redness Reliever (Ross) p 304
Gonak Ophthalmic Demulcent Solution (Akorn) p 209
Goniosol Ophthalmic Solution (IOLAB Pharmaceuticals) p 271
Lacril Lubricant Ophthalmic Solution (Allergan Pharmaceuticals) p 248
Liquifilm Forte Lubricant Ophthalmic Solution (Allergan Pharmaceuticals) p 249
Liquifilm Tears Lubricant Ophthalmic Solution (Allergan Pharmaceuticals) p 249
Murine Eye Lubricant (Ross) p 305
Murine Plus Lubricating Eye Redness Reliever (Ross) p 305
Murocel (Bausch & Lomb Pharmaceuticals) p 259
Prefrin Liquifilm Vasoconstrictor and Lubricant Eye Drops (Allergan Pharmaceuticals) p 254
Refresh Lubricant Ophthalmic Solution (Allergan Pharmaceuticals) p 256
Relief Vasoconstrictor and Lubricant Eye Drops (Allergan Pharmaceuticals) p 256
Tears Plus Lubricant Ophthalmic Solution (Allergan Pharmaceuticals) p 256
Visine EXTRA Eye Drops (Pfizer Consumer) p 104, 303
Visine L.R. Eye Drope (Pfizer Consumer) p 104, 303

DIAGNOSTICS

LACRIMAL GLAND FUNCTION
Color Bar Schirmer Tear Test (Eagle Vision) p 269

OPHTHALMICS
AK-Fluor Injection 10% and 25% (Akorn) p 204
EV Rose Bengal (Eagle Vision) p 269
Fluoracaine (Akorn) p 208
Fluorescein Sodium 2% Dropperettes (IOLAB Pharmaceuticals) p 271
Fluorescite Injection (Alcon Laboratories) p 217
Fluorescite Syringe (Alcon Laboratories) p 217
Fluorets Ophthalmic Strips (Akorn) p 208
Fluor-I-Strip (Wyeth-Ayerst) p 105, 314
Fluor-I-Strip A.T. (Wyeth-Ayerst) p 105, 314
Funduscein 10% and Funduscein 25% (IOLAB Pharmaceuticals) p 271
Lactoplate (Eagle Vision) p 269
Rose Bengal 1% (Akorn) p 209
Sno Strips Tear Flow Test Strips (Akorn) p 209

DIURETICS

CARBONIC ANHYDRASE INHIBITORS
Diamox Parenteral (Storz Ophthalmics) p 308
Diamox Sequels (Sustained Release) (Storz Ophthalmics) p 105, 310
Diamox Tablets (Storz Ophthalmics) p 105, 308

DRY EYE DEVICES
Collagen Implants (Intracanalicular) for Lacrimal Efficiency Test (Lacrimedics) p 281
EV Monocanalicular Stent (Eagle Vision) p 269
EV Rose Bengal (Eagle Vision) p 269
Eagle Vision-Freeman Punctum Plug (Eagle Vision) p 269
Herrick Lacrimal Plug (Lacrimedics) p 281
Intracanalicular Collagen Implants-Temporary (Eagle Vision) p 269
Lactoplate (Eagle Vision) p 269
Moist Eye Moisture Panels for the Eye (Eagle Vision) p 269

E

EMOLLIENTS, OPHTHALMIC
Lacri-Lube NP Lubricant Ophthalmic Ointment (Allergan Pharmaceuticals) p 249
Lacri-Lube S.O.P. Sterile Ophthalmic Ointment (Allergan Pharmaceuticals) p 249
Refresh P.M. Lubricant Ophthalmic Ointment (Allergan Pharmaceuticals) p 256

EYELID CLEANSER
EV Lid-Cleanser Kit II (Eagle Vision) p 269
EYEscrub Eyelid Cleanser (CooperVision) p 269

EYEWASHES
Allergan Eyewash (Allergan Pharmaceuticals) p 238
Collyrium for Fresh Eyes (Wyeth-Ayerst) p 105, 314
Eye Wash (Bausch & Lomb Personal) p 258
Eye Wash (Bausch & Lomb Pharmaceuticals) p 259
Iri-Sol Sterile Isotonic Buffered Solution (Ocumed) p 297

F

FUNGAL AGENTS

SYSTEMIC
(see under ANTIBIOTICS)

G

GLAUCOMA
(see under ANTIGLAUCOMATOUS AGENTS)

GONIOSCOPIC SOLUTION
Gonak Ophthalmic Demulcent Solution (Akorn) p 209
Gonioscopic Prism Solution (Alcon Laboratories) p 218

H

HERPES TREATMENT
Viroptic Ophthalmic Solution, 1% Sterile (Burroughs Wellcome) p 267

HYPEROSMOTIC OINTMENT & SOLUTION

TOPICAL HYPERTONIC AGENT
Adsorbonac 2% and 5% (Alcon Laboratories) p 210
AK-NaCl 5% Ointment & Solution (Akorn) p 204
Muro 128 Sodium Chloride Ophthalmic Ointment (Bausch & Lomb Pharmaceuticals) p 103, 260
Muro 128 Solution 2% and 5% (Bausch & Lomb Pharmaceuticals) p 103, 260
Ophthalgan (Wyeth-Ayerst) p 105, 315

I

INTRAOCULAR MIOTIC
Miochol with Iocare Steri-Tags, Miochol System Pak and Miochol System Pak Plus (IOLAB Pharmaceuticals) p 103, 274
MIOSTAT (Alcon Surgical) p 233
Rēv-Eyes Ophthalmic Eyedrops 0.5% (Storz Ophthalmics) p 312

IRRIGATING SOLUTION, OPHTHALMIC

FOR EXTERNAL USE
Balanced Salt Solution (Bausch & Lomb Pharmaceuticals) p 259
Collyrium for Fresh Eyes (Wyeth-Ayerst) p 105, 314
Dacriose (IOLAB Pharmaceuticals) p 271

PHYSIOLOGIC
BSS (15 mL & 30 mL) Sterile Irrigation Solution (Alcon Surgical) p 230
BSS (250 mL) Sterile Irrigation Solution (Alcon Surgical) p 231
BSS (500 mL) Sterile Irrigation Solution (Alcon Surgical) p 231
BSS PLUS (500 mL) Sterile Irrigation Solution (Alcon Surgical) p 231
Balanced Salt Solution (Allergan Pharmaceuticals) p 239
Eye-Stream (Alcon Laboratories) p 217
Iocare Balanced Salt Solution 15 ml (IOLAB Pharmaceuticals) p 271
Iocare Balanced Salt Solution 500 ml (IOLAB Pharmaceuticals) p 271
Iri-Sol Sterile Isotonic Buffered Solution (Ocumed) p 297

L

LUBRICANTS, OPHTHALMIC
AKWA Tears Ointment (Akorn) p 208
AKWA Tears Solution (Akorn) p 208
AMVISC Plus (IOLAB) p 323
Boston Advance Rewetting Drops (Polymer Technology) p 348
Cellufresh Lubricant Ophthalmic Solution (Allergan Pharmaceuticals) p 243
Celluvisc Lubricant Ophthalmic Solution (Allergan Pharmaceuticals) p 243
Clear Eyes ACR (Ross) p 105, 305
Clear Eyes Lubricating Eye Redness Reliever (Ross) p 304
Collyrium Fresh (Wyeth-Ayerst) p 105, 314
Dry Eyes Solution (Bausch & Lomb Pharmaceuticals) p 259
Dry Eye Therapy (Bausch & Lomb Personal) p 258
Duolube Eye Ointment (Bausch & Lomb Personal) p 258
Duratears Naturale (Alcon Laboratories) p 216
HypoTears Lubricating Eye Drops (IOLAB Pharmaceuticals) p 273
HypoTears Ointment (IOLAB Pharmaceuticals) p 273
HypoTears PF Preservative-Free Lubricating Eye Drops (IOLAB Pharmaceuticals) p 273
Lacril Lubricant Ophthalmic Solution (Allergan Pharmaceuticals) p 248
Lacri-Lube NP Lubricant Ophthalmic Ointment (Allergan Pharmaceuticals) p 249
Lacri-Lube S.O.P. Sterile Ophthalmic Ointment (Allergan Pharmaceuticals) p 249
Lacrisert (Merck Sharp & Dohme) p 104, 289
Liquifilm Forte Lubricant Ophthalmic Solution (Allergan Pharmaceuticals) p 249
Liquifilm Tears Lubricant Ophthalmic Solution (Allergan Pharmaceuticals) p 249
LubriTears Ointment (Bausch & Lomb Pharmaceuticals) p 259
Moisture Drops (Bausch & Lomb Personal) p 258
Murine Eye Lubricant (Ross) p 305
Murine Plus Lubricating Eye Redness Reliever (Ross) p 305
Murocel (Bausch & Lomb Pharmaceuticals) p 259
Ocu-Lube Sterile Ophthalmic Ointment (Ocumed) p 297
Ocu-Tears Sterile Ophthalmic Solution (Ocumed) p 297
Petrolatum Ointment (Bausch & Lomb Pharmaceuticals) p 259
Prefrin Liquifilm Vasoconstrictor and Lubricant Eye Drops (Allergan Pharmaceuticals) p 254
Refresh Lubricant Ophthalmic Solution (Allergan Pharmaceuticals) p 256
Refresh P.M. Lubricant Ophthalmic Ointment (Allergan Pharmaceuticals) p 256
Relief Vasoconstrictor and Lubricant Eye Drops (Allergan Pharmaceuticals) p 256
Tearisol Ophthalmic Solution (IOLAB Pharmaceuticals) p 271
Tears Naturale II Lubricant Eye Drops (Alcon Laboratories) p 228
Tears Naturale Free (Alcon Laboratories) p 228
Tears Plus Lubricant Ophthalmic Solution (Allergan Pharmaceuticals) p 256
Tears Renewed Ointment (Akorn) p 209
Tears Renewed Solution (Akorn) p 209
Visine EXTRA Eye Drops (Pfizer Consumer) p 104, 303
Visine L.R. Eye Drope (Pfizer Consumer) p 104, 303

M

MAST CELL STABILIZER
Opticrom 4% Ophthalmic Solution (Fisons) p 103, 270

MOISTURIZING AGENT, OPHTHALMIC
AKWA Tears Ointment (Akorn) p 208
Moisture Drops (Bausch & Lomb Personal) p 258
Tears Renewed Ointment (Akorn) p 209

MYDRIATICS
AK-Dilate Solution 2.5% and 10% (Akorn) p 203
Mydfrin 2.5% (Alcon Laboratories) p 224
Phenylephrine HCl 10% (Rfg.) Dropperettes (IOLAB Pharmaceuticals) p 271

MYDRIATICS & CYCLOPLEGICS
AK-Pentolate (Akorn) p 204
Atropine Sulfate Ophthalmic Ointment, Sterile (Bausch & Lomb Pharmaceuticals) p 259
Atropine Sulfate Ophthalmic Solution, Sterile (Bausch & Lomb Pharmaceuticals) p 259
Atropine Sulfate Sterile Ophthalmic Solution and S.O.P. Sterile Ophthalmic Ointment (Allergan Pharmaceuticals) p 239
Atropisol Dropperettes ½%, 1% and 2% (IOLAB Pharmaceuticals) p 271
Cyclogyl (Alcon Laboratories) p 215
Cyclomydril (Alcon Laboratories) p 216
Homatropine Hydrobromide 2% and 5% Dropperettes (IOLAB Pharmaceuticals) p 271
Homatropine Hydrobromide Ophthalmic Solution 2% and 5% (IOLAB Pharmaceuticals) p 271
Isopto Atropine (Alcon Laboratories) p 218
Isopto Homatropine (Alcon Laboratories) p 221
Isopto Hyoscine (Alcon Laboratories) p 222
Murocoll-2 Sterile Ophthalmic Solution (Bausch & Lomb Pharmaceuticals) p 261
Mydriacyl (Alcon Laboratories) p 225
Ocu-Pentolate Sterile Ophthalmic Solution (Ocumed) p 297
Ocu-Tropic Sterile Ophthalmic Solution (Ocumed) p 297
Ocu-Tropine Sterile Ophthalmic Ointment (Ocumed) p 297
Ocu-Tropine Sterile Ophthalmic Solution (Ocumed) p 297
Pentolair Solution (Bausch & Lomb Pharmaceuticals) p 259
Tropicacyl (Akorn) p 209
Tropicamide Ophthalmic Solution, Sterile (Bausch & Lomb Pharmaceuticals) p 259

MYDRIATICS, INTRAOPERATIVE
Profenal Sterile Ophthalmic Solution (Alcon Surgical) p 234

O

OPTIC OPACITIES

SYMPTOMATIC RELIEF
Succus Cineraria Maritima (SCM-Walker) (Walker Pharmacal) p 313

P

PROTEOLYTIC ENZYMES, OPHTHALMIC
Catarase 1:5000 (IOLAB Pharmaceuticals) p 271
Zolyse (Alcon Surgical) p 236

S

SPECTACLE LENSES
Colormatic Hard Resin Spectacle Lenses (Rodenstock) p 349
Cosmolit Bifo 28 Spectacle Lenses (Rodenstock) p 349
Cosmolit Single Vision Spectacle Lenses (Rodenstock) p 349
Photocolor Hard Resin Spectacle Lenses (Rodenstock) p 349

SPECTACLE LENSES, PROGRESSIVE
Progressiv R Spectacle Lenses (Rodenstock) p 349
Progressiv S Spectacle Lenses (Rodenstock) p 349

SURGICAL AID, OPHTHALMIC
AMO Vitrax Solution (Allergan Medical Optics) p 236
AMVISC Plus (IOLAB) p 323
Basol-S Sterile Surgical Solution (Ocumed) p 297
Healon (Kabi Pharmacia Ophthalmics) p 279
IOPIDINE (Alcon Surgical) p 232
Ocufen (Allergan Medical Optics) p 237
Orcolon (Optical Radiation) p 325
Viscoat Sterile Viscoelastic Ophthalmic (Alcon Surgical) p 235

SURGICAL STERILE UNITS
Dropperettes (1mL) (IOLAB Pharmaceuticals) p 271
STERI-UNITS (Alcon Surgical) p 235

V

VASOCONSTRICTOR
AK-Con (Akorn) p 202
Albalon Solution with Liquifilm (Allergan Pharmaceuticals) p 238
Albalon-A Liquifilm (Allergan Pharmaceuticals) p 238
Clear Eyes ACR (Ross) p 105, 305
Clear Eyes Lubricating Eye Redness Reliever (Ross) p 304
Murine Plus Lubricating Eye Redness Reliever (Ross) p 305
Naphcon (Alcon Laboratories) p 226

Naphcon Forte (Alcon Laboratories) p 226
OcuClear Eye Drops (Schering) p 306
Opcon Ophthalmic Solution (Bausch & Lomb Pharmaceuticals) p 259
Prefrin Liquifilm Vasoconstrictor and Lubricant Eye Drops (Allergan Pharmaceuticals) p 254
Prefrin-A (Allergan Pharmaceuticals) p 255
Relief Vasoconstrictor and Lubricant Eye Drops (Allergan Pharmaceuticals) p 256
Visine EXTRA Eye Drops (Pfizer Consumer) p 104, 303

VIRAL AGENTS, OPHTHALMOLOGICAL

Herplex Liquifilm (Allergan Pharmaceuticals) p 248
Vira-A Ophthalmic Ointment, 3% (Parke-Davis) p 104, 302
Viroptic Ophthalmic Solution, 1% Sterile (Burroughs Wellcome) p 267

VISCOELASTIC AGENT

AMO Vitrax Solution (Allergan Medical Optics) p 236
AMVISC Plus (IOLAB) p 323
Healon (Kabi Pharmacia Ophthalmics) p 279
Occucoat (Storz Ophthalmics) p 105, 312
Orcolon (Optical Radiation) p 325

VITAMINS

MULTIVITAMINS WITH MINERALS

ICAPS Plus (La Haye) p 280
Ocuvite Vitamin and Mineral Supplement (Storz Ophthalmics) p 312
Ophthalmic Nutrients (Health Maintenance) p 270

Part 4—Active Ingredients Index

A

ACETAZOLAMIDE
Diamox Parenteral (Storz Ophthalmics) p 308
Diamox Sequels (Sustained Release) (Storz Ophthalmics) p 105, 310
Diamox Tablets (Storz Ophthalmics) p 105, 308

ACETYLCHOLINE CHLORIDE
Miochol with Iocare Steri-Tags, Miochol System Pak and Miochol System Pak Plus (IOLAB Pharmaceuticals) p 103, 274

ALKYL ETHER SULFATE
Boston Advance Cleaner (Polymer Technology) p 104, 348

ALPHA CHYMOTRYPSIN
Zolyse (Alcon Surgical) p 236

AMPHOTERIC 10
MiraFlow Extra-Strength Cleaner (CIBA Vision Corp.) p 346

ANHYDROUS LIQUID LANOLIN
LubriTears Ointment (Bausch & Lomb Pharmaceuticals) p 259

ANTAZOLINE PHOSPHATE
Albalon-A Liquifilm (Allergan Pharmaceuticals) p 238
Vasocon-A (IOLAB Pharmaceuticals) p 278

APRACLONIDINE HYDROCHLORIDE
IOPIDINE (Alcon Surgical) p 232

ATROPINE SULFATE
Atropine Sulfate Ophthalmic Ointment, Sterile (Bausch & Lomb Pharmaceuticals) p 259
Atropine Sulfate Ophthalmic Solution, Sterile (Bausch & Lomb Pharmaceuticals) p 259
Atropine Sulfate Sterile Ophthalmic Solution and S.O.P. Sterile Ophthalmic Ointment (Allergan Pharmaceuticals) p 239
Atropisol Dropperettes ½%, 1% and 2% (IOLAB Pharmaceuticals) p 271
Isopto Atropine (Alcon Laboratories) p 218
Ocu-Tropine Sterile Ophthalmic Ointment (Ocumed) p 297
Ocu-Tropine Sterile Ophthalmic Solution (Ocumed) p 297

B

BACITRACIN
Bacitracin Ophthalmic Ointment-Sterile (Bausch & Lomb Pharmaceuticals) p 259

BACITRACIN ZINC
AK-Poly-Bac Ointment (Akorn) p 205
AK-Spore H.C. Ointment (Akorn) p 206
AK-Spore Ointment (Akorn) p 205
Bacitracin Zinc and Polymyxin B Sulfate Ophthalmic Ointment, Sterile (Bausch & Lomb Pharmaceuticals) p 259
Cortisporin Ophthalmic Ointment Sterile (Burroughs Wellcome) p 263
Neosporin Ophthalmic Ointment Sterile (Burroughs Wellcome) p 265
Ocutricin HC Ointment (Bausch & Lomb Pharmaceuticals) p 259
Ocutricin Ointment (Bausch & Lomb Pharmaceuticals) p 259
Polysporin Ophthalmic Ointment Sterile (Burroughs Wellcome) p 266

BALANCED SALT SOLUTION
BSS (15 mL & 30 mL) Sterile Irrigation Solution (Alcon Surgical) p 230
BSS (250 mL) Sterile Irrigation Solution (Alcon Surgical) p 231
BSS (500 mL) Sterile Irrigation Solution (Alcon Surgical) p 231
BSS PLUS (500 mL) Sterile Irrigation Solution (Alcon Surgical) p 231
Balanced Salt Solution (Allergan Pharmaceuticals) p 239
Balanced Salt Solution (Bausch & Lomb Pharmaceuticals) p 259
Basol-S Sterile Surgical Solution (Ocumed) p 297
Eye-Stream (Alcon Laboratories) p 217
Iocare Balanced Salt Solution 15 ml (IOLAB Pharmaceuticals) p 271
Iocare Balanced Salt Solution 500 ml (IOLAB Pharmaceuticals) p 271

BENZALKONIUM CHLORIDE
Enuclene (Alcon Surgical) p 232
Soakare Hard Contact Lens Soaking Solution (Allergan Optical) p 340
Total All-In-One Hard Contact Lens Solution (Allergan Optical) p 340
Wet-N-Soak Wetting and Soaking Solution (Allergan Optical) p 342
Wet-N-Soak Plus Wetting and Soaking Solution (Allergan Optical) p 342

BETA CAROTENE
Ophthalmic Nutrients (Health Maintenance) p 270

BETAXOLOL HYDROCHLORIDE
Betoptic Sterile Ophthalmic Solution (Alcon Laboratories) p 211
Betoptic S Sterile Ophthalmic Suspension (Alcon Laboratories) p 212

BORIC ACID
CIBA Vision Saline Solution (CIBA Vision Corp.) p 344
Clear Eyes ACR (Ross) p 105, 305
Collyrium for Fresh Eyes (Wyeth-Ayerst) p 105, 314
Eye Wash (Bausch & Lomb Personal) p 258
Lens Plus Rewetting Drops (Allergan Optical) p 336
Lensept Disinfection System (CIBA Vision Corp.) p 345
Lensept Neutralizer & Rinsing/Storage Solution (CIBA Vision Corp.) p 345

BOVINE CATALASE
Lensept Disinfection System (CIBA Vision Corp.) p 345
Lensept Neutralizer & Rinsing/Storage Solution (CIBA Vision Corp.) p 345

C

CARBACHOL
Isopto Carbachol (Alcon Laboratories) p 219
MIOSTAT (Alcon Surgical) p 233

CARBAMYL CHOLINE CHLORIDE
MIOSTAT (Alcon Surgical) p 233

CARBOXYMETHYLCELLULOSE SODIUM
Cellufresh Lubricant Ophthalmic Solution (Allergan Pharmaceuticals) p 243
Celluvisc Lubricant Ophthalmic Solution (Allergan Pharmaceuticals) p 243

CATALASE
Lens Plus Oxysept Disinfection System (Allergan Optical) p 332
Lens Plus Oxysept 2 Rinse & Neutralizer (Allergan Optical) p 334

CHLORAMPHENICOL
AK-Chlor Sterile Ophthalmic Ointment & Solution (Akorn) p 201
Chloramphenicol Ophthalmic Ointment, Sterile (Bausch & Lomb Pharmaceuticals) p 259
Chloramphenicol Ophthalmic Solution, Sterile (Bausch & Lomb Pharmaceuticals) p 259
Chloromycetin Hydrocortisone Ophthalmic (Parke-Davis) p 104, 298
Chloromycetin Ophthalmic Ointment, 1% (Parke-Davis) p 104, 299
Chloromycetin Ophthalmic Solution (Parke-Davis) p 104, 300
Chloroptic S.O.P. (Allergan Pharmaceuticals) p 243
Chloroptic Sterile Ophthalmic Solution (Allergan Pharmaceuticals) p 243
Ocu-Chlor Sterile Ophthalmic Solution (Ocumed) p 297
Ocu-Chlor Sterile Ophthalmic Ointment (Ocumed) p 297
Ophthochlor Ophthalmic Solution (Parke-Davis) p 104, 300
Ophthocort (Parke-Davis) p 104, 301

CHLORTETRACYCLINE HYDROCHLORIDE
Auroemycin Ophthalmic Ointment 1.0% (Storz Ophthalmics) p 308

CHYMOTRYPSIN
Catarase 1:5000 (IOLAB Pharmaceuticals) p 271

CIPROFLOXACIN HYDROCHLORIDE
Ciloxan Sterile Ophthalmic Solution (Alcon Laboratories) p 214

COCOAMPHOCARBOXYGLYCINATE
EasyClean/GP Daily Cleaner (Allergan Optical) p 328
Lens Clear Soft Lens Cleaner (Allergan Optical) p 331
Lens Plus Daily Cleaner (Allergan Optical) p 332
Resolve/GP Daily Cleaner (Allergan Optical) p 339

COLLAGEN
BIO-COR 12, 24, and 72 Collagen Corneal Shield (Bausch & Lomb Pharmaceuticals) p 103, 260
Collagen Implants (Intracanalicular) for Lacrimal Efficiency Test (Lacrimedics) p 281
Intracanalicular Collagen Implants-Temporary (Eagle Vision) p 269

CROMOLYN SODIUM
Opticrom 4% Ophthalmic Solution (Fisons) p 103, 270

CYCLOPENTOLATE HYDROCHLORIDE
AK-Pentolate (Akorn) p 204
Cyclogyl (Alcon Laboratories) p 215
Cyclomydril (Alcon Laboratories) p 216
Ocu-Pentolate Sterile Ophthalmic Solution (Ocumed) p 297
Pentolair Solution (Bausch & Lomb Pharmaceuticals) p 259

D

DAPIPRAZOLE HYDROCHLORIDE
Rēv-Eyes Ophthalmic Eyedrops 0.5% (Storz Ophthalmics) p 312

DEMECARIUM BROMIDE
Humorsol Ophthalmic Solution (Merck Sharp & Dohme) p 103, 287

DEXAMETHASONE
AK-Trol Ointment & Suspension (Akorn) p 207
Dexacidin Ointment (IOLAB Pharmaceuticals) p 272
Dexacidin Suspension (IOLAB Pharmaceuticals) p 272
Dexasporin Ointment (Bausch & Lomb Pharmaceuticals) p 259
Dexasporin Suspension (Bausch & Lomb Pharmaceuticals) p 259
Maxidex Sterile Ophthalmic Suspension (Alcon Laboratories) p 223
Maxitrol Ophthalmic Ointment/Suspension (Alcon Laboratories) p 223
Ocu-Trol Sterile Ophthalmic Ointment (Ocumed) p 297
Ocu-Trol Sterile Ophthalmic Suspension (Ocumed) p 297
TobraDex Ophthalmic Suspension and Ointment (Alcon Laboratories) p 228

DEXAMETHASONE SODIUM PHOSPHATE
AK-Dex 0.05% Ointment (Akorn) p 203
AK-Dex 0.1% Solution (Akorn) p 203
Decadron Phosphate Sterile Ophthalmic Ointment (Merck Sharp & Dohme) p 103, 285
Decadron Phosphate Sterile Ophthalmic Solution (Merck Sharp & Dohme) p 103, 285
Dexamethasone Sodium Phosphate Injection, USP (IOLAB Pharmaceuticals) p 271
Dexamethasone Sodium Phosphate Ophthalmic Ointment, Sterile (Bausch & Lomb Pharmaceuticals) p 259
Dexamethasone Sodium Phosphate Ophthalmic Solution, Sterile (Bausch & Lomb Pharmaceuticals) p 259
Dexamethasone Sodium Phosphate Ophthalmic Solution, USP (IOLAB Pharmaceuticals) p 271
Maxidex Sterile Ophthalmic Ointment (Alcon Laboratories) p 222
Neo-Dexair Ophthalmic Solution (Bausch & Lomb Pharmaceuticals) p 259
NeoDecadron Sterile Ophthalmic Ointment (Merck Sharp & Dohme) p 104, 290
NeoDecadron Sterile Ophthalmic Solution (Merck Sharp & Dohme) p 104, 291
Neomycin Sulfate-Dexamethasone Sodium Phosphate Ophthalmic Solution, USP (IOLAB Pharmaceuticals) p 271
Ocu-Dex Sterile Ophthalmic Ointment (Ocumed) p 297
Ocu-Dex Sterile Ophthalmic Solution (Ocumed) p 297

DEXTRAN
Tears Naturale II Lubricant Eye Drops (Alcon Laboratories) p 228
Tears Naturale Free (Alcon Laboratories) p 228
Tears Renewed Solution (Akorn) p 209

DEXTRAN 70
LubriTears Solution (Bausch & Lomb Pharmaceuticals) p 259
Moisture Drops (Bausch & Lomb Personal) p 258

DICHLORPHENAMIDE
Daranide Tablets (Merck Sharp & Dohme) p 103, 284

DICLOFENAC SODIUM
Voltaren Ophthalmic Sterile Ophthalmic Solution (CIBA Vision Ophthalmics) p 103, 268

DIPIVEFRIN HYDROCHLORIDE
Propine with C Cap Compliance Cap (Allergan Pharmaceuticals) p 255

DISODIUM LAURETH SULFOSUCCINATE
EYEscrub Eyelid Cleanser (CooperVision) p 269

E

ECHOTHIOPHATE IODIDE
Phospholine Iodide (Wyeth-Ayerst) p 105, 315

EDETATE DISODIUM
Soakare Hard Contact Lens Soaking Solution (Allergan Optical) p 340
Total All-In-One Hard Contact Lens Solution (Allergan Optical) p 340
Wet-N-Soak Wetting and Soaking Solution (Allergan Optical) p 342
Wet-N-Soak Plus Wetting and Soaking Solution (Allergan Optical) p 342

EPINEPHRINE
Epinephrine 1:1000 Dropperettes (IOLAB Pharmaceuticals) p 271

EPINEPHRINE BITARTRATE
E-Pilo-1, E-Pilo-2, E-Pilo-3, E-Pilo-4, E-Pilo-6 (IOLAB Pharmaceuticals) p 271

EPINEPHRINE HYDROCHLORIDE
Epifrin (Allergan Pharmaceuticals) p 244
Glaucon (Alcon Laboratories) p 218

ERYTHROMYCIN
AK-Mycin Ointment (Akorn) p 204
Erythromycin Ophthalmic Ointment, Sterile (Bausch & Lomb Pharmaceuticals) p 259

ESERINE SULFATE
Eserine Sulfate Ophthalmic Ointment 0.25% (IOLAB Pharmaceuticals) p 271

ETAFILCON A
Acuvue Contact Lenses (Vistakon) p 321
SureVue Contact Lenses (Vistakon) p 322

ETHYL AMINOBENZOATE (see under BENZOCAINE)

F

FLUORESCEIN SODIUM
AK-Fluor Injection 10% and 25% (Akorn) p 204
Fluoracaine (Akorn) p 208
Fluorescein Sodium 2% Dropperettes (IOLAB Pharmaceuticals) p 271
Fluorescite Injection (Alcon Laboratories) p 217
Fluorescite Syringe (Alcon Laboratories) p 217
Fluorets Ophthalmic Strips (Akorn) p 208
Fluor-I-Strip (Wyeth-Ayerst) p 105, 314
Fluor-I-Strip A.T. (Wyeth-Ayerst) p 105, 314
Funduscein 10% and Funduscein 25% (IOLAB Pharmaceuticals) p 271
Proparacaine Hydrochloride and Fluorescein Sodium Ophthalmic Soluton, Sterile (Bausch & Lomb Pharmaceuticals) p 259

FLUOROMETHOLONE
FML Forte Liquifilm (Allergan Pharmaceuticals) p 245
FML Liquifilm (Allergan Pharmaceuticals) p 244
FML S.O.P. (Allergan Pharmaceuticals) p 245
FML-S Sterile Ophthalmic Suspension (Allergan Pharmaceuticals) p 246
Fluor-Op Ophthalmic Suspension (IOLAB Pharmaceuticals) p 272

FLURBIPROFEN SODIUM
Ocufen (Allergan Medical Optics) p 237

G

GELATIN A
Lacril Lubricant Ophthalmic Solution (Allergan Pharmaceuticals) p 248

GENTAMICIN SULFATE
Garamycin Ophthalmic Ointment—Sterile (Schering) p 305
Garamycin Ophthalmic Solution—Sterile (Schering) p 305
Genoptic Liquifilm Sterile Ophthalmic Solution (Allergan Pharmaceuticals) p 247
Genoptic S.O.P. Sterile Ophthalmic Ointment (Allergan Pharmaceuticals) p 247
Gentacidin Ointment (IOLAB Pharmaceuticals) p 273
Gentacidin Solution (IOLAB Pharmaceuticals) p 273
Gentak Ointment & Solution (Akorn) p 208
Gentamicin Ointment (Bausch & Lomb Pharmaceuticals) p 259
Gentamicin Solution (Bausch & Lomb Pharmaceuticals) p 259
Gentamicin Sulfate Injection, USP (IOLAB Pharmaceuticals) p 271
Ocu-Mycin Sterile Ophthalmic Ointment (Ocumed) p 297
Ocu-Mycin Sterile Ophthalmic Solution (Ocumed) p 297
Pred-G Liquifilm Sterile Ophthalmic Suspension (Allergan Pharmaceuticals) p 252
Pred-G S.O.P. Sterile Ophthalmic Ointment (Allergan Pharmaceuticals) p 253

GLUTATHIONE
Ophthalmic Nutrients (Health Maintenance) p 270

GLYCERIN
Clear Eyes ACR (Ross) p 105, 305
Clear Eyes Lubricating Eye Redness Reliever (Ross) p 304
Collyrium Fresh (Wyeth-Ayerst) p 105, 314
Dry Eye Therapy (Bausch & Lomb Personal) p 258
Moisture Drops (Bausch & Lomb Personal) p 258
Ophthalgan (Wyeth-Ayerst) p 105, 315
OSMŌGLYN (Alcon Surgical) p 234

GRAMICIDIN
AK-Spore Solution (Akorn) p 205
Neomycin and Polymyxin B Sulfates and Gramicidin Ophthalmic Solution (IOLAB Pharmaceuticals) p 271
Neosporin Ophthalmic Solution Sterile (Burroughs Wellcome) p 266
Ocu-Spor-G Sterile Ophthalmic Solution (Ocumed) p 297
Ocutricin Solution (Bausch & Lomb Pharmaceuticals) p 259

H

HEXYLENE GLYCOL
Resolve/GP Daily Cleaner (Allergan Optical) p 339

HOMATROPINE HYDROBROMIDE
Homatropine Hydrobromide 2% and 5% Dropperettes (IOLAB Pharmaceuticals) p 271
Homatropine Hydrobromide Ophthalmic Solution 2% and 5% (IOLAB Pharmaceuticals) p 271
Isopto Homatropine (Alcon Laboratories) p 221

HYDROCORTISONE
AK-Spore H.C. Ointment (Akorn) p 206

AK-Spore H. C. Suspension (Akorn) p 206
Cortisporin Ophthalmic Ointment Sterile (Burroughs Wellcome) p 263
Cortisporin Ophthalmic Suspension Sterile (Burroughs Wellcome) p 264
Neomycin and Polymyxin B Sulfates and Hydrocortisone Ophthalmic Suspension (IOLAB Pharmaceuticals) p 271
Ocu-Cort Sterile Ophthalmic Ointment (Ocumed) p 297
Ocutricin HC Ointment (Bausch & Lomb Pharmaceuticals) p 259
Ocutricin HC Suspension (Bausch & Lomb Pharmaceuticals) p 259

HYDROCORTISONE ACETATE
Chloromycetin Hydrocortisone Ophthalmic (Parke-Davis) p 104, 298
Ophthocort (Parke-Davis) p 104, 301

HYDROGEN PEROXIDE
AOSEPT Disinfection/Neutralization Solution (CIBA Vision Corp.) p 343
Lens Plus Oxysept Disinfection System (Allergan Optical) p 332
Lens Plus Oxysept 1 Disinfecting Solution (Allergan Optical) p 335
Lensept Disinfection Solution (CIBA Vision Corp.) p 345
Lensept Disinfection System (CIBA Vision Corp.) p 345

HYDROPHYLIC POLYELECTROLYTE
Boston Advance Conditioning Solution (Polymer Technology) p 348
Boston Advance Rewetting Drops (Polymer Technology) p 348

HYDROXYETHYLCELLULOSE
Adsorbotear (Alcon Laboratories) p 210
Gonioscopic Prism Solution (Alcon Laboratories) p 218
Lens Fresh Lubricating & Rewetting Drops (Allergan Optical) p 331

HYDROXYPROPYL CELLULOSE
Lacrisert (Merck Sharp & Dohme) p 104, 289

HYDROXYPROPYL METHYLCELLULOSE
Gonak Ophthalmic Demulcent Solution (Akorn) p 209
Goniosol Ophthalmic Solution (IOLAB Pharmaceuticals) p 271
Lacril Lubricant Ophthalmic Solution (Allergan Pharmaceuticals) p 248
LubriTears Solution (Bausch & Lomb Pharmaceuticals) p 259
Moisture Drops (Bausch & Lomb Personal) p 258
Occucoat (Storz Ophthalmics) p 105, 312
Tears Naturale II Lubricant Eye Drops (Alcon Laboratories) p 228
Tears Naturale Free (Alcon Laboratories) p 228
Tears Renewed Solution (Akorn) p 209

I

IDOXURIDINE
Herplex Liquifilm (Allergan Pharmaceuticals) p 248

IRON POLYSACCHARIDE COMPLEX (see under POLYSACCHARIDE-IRON COMPLEX)

ISOFLUROPHATE
Floropryl Sterile Ophthalmic Ointment (Merck Sharp & Dohme) p 103, 286

ISOPROPYL ALCOHOL
MiraFlow Extra-Strength Cleaner (CIBA Vision Corp.) p 346

ISOSORBIDE
ISMOTIC (Alcon Surgical) p 233

ISOTONIC SOLUTION
Allergan Eyewash (Allergan Pharmaceuticals) p 238
CIBA Vision Saline Solution (CIBA Vision Corp.) p 344
Eye Wash (Bausch & Lomb Pharmaceuticals) p 259
Iri-Sol Sterile Isotonic Buffered Solution (Ocumed) p 297

L

LANOLIN
AKWA Tears Ointment (Akorn) p 208

LEVOBUNOLOL HYDROCHLORIDE
Betagan Liquifilm (Allergan Pharmaceuticals) p 239
Betagan Liquifilm with C Cap Compliance Cap (Allergan Pharmaceuticals) p 239

M

MEDRYSONE
HMS Liquifilm (Allergan Pharmaceuticals) p 247

METHAZOLAMIDE
Neptazane Tablets (Storz Ophthalmics) p 105, 311

METHYLCELLULOSE
Murocel (Bausch & Lomb Pharmaceuticals) p 259

METIPRANOLOL HYDROCHLORIDE
OptiPranolol Sterile Ophthalmic Solution (Bausch & Lomb Pharmaceuticals) p 103, 261

MINERAL OIL
AKWA Tears Ointment (Akorn) p 208
Duolube Eye Ointment (Bausch & Lomb Personal) p 258
Duratears Naturale (Alcon Laboratories) p 216
Lacri-Lube NP Lubricant Ophthalmic Ointment (Allergan Pharmaceuticals) p 249
Lacri-Lube S.O.P. Sterile Ophthalmic Ointment (Allergan Pharmaceuticals) p 249
LubriTears Ointment (Bausch & Lomb Pharmaceuticals) p 259
Petrolatum Ointment (Bausch & Lomb Pharmaceuticals) p 259
Refresh P.M. Lubricant Ophthalmic Ointment (Allergan Pharmaceuticals) p 256
Tears Renewed Ointment (Akorn) p 209

N

NAPHAZOLINE HYDROCHLORIDE
AK-Con (Akorn) p 202
AK-Con-A (Akorn) p 203
Albalon Solution with Liquifilm (Allergan Pharmaceuticals) p 238
Albalon-A Liquifilm (Allergan Pharmaceuticals) p 238
Allergy Drops (Bausch & Lomb Personal) p 258
Clear Eyes ACR (Ross) p 105, 305
Clear Eyes Lubricating Eye Redness Reliever (Ross) p 304
Naphcon (Alcon Laboratories) p 226
Naphcon Forte (Alcon Laboratories) p 226
Naphcon-A Ophthalmic Solution (Alcon Laboratories) p 226
Ocu-Zoline Sterile Ophthalmic Solution (Ocumed) p 297
Opcon Ophthalmic Solution (Bausch & Lomb Pharmaceuticals) p 259
Opcon-A Ophthalmic Solution (Bausch & Lomb Pharmaceuticals) p 262
Vasocon Regular (IOLAB Pharmaceuticals) p 271
Vasocon-A (IOLAB Pharmaceuticals) p 278

NATAMYCIN
Natacyn (Alcon Laboratories) p 227

NEOMYCIN SULFATE
AK-Spore H.C. Ointment (Akorn) p 206
AK-Spore H. C. Suspension (Akorn) p 206
AK-Spore Ointment (Akorn) p 205
AK-Spore Solution (Akorn) p 205
AK-Trol Ointment & Suspension (Akorn) p 207
Cortisporin Ophthalmic Ointment Sterile (Burroughs Wellcome) p 263
Cortisporin Ophthalmic Suspension Sterile (Burroughs Wellcome) p 264
Dexacidin Ointment (IOLAB Pharmaceuticals) p 272
Dexacidin Suspension (IOLAB Pharmaceuticals) p 272
Dexasporin Ointment (Bausch & Lomb Pharmaceuticals) p 259
Dexasporin Suspension (Bausch & Lomb Pharmaceuticals) p 259
Maxitrol Ophthalmic Ointment/Suspension (Alcon Laboratories) p 223
Neo-Dexair Ophthalmic Solution (Bausch & Lomb Pharmaceuticals) p 259
NeoDecadron Sterile Ophthalmic Ointment (Merck Sharp & Dohme) p 104, 290
NeoDecadron Sterile Ophthalmic Solution (Merck Sharp & Dohme) p 104, 291
Neomycin and Polymyxin B Sulfates and Gramicidin Ophthalmic Solution (IOLAB Pharmaceuticals) p 271
Neomycin and Polymyxin B Sulfates and Hydrocortisone Ophthalmic Suspension (IOLAB Pharmaceuticals) p 271
Neomycin Sulfate-Dexamethasone Sodium Phosphate Ophthalmic Solution, USP (IOLAB Pharmaceuticals) p 271
Neosporin Ophthalmic Ointment Sterile (Burroughs Wellcome) p 265
Neosporin Ophthalmic Solution Sterile (Burroughs Wellcome) p 266
Ocu-Cort Sterile Ophthalmic Ointment (Ocumed) p 297
Ocu-Spor-B Sterile Ophthalmic Ointment (Ocumed) p 297
Ocu-Spor-G Sterile Ophthalmic Solution (Ocumed) p 297
Ocutricin HC Ointment (Bausch & Lomb Pharmaceuticals) p 259
Ocutricin HC Suspension (Bausch & Lomb Pharmaceuticals) p 259
Ocutricin Ointment (Bausch & Lomb Pharmaceuticals) p 259
Ocutricin Solution (Bausch & Lomb Pharmaceuticals) p 259
Ocu-Trol Sterile Ophthalmic Ointment (Ocumed) p 297
Ocu-Trol Sterile Ophthalmic Suspension (Ocumed) p 297
Poly-Pred Liquifilm (Allergan Pharmaceuticals) p 250

NORFLOXACIN
Chibroxin Sterile Ophthalmic Solution (Merck Sharp & Dohme) p 103, 282

O

OXYMETAZOLINE HYDROCHLORIDE
OcuClear Eye Drops (Schering) p 306
Visine L.R. Eye Drope (Pfizer Consumer) p 104, 303

P

PEG-200 GLYCERYL TALLOWATE
EYEscrub Eyelid Cleanser (CooperVision) p 269

PAPAIN

Allergan Enzymatic Contact Lens Cleaner (Allergan Optical) p 327
Extenzyme Protein Cleaner (Allergan Optical) p 329
ProFree/GP Weekly Enzymatic Cleaner (Allergan Optical) p 339

PETROLATUM

Duratears Naturale (Alcon Laboratories) p 216
HypoTears Ointment (IOLAB Pharmaceuticals) p 273
Lacri-Lube NP Lubricant Ophthalmic Ointment (Allergan Pharmaceuticals) p 249
Lacri-Lube S.O.P. Sterile Ophthalmic Ointment (Allergan Pharmaceuticals) p 249
Ocu-Lube Sterile Ophthalmic Ointment (Ocumed) p 297
Refresh P.M. Lubricant Ophthalmic Ointment (Allergan Pharmaceuticals) p 256

PHENIRAMINE MALEATE

AK-Con-A (Akorn) p 203
Naphcon-A Ophthalmic Solution (Alcon Laboratories) p 226
Opcon-A Ophthalmic Solution (Bausch & Lomb Pharmaceuticals) p 262

PHENYLEPHRINE HYDROCHLORIDE

AK-Dilate Solution 2.5% and 10% (Akorn) p 203
Cyclomydril (Alcon Laboratories) p 216
Murocoll-2 Sterile Ophthalmic Solution (Bausch & Lomb Pharmaceuticals) p 261
Mydfrin 2.5% (Alcon Laboratories) p 224
Ocu-Phrin Sterile Eye Drops (Ocumed) p 297
Ocu-Phrin Sterile Ophthalmic Solution (Ocumed) p 297
Phenylephrine HCl 10% (Rfg.) Dropperettes (IOLAB Pharmaceuticals) p 271
Phenylephrine Hydrochloride Ophthalmic Solution 2.5%, Sterile (Bausch & Lomb Pharmaceuticals) p 259
Phenylephrine Hydrochloride 2.5% Ophthalmic Solution, USP (IOLAB Pharmaceuticals) p 271
Prefrin Liquifilm Vasoconstrictor and Lubricant Eye Drops (Allergan Pharmaceuticals) p 254
Prefrin-A (Allergan Pharmaceuticals) p 255
Relief Vasoconstrictor and Lubricant Eye Drops (Allergan Pharmaceuticals) p 256
Vasosulf (IOLAB Pharmaceuticals) p 279
Zincfrin (Alcon Laboratories) p 230

PILOCARPINE

Ocusert Pilo-20 and Pilo-40 Ocular Therapeutic Systems (Alza) p 256

PILOCARPINE HYDROCHLORIDE

Akarpine Ophthalmic Solution (Akorn) p 201
E-Pilo-1, E-Pilo-2, E-Pilo-3, E-Pilo-4, E-Pilo-6 (IOLAB Pharmaceuticals) p 271
Isopto Carpine (Alcon Laboratories) p 219
Ocu-Carpine Sterile Ophthalmic Solution (Ocumed) p 297
Pilocar (IOLAB Pharmaceuticals) p 103, 275
Pilocar Dropperettes 1%, 2% and 4% (IOLAB Pharmaceuticals) p 103, 271
Pilocar Twin Pack (IOLAB Pharmaceuticals) p 103, 275
Pilopine HS Gel (Alcon Laboratories) p 227
Pilostat Sterile Ophthalmic Solution 0.5%, 1%, 2%, 3%, 4%, 5%, 6% (Bausch & Lomb Pharmaceuticals) p 263

PILOCARPINE NITRATE

Pilagan Liquifilm Sterile Ophthalmic Solution (Allergan Pharmaceuticals) p 250
Pilagan Liquifilm Sterile Ophthalmic Solution with C Cap Compliance Cap (Allergan Pharmaceuticals) p 250

POLOXAMER 407

MiraFlow Extra-Strength Cleaner (CIBA Vision Corp.) p 346

POLYACRYLAMIDE

Orcolon (Optical Radiation) p 325

POLYETHYLENE GLYCOL

Allergy Drops (Bausch & Lomb Personal) p 258
Blink-N-Clean Contact Lens Solution (Allergan Optical) p 328
Visine EXTRA Eye Drops (Pfizer Consumer) p 104, 303

POLYMACON

Bausch & Lomb Medalist Tinted Contact Lenses (Bausch & Lomb Contact Lens) p 317
Bausch & Lomb NaturalTint Hydrophilic Contact Lenses (Bausch & Lomb Contact Lens) p 317
Bausch & Lomb P.A.1 Bifocal Hydrophilic Contact Lenses (Bausch & Lomb Contact Lens) p 317
Bausch & Lomb Soflens Hydrophilic Contact Lenses (Bausch & Lomb Contact Lens) p 317
Polymacon Hydrophilic Contact Lenses (Bausch & Lomb Contact Lens) p 317

POLYMYXIN B SULFATE

AK-Poly-Bac Ointment (Akorn) p 205
AK-Spore H.C. Ointment (Akorn) p 206
AK-Spore H. C. Suspension (Akorn) p 206
AK-Spore Ointment (Akorn) p 205
AK-Spore Solution (Akorn) p 205
AK-Trol Ointment & Suspension (Akorn) p 207
Bacitracin Zinc and Polymyxin B Sulfate Ophthalmic Ointment, Sterile (Bausch & Lomb Pharmaceuticals) p 259
Cortisporin Ophthalmic Ointment Sterile (Burroughs Wellcome) p 263
Cortisporin Ophthalmic Suspension Sterile (Burroughs Wellcome) p 264
Dexacidin Ointment (IOLAB Pharmaceuticals) p 272
Dexacidin Suspension (IOLAB Pharmaceuticals) p 272
Dexasporin Ointment (Bausch & Lomb Pharmaceuticals) p 259
Dexasporin Suspension (Bausch & Lomb Pharmaceuticals) p 259
Maxitrol Ophthalmic Ointment/Suspension (Alcon Laboratories) p 223
Neomycin and Polymyxin B Sulfates and Gramicidin Ophthalmic Solution (IOLAB Pharmaceuticals) p 271
Neomycin and Polymyxin B Sulfates and Hydrocortisone Ophthalmic Suspension (IOLAB Pharmaceuticals) p 271
Neosporin Ophthalmic Ointment Sterile (Burroughs Wellcome) p 265
Neosporin Ophthalmic Solution Sterile (Burroughs Wellcome) p 266
Ocu-Cort Sterile Ophthalmic Ointment (Ocumed) p 297
Ocu-Spor-B Sterile Ophthalmic Ointment (Ocumed) p 297
Ocu-Spor-G Sterile Ophthalmic Solution (Ocumed) p 297
Ocutricin HC Ointment (Bausch & Lomb Pharmaceuticals) p 259
Ocutricin HC Suspension (Bausch & Lomb Pharmaceuticals) p 259
Ocutricin Ointment (Bausch & Lomb Pharmaceuticals) p 259
Ocutricin Solution (Bausch & Lomb Pharmaceuticals) p 259
Ocu-Trol Sterile Ophthalmic Ointment (Ocumed) p 297
Ocu-Trol Sterile Ophthalmic Suspension (Ocumed) p 297
Ophthocort (Parke-Davis) p 104, 301
Poly-Pred Liquifilm (Allergan Pharmaceuticals) p 250
Polysporin Ophthalmic Ointment Sterile (Burroughs Wellcome) p 266
Polytrim Ophthalmic Solution Sterile (Allergan Pharmaceuticals) p 251

POLYOXYL STEARATE

Blink-N-Clean Contact Lens Solution (Allergan Optical) p 328

POLYVINYL ALCOHOL

AKWA Tears Solution (Akorn) p 208
Dry Eyes Solution (Bausch & Lomb Pharmaceuticals) p 259
HypoTears Lubricating Eye Drops (IOLAB Pharmaceuticals) p 273
HypoTears PF Preservative-Free Lubricating Eye Drops (IOLAB Pharmaceuticals) p 273
Lens-Wet Lubricating & Rewetting Solution (Allergan Optical) p 338
Liquifilm Forte Lubricant Ophthalmic Solution (Allergan Pharmaceuticals) p 249
Liquifilm Tears Lubricant Ophthalmic Solution (Allergan Pharmaceuticals) p 249
Liquifilm Wetting Solution (Allergan Optical) p 338
Murine Eye Lubricant (Ross) p 305
Murine Plus Lubricating Eye Redness Reliever (Ross) p 305
Ocu-Tears Sterile Ophthalmic Solution (Ocumed) p 297
Prefrin Liquifilm Vasoconstrictor and Lubricant Eye Drops (Allergan Pharmaceuticals) p 254
Refresh Lubricant Ophthalmic Solution (Allergan Pharmaceuticals) p 256
Relief Vasoconstrictor and Lubricant Eye Drops (Allergan Pharmaceuticals) p 256
Tears Plus Lubricant Ophthalmic Solution (Allergan Pharmaceuticals) p 256
Total All-In-One Hard Contact Lens Solution (Allergan Optical) p 340
Wet-N-Soak Wetting and Soaking Solution (Allergan Optical) p 342
Wet-N-Soak Plus Wetting and Soaking Solution (Allergan Optical) p 342

POLYVINYLPYRROLIDONE (see under POVIDONE)

POVIDONE

Adsorbotear (Alcon Laboratories) p 210
Murine Eye Lubricant (Ross) p 305
Murine Plus Lubricating Eye Redness Reliever (Ross) p 305
Refresh Lubricant Ophthalmic Solution (Allergan Pharmaceuticals) p 256
Tears Plus Lubricant Ophthalmic Solution (Allergan Pharmaceuticals) p 256

PREDNISOLONE ACETATE

AK-Cide Sterile Ophthalmic Ointment & Suspension (Akorn) p 202
Blephamide Liquifilm (Allergan Pharmaceuticals) p 242
Blephamide S.O.P. (Allergan Pharmaceuticals) p 242
Cetapred Ointment (Alcon Laboratories) p 220
⅛% Econopred & 1% Econopred Plus (Alcon Laboratories) p 217
Isopto Cetapred Suspension (Alcon Laboratories) p 220

Metimyd Ophthalmic Ointment—Sterile (Schering) p 306
Metimyd Ophthalmic Suspension—Sterile (Schering) p 306
Ocu-Lone-C Sterile Ophthalmic Ointment (Ocumed) p 297
Ocu-Lone-C Sterile Ophthalmic Suspension (Ocumed) p 297
Ocu-Pred-A Sterile Ophthalmic Suspension (Ocumed) p 297
Poly-Pred Liquifilm (Allergan Pharmaceuticals) p 250
Pred Forte (Allergan Pharmaceuticals) p 252
Pred Mild (Allergan Pharmaceuticals) p 254
Pred-G Liquifilm Sterile Ophthalmic Suspension (Allergan Pharmaceuticals) p 252
Pred-G S.O.P. Sterile Ophthalmic Ointment (Allergan Pharmaceuticals) p 253
Sulphrin Ointment (Bausch & Lomb Pharmaceuticals) p 259
Sulphrin Suspension (Bausch & Lomb Pharmaceuticals) p 259
Sulpred Suspension (Bausch & Lomb Pharmaceuticals) p 259
Vasocidin Ointment (IOLAB Pharmaceuticals) p 275

PREDNISOLONE SODIUM PHOSPHATE
AK-Pred (Akorn) p 103, 205
Inflamase Forte 1% (IOLAB Pharmaceuticals) p 274
Inflamase Mild ⅛% (IOLAB Pharmaceuticals) p 274
Ocu-Pred Forte Sterile Ophthalmic Solution (Ocumed) p 297
Ocu-Pred Sterile Ophthalmic Solution (Ocumed) p 297
Prednisolone Sodium Phosphate Ophthalmic Solution, Sterile (Bausch & Lomb Pharmaceuticals) p 259
Vasocidin Ophthalmic Solution (IOLAB Pharmaceuticals) p 276

PROPARACAINE HYDROCHLORIDE
AK-Taine (Akorn) p 207
Alcaine (Alcon Laboratories) p 210
Fluoracaine (Akorn) p 208
Ocu-Caine Sterile Ophthalmic Solution (Ocumed) p 297
Ophthetic (Allergan Pharmaceuticals) p 249
Proparacaine Hydrochloride Ophthalmic Solution, Sterile (Bausch & Lomb Pharmaceuticals) p 259
Proparacaine Hydrochloride and Fluorescein Sodium Ophthalmic Soluton, Sterile (Bausch & Lomb Pharmaceuticals) p 259

PYRILAMINE MALEATE
Prefrin-A (Allergan Pharmaceuticals) p 255

R

RESIN
Colormatic Hard Resin Spectacle Lenses (Rodenstock) p 349
Cosmolit Bifo 28 Spectacle Lenses (Rodenstock) p 349
Cosmolit Single Vision Spectacle Lenses (Rodenstock) p 349
Photocolor Hard Resin Spectacle Lenses (Rodenstock) p 349

RIBOFLAVIN
(see under VITAMIN B_2)

ROSE BENGAL
EV Rose Bengal (Eagle Vision) p 269
Rose Bengal 1% (Akorn) p 209

S

SALINE SOLUTION
Allergan Hydrocare Preserved Saline Solution (Allergan Optical) p 326
Allergan Sorbi-Care Saline Solution (Allergan Optical) p 327
Lens Plus Sterile Saline Solution (Preservative Free) (Allergan Optical) p 336
Lensrins Preserved Saline Solution (Allergan Optical) p 337
SoftWear Sterile Saline Solution for Sensitive Eyes (CIBA Vision Corp.) p 347

SCOPOLAMINE HYDROBROMIDE
Isopto Hyoscine (Alcon Laboratories) p 222
Murocoll-2 Sterile Ophthalmic Solution (Bausch & Lomb Pharmaceuticals) p 261

SELENIUM
Ocuvite Vitamin and Mineral Supplement (Storz Ophthalmics) p 312

SENECIO CINERARIA EXTRACTS
Succus Cineraria Maritima (SCM-Walker) (Walker Pharmacal) p 313

SILICA
Boston Advance Cleaner (Polymer Technology) p 104, 348

SILICONE
EV Monocanalicular Stent (Eagle Vision) p 269
Herrick Lacrimal Plug (Lacrimedics) p 281

SILVER PROTEIN
Argyrol S.S. 10% (IOLAB Pharmaceuticals) p 271
Argyrol S.S. 20% Dropperettes (IOLAB Pharmaceuticals) p 271

SODIUM BORATE
Collyrium for Fresh Eyes (Wyeth-Ayerst) p 105, 314
Eye Wash (Bausch & Lomb Personal) p 258

SODIUM CHLORIDE
AOSEPT Disinfection/Neutralization Solution (CIBA Vision Corp.) p 343
Adsorbonac 2% and 5% (Alcon Laboratories) p 210
AK-NaCl 5% Ointment & Solution (Akorn) p 204
CIBA Vision Saline Solution (CIBA Vision Corp.) p 344
Lens Fresh Lubricating & Rewetting Drops (Allergan Optical) p 331
Lens Plus Rewetting Drops (Allergan Optical) p 336
Lensept Disinfection System (CIBA Vision Corp.) p 345
Lensept Neutralizer & Rinsing/Storage Solution (CIBA Vision Corp.) p 345
Muro 128 Sodium Chloride Ophthalmic Ointment (Bausch & Lomb Pharmaceuticals) p 103, 260
Muro 128 Solution 2% and 5% (Bausch & Lomb Pharmaceuticals) p 103, 260

SODIUM CHRONDROITIN SULFATE
Viscoat Sterile Viscoelastic Ophthalmic (Alcon Surgical) p 235

SODIUM HYALURONATE
AMO Vitrax Solution (Allergan Medical Optics) p 236
AMVISC (IOLAB) p 324
AMVISC Plus (IOLAB) p 323
Healon (Kabi Pharmacia Ophthalmics) p 279
Healon Yellow (Kabi Pharmacia Ophthalmics) p 280
Viscoat Sterile Viscoelastic Ophthalmic (Alcon Surgical) p 235

SODIUM LAURYL SULFATE
Lens Plus Daily Cleaner (Allergan Optical) p 332
Resolve/GP Daily Cleaner (Allergan Optical) p 339

SUBTILISIN A
Ultrazyme Enzymatic Cleaner (Allergan Optical) p 340

SULFACETAMIDE SODIUM
AK-Cide Sterile Ophthalmic Ointment & Suspension (Akorn) p 202
AK-Sulf (Akorn) p 103, 207
Bleph-10 Ophthalmic Solution with Liquifilm (Allergan Pharmaceuticals) p 241
Bleph-10 Ophthalmic Ointment (Allergan Pharmaceuticals) p 241
Blephamide Liquifilm (Allergan Pharmaceuticals) p 242
Blephamide S.O.P. (Allergan Pharmaceuticals) p 242
Cetamide Ointment (Alcon Laboratories) p 220
Cetapred Ointment (Alcon Laboratories) p 220
FML-S Sterile Ophthalmic Suspension (Allergan Pharmaceuticals) p 246
Isopto Cetamide Solution (Alcon Laboratories) p 220
Isopto Cetapred Suspension (Alcon Laboratories) p 220
Metimyd Ophthalmic Ointment—Sterile (Schering) p 306
Metimyd Ophthalmic Suspension—Sterile (Schering) p 306
Ocu-Lone-C Sterile Ophthalmic Ointment (Ocumed) p 297
Ocu-Lone-C Sterile Ophthalmic Suspension (Ocumed) p 297
Ocu-Sul-10 Sterile Ophthalmic Ointment (Ocumed) p 297
Ocu-Sul-10, -15, -30 Sterile Ophthalmic Solution (Ocumed) p 297
Sodium Sulamyd Ophthalmic Ointment 10%-Sterile (Schering) p 307
Sodium Sulamyd Ophthalmic Solution 10%-Sterile (Schering) p 307
Sodium Sulamyd Ophthalmic Solution 30%-Sterile (Schering) p 307
Sulf-10 Dropperettes 10% (IOLAB Pharmaceuticals) p 271
Sulf-10 Ophthalmic Solution 10% (IOLAB Pharmaceuticals) p 271
Sulfacetamide Sodium Ophthalmic Ointment 10%, Sterile (Bausch & Lomb Pharmaceuticals) p 259
Sulfacetamide Sodium Ophthalmic Solution, 10%, 15% and 30%, Sterile (Bausch & Lomb Pharmaceuticals) p 259
Sulphrin Ointment (Bausch & Lomb Pharmaceuticals) p 259
Sulphrin Suspension (Bausch & Lomb Pharmaceuticals) p 259
Sulpred Suspension (Bausch & Lomb Pharmaceuticals) p 259
Vasocidin Ointment (IOLAB Pharmaceuticals) p 275
Vasocidin Ophthalmic Solution (IOLAB Pharmaceuticals) p 276
Vasosulf (IOLAB Pharmaceuticals) p 279

SULFISOXAZOLE DIOLAMINE
Gantrisin Ophthalmic Ointment/Solution (Roche) p 105, 304

SUPROFEN
Profenal Sterile Ophthalmic Solution (Alcon Surgical) p 234

T

TETRACAINE HYDROCHLORIDE
Tetracaine HCl Dropperettes ½% (IOLAB Pharmaceuticals) p 271

Tetracaine Hydrochloride Ophthalmic Solution, Sterile (Bausch & Lomb Pharmaceuticals) p 259

TETRACYCLINE HYDROCHLORIDE

Achromycin Ophthalmic Ointment 1% (Storz Ophthalmics) p 307
Achromycin Ophthalmic Suspension 1% (Storz Ophthalmics) p 105, 308

TETRAHYDROZOLINE HYDROCHLORIDE

Collyrium Fresh (Wyeth-Ayerst) p 105, 314
Eye Drops (Bausch & Lomb Pharmaceuticals) p 259
Eye-Zine Sterile Eye Drops (Ocumed) p 297
Murine Plus Lubricating Eye Redness Reliever (Ross) p 305
Visine A.C. Eye Drops (Pfizer Consumer) p 104, 303
Visine EXTRA Eye Drops (Pfizer Consumer) p 104, 303
Visine Eye Drops (Pfizer Consumer) p 104, 303

TIMOLOL MALEATE

Timoptic in Ocudose (Merck Sharp & Dohme) p 104, 294
Timoptic Sterile Ophthalmic Solution (Merck Sharp & Dohme) p 104, 292

TOBRAMYCIN

TobraDex Ophthalmic Suspension and Ointment (Alcon Laboratories) p 228
Tobrex Ophthalmic Ointment and Solution (Alcon Laboratories) p 229

TRIFLURIDINE

Viroptic Ophthalmic Solution, 1% Sterile (Burroughs Wellcome) p 267

TRIMETHOPRIM SULFATE

Polytrim Ophthalmic Solution Sterile (Allergan Pharmaceuticals) p 251

TROPICAMIDE

Mydriacyl (Alcon Laboratories) p 225
Ocu-Tropic Sterile Ophthalmic Solution (Ocumed) p 297
Tropicacyl (Akorn) p 209
Tropicamide Ophthalmic Solution, Sterile (Bausch & Lomb Pharmaceuticals) p 259

TYLOXAPOL

Enuclene (Alcon Surgical) p 232

V

VIDARABINE

Vira-A Ophthalmic Ointment, 3% (Parke-Davis) p 104, 302

VITAMIN A

Ocuvite Vitamin and Mineral Supplement (Storz Ophthalmics) p 312

VITAMIN B_2

ICAPS Plus (La Haye) p 280

VITAMIN C

ICAPS Plus (La Haye) p 280
Ocuvite Vitamin and Mineral Supplement (Storz Ophthalmics) p 312
Ophthalmic Nutrients (Health Maintenance) p 270

VITAMIN E

Ocuvite Vitamin and Mineral Supplement (Storz Ophthalmics) p 312
Ophthalmic Nutrients (Health Maintenance) p 270

VITAMINS WITH MINERALS, THERAPEUTIC

ICAPS Plus (La Haye) p 280

W

WHITE PETROLATUM

AKWA Tears Ointment (Akorn) p 208
Duolube Eye Ointment (Bausch & Lomb Personal) p 258
LubriTears Ointment (Bausch & Lomb Pharmaceuticals) p 259
Petrolatum Ointment (Bausch & Lomb Pharmaceuticals) p 259
Tears Renewed Ointment (Akorn) p 209

Z

ZINC

Ocuvite Vitamin and Mineral Supplement (Storz Ophthalmics) p 312

ZINC BACITRACIN

Ocu-Cort Sterile Ophthalmic Ointment (Ocumed) p 297
Ocu-Spor-B Sterile Ophthalmic Ointment (Ocumed) p 297

ZINC SULFATE

Clear Eyes ACR (Ross) p 105, 305
Visine A.C. Eye Drops (Pfizer Consumer) p 104, 303
Zincfrin (Alcon Laboratories) p 230

Part 5—Instrumentation, Equipment, Lenses and Sutures

CAMERAS
Fundus/Retinal
Allergan Humphrey p 352
Canon U.S.A. p 354
Topcon p 357

CAUTERY, DISPOSABLE
Alcon Surgical p 351

COMPUTER SYSTEMS
Allergan Humphrey p 352

CONTACT LENS INSTRUMENTS
Ophthalmometer
Topcon p 357

CRYOSURGICAL SYSTEMS
Disposable
Alcon Surgical p 351

EXAMINING UNITS
Chairs
Marco Equipment p 355
Topcon p 357
Chairs with Instrument Stand
Marco Equipment p 355
Topcon p 357

INSTRUMENTS
Cleaning Systems
Alcon Surgical p 351
Knife Protector
Alcon Surgical p 351
Knives, Disposable
Alcon Surgical p 351
IOLAB Intraocular p 323
Microsurgical
Alcon Surgical p 351
IOLAB Intraocular p 323
SITE p 357
Surgical Systems
Alcon Surgical p 351
IOLAB Intraocular p 323
SITE p 357
Anterior Segment Vitrectory
Alcon Surgical p 351
SITE p 357
Posterior Segment Vitrectomy
Alcon Surgical p 351
SITE p 357
Trays, Storage & Sterilizing
Alcon Surgical p 351
Visual Electrodiagnostic
Canon U.S.A. p 354

LASERS
Argon
Allergan Humphrey p 352
Yag
Marco Technologies p 356

LENS MEASURING INSTRUMENTS
Lensmeter
Allergan Humphrey p 352
Marco Equipment p 355
Topcon p 357
Radius Gauge
Marco Equipment p 355

LENSES
Aspheric Indirect Ophthalmoscopic Lenses
Topcon p 357
Volk Optical p 358
Fundus Laser Lenses
Volk Optical p 358
Intraocular
Alcon Surgical p 323
IOLAB Intraocular p 323
Optical Radiation p 325
Trial Lens Set
Marco Equipment p 355
Topcon p 357

MICROSCOPE SYSTEMS, OPERATING TYPE
Marco Equipment p 355
SITE p 357
Topcon p 357

NEEDLES
Irrigating
Alcon Surgical p 359
Reverse Cutting
Alcon Surgical p 359
Spatula
Alcon Surgical p 359
Taper Cut
Alcon Surgical p 359
Taper Point
Alcon Surgical p 359

OFFICE COMPUTER SYSTEMS
Allergan Humphrey p 352

OPERATING ROOM ACCESSORIES
Sterile Drapes, Disposable
Alcon Surgical p 351

OPHTHALMOMETER/KERATOMETER
Keratometer
Allergan Humphrey p 352
Canon U.S.A. p 354
Marco Equipment p 355
Marco Technologies p 356
Topcon p 357
Surgical Keratometer
Alcon Surgical p 351
Canon U.S.A. p 354
Marco Technologies p 356

OPHTHALMOSCOPES
Binocular
Alcon Surgical p 351
Topcon p 357
Indirect Type
Alcon Surgical p 351
Topcon p 357

PERIMETERS
Allergan Humphrey p 352
Canon U.S.A. p 354
Marco Equipment p 355
Marco Technologies p 356
Topcon p 357

PERIMETERS, AUTOMATED
Allergan Humphrey p 352
Marco Technologies p 356
Topcon p 357

RADIUS GAUGE
Marco Equipment p 355

REFRACTIVE SURGERY INSTRUMENTS
SITE p 357

REFRACTOMETERS
Accessories
Topcon p 357
Objective Automated Refractors
Allergan Humphrey p 352
Canon U.S.A. p 354
Marco Equipment p 355
Marco Technologies p 356
Topcon p 357
Subjective Automated Refractors
Allergan Humphrey p 352
Marco Equipment p 355
Marco Technologies p 356
Topcon p 357

REFRACTORS
Allergan Humphrey p 352
Canon U.S.A. p 354
Marco Equipment p 355
Marco Technologies p 356
Topcon p 357

RETINAL ANALYZER (COMPUTER)
Allergan Humphrey p 352

RETINOSCOPE
Allergan Humphrey p 352

SLIT LAMPS
Marco Equipment p 355
Volk Optical p 358
Biomicroscopes
Marco Equipment p 355
Topcon p 357
Volk Optical p 358

SPECULAR MICROSCOPES & ACCESSORIES
Topcon p 357

SPONGES
Sterile Micro Type, Disposable
Alcon Surgical p 351

SURGICAL KIT SYSTEMS
Alcon Surgical p 351
SITE p 357

SUTURES
Non-Absorbable
Black Braided Silk
Alcon Surgical p 359
Dacron
Alcon Surgical p 359
Monofilament Nylon
Alcon Surgical p 359
Polypropylene
Alcon Surgical p 359
Virgin Silk
Alcon Surgical p 359
White Braided Silk
Alcon Surgical p 359

TONOMETRIC/TONOGRAPHIC SYSTEMS

Applanation Type
Alcon Surgical p 351
Topcon p 357

Non-Contact
Topcon p 357

TRIAL FRAMES

Marco Equipment p 355
Topcon p 357

TRIAL SET

Marco Equipment p 355
Topcon p 357

ULTRASOUND

Allergan Humphrey p 352
Canon U.S.A. p 354
Marco Technologies p 356

Diagnostic
Allergan Humphrey p 352
Canon U.S.A. p 354
Marco Technologies p 356

VISCOELASTIC MATERIAL FOR SURGERY

IOLAB Intraocular p 323

VISUAL ACUITY CHART PROJECTORS

Automatic
Marco Equipment p 355
Topcon p 357

Manual
Marco Equipment p 355
Topcon p 357

VISUAL ACUITY TEST SYSTEM

Allergan Humphrey p 352
Canon U.S.A. p 354
Topcon p 357

SECTION 2

PHARMACEUTICALS IN OPHTHALMOLOGY

By: Joseph B. Walsh, M.D., Arthur Gold, M.D. and Howard Charles, M.D. with a section on Ocular Toxicology by F.T. Fraunfelder, M.D.

The section of Pharmaceuticals in Ophthalmology has been revised and expanded from the previous edition. Proprietary or trade names appear in the text and in the product section, with indices relating to the product information.

The ocular side effects of systemic medications have only nonproprietary names for medications but ample space is left for the reader to write in the brand names of the various drugs.

There are numerous sources which contain useful material on pharmacology in general and as it pertains to ophthalmology. Included below are some of the more useful volumes.

GENERAL REFERENCES:

1. A.M.A. Drug Evaluations 5th ed. *Am. Med. Assoc.,* 1983.
2. Baum, J.L. in Duane, T.D. *Clinical Ophthalmology,* Vol. 4, Chapter 26. Phila: J.B. Lippincott
3. Boyd, J.R., ed., *Facts and Comparisons,* St. Louis: Lippincott, 1984.
4. Ellis, P., *Ocular Therapeutics and Pharmacology,* 7th ed., St. Louis: Mosby, 1 985.
5. Fraunfelder, F.T. and Roy, F.H. *Current Ocular Therapy,* 2nd ed., Phila: W.B. Saunders, 1985.
6. Goodman, L.S. and Gilman, A., *The Pharmacology Basis of Therapeutics,* 6th ed., New York: Macmillan, 1980.
7. Grant, M. *Toxicology of the Eye,* 2nd ed., Springfield, 11, Thomas, 1 974.
8. Havener, W.H., *Ocular Pharmacology,* 5th ed., St. Louis: Mosby 1 983.
9. Lamberts, D.W. and Potter, D.E. *Clinical Ophthalmic Pharmacology,* Boston: Little Brown & Co. 1987 10 Leopold, 1, ed., Symposium on Ocular Therapy, Vol. 3-7, St. Louis: Mosby, 1968-1 974.
10. Leopold, I, ed., *Symposium on Ocular Therapy,* Vol. 3-7, St. Louis: Mosby, 1968-1974.

1. MYDRIATICS AND CYCLOPLEGICS

The topically applied autonomic drugs which produce mydriasi (pupillary dilatation) and cycloplegia (paralysis of accommodation) are among the most useful pharmacologic agents in ophthalmic practice. The common mydriatics comprise two groups of drugs: (A) Sympathomimetics; and (B) Parasympatholytics.

Sympathomimetic agents imitate (direct acting) or potentiate (indirect acting) the action of adrenaline, and their effect is upon the dilator muscle of the iris. They do not, with the exception of cocaine, cause cycloplegia. **Table 1** lists their generic and trade names and duration of action.

Parasympatholytic drugs produce pupil dilatation and paralysis of accommodation by rendering the pupillary sphincter and ciliary muscles insensitive to acetylcholine. **Table 2** lists their names and duration of action.

It is important to remember that the effect of the autonomic drugs listed below depends upon many factors such as the age of the patient, the color of his iris and his race. For example, the mydriatics and cycloplegics tend to be less effective at the same dose levels in dark-eyed individuals as compared to blue-eyed ones.

REFERENCE:

1. AMA Drug Evaluations. Fifth Edition. Chapter 20/Mydriatics and Cycloplegics. Chicago. American Medical Association. pp. 467-479, 1983.

TABLE 1

SYMPATHOMIMETIC DRUGS

U.S.P. OR N.F. NAME	TRADE NAME	PERCENT	MAXIMUM MYDRIASIS/DURATION
Phenylephrine HCl[(a)]	Ak-Dilate Efricel Mydfrin Neo-Synephrine HCl Phenoptic	2.5 & 10*	~20 minutes/~3 hours
Hydroxyamphetamine HBr[(b)]	Paredrine	1	~40 minutes
Cocaine[(b)]		2-4	~20 minutes ~2 hours

(a) Direct acting (b) Indirect acting sympathomimetic

*10% rarely used because of systemic effects

TABLE 2

PARASYMPATHOLYTIC DRUGS

U.S.P. OR N.F. NAME	TRADE NAME	PERCENT	MAX. MYD/MAX CYCL	DURATION
Atropine Sulfate*	Many	5-3.0	~30-40 min hours	~1-2 weeks
Cyclopentolate HCl	Ak-Pentolate Cyclogyl	5-2.0	~15-30 min 15-45 min	~1 day
Homatropine HBr	Homatrocel Isopto Homatropine	2 & 5	~10-30 min 30-90 min	~Several days
Scopolamine	Isopto Hyoscine Mydramide	.25	~15-30 min 30-45 min	~days to 1 week
Tropicamide	Mydriacyl Tropicacyl	.5 & 1.0	~20-30 min 20-30 min	~4-6 hours

*Possible exaggerated pupil response or systemic reaction in Down's syndrome.

Figures for mydriasis, cycloplegia and duration of effect are only approximate.

2. MIOTICS

The primary use for parasympathomimetics (miotics) is the treatment of glaucoma by the topical route. A secondary use is the control of accommodative esotropia. This class of agents mimics the effect of acetylcholine on parasympathomimetic post-ganglionic nerve endings within the eye. These agents are subdivided into direct-acting (cholinergic agents) or indirect-acting (anticholinesterase agents) based on their ability to bind acetylcholine receptors or inhibit the enzymatic hydrolysis of acetylcholine respectively. **Table 3** lists the parasympathomimetics approved for topical use in this country. In addition, two agents are available for intraocular use: Miochol, a 1% solution of acetylcholine and Miostat, a 0.01% solution of carbachol .

TABLE 3

TOPICAL MIOTIC AGENTS

U.S.P. OR N.F. NAME	TRADE NAME	PERCENT	DURATION OF MIOSIS
CHOLINERGICS			
Carbachol	Carbacel, Isopto Carbachol	0.75-3.0	~2 hours
Pilocarpine Hydrochloride	Adsorbocarpine, Akarpine, Almocarpine, Isopto Carpine, Pilocar, Pilocel, Pilomiotin Ocusert Pilo-20 Ocusert Pilo-40	0.5-10 (20 µg/hr) (40 µg/hr)	~4-8 hours 1 week 1 week
Pilocarpine Nitrate	Piloptic, Pilagan	0.5-6.0	~4-8 hours
ANTICHOLINESTERASES			
Short-acting			
Physostigmine Sulfate[(a)]	Eserine Sulfate	0.25	~12-36 hours
Physostigmine Salicylate	Isopto Eserine	0.25-0.5	~12-36 hours
Long-acting			
Demecarium Bromide[(b)]	Humorsol	0.125-0.25	~days to weeks
Echothiophate Iodide[(b)]	Echodide, Phospholine Iodide	0.03-0.25	~days to weeks ~days to weeks
Isoflurophate (DFP)[(b)]	Floropryl	0.025	

(a) Reversible anticholinesterase

(b) Irreversible anticholinesterases. Pralidoxime Chloride (Protopam Chloride) and atropine may counteract the effect of these drugs.

3. ANTIMICROBIAL THERAPY

Proper treatment of an ocular infection depends on determining the inciting agent (i.e. bacteria, fungi, virus, helminth, etc). Many agents are available for the treatment of external and intraocular infections **(Tables 4-10).** Most practitioners develop a preference for one or another of the topical agents (See Product Information Section), and some utilize combinations of antibiotics and/or antibiotic-steroid mixtures. It is recommended that therapy be initiated based on experience but only after slides for a Gram and Giemsa stain and aerobic and anerobic cultures are secured to guide in treatment. When fungal involvement is considered, additional stains to consider are methenamine silver, acridine orange and calcflour white.

Corneal ulcers and intraocular infections require vigorous and appropriate management. D.B. Jones[9] has provided an excellent article on the management of the former condition and Baum et al[2] and Mandelbaum et al[10] useful regimens for endophthalmitis. **Tables 4 and 5** list concentrations and dosages of principal antibiotics for ocular use. The essential routes of drug delivery in bacterial corneal ulcers are topical, subconjunctival, and intravenous administration. The latter route is generally reserved for severe cases such as impending or actual perforation and scleral extension. Collagen shields and hydrogel contact lenses may be helpful as a drug delivery system. Drops are preferred over ointment. "Fortified" antibiotics are preferred with cefazolin (50 mg/ml) for gram positive and gentamicin (13.6 mg/ml) for gram negative organisms. Gentamicin can be fortified by adding 2.0 ml of the parenteral preparation to the 5.0 ml drop bottle. Drops are usually given every 30 minutes. "Ciprofloxacin HCL 03% may be used without fortified topical or subconjunctival antibiotics for Staph spp, Strep spp, pseudomonas and serratia.[4, 7]

Fungal keratitis (keratomycosis) is relatively uncommon, but should be suspected in patients who have previously received topical steroids and/or antibiotics, and in patients whose corneal ulcer does not respond to antibiotics. Corneal scraping often permits correct clinical diagnosis. Pimaricin[8] (Natamycin) 5%, is recognized as the most potent broad-spectrum anti-fungal agent. Protozoa acanthamoeba may cause keratitis especially in soft contact lens wearers. Current treatment includes topical neosporin and Propamidine Isethionate. Additional medications for Acanthomeba are dibromoprapamide, clortrimazole and systemic ketoconazole.[1, 13] Penetrating keratoplasty is still an acceptable treatment.

In the treatment of endogenous fungal endophthalmitis **(Table 8),** we have utilized Amphotericin B subconjunctivally, intravenously and, where indicated, intravitreally. When administered intravitreally, we utilize sterile operating room technique and a coaxially illuminated operating microscope. Prior to intravitreal instillation of Amphotericin B (5-10 m), we aspirate a portion of the vitreous abscess for microbiological study. Flucytosine, topically and systemically, is of value in treating fungal endophthalmitis.

In bacterial endophthalmitis, the use of intraocular and periocular antimicrobial therapy has significantly improved the final visual function. The diagnosis of bacterial endophthalmitis should be strongly suspected in a patient who is post-operative, post-traumatic, or when the intraocular inflammation is out of proportion to what would be expected for the specific situation. Ocular pain is often present before obvious inflammation. Preoperative antibiotics may decrease the incidence of postoperative endophthalmitis.[18]

Once the diagnosis is suspected, prompt intervention is necessitated. Samples of the aqueous and vitreous must be promptly secured and treatment initiated depending on the suspected organism(s). In inflammation occurring several weeks or more after surgery or trauma or in immunosuppressed patients, fungal or an anaerobic (e.g. Propionibacterium Acenes) infections should be considered. Propionobacterium acnes endophthalmitis can have a delayed onset from a few weeks to 2 years following cataract surgery. These organisms have been cultured three years after implantation. The characteristic features are white plaques in the capsular bag, granulomatous deposits on the lens surface and corneal endothelium, and an initial response to steroids. The organism is sensitive to clindamycin, penicillin and cefazolin.

Once the aqueous and vitreous are cultured, antimicrobial agents should be directly injected into these cavities.[2] To prevent retinal toxicity, drugs should be injected slowly into the anterior vitreous cavity with particular caution after vitrectomy. (See **Table 10** for dosages). Because of the retinal toxicity of intravitreal gentamycin, amikacin may be a safer choice for treatment.

The use of topical subconjunctival antibiotics should be utilized for at least 7-10 days. Atropine 1%, 3-4 times daily may be utilized. The role of vitrectomy in the management of endophthalmitis is an important modality and is utilized as follows: first, as a means of securing a vitreous sample for analysis, second in trauma cases where severe disorganization of the anterior segment and/or a contaminated foreign body is present (if found the foreign body should be cultured), third when there is no response to treatment over 48-72 hours or marked deterioration over 24 hours and finally as a primary therapeutic modality.[12] Peyman recommends adding antibiotics to the vitrectomy infusion, e.g. gentamycin, 4 mg/ml. **Table 9** lists the suggested maximal non-toxic dose of antibiotic and antifungal drugs that might be used in the intravitreal infusions. When vitrectomy and intravitreal antibiotics are used, systemic antibiotics appear not to be necessary.[14, 16]

The place of corticosteroids in endophthalmitis has yet to be established but the tendency is to wait 24-48 hours after starting antimicrobial therapy before steroids are initiated.

REFERENCES:

1. Auran, JD, Starr, MB and Jakobiec, FA Acanthamoeba keratitis: a review of the literature. *Cornea* 6:2-26, 1987
2. Baum, J., Peyman, G.A., and Barza, M.: Intravitreul administration of antibiotics,in the treatment of bacterial endophthalmitis. *Surv. Ophthl* 26:204, 1982.
3. Blumekranz, M.S.. Culberson, W.W.. Clarkson, T.G., et al: Treatment of the Acute Retinal Necrosis Syndrome with Intravenous Acyclovir. *Opthalmology,* 93:296, 1986.
4. Boorman LR and Leopold, IH The potential use of quinolones in future antimicrobial therapy *AJO* 106: 227-229, 1988
5. Cohen, E.J., Perlato, C.J., Arensten, J.J.: Medical and Surgical Treatment of Acanthamoeba Keratitis. *American Journal of Ophthalmology.* Volume 103:615, 1987.
6. Driebe, W.T. Jr., Mandelbaum. S., Forster, R.K., Schwanz, L.K., Culbenson, W.W.: Pseudophakic Endophthalmitis: Diagnosis and Management. *Ophthalmology* 93:441-448, 1986 .
7. Hooper, DG and Wolfson, JS Fluoroquinotone antimicrobial agents *NEJM* 324: 3384-394, 1991
8. Jones, D.B. Chemotherapy of fungal infections. Chapt. 4. In Srinivasin, B.D. *Ocular Therapeutics,* New York. Masson USA, 1980.
9. Jones, D.B.: Early diagnosis and therapy of bacterial corneal ulcers. *Int. Ophthal. Clin.* 13:1, 1973.
10. Mandelbaum, S. and Forster. R.K.: Endophthalmitis, Focal Points; Clinical Modules For Ophthalmologists. *Module* 9 1983 .
11. Mandelbaum, S., Forster, R.K., Gelender, H., and Culbertson, W.: Late onset Endophthalmitis Associated with Filtering Blebs. *Ophthalmology* 92:964-972, 1985.
12. Meridith, TA, Aguilar, HE, Miller, MJ, Gardner, SK, Trablesi, A and Wilson, LA Comparative treatment of experimental *staphylococcus epidermidis* endophthalmitis *Arch Ophthal* 108:857-860
13. Moore, MB and McCully, JP Acanthamoeba keratitis associated with contact lenses six consecutive cases of successful management *BJO* 73:271-275, 1989
14. Pavan, P.R., Brinser, J.H.: Exogenous Bacterial Endophthalmitis Treated without Systemic Antibiotics. *American Journal of Ophthalmology,* Volume 104:121, 1987.
15. Peyman, G.A., Carroll, C.P. and Raichand, M.L.: Prevention and management of traumatic endophthalmitis. *Ophthalmology* 87:320-324, 1980.
16. Peyman, G.A.: Antibiotic Administration in the Treatment of Bacterial Endophthalmitis II Intravitreal Injections. *Survey of Ophthalmology.* Line 21:332, 239, 1987
17. Rhodes, H.K.: Antibiotic therapy for severe infections in infants and children. *Mayo Clin. Proc.* 52:707, 1977.
18. Starr, M.B.: Prophylactic antibiotics for ophthalmic surgery. *Survey of Ophthalmology* 26:353-373, 1983.
19. Tabbara, K.F. and O'Conor, G.R.: Treatment of ocular toxoplasmosis with clindamycin and sulfadiazine . *Ophthalmology* 87:129, 1980.
20. Ussery, F.M., Gibson, S.R., Conklin, R.H., et al: Intravitreal Ganciclovir in the Treatment of AIDS-Associated Cytomeglovirus Retinitis. *Ophthalmology* 95:640 1988.

TABLE 4

TOPICAL ANTIBACTERIAL AGENTS

U.S.P. OR N.F. NAME	TRADE NAME	CONCENTRATION/ DROPS	OINTMENT
INDIVIDUAL AGENTS			
Bacitracin	Various		500 units/g
Chloramphenicol	Ak-Chlor		10 mg/g
	Chlorofair	5 mg/g	10 mg/g
	Chloromycetin Ophthalmic		10 mg/g
	Chloroptic SOP	5 mg/g	10 mg/g
	Various	5 mg/g	
	Chloracol 0.5%	5 mg/g	
	I Cholor	5 mg/g	
	Ophthochlor	5 mg/g	
Colistin Sulfate	Coly-Mycin C	Powder for solution	
Erythromycin	Ak-Mycin		5 mg/g
	Ilotycin		5 mg/g
Gentamicin	Gentafair	3 mg/ml	3 mg/g
	Gentak	3 mg/ml	3 mg/g
	Gentacidin	3 mg/ml	3 mg/g
	Garamycin	3 mg/ml	3 mg/g
	Genoptic SOP	3 mg/ml	3 mg/g
Polymyxin B Sulfate		Powder for solution	
Silver Nitrate		1%	
Sulfacetamide Sodium	Ak-Sulf	10, 15 and 30%	10%
	Bleph-10	10%	10%
	Ophthacet	10%	
	Sodium Sulamyd	10 and 30%	10%
	Sulf-10	10%	
	Sulfamide 10%	10%	
	Isopto Cetamide	15%	10%
	Sulfair 15	15%	
	Vasosulf	15%	
Sulfisoxazole Diolamine	Gantrisin	4%	4%
Tetracycline	Achromycin	1%	1%
	Aureomycin		1%
Tobramycin	Tobrex	3 mg/ml	3 mg/g
MIXTURES			
Polymyxin B + bacitracin	Ak-Poly-Bac		10,000 units + 500 units/g
	Polysporin		same as above
Polymyxin B + neomycin	Statrol	16,250 + 3.5 mg/ml	10,000 units + 3.5 mg/g
Polymyxin B + oxytetracycline	Terramycin w/ polymyxin B		10,000 units + 5 mg/g
Polymyxin B + neomycin + bacitracin	Neonatal Ophthalmic		5,000 units + 5 mg + 400 units/g
Polymyxin B + neomycin + bacitracin	Ak-Spore		10,000 units + 3.4 mg + 500 units/g
	Neosporin Ophthalmic		same as above
	Mycitracin Ophthalmic		same as above
Polymyxin B + neomycin + gramicidin	Ak-Spore	10,000 units + 1.75 mg + 0.025 mg/ml	
	Neocidin	same as above	
	Neosporin Ophthalmic	same as above	
Polymyxin B + Trimethoprim	Polytrim	10,000 + 1 mg/ml	

+ Neosporin drops contain polymxyin B sulfate 5,000 units + neomycin sulfate 2.5 mg + gramicidin 0.025 mg/ml

TABLE 5

CONCENTRATIONS AND DOSAGES OF PRINCIPAL ANTIBIOTIC AGENTS

	TOPICAL	SUBCONJUNCTIVAL	INTRAVITREAL	INTRAVENOUS*
Amikacin	....	....	400 ug	....
Ampicillin	....	50-250 mg	500 ug	2.0-4.0 gm/4 hr
Bacitracin	10,000 units/ml	10,000 units	....	....
Carbenicillin**	4.0 mg/ml	100 mg	250 ug-2.0 mg	2.0-6.0 gm/4 hr
Cefazolin	50 mg/ml	100 mg	2.25 mg	0.5-1.0 gm/6 hr
Cephalothin	50 mg/ml	50-100 mg	....	1.0 gm/4 hr
Chloramphenicol	5 mg/ml	1-2 mg	2 mg	50 mg/kg/dy
Clindamycin	....	15-40 mg	1.0 mg	300-600 mg/8 hr
Colistin	5-10 mg/ml	15-37.5 mg	....	5.0 mg/kg/dy
Erythromycin	50 mg ml	100 mg	500 ug	....
Gentamicin**	8-15 mg/ml	10 -20 mg	100-200 ug	5.0 mg/kg/dy
Lincomycin	....	150 mg	1.5 mg	600 mg/8 hr
Methicillin	....	20-100 mg	2.0 mg	2.0 gm/4 hr
Neomycin	5-8 mg/ml	250-500 mg	....	....
Penicillin G	100,000 units/ml	0.5-1.0 million units	....	2.0-6.0 mega units/4 hr
Polymyxin B	16,250 units/ml	10 mg	....	....
Sulfacetamide	100-300 mg/ml	....	....	4-8 gm/day
Tobramycin	3 mg/ml	....	0.2-0.4 mg	3-5 mg/kg/dy
Vancomycin	50 mg/ml	25 mg	1.0 mg	1.0 gm/12 hr

*Adult Doses, see reference 13 for pediatric doses. **Incompatible mixture for I.V. administration.

TABLE 6

TOPICAL ANTIVIRAL AGENTS

U.S.P. OR N.F. NAME	TRADE NAME	CONCENTRATION DROP	CONCENTRATION OINTMENT	SYSTEMIC
Idoxuridine (IDU)	Dendrid	0.1%		
	Herplex Liquifilm	0.1%		
	Stoxil	0.1%	0.5%	
Trifluridine	Viroptic	1.0%		
Vidarabine (Adenine Arabinoside, ARA-A)	Vira-A		3.0%	
Acyclovir (Acycloguanosine)*	Zovirax			200 mg po 5Xs/dy I.V. 5mg/kg/dy t.i.d. for 7-10 days.
Gancyclovir**	Cytovene			I.V. 10-15mg/kg/dy

* May be used orally in cases of herpes simplex heratitis and systemically in herpes retinitis and some cases of retinal necrosis. The course of treatment is 7-10 days. Experimental drugs such as DHPG has shown promising results in cytomegalic retinitis in immunosuppressed patients.

** Used in cytomagalic retinitis in AIDS. Because of the high relapse rate maintenance therapy is needed.Weekly intravitreal injections of the drug at the dosage of 200 ug may suffice. Randomized trials are underway using IV Forscanet as an alternative to Gancyclovir in these cases.

TABLE 7

ANTI-PROTOZOAL AGENTS

ORGANISM	DRUG	INDICATION FOR TREATMENT	ORAL MEDICATION
Toxoplasma gondii	Pyrimethamine†	Vision-threatening uveitis	Initial dose 100 mg followed by 25 mg 1 or 2/dy.
	Sulfadiazine	Uveitis	1-2 gm q.i.d. x 3-4 weeks.
	Corticosteroid preparation	Uveitis	40 mg daily orally
	Clindamycin[10]**	Uveitis	Subconjunctival Clindamycin Phosphate (40 mg/ml) diluted 1:3 in Normal saline. Dose 15-40 mg. Or oral Clindamycin Hydrochloride 300 mg QID/4 weeks

Pyrimethamine should be used in conjunction with sulfa and not alone. Hemogram must be monitored.

Corticosteroids should be used with caution and in conjunction with anti-protozoal agents.

† Folinic acid 10 mg/2-3x week I.M. can be added to prevent hematologic toxicity from Pyrimethamine, e.g bone marrow suppression, especially thrombocytopenia. Folinic acid can also be given by the oral route.

** Oral Clindamycin and its parent compound Lincomycin have been associated with Pseudomembranous Colitis.

TABLE 8

ANTIFUNGAL AGENTS

U.S.P. OR N.F. NAME	DOSAGE	SPECTRUM	TOXICITY
1. Amphotericin B (Topical solution)	2.5-10 mg/ml of diluent (distilled water or 5% dextrose solution)	Blastomyces Candida Coccidioides Histoplasma	
(Subconjunctival injection)	750 mcg/ml of diluent (as above) every other day		
2. Amphotericin B (Intravenous)	Start with 0.25 mg/Kg body weight and increase to 1-1.5, utilizing a preparation of 0.1 mg Amphotericin B/ml solution obtained by diluting 50 mg of powder in 10 ml sterile water and then diluting final concentration 0.1 mg/dl		Chills; fever; nausea; vomiting; renal impairment; hematuria; albuminuria; increased BUN; bone marrow depression; thrombophlebitis at site of injection
3. Amphotericin B (Intravitreal)	0.005-0.01 mg		
4. Nystatin (Topical)	a) Ointment 100,000 units/Gm	Aspergillus Candida	
5. Flucytosine	a) PO: 150 mg/Kg body weight b) Topical: 1% solution	Candida Cryptococcus	Diarrhea; nausea; bone marrow suppression
6. Natamycin* (Topical suspension)	5% Suspension	Candida Aspergillus Cephalosporium Fusarium Penicillium	
7. Miconazole	a) PO (IV) 0.3 Gm/day b) Topical, 1% solution c) Subconjunctival Inj., 5-10 mg d) Intravitreal, 0.25 mg	Candida Aspergillus	Phlebitis; GI disturbance; enhances coumadin effect
8. Ketoconazole	PO 200-400 mg/day PO 400-600 mg/day	Candida Histoplasmosis Cryptococcus P. Lilacinus endophthalmitis	

*Only drug available as ophthalmic preparation (Natacyn). Others must be mixed by pharmacy or physician.

TABLE 9*

MAXIMUM NON-TOXIC DOSE OF ANTIBIOTIC AND ANTIFUNGAL AGENTS FOR VITRECTOMY INFUSION FOR ENDOPHTHALMITIS*

SINGLE				COMBINATION	
	NONTOXIC DOSE (MG/ML)		NONTOXIC DOSE (MG/ML)		NONTOXIC DOSE (MG/ML)
Chloramphenicol	10	Lincomycin	10	1) Gentamicin	8
Clindamycin	9	Oxacillin	10	Oxacillin	10
Amikacin	10	Penicillin	10	2) Clindamycin	9
Tobramycin	10	Amphotericin B		Gentamicin	8
Gentamicin	8	methyl ester	75	3) Methicillin	20
Methicillin	20	**(Recommended dose IO mg/ml.)**		Gentamicin	8

*from Peyman, Carroll, Raichand[9].

TABLE 10

AN INTRAOCULAR THERAPEUTIC REGIMEN FOR ENDOPHTHALMITIS

1. Diagnostic anterior chamber and vitreous aspiration; diagnostic vitrectomy when liquid vitreous fails to aspirate or in cases of suspected fungal endophthalmitis.

2. Initial therapy (in operating room after diagnostic technique).
   A. Intraocular
   gentamycin 100 µg or Amikacin 400 µg *and*
   vancomycin 1.0 mg or cefazolin 2.25 mg
   B. Subconjunctival
   gentamicin 40 mg *and*
   triamcinolone diacetate (Aristocort) 40 mg**
   C. Topical
   gentamicin 9.1 or 13.4 mg/ml *and*
   cefazolin 50 mg/ml *and*
   prednisolone acetate 1%
   D. Systemic
   cefazolin (Ancef or Kefzol) 1000 mg every 6 to 8 hours (Ceftriaxone has good penetration of the blood ocular barrier and may be used as an alternative).

3. If cultures are *positive* for a virulent bacteria consider repeating the above intraocular injections at the bedside on the second and fourth postoperative days. Continue topical treatment every half hour, subconjunctival treatment daily and systemic therapy. Consider therapeutic vitrectomy with repeat intraocular antibiotics.

4. If cultures are negative after 48 hours, do not repeat intraocular antibiotics. Consider tapering topical, subconjunctival and systemic antibiotic therapy while continuing topical and subconjunctival corticosteroids.

5. If the endophthalmitis presents as a *delayed inflammation* in which a fungal etiology is considered, the vitreous sample should be obtained by a vitreous instrument utilizing membrane filters; intraocular amphotericin B (Fungizone) at a dosage of 0.005 to 0.01 mg or miconazole at a dosage of 0.025 mg should be considered.

* from Mandelbaum, S. and Forster, R.K.[9]

** Subconjunctival corticosteroids should be deferred 48 to 72 hours to await culture growth and confirmation if a fungal etiology is suspected or the inflammation is delayed.

4. OCULAR ANTI-INFLAMMATORY THERAPY

A wide variety of agents is available to treat ocular inflammation. The most commonly used drugs are the natural and synthetic corticosteroid preparations. **Table 11** lists the available ophthalmic corticosteroid preparations. Many of these are available in combination with antibiotics or other medications.

At one time it was felt that corticosteroids were contraindicated in infectious disease states. However, it is now appreciated that steroids, when used in conjunction with appropriate antimicrobial or antiviral agents, may help to prevent serious ocular damage.

Steroids may be administered by four different routes in the treatment of ocular inflammation. **Table 12** lists the preferred routes in various conditions.

Topical corticosteroids can elevate intraocular pressure, and in susceptible individuals can induce glaucoma. They can also cause cataract formation, a situation more likely with high dosage systemic corticosteroids.

Other useful agents include 4% sodium cromolyn (Opcrom 4%) to treat vernal conjunctivitis or allergic keratoconjunctivitis and 0.03% Sodium Flurbiprofen (Ocufen) for inhibition of intraoperative miosis. Tetracycline p.o. 250 mg q.i.d./4 weeks then 250 mg/day is useful in treating ocular rosacea.

Immunosuppressive therapy may be useful in some cases of severe, corticosteroid unresponsive ocular inflammation, but the medication should be supervised by a physician well versed in its use. Topical Cyclosporin, a 2% in olive oil, has been used postoperatively in high risk cornea transplants. Also, 5-Fluorouracil is being used subconjunctivally (e.g. 5 mg QD for a week) to improve the success of glaucoma filtering procedures. Mitomycin C topically post-pterygia surgery has been reported to decrease recurrence and in glaucoma surgery.

TABLE 12

USUAL ROUTE OF STEROID ADMINISTRATION IN OCULAR INFLAMMATION

CONDITION	ROUTE
Blepharitis	Topical
Conjunctivitis	Topical
Episcleritis	Topical
Scleritis	Topical and/or Systemic
Keratitis	Topical
Anterior Uveitis	Topical and/or Depot
Posterior Uveitis	Systemic and/or Depot
Endophthalmitis	Systemic/Depot, Intravitreal
Optic neuritis	Systemic or Depot
Cranial arteritis	Systemic
Sympathetic Ophthalmia	Systemic and Topical

TABLE 11

OPHTHALMIC CORTICOSTEROID PREPARATIONS

GENERIC NAME	TRADE NAME	CONCENTRATION %
I. Hydrocortisone		
— acetate suspension	Hydrocortone acetate	2.5
— acetate ointment	Hydrocortone acetate	1.5
— solution	Optef drops	0.2
II. Prednisolone		
— acetate suspension	Pred Mild/Pred Forte	0.12/1.0
— acetate suspension	Econopred/Econopred Plus	0.125/1.0
— acetate suspension	Ak-Tate	1.0
— acetate suspension	Predulose	0.25
— sodium phosphate solution	Inflamase/Inflamase forte	0.12/1.0
— sodium phosphate solution	B-H™ Prednisolone	0.125/1 0
— sodium phosphate solution	Ak-Pred	0.125/1.0
— phosphate solution	Hydeltrasol	0.5
— phosphate solution	Metreton	0.5
— phosphate ointment	Hydeltrasol	0.25
III. Dexamethasone		
— phosphate solution	Ak-Dex	0.1
— phosphate ointment	Ak-Dex	0.05
— phosphate solution	Decadron	0.1
— phosphate ointment	Decadron	0.05
— suspension	Maxidex	0.1
IV. Progesterone-like Compounds		
— medrysone	HMS	1.0
— fluorometholone suspension	FML/FML Forte	0.1/0.25
— fluorometholone ointment	FML	0.1

5. ANESTHETIC AGENTS

A. Topical anesthetics

Topical anesthetics (Table 13) permit the clinician to perform ocular procedures such as tonometry, removal of foreign bodies from the surface of the eye, and lacrimal canalicular manipulation and irrigation. Cocaine, the prototype topical anesthetic, is a natural compound: the other agents are synthetics.

Cocaine is rarely used as an anesthetic agent because it causes damage to the corneal epithelium, produces pupillary dilatation, and it may affect the intraocular pressure. It is a useful agent when it is desired to remove the corneal epithelium, as in the case of epithelial debridement for dendritic keratitis.

The table lists the various agents and the concentrations which are available. Most of the agents work within a minute and their duration of action is between 10 and 20 minutes. A transient, superficial punctate keratitis may develop rapidly after the instillation of the agent.

B. Regional anesthetics

The actions and usefulness of the most commonly utilized regional anesthetic agents in ophthalmic surgery are summarized in Table 14.

REFERENCES:

1. Everett, W. G., Vey, E. K. and Finlay, J. W. Duration of oculomotor akinesia of injectable anesthetics. *Trans. Am. Acad. Ophth.* 65: 308, 1961.
2. Holekamp, T.L.R., Arribas, N.P., and Boniuk. I.: Bupivacaine anesthesia in retinal detachment surgery. *Arch. Ophth.* 97:109, 1979.

TABLE 13

TOPICAL ANESTHETIC AGENTS

U.S.P. OR N.F. NAME	TRADE NAME	CONCENTRATION
Cocaine Hydrochloride		1 to 4%
Proparacaine Hydrochloride	Ak-Taine	0.5%
	Alcaine	0.5%
	Ophthaine	0.5%
	Ophthetic	0.5%
Tetracaine Hydrochloride	Anacel	0.5%
	Pontocaine	0.5%

TABLE 14

REGIONAL ANESTHETICS ***

U.S.P. OR N.F. NAME	CONCENTRATION USED MAXIMUM DOSE	ONSET OF ACTION	DURATION OF ACTION	MAJOR ADVANTAGES/ DISADVANTAGES
Procaine*	1-4%/500 mg	7-8 mins.	30-45 mins. 60 mins. (with epinephrine)	Short duration. Poor absorption from mucous membranes
Tetracaine*	0.25%	5-9 mins.	120-140 mins (with epinephrine)	
Hexylcaine*	1-2%	5-10 mins.	60 mins.	
Bupivacaine** (1)	0.25-0.75%	5-11 mins.	480-720 mins. (with epinephrine)	
Lidocaine**	1-2%/500 mg	4-6 mins.	40-60 mins. 120 mins. (with epinephrine)	Spreads readily without hyaluronidase
Mepivacaine**	1-2%/500 mg	3-5 mins.	120 mins.	Duration of action greater without epinephrine (Everett et al[1])
Prilocaine**	1-2%/600 mg	3-4 mins.	90-120 mins. (with epine-phrine)	As effective as lidocaine
Etidocaine**	1%	3 mins.	300-600 mins.	

*Ester type compound **Amide type compound ***Retrobulbar injection has been reported to cause apnea.

(1) a mixture of bupivacaine, lidocaine, and epinephrine has been shown to be effective in retinal detachment surgery under local anesthesia.[2]

6. AGENTS FOR THE TREATMENT OF GLAUCOMA

A. Parasympathomimetics, See page 3, **Table 3.** These agents increase aqueous outflow.

B. Sympathomimetics. (Table 15) This class of agents has a complex prior exposure and time dependent effect on aqueous dynamics. These effects include changes from baseline aqueous secretion rates, an increase in "Clearance" values, and an increase in uvea-scleral outflow. The net effect of a topical application of an adrenergic agent is usually a decrease in intraocular pressure. **Table 15** lists the agents of this class available for the treatment of glaucoma.

C. Adrenergic Antagonists. (Table 15) Blockade of the beta adrenergic receptors found in the ciliary body lowers intra ocular pressure by decreasing aqueous humor secretion.

D. Hyperosmotic agents (Table 16) These agents decrease intraocular pressure by decreasing intraocular volume through a blood-ocular osmotic gradient.

E. Carbonic anhydrase inhibitors (Table 17) Carbonic anhydrase catalyzes the formation of bicarbonate in a multitude of tissues. The inhibition of this enzyme in ciliary processes decreases aqueous humor secretion and intraocular pressure.

REFERENCE:

Glaucoma: Applied Pharmacology in Medical Treatment, Sears, M Grune & Stratton Inc 1984

TABLE 15

TOPICAL ADRENERGIC AGENTS IN GLAUCOMA TREATMENT

U.S.P. OR N.F. NAME	TRADE NAME	CONCENTRATION
Epinephrine Bitartrate	E	1 & 2%
	Epitrate	2%
	Mytrate	1 & 2%
	Murocoll	1 & 2%
Epinephrine Hydrochloride	Epifrin	0.25-2.0%
	Glaucon	0.5-2.0%
Epinephrine Borate	Epinal	0.25-1.0%
	Eppy/N	0.5 & 1.0%
Dipivefrin Hydrochloride (Dipivalyl Epinephrine)	Propine	0.1%
Timolol Maleate	Timoptic	0.25 & 0.5%
Levobunolol	Betagan	0. 5%
Betaxolol	Betoptic	0. 5%
Apraclonidine*	lopidine	1%

* Use only pre and post anterior segment laser to control intraocular pressure.

TABLE 16

HYPEROSMOTIC AGENTS

U.S.P. OR N.F. NAME	TRADE NAME	PREPARATION	DOSE/ROUTE	ACTION ONSET/DURATION
Glycerin	Glyrol	75%	1-1.5 g/kg oral	10-30 min/4-5 hr
	Osmoglyn	50%	1-1.5 g/kg oral	
Isosorbide*	Ismotic	45%	1.5 g/kg oral	30 min/5-6 hr
Mannitol**	Osmitrol	5-20%	0.5-2 g/kg I.V.	30-60 min/6 hr
Urea	Ureaphil	Powder 40g	0.5-2 g/kg of 30% soln. I.V.	30-45 min/5-6 hr

* Do not confuse with isosorbide dinitrate, an antianginal agent.

** Do not confuse with mannitol hexanitrate, an antianginal agent.

TABLE 17

CARBONIC ANHYDRASE INHIBITORS

U.S.P. OR N.F. NAME	TRADE NAME	PREPARATION	ACTION ONSET/DURATION
Acetazolamide	Ak-Zol	Tablets 250 mg	2 hr/4-6 hr
	Cetazol		
	Diamox	Tablets 125 & 250 mg Capsules 500 mg (timed-release)	
Acetazolamide Sodium	Diamox (parenteral)	500 mg	5-10 min/2 hr
Dichlorphenamide	Daranide	Tablets 50 mg	30 min/6 hr
	Oratrol	Tablets 50 mg	
Methazolamide	Neptazane	Tablets 50 mg	2 hr/4-6 hr

7. MEDICATIONS FOR THE DRY EYE

The dry eye refers to a condition in which the eye may be deficient in either the aqueous or mucin components of the precorneal tear film. The most commonly encountered aqueous deficient dry eye in the United States is kerato conjunctivitis sicca while mucin deficient dry eyes may be seen in hypovitaminosis A. Stevens-Johnson syndrome, ocular pemphigoid, extensive trachoma and after chemical burns.

Artificial tear preparations (demulcents) are available for treatment of dry eyes **(Table 18)**.

Emollients form an occlusive film over the ocular surface and lubricate and protect the eye from drying. They are useful to protect patients with dry-eyes and those suffering from recurrent corneal erosions. They are used as a nighttime medication **(Table 19)**.

TABLE 18

ARTIFICIAL TEAR PREPARATIONS (DEMULCENTS)

MAJOR COMPONENT	TRADE NAME	ADDITIONAL COMPONENTS
Carboxymethylcellulose	Celluvisc	
Hydroxyethylcellulose	Clerz	thimerosal + edetate disodium
	Lyteers	benzalkonium chloride + edetate disodium
	TearGard	sorbic acid + ededate disodium
Hydroxypropyl cellulose	Lacrisert* (Water soluble insert)	
Hydroxypropyl methylcellulose	Isopto Alkaline	benzalkonium chloride
	Isopto Plain	benzalkonium chloride
	Isopto Tears	benzalkonium chloride
	Lacril	chlorobutanol
	Muro Tears	benzalkonium chloride + edetate disodium
	Tearisol	benzalkonium chloride
Methylcellulose	Methopto	benzalkonium chloride
	Methulose	benzalkonium chloride
	Murocel	methylparaben & propylparaben
	Visculose	benzalkonium chloride
Polyvinyl alcohol	Akwa Tears	benzalkonium chloride + edetate sodium
	Liquifilm Tears	chlorobutanol
	Liquifilm Forte	thimerosal + edetate disodium
	Tears Plus	chlorobutanol
Polyvinyl alcohol and cellulose ester	aqua-FLOW	benzalkonium chloride + edetate disodium
	Neo-Tears	thimerosal + edetate disodium
Polyvinyl alcohol and povidone	Refresh	
Polyvinyl alcohol and lipiden™	Hypotears PF	
Other Polymeric Systems	Adapettes	thimerosal + edetate disodium
	Adsorbotear	thimerosal + edetate disodium
	Comfort Drops	benzalkonium chloride + edetate disodium
	Dual Wet	benzalkonium chloride + edetate disodium
	Hypotears	benzalkonium chloride
	Tears Naturale	benzalkonium chloride
	Tears Naturale II	benzalkonium chloride
	Tears Naturale Free	benzalkonium chloride
	Tears Renewed	benzalkonium chloride + edetate disodium

* Prescription medication; all the other preparations are nonprescription.

TABLE 19

OCULAR EMOLLIENTS

TRADE NAME	COMPOSITION
Akwa Tears Ointment (Akorn)	Petrolatum, Liquid Lanolin, Mineral Oil—sterile
Duolube (Muro)	Sterile ointment containing white petrolatum and mineral oil.
Duratears (Alcon)	Sterile ointment with white petrolatum, liquid lanolin, mineral oil, methylparaben and polyparaben.
Hypotears (Iolab)	Sterile ointment containing white petrolatum and light mineral oil.
Lacri-Lube S.O.P. (Allergan)	Sterile ointment with 42.5% mineral oil, 55% white petrolatum (and) lanolin alcohol, and chlorobutanol.
Refresh P.M.	Sterile ointment with 41.5% mineral oil, 55% white petrolatum, petrolatum (and) lanolin alcohol with no preservatives
Tears Renewed Ointment (Akon)	Sterile ointment with white petrolatum and light mineral oil. Preservative-free and lanolin-free.

8. OCULAR DECONGESTANTS

These topically applied adrenergic medications are commonly used to whiten the eye. Four types of agents are available with those containing naphazoline and tetrahydrozoline being more stable than phenylephrine. They are usually applied one or two drops no more than four times a day **(Table 20).**

TABLE 20

OCULAR DECONGESTANTS

DRUG	TRADE NAME	ADDITIONAL COMPONENTS
Naphazoline Hydrochloride	Ak-Con*	Benzalkonium chloride + edetate disodium
	Albalon*	Benzalkonium chloride + edetate disodium
	Clear Eyes*	Benzalkonium chloride + edetate disodium
	Degest 2	Benzalkonium chloride + edetate disodium
	Muro's Opcon*	Benzalkonium chloride + edetate disodium
	Naphcon*	Benzalkonium chloride + edetate disodium
	Vasoclear	Benzalkonium chloride + edetate disodium
	Vasocon Regular*	Phenylmercuric acetate
Phenylephrine Hydrochloride	Ak-Nefrin	Benzalkonium chloride + edetate disodium
	Efricel	Benzalkonium chloride + edetate disodium
	Eye Cool	Thimerosal + edetate disodium
	Isopto Frin	Benzalkonium chloride + edetate disodium
	Prefrin Liquifilm	Benzalkonium chloride + edetate disodium
	Relief	—
	Tear-Efrin	Benzalkonium chloride + edetate disodium
	Velva-Kleen	Thimerosal + edetate disodium
Tetrahydrozoline Hydrochloride	Collyrium	Benzalkonium chloride + edetate disodium
	Murine Plus	Benzalkonium chloride + edetate disodium
	Soothe*	Benzalkonium chloride + edetate disodium
	Tetracon	Benzalkonium chloride + edetate disodium
	Visine	Benzalkonium chloride + edetate disodium
	Decongestant/Astringent Combinations	
Phenylephrine Hydrochloride plus Zinc Sulfate	Prefrin-Z	Thimerosal
	Zincfrin	Benzalkonium chloride
Tetrahydrozoline plus Zinc Sulphate	Visine A.C.	Benzalkonium chloride + edetate disodium

* Prescription medication

9. OPHTHALMIC IRRIGATING SOLUTIONS

Table 21 lists sterile isotonic solutions for general ophthalmic use. These products are all over the counter medications. There are also intraocular irrigating solutions available for use during surgical procedures. These include Akorn Balanced Salt Solution, BSS, BSS Plus, IO Care Balanced Salt Solution, and Nutrisol, and they are prescription medications.

TABLE 21

TRADE NAME	COMPONENTS	ADDITIONAL COMPONENTS
Ak-Rinse	Sodium, potassium, calcium, & magnesium chlorides & sodium acetate & citrate	benzalkonium chloride
Aqua-Flow	Sodium bicarbonate, sodium & potassium chlorides, polyvinyl alcohol & hydroxyethylcellulose	benzalkonium chloride + edetate disodium
Blinx	Boric acid and sodium borate	phenylmercuric acetate
Collyrium	Antipyrine, boric acid, & borax	thimerosal
Dacriose	Sodium chloride, potassium chloride & sodium phosphate	benzalkonium chloride + edetate disodium
Eye-Stream	Sodium, potassium, magnesium & calcium chloride. Sodium acetate and citrate	benzalkonium chloride
Irigate	Boric acid, potassium chloride, sodium carbonate	benzalkonium chloride + edetate disodium
Lauro	Boric acid and sodium chloride	
Lavoptik Eye Wash	Sodium chloride, biphosphate & phosphate	benzalkonium chloride
M/Rinse	Sodium & potassium chloride, sodium borate, boric acid	thimerosal + edetate disodium
Neo-Flow	Boric acid, sodium & potassium chloride, and sodium carbonate	benzalkonium chloride
Trisol	Borax, boric acid, sodium chloride	

10. HYPEROSMOLAR AGENTS

Hyperosmolar (hypertonic) agents are used to reduce corneal edema therapeutically or for diagnostic purposes. They osmotically attract water through the semi-permeable corneal epithelium.

TABLE 22

	TRADE NAME	PERCENT
A. Therapeutic Preparations		
Sodium Chloride:	Adsorbonac Ophthalmic	2 or 5%
	AK-NaCl 5%	5% (solution and ointment)
	Hypersal Ophthalmic	5%
	Muro-128	5% (solution or ointment)
Glucose:	Glucose 40% Ophthalmic	40%
B. Diagnostic Preparation		
Glycerin:	Ophthalgan	

11. DIAGNOSTIC AGENTS

Some of the more common diagnostic agents and tests used in ophthalmologic practice are listed below.

A. Examination of Conjunctiva, Cornea and Lacrimal Apparatus

Fluorescein and rose bengal are two of the more commonly used dyes which aid in the diagnosis of external ocular disorders.

Fluorescein, used primarily as a 2% alkaline solution, and in the form of impregnated paper strips, is used to examine the integrity of the conjunctival and corneal epithelium. Defects in the corneal epithelium will show up bright green by ordinary light or bright yellow if a cobalt blue filter is used in the light path. Similar lesions of the conjunctiva appear bright orange-yellow by ordinary illumination. Fluorescein has also come into wide use in the fitting of contact lenses.* The assessment of a proper fit is often determined by examining the pattern of fluorescein beneath the contact lens. In addition, fluorescein dye is used in performing applanation tonometry. One test of lacrimal apparatus patency (Jones test) uses one drop of 1 per cent fluorescein instilled into the conjunctival sac. The presence of the dye appearing in the nose indicates normal functioning of the drainage apparatus.[2]

Rose bengal, as a 1% solution, is particularly useful for demonstrating abnormal conjunctival or corneal epithelium. Devitalized cells will stain bright red, but normal cells will not stain. The abnormal epithelial cells present in "dry eye" disorders are effectively demonstrated by this stain.

The *Schirmer test* is a valuable method of assessing tear production. Prepared filter paper strips 5 x 30 mm in dimension are available for performing this test. The strips are inserted into the topically anesthetized conjunctival sac at the junction of the middle and outer third of the lower lid with approximately 25 mm of paper exposed. After 5 minutes the strip is removed and the amount of moistening measured. The normal range is 10 to 25 mm. If inadequate production of tears is found on the initial test, a Schirmer 11 test can be performed by repeating the procedure while stimulating the nasal mucosa.[1] A number of variations of the Schirmer test can be found in textbooks and articles.

B. Examination Or Acquired Ptosis or Extraocular Muscle Palsy

Edrophonium chloride may be injected intravenously when myasthenia gravis is suspected as the cause of the ptosis or muscle palsy. The test is performed by injecting 2 mg of edrophonium intravenously, followed 45 seconds later by an additional 8 mg if there was no response to the first dose. (In case of a severe reaction to the edrophonium one should immediately give atropine sulfate, 0.6 mg intravenously.)

* Not to be used in fitting soft lenses which absorb fluorescein.

C. Examination of the Retina and Choroid

Sodium fluorescein solution in concentrations of 5%, 10% and 25%, is injected intravenously to study the retinal and choroidal circulation. Its primary use has been to examine lesions at the posterior pole of the eye, but anterior segment fluorescein angiography (wherein the iris scleral and conjunctival vessels can be studied) is a useful clinical tool.

Intravascular fluorescein is normally prevented from entering the retina by the intact retinal vascular endothelium (blood-retinal barrier) and the intact retinal pigment epithelium. Defects in either the retinal vessels or the pigment epithelium will permit leakage of fluorescein which can then be studied either by direct observation or photographically. The primary requirement for good observation or photography is the provision of appropriate filters to excite the fluorescein and to exclude unwanted wavelengths. The peak frequencies for excitation lie between 485 and 500 mu and for emission between 520 and 530 mu.

Fluorescein has proven to be a safe diagnostic agent, the most common side effect being nausea and vomiting. Occasional allergic reactions and vagal reactions occur and oxygen and emergency equipment should be readily available when angiography is performed. Patients should also be alerted that there will be staining of their skin and urine by the dye: in the average patients this lasts no more than a day.

D. Examination of Abnormal Pupillar Responses

Methocholine, as a 2.5% solution instilled into the conjunctival sac, will cause the tonic pupil (Adie's pupil) to contract, but will not cause contraction of a normal pupil. A similar pupillary response is seen following instillation of 2.5% methacholine in patients with familial dysautonomia (Riley-Day Syndrome).

Table 23 shows the effects of several drugs on the miotic pupil occurring after the interruption of the sympathetic system (Horner's syndrome). The effect depends on the location of the lesion involving the sympathetic chain.

TABLE 23

HORNER'S SYNDROME

TOPICAL DROP	NEURON III (POST-GANGLIONIC)	NEURON II (PRE-GANGLIONIC)	NEURON I (CENTRAL)
Cocaine 5%	–	–	+/–
Adrenaline 1/1000**	+++	–	–
Atropine	+	+	+
Hydroxy-amphetamine(2)	–	+	+

**Adrenaline l/1000 does not dilate a normal pupil

Pilocarpine may be utilized in determining whether a fixed dilated pupil is due to an atropine-like drug or interruption of its parasympathetic innervation.[3] The dilated pupil due to instillation of an atropine-like drug fails to constrict to pilocarpine while the dilated pupil due to interruption of its parasympathetic innervation (compression by aneurysm, Adie's tonic pupil) constricts, after instillation of pilocarpine.

REFERENCES:

1. Hecht, S.D.: Evaluation of the lacrimal drainage system. *Ophthalmology.* 85:1250,1978.
2. Thompson, H.S. and Mensher, J.H. Adrenergic mydriasis in Homer's syndrome: Hydroxyamphetamine test for diagnosis of post-ganglionic defects. *Amer. J. Ophth.* 72:472, 1971.
3. Thompson, H.S., Newsome, D.A. and Lowenfeld, 1. E. The fixed dilated pupil. Sudden iridoplegia or mydriatic drops; A simple diagnostic test. *Arch. Ophthal.* 86:12, 1971.

12. OTHER AGENTS

A. Adjuncts to surgery

1. *Alpha-chymotrypsin*—A proteolytic enzyme prepared from mammalian pancreas. Primary use is enzymatic zonulysis during cataract extraction. A 1:5,000 dilution contains 150 APA (Armour Proteolytic Activity) units/ml. Solutions are prepared fresh just prior to instillation into the eye. The major complication arising from its use is a transient postoperative rise in intraocular tension due to the blockage of the trabecular meshwork by products of enzyme digestion.

2. *Hyaluronidase*—A hydrolytic enzyme whose action is to depolymerize tissue hyaluronic acid and thus increase tissue permeability. The optimal dosage in ophthalmic surgery is 5-7 turbidity reducing units per ml of anesthetic solution. The duration of local anesthesia may be reduced by hyaluronidase alone but the addition of epinephrine maintains the usual duration of anesthesia.

3. Sodium hyaluronadate (Healon®, Amvisc®) — A purified viscoelastic gel with a viscosity 400,000 times greater than that of balanced salt, yet is 98% water. The inertness of this purified derivative averts the problem of immunologic reaction. The chief complication presently is transient post-operative rise of intraocular pressure. This is especially true if the sodium hyaluronadate mixes with blood, cortical material, or alpha-chymotrypsin. To diminish the pressure rise, a minimal amount of the substance should be used during surgery.[1,2] Other similar compounds include:

A. Sodium chondrotin sulfate and sodium hyluronate (Viscot R)

B. Hydroxypropylmethylcellulose (Occucoat R)[3]

B. Chelating agents

1. *Ethylenediamine tetra-acetate (EDTA)*—A useful chelating agent in the treatment of band keratopathy and lime injury. The disodium salt in 0.37% solution is useful after removal of the corneal epithelium in removing calcium from Bowman's membrane. Lime injury (e.g., painter's plaster) is treated with a similar EDTA preparation.

2. *Deferoxamine*—Superficial corneal iron deposits may be removed by treatment with a 10% solution (in 1% methylcellulose) four times daily for several weeks.

REFERENCES:

1. Pape, L.G. and Balazs. E.A., The use of sodium hyaluronadate (Healon®) in human anterior segment surgery. *Ophthalmology* 87:699, 1980.
2. Polack, F.M., DeMong, J. and Santella, H., Sodium hyaluronadate (Healon®) in keratoplasty and intraocular lens implantation. *Ophthalmology* 88:425,1981.
3. Liesegang T.J., Viscoelastic *Substances in Ophthalmology Surv Ophthal* 34: 268-293, 1990.

13. OCULAR TOXICOLOGY

by F. T. Fraunfelder, M.D.

The intent of the section is not to list the common ocular or systemic side effects of drugs, since the data would be too lengthy for this format. It is primarily to mention some of the more recently published, or to be published, adverse drug effects of medications involving the eye or drugs commonly used by ophthalmologists.

The clinician is overwhelmed by the volume of ocular toxicology in the medical literature. However, much of the clinical toxicology is only on soft data, since few physicians have the volume of patients on a particular drug necessary for an adequate sample. Even in a controlled experimental environment, it is often difficult to prove a cause and effect drug relationship and in clinical practice with a multitude of variables. this may be impossible in many instances. In an attempt to alleviate this problem, the National Registry was formed.

The National Registry of Drug-Induced Ocular Side Effects was established by the Federal Food and Drug Administration, with the endorsement of the American Academy of Ophthalmology. It is based on the supposition that the suspicions of the practicing clinician. if sought, could be pooled to increase the data base, and may act as a flagging system to decrease the lag time in recognizing a possible adverse ocular drug response. The Registry does the following for the clinician:

1. Accumulates reports from ophthalmologists as to their suspicions of a possible drug-related event,
2. Keeps an ongoing file of any report in the world literature of a possible drug-related ocular event,
3. Prepares publications of adverse drug related ocular events, and
4. Provides bibliographies or consultation on possible drug-related events.

If you would like to report a suspected drug response or are interested in the reference for the material cited here, please contact F.T. Fraunfelder, M.D. Director, National Registry of Drug-Induced Ocular Side Effects, Department of Ophthalmology. University of Oregon Health Science Center, 3181 S.W. Sam Jackson Park Road, Portland, Oregon 97201 .

REFERENCE:

Fraunfelder, F.T.: *Drug-Induced Ocular Side Effects and Drug Interactions.* 3rd ed., Philadelphia, W.B. Saunders, 1989.

ADVERSE DRUG EFFECTS

I. MEDICATION BY INJECTION

GENERIC NAME	PRINCIPAL GENERAL USE	POSSIBLE ADVERSE EFFECTS
a. Adrenal Corticosteroids		
Depo-steroids	Allergic disorders Anti-inflammatory disorders	If injected into a blood vessel, i.e. the tonsilar fossa, may cause unilateral or bilateral retinal arterial occulsions due to emboli of depo-steroid. Permanent bilateral blindness may ensue.
Triamcinolone	Allergic disorders Anti-inflammatory disorders	Fatty atrophy in area of injection, i.e. enophthalmus if given retrobulbar or if given in periocular skin, some deformity can occur in area of injection due to loss of fat.
b. Anesthetics		
Ketamine	Adjunct to anesthesia Short-term diagnostic or surgical procedures	Reversible nystagmus
c. Antifungals		
Amphotericin B	Aspergillosis Blastomycosis Candidiasis Coccidioidiomycosis Histoplasmosis	Ischemic necrosis after subconjunctival injection Subconjunctival nodule
d. Antineoplastics		
Carmustine	Brain tumors Multiple myeloma	Optic neuritis Retinal vascular disorders
Cisplatin	Metastatic testicular or ovarian tumors Advanced bladder carcinoma	Cortical blindness Papilledema Retrobulbar or optic neuritis
Fluorouracil	Carcinoma of the colon, rectum, breast, stomach and pancreas	Ocular irritation with tearing Conjunctival hyperemia Canalicular fibrosis
e. Miscellaneous		
Skin Tests	Tests for allergies	Recurrence or aggravation of episcleritis or scleritis
f. Ophthalmic Dyes		
Fluorescein	Ocular diagnostic tests	Nausea, vomiting, urticaria, rhinorrhea. dizziness, hypotension, pharyngo-edema, anaphylactic reaction
g. Parasympathomimetics		
Acetylcholine	Produces prompt, short-term miosis	Hypotension and bradycardia with intraocular injection
II. ORAL		
a. Ameobicides		
5 Iodochlorhydroxyquin	Acrodermatitis enteropathica *Entamoeba histolytia*	Optic atrophy—may be due to a zinc deficiency of the optic nerve

GENERIC NAME	PRINCIPAL GENERAL USE	POSSIBLE ADVERSE EFFECTS
b. Antihelminthics		
Levamisol	Connective tissue disorders Ascaris infestation	Patients with Sjogren's syndrome and possibly keratitis sicca have marked increase in systemic side effects, including pruritis and muscle weakness
c. Antianxiety Agents		
Diazepam	Acute alcohol withdrawal Preoperative medication Psychoneurotic anxiety, depression, tension. or agitation Skeletal muscle spasms	Allergic conjunctivitis Extraocular muscle paresis Nystagmus
d. Antiarrhythmics		
Amiodarone	Cardiac abnormalities Ventricular arrhythmias	Keratopathy Lens opacities, Optic Neuropathy Optic neuritis
Oxprenolol	Cardiovascular abnormalities Certain hypertensive states	Conjunctival hyperemia Decreased lacrimation Nonspecific ocular irritation Photophobia
Propranolol	Cardiovascular abnormalities Certain hypertensive states	May precipitate latent myotonia May mask hyperthyroidism; when taken off drug thyroid stare and exophthalmos may occur
e. Antibiotics and Antituberculars		
Chloramphenicol		Aplastic anemia
Ethambutol	Pulmonary tuberculosis	Optic neuropathy
Rifampin	Asymptomatic carriers of meningococcus Many gram-negative and gram-positive cocci, including Neisseria and Hemophilus influenza Pulmonary tuberculosis	Conjunctival hyperemia Exudative conjunctivis Increased lacrimation
Tetracycline	Useful against gram-negative and gram-positive bacteria Members of lymphogranuloma-psittacosis group Mycoplasma	Pseudotumor cerebri and papilledema as early as 3 days after onset of medication in infants and in young adults Transient myopia
f. Antihypertension Agents		
Nitroprusside	Provides controlled hypertension during anesthesia Management of severe hypertension	Contraindicated in Leber's hereditary optic atrophy and tobacco ambylopia
g. Antileprotics		
Clofazimine	Dermatological diseases-psoriasis, pyoderma gangrenosum Leprosy	Conjunctival, corneal, and macular pigmentation
h. Antimalarial and anti-inflammatory		
Hydroxychloroquine	Malaria Lupus erythematosus Rheumatoid arthritis	Disturbance of accommodation Corneal changes "Bull's Eye" maculopathy central, pericentral, or paracentral scotomas
i. Antineoplastlcs		
Busulfan	Chronic myelogenous leukemia	Cataracts Decreased lacrimation
Tamoxifen	Metastatic breast carcinoma	Corneal opacities Refractile retinal deposits
j. Antipsychotics		
Haloperidol	Acute and chronic schizophrenia Manic/depressive psychosis	Capsular cataracts with chronic use Cycloplegia and mydriacis
Lithium Carbonate	Manic phase of manic/depressiveExophthalmos psychosis	Oculogyric crisis Myoclonus
k. Antispasmodics		
Baclofen	Muscle spasms in multiple sclerosis and disorders associated with increased muscular tone	Blurred vision Hallucinations
l. Carbonic Anhydrase Inhibitors		
Acetazolamide Dichlorophenamide Ethoxzolamide Methazolamide	Centracephalic epilepsies Congestive heart failure edema Drug-induced edema Glaucoma	Aggravation of metabolic acidosis, primarily in known CO_2 retaining diseases such as emphysema, bronchiectasis, and patients with poor vital capacity. Aplastic anemia Decreased libido Impotency
m. Chelatlng Agents		
Penicillamine	Cystinuria Heavy metal antagonist-iron. lead, copper, mercury poisoning Wilson's disease	Facial or ocular myasthenia, including extraocular muscle paralysis, ptosis. and diplopia Ocular pemphigoid Optic neuritis and color vision problems

GENERIC NAME	PRINCIPAL GENERAL USE	POSSIBLE ADVERSE EFFECTS
n. Hormonal Agents		
Oral Contraceptives	Amenorrhea Dysfunctional uterine bleeding Dysmenorrhea Hypogonadism Oral contraception Premenstrual tension	Contraindicated in patients with pre-existing retinal vascular diseases Decrease in color vision with chronic use Macular edema
o. Hydantoins		
Phenytoin	Chronic epilepsy	Optic nerve hypoplasia in infants with epileptic mothers on the drug Ocular teratogenic effects, including strabismus, ptosis, hypertelorism, epicanthus
p. Nonsteroidal Anti-inflammatory Agents		
Ibuprofen	Rheumatoid arthritis Osteoarthritis	Decreased color vision Optic neuritis Visual field defects
Naproxen	Rheumatoid arthritis Osteoarthritis Ankylosing spondylitis	Corneal opacity Periorbital edema
Sulindac	Rheumatoid arthritis Osteoarthritis Ankylosing spondylitis	Keratitis Stevens-Johnson syndrome
q. Psychedelics		
Marijuana	Cerebral sedative or narcotic	Conjunctival hyperemia Decreased lacrimation Decreased intraocular pressure Dyschromatopsia with chronic long-term use
r. Red Blood Cell Sickling Inhibitors		
Sodium Cyanate	Sickle cell hemoglobinopathy	Partially reversible posterior subcapsular cataracts
s. Sedatives and Hypnotics		
Ethanol	Antiseptic Used as a beverage	Fetal Alcohol syndrome: offspring of alcoholic mothers may have epicanthus, small palpebral fissures, and microphthalmia
t. Synthetic retinoids		
Etretinate Isotretinoin	Cystic acne and other keratinizing skin disorders	Dark eye, abnormal dark adaptation. EOG and ERG, cataracts, optic neuritis, pseudotumor, cerebri and papilledema
III. TOPICAL		
a. Anticholinergics		
Cyclopentolate	Used as a cycloplegic and mydriatic	Central nervous toxicity, including slurred speech, ataxia, hallucinations, hyperactivity, seizures and syncope, paralytic ileus
Tropicamide	Used as a cycloplegic and mydriatic	Cyanosis, muscle rigidity, nausea, pallor, vomiting, vasomotor collapse
b. Parasympathomimetics or Anticholinesterases		
Demecarium Echotiophate Isofluorphate Pilocarpine	Glaucoma	Retinal detachments primarily in eyes with peripheral retinal or retinal-vitreal disease. (Patients need to be warned of this possible effect when first placed on this medication.) Miotic URI—Rhinorrhea, sensation of chest constriction, cough, conjunctival hyperemia, seen primarily in young children on anti-cholinesterase agents.
c. Sympathomimetics		
Dipivefrin	Open-angle glaucoma	Follicular blepharo-conjunctivitis Keratitis
Epinephrine	Used as a bronchodilator Open-angle glaucoma Used as a vasoconstrictor to prolong anesthetic action	Cicatrical pemphigoid Stains soft contact lenses black Hypertension, headache
10% Phenylephrine	Used as a mydriatic and vasoconstrictor	Cardiac arrhythmias and cardiac arrests with pledget form or subconjunctival injection Possible myocardial infarcts Systemic hypertension
Betaxolol Levobunolol Timolol	Glaucoma	Cardiac syncope, bradycardia, lightheadedness, fatigue Congestive heart failure In diabetics—hyperglycemia In myasthenia gravis—severe dysarthia

SECTION 3

SUTURE MATERIALS

Perhaps no other surgical discipline requires as many specialized needles and suture material as ophthalmic surgery. To meet this need, manufacturers of surgical needles and sutures offer the ophthalmologist a comprehensive array of precisely manufactured reverse cutting and spatula needles swaged to suture materials of collagen (plain and chromic), silk (black and white braided), virgin silk (black and white twisted), Nylon*, Dacron* synthetics and synthetic absorbables. Suture material intended for use in ophthalmic surgery can be either non-absorbable or absorbable. The following is a list of various suture materials available for ophthalmology with a brief description of each:

Absorbable:

Plain Catgut—suture material prepared from the submucosal or mucosal layers of sheep or beef intestine respectively, which consists primarily of collagen—a fibrous protein—and is absorbed by the body.This material is chemically purified to minimize tissue reaction. Available in sizes 4-0 through 6-0.

Chromic Catgut—same as plain catgut except additionally treated by chromium salts to delay the absorption time. Available in sizes 4-0 through 7-0.

Plain Collagen—prepared from bovine deep flexor tendon. The tendon is purified and converted to a uniform suspension of collagen fibril. This fibrillar suspension is then extruded into suture strands and chemically treated to accurately control absorption rate. Available in sizes 4-0 through 7-0.

Chromic Collagen—prepared in the same way as plain collagen except chromium salts are added during the chemical treatment to further delay absorption. Available in sizes 4-0 through 8-0.

TABLE 24

COMPARISON OF OPHTHALMIC SUTURE MATERIALS

SUTURE MATERIAL	RELATIVE TENSILE STRENGTH**	RELATIVE HOLDING DURATION†	RELATIVE TISSUE REACTION†	EASE OF HANDLING	SPECIAL KNOT REQUIRED	BEHAVIOR OF EXPOSED ENDS	AVAILABLE SIZES***
Surgical gut or collagen							
Plain	6	1 week	4+	Fair	No	Stiff	4-0 to 6-0
Chromic	6	< 2 weeks	3+	Fair	No	Stiff	4-0 to 8-0
Polyglactin 910							
Braided	9	2 weeks	2+	Good	Yes	Stiff	4-0 to 9-0
Monofilament	9	2 weeks	2+	Good	Yes	Stiff	9-0 to 10-0
Polyglycolic acid	9	2 weeks	2+	Good	Yes	Stiff	
Silk							
Virgin	7	2 months	3+	Excellent	No	Softest	8-0 to 9-0
Braided	8	2 months	3+	Good	No	Soft	4-0 to 9-0
Polyamide (Nylon)	9	6 months	1+	Fair	Yes+	Stiff & sharp	8-0 to 11-0
Polypropylene	10	> 12 months	1+	Fair	Yes	Stiff & sharp	4-0 to 6-0 9-0 to 10-0

* Adapted from Spaeth, G.L., *Ophthalmic Surgery, Principles and Practice,* Phila. Saunders, 1982 p 64.

** The higher the number, the greater the relative tensile strength. Strength varies with size of material; estimates apply mainly to size 8-0 sutures.

† Holding duration will vary with location and size of suture, health of patient, medications employed, etc. The time given in this table is an average of the time at which about 30 per cent of tensile strength is lost.

‡ 1+ indicates least inflammatory response; 4+ greatest.

*** With needles appropriate for ophthalmic use. Sizes available will vary from time to time.

Synthetic Absorbable Sutures: Vicryl* (Polyglactin 910, a copolymer of lactide and glycolide) and Dexon* (Polyglycolic acid). These materials offer high tensile strength during critical postoperative healing with minimal tissue reaction followed by predictable absorption. This is also available as coated Vicryl*. Available in size 4-0 through 10-0 and coated 4-0 through 8-0.

It is interesting to note that the absorption of sutures may be considered to occur in two distinct phases. After the suture is implanted, the tensile strength diminishes during the early postoperative period. After most of the strength is lost, the remaining suture mass, which is still present, begins to decrease in what may be termed the second phase of absorption. The mass loss phase then proceeds until the entire suture has been absorbed.

Non-Absorbable:

Monofilament Nylon Sutures (Ethilon*, Dermalon Supramid*) high tensile strength and minimal tissue reaction. Nylon has been reported to lose tensile strength post-operatively at a rate of approximately 15% per year. Available in sizes 8-0 through 14-0.

Polypropylene Suture (Prolene*)—monofilament suture with high tensile strength and minimal tissue reaction. Sutures are not degraded or weakened by tissue enzymes. Available in sizes 5-0 and 9-0 and 11-0.

Black Braided Silk Suture—braided under controlled conditions to maximize strength and assure resistance to breaking during knot tying. Gums and other impurities are removed, resulting in a suture that remains tightly braided with virtually no loose filaments and minimal tendency to broom. Available in sizes 4-0 and 6-0 through 9-0.

Virgin Silk—twisted with the individual silk filaments still embedded in the natural sericin coating, providing a smooth, uniform suture in very fine sizes. They are offered in black and white for selection of optimum contrast with tissues. Available in sizes 8-0 and 9-0.

Polyester Fiber Sutures (Mersilene*, Ti Cron*)—exhibit minimal tissue reaction and are braided by a special method for tightness, uniformity and a smooth surface that minimizes trauma. Available in sizes 4-0 through 6-0.

A variety of physical characteristics of different sutures has been published. In addition, the United States Pharmacopeia has established specifications for various suture materials. Some of the useful parameters measured have been: l) tensile strength, 2) elasticity; 3) suture diameters; 4) weight per unit length. Data is summarized in Tables 24-26.

REFERENCES:

1. Middleton, D. G. and McCulloch, C.: An enquiry into characteristics of sutures, particularly fine sutures. *Adv. Ophthal.* 22:35, 1970

*Trademark

TABLE 25

ELASTICITY OF SUTURES*

SUTURE MATERIAL	ELONGATION OF A STANDARD 30.5 CM SEGMENT IN CM.	INCREASE IN LENGTH %—WEIGHT AT BREAKING POINT (GM)
6-0 plain gut	4.7 cm	15.4%—264
6-0 chromic gut	4.3 cm	14.1%—257
6-0 mersilene	1.9 cm	6.3%—254
6-0 braided silk	1.2 cm	3.9%—237
7-0 chromic gut	3.6 cm	1.8%—118
7-0 braided silk	0.9 cm	3.0%—126
8-0 virgin silk	0.8 cm	2.6%— 53
10-0 nylon	8.7 cm	28.5%— 23

*From Middleton and McCulloch. *Adv. Ophthal.* 22:35, 1970.

TABLE 26

WEIGHT OF SUTURE MATERIAL PER UNIT LENGTH MG/CM

SUTURE MATERIAL	WEIGHT /LENGTH
6-0 plain gut (wet)	0.170 mg/cm
6-0 chromic gut (wet)	0.176 mg/cm
6-0 mersilene	0.116 mg/cm
6-0 braided silk	0.165 mg/cm
7-0 chromic gut (wet)	0.062 mg/cm
7-0 braided silk	0.065 mg/cm
8-0 virgin silk	0.025 mg/cm
10-0 nylon	0.007 mg/cm

SECTION 4

OPHTHALMIC LENSES

by Arthur Gold, M.D.

The processes, the materials used in producing ophthalmic lenses are changing. Glass still is in use but there is an ever-increasing shift toward the use of plastics, particularly the CR39, the polycarbonates, and high-index plastic.

Scratch resistant coatings have been developed by manufacturers for the CR39 and polycarbonate lenses. Anti-reflection coatings have also been developed.

Many lenses will provide UV blocking protection ranging from 395 to 400nm. Some tints that may be applied to existing spectacle lenses in order to provide UV protection are also being presented.

1.80 index glass and similar high index plastic will provide lenses of lighter weight, reduced thickness, be tintable and greatly impact resistant.

CR39 Aphakic lens corrections will provide wider fields, reduced magnification, and be much thinner.

Polarized glass and plastic lenses are becoming available in single vision, multifocal and progressive lens form. Progressive lens designs are being modified to reduce distortions and provide wider progressive corridots.

Though glass will still be available for some time, the use of plastics is expected to increase. As these new products become available new efficiency will be added to the filled prescription.

1. ABSORPTIVE AND TINTED LENSES

These lenses provide protection against radiation, generally against an excess of light or, preferentially, against harmful wave lengths in the long and short wave bands of spectrum. A variety of absorptive and tinted lenses are available and **Tables 27-28** summarize the types and functions of some of them.

TABLE 27

ABSORPTIVE AND TINTED LENSES
(AFTER BORISH AND MANUFACTURER'S DATA)

TYPE (TRANSMISSION)	PURPOSE
1. Ordinary Tint lighter shades—	Cosmetic, slight reduction in light intensity
2. Sunglasses	
a. Neutral Gray (20%-30%)—	Reduce intensity of light (designed to transmit the spectrum non-selectively, i.e. without altering the relative proportions of the various wave lengths.)
b. Colored Green (30%-70%)—	Transmission curve follows sensitivity curve of the eye: absorbs most of ultraviolet and nearly all of the infrared in heat producing range.
c. Yellow (77%)—	Minimize haze, no effect on glare. Filter out blue light. Absorbs ultraviolet. No effect on infrareds.
d. Brown Polaroid™ (21%)—	Absorbs blue light. Transmission of plane polarized light.
e. Photochromic—	Change density by decomposition of a silver halide crystal in the presence of ultraviolet or deep ultraviolet light.
3. Anti-reflecting (approx. 6%)—	Increase transmission
4. Special use lenses	
a. Ultraviolet absorption—	Almost all glass absorptive lenses absorb strongly in the ultraviolet. (Neutral gray and green absorb strongly throughout the spectrum and in the ultraviolet)
b. Infrared absorption—	Relatively few glass absorptive lenses are good absorbers of infrared radiation alone. (Green absorbs large amounts of visible and infrared)
c. Laser Protection—	Didymium
d. X-ray protection—	Radiglasses™ offer significant protection to the eye lens of the physician, technologist, and other personnel against direct and scattered radiation during the use of X-ray equipment. Shielding is equivalent to 0.25 mm of lead, and provides radiation dose reduction up to 90%. Optically clear optional side-shields provide protection from scatter radiation without restricting peripheral vision. Range of available foci: Plano to + and -8.00 +0.25 to +8.00 ≈ -0.25 to -5.00 Cyl. –0.25 to -8.00 ≈ -0.25 to -5.00 Cyl. Bifocals (Flat-Top), (laminated), 22 mm. seg. Additions to 4.00

Foci beyond standard range may be obtained by inquiry from Nuclear Associates, Carle Place, NY 11514

TABLE 28

INDUSTRIAL USES

SHADE NUMBER	USE	LUMINOUS TRANSMITTANCE	MAXIMUM INFRARED	MAXIMUM ULTRAVIOLET (% AT 365 NM)
14	Carbon arc welding, furnace operation	0.00027	0.3	0.05
12	Metallic electric arc welding over 250 amps	0.0019	0.5	0.5
10	Metal arc welding 75-250 amps	0.0139	0.6	0.1
8	Heavy acetylene cutting and welding	0.1	1.0	0.1
6	Acetylene welding, Electrical welding, fire-box observation	0.72	1.5	0.1
5	Acetylene buming, brazing, cutting	1.93	2.5	0.2
3	Light brazing	13.9	9.0	0.5

Adapted from Borish I.M. clinical Refraction 3rd ed. The Professional Press, 1970, p. 1123.

2. MULTIFOCAL LENSES

TABLE 29

MULTIFOCAL LENSES, PRINCIPAL TYPES

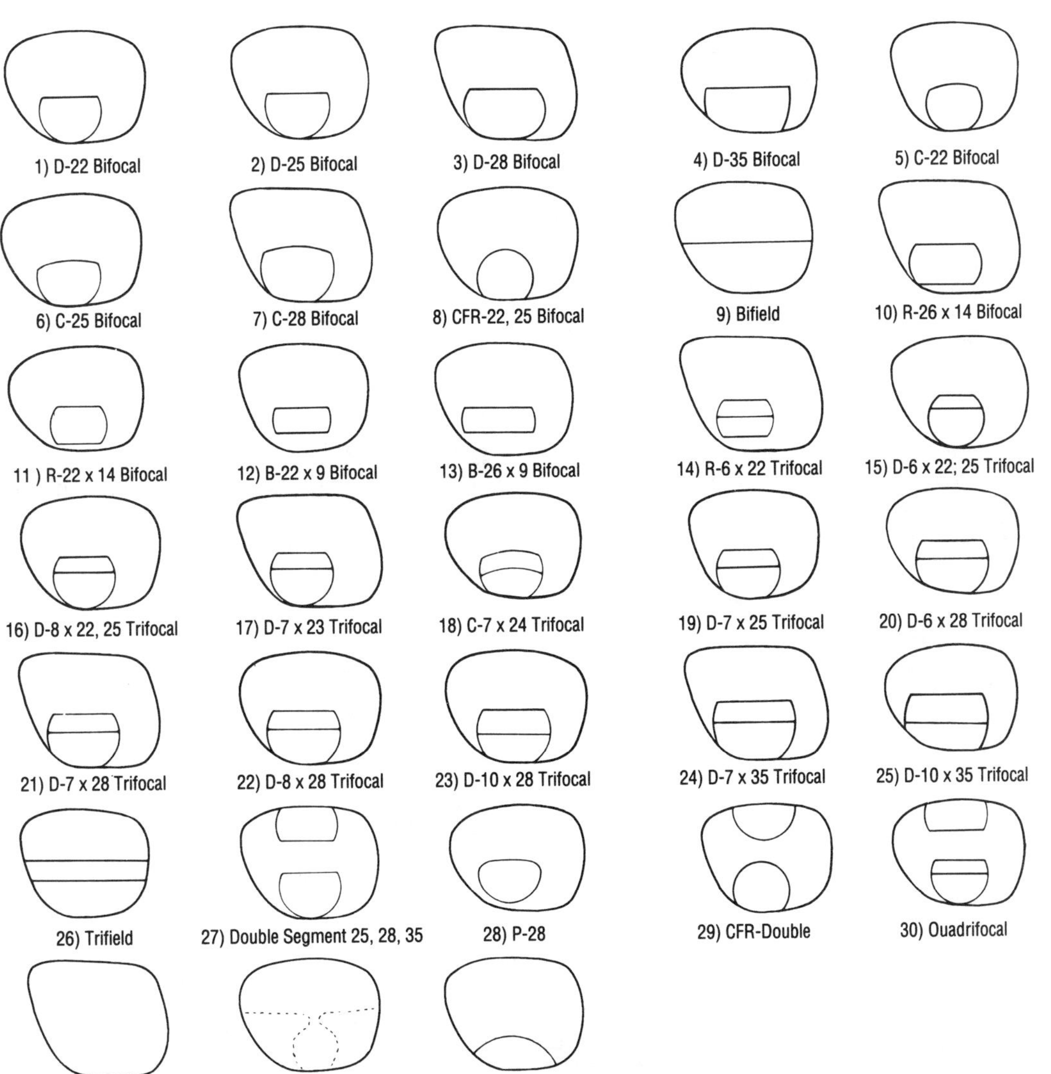

3. NON-VISIBLE SEGMENT LENSES

NON-VISIBLE MULTIFOCALS

Non-visible multifocals are made in bifocal form, providing both distance and near powers, and in progressive power lenses providing distance, intermediate and near corrections. One of the reasons for prescribing these lenses is cosmetic. Many patients object to the visible segment and dividing line of the bifocals, the several segment areas and dividing lines of the trifocals. Improved optics are not always obtained along with improved appearance.

The bifocals have a blend area surrounding the reading area which reduces the area of clear vision and can be apparent to the patient in use. The progressive power lenses have, in most cases, a distance prescription area, a progressive power corridor, and a reading area roughly resembling the round seg bifocal. To either side of the corridor and reading areas varying amounts of astigmatism can cause distortions. Through new design, the corridor effect and peripheral distortions have, according to the manufacturer of the Varilux 2®, been minimized.

Non-visible bifocals are fitted in the manner of ordinary bifocals. The progressive power lenses require extreme care in fitting. Pupillary distance measurements must be precise in both the horizontal and vertical meridians. Rx must be fitted as close as possible with proper pantascopic tilt. The range of available foci for non-visible bifocals and progressive power lenses is generally less than that of the standard multifocals.

Advantages of Progressive Power Lenses

Clear vision at all distances without abrupt power changes; absence of visible segment lines.

Disadvantages of Progressive Power Lenses

Optical aberrations; Rx limitations; fitting difficulties.

Contraindications

Patient cannot turn eye properly; convergence difficulty; cannot be fully corrected; occupation requiring unusually wide field of vision. Non-Visible Bifocals Distance portion similar to standard bifocals. Round reading area diminished by blend area (cross-hatched area of diagrams).

E-Z 2 Vue Invisible Bifocal® (Coburn Optical)
Plastic
+0.25 to +4.00 ≈ -0.25 to -4.00 Cyl.
-0.25 to -5.00 ≈ -0.25 to -3.00 Cyl

Additions +0.75 to +3.00 in 0.25 Diopter steps,
Reading area 25 mm., blend area 1.5 mm.

Super Blend (Silor Optical)
Plastic
Plano to + 2.00
Adds + 1.00 to + 2.50

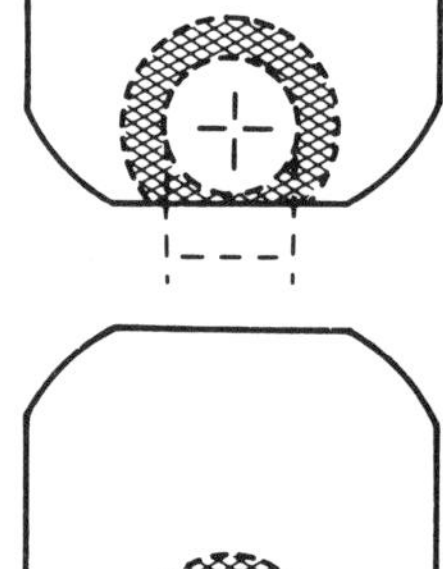

Plano to + 6.00
- 0.25 to - 5.50
Cyl. to -6.00
Adds + 1.00 to + 2.50

Younger Seamless™ (Younger Optics) **Glass**
+0.25 to +7.00 ≈ -0.25 to -4.00 Cyl.
-0.25 to -7.00 ≈ -0.25 to -4.00 Cyl.
Additions + 0.75 to +3.00 in 0.25 Diopter steps
Reading area 22 mm., blend area 3 to 5 mm depending on strength of addition.

Younger Seamless™ (Younger Optics)
Plastic
+ 0.25 to + 10.00 ≈ Full - Cyl. range
– 0.25 to – 7.00 ≈ Full - Cyl. range
Additions + 0.75 to + 3.00 in 0.25 Diopter steps
Reading area 22 mm., blend area 3 to 5 mm depending on strength of addition.

Note: American Optical Company claims to now produce the new Ultravue blended bifocal (adds + 0.50 to + 1.50) which has a 2 mm blend zone and 26% larger reading area than comparable lenses.

Non-Visible Progressive Power Lenses

Non-visible progressive power lenses have a distance Rx zone . A region of increasing power progressing to full reading strength forming either a progressive corridor or intermediate zone. To the periphery of the progressive corridor and the reading areas, areas of astigmatic distortion occur in some types. This is indicated in the cross-hatched areas of the diagrams.

AMERICAN OPTICAL

SEMI-FINISHED

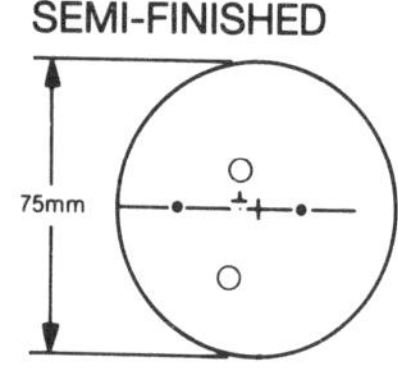

Permalite®
TruVision® Omni

Blank Sizes: 75mm
Base Curves: 4.00D, 6.00D, 8.00D
Segment Placement: Decentered 7.5mm right and left
Additions: 1.00D to 3.00D in 0.25D steps
Material: Scratch-resistant CR-39®

ORCOLITE

SEMI-FINISHED

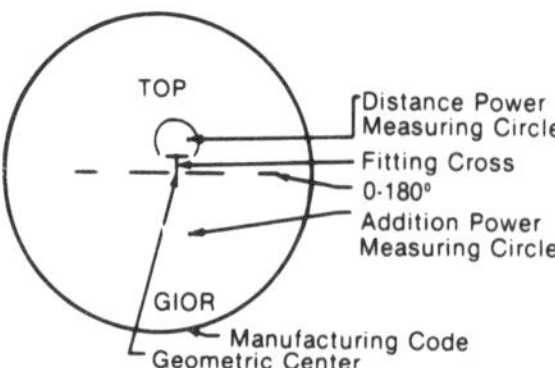

Line Free Progressive

Blank Sizes: 80mm, decentered; 5mm
Base Curves: 4.50D, 6.50D, 8.50D
Center Thickness: 4.50D-12.0mm; 6.50D.-11.00mm, 8.50D-15.00mm
Segment Placement: 12mm down, 5mm in
Additions: 0.75D to 3.00D in 0.25D steps
Colors: Clear
Material: CR-39 with Abrasion Resistant Coating (ARC-901)

SELEX

SEMI-FINISHED

The Affordable

Blank Sizes: 75mm
Base Curves 4.25D 6.25D, 8.25D
Additions: 1.00D to 3.00D in 0.25D steps
Colors: Clear

SILOR

SEMI-FINISHED

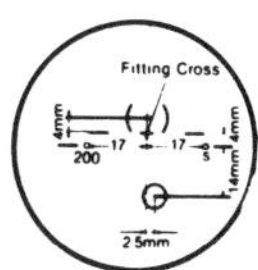

Super No-Line

Photochromic
Blank Sizes: 70/75mm
Base Curves: 5.00D, 6.50D
Additions: 0.75D to 3.50D in 0.25D steps
Material: Clear Glass, Photogray Extra

SILOR

FINISHED/UNCUT

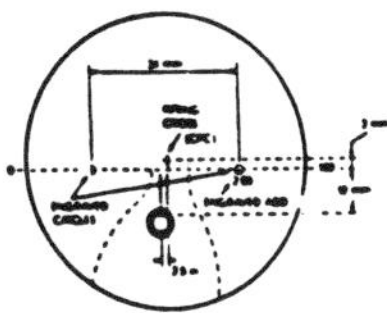

80mm SUPER NO-LINE

Blank Sizes: 80mm
Base Curves: 2.50D, 4.50D, 6.00D. 7.50D, 8.75D
Additions: 0.75D to 3.50D in 0.25D steps; 8.75D Base: 1.00D to 3.00D in 0.25D steps
Material: Hard Resin

SOLA

SEMI-FINISHED

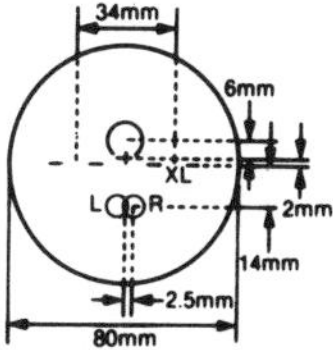

XL w/Perma-Gard™

Blank Sizes: 80mm fully useable
Base Curves: 2.50D, 4.00D, 6.00D 8.00D
Segment Placement: 2.5mm in
Additions: 2.50D: 0.75D to 3.00D in 0.25D steps; 4.00D 6.00D, 8.00D: 0.75D to 3.50D in 0.25D steps
Material: Scratch Resistant, Tintable, Front Side Coated

TITMUS

SEMI-FINISHED

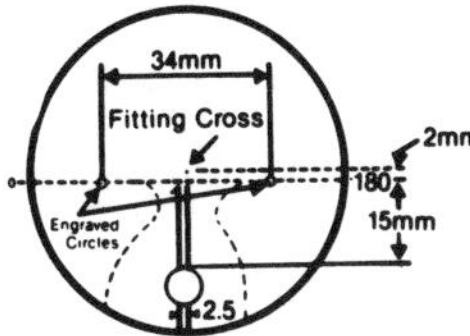

Natural Vue

Blank Sizes: 80mm
Base Curves: 4.00D, 6.00D, 8.00D
Additions: 0.75DD to 3.00D in 0.25D steps
Colors: White, Scratch Coated,
Material: CR-39

VARILUX CORP.

SEMI-FINISHED

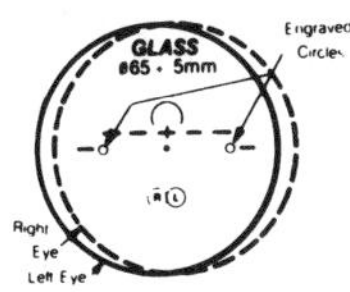

Varilux High Index

Blank Sizes: 65/70mm
Base Curves: 3.00D
Segment Size: Due to aspheric curve design, the entire lower area is usable at varying distances.
Segment Placement: Separate right and left eyes. Near Vision area is inset 2.5mm.
Additions: 1.00D to 3.50D in 0.25D steps
Intermediate Powers: Progressive
Colors: White
Material: High Index Glass, N=1.706

VISION-EASE

SEMI-FINISHED

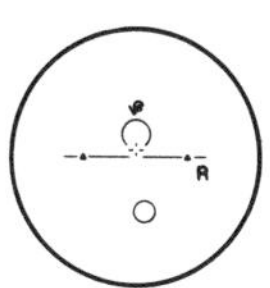

Delta

Blank Sizes: 75mm
Base Curves: 2.75D, 5.25D, 7.25D, 8.25D
Center Thickness: 2.75D: 5.0mm; 5.25D: 5.8mm; 7.25D; 6.8mm
Segment Placement: 2.5mm in
Additions: 0.75D to 3.00D in 0.25D steps, 3.5OD in all but 8.25D base
Colors: White, Photogray Extra
Material: Crown Glass

X-CEL

SEMI-FINISHED

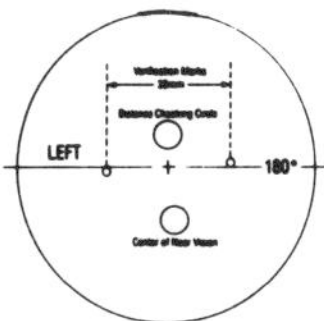

X-Celite Progressive

Blank Sizes: 81mm
Base Curves: 4.50D, 6.00D, 8.00D
Center Thickness: 7.5mm to 12.4mm
Segment Placement: 13mm down, 3.5mm in
Additions: 1.00D to 3.00D in 0.25D steps
Colors: Clear
Material: Hard Resin, Hard Coated

YOUNGER OPTICS

SEMI-FINISHED

C.P.S.

Blank Sizes: 71 mm, 75mm, 80mm
Base Curves: 2.25D, 4.25D, 6.25D, 8.25D; 71mm: 2.25D,10.25D
Additions: 0.75 to 3.00D in 0.25D steps
Colors: Clear, PLS 400, 530, 540, 550
Material: CR-39

Fully spherical distance area; lower portion aspherical vertically and horizontally; 12.5mm transition.

CARL ZEISS

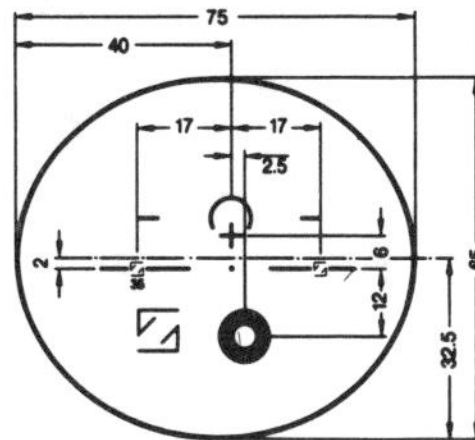

Gradal HS

Blank: 65 mm, 75mm, and 80mm
Base Curves: The Zeiss Punktal Curvature Theory applied
Additions: +.50 to +3.50
Colors: Clear Glass, Photobrown, Photogray, umbra 35, 65, 85%.
Material: High-crown glass, High Index glass, and CR-39.

Non-Visible Progressive Power Lenses continued

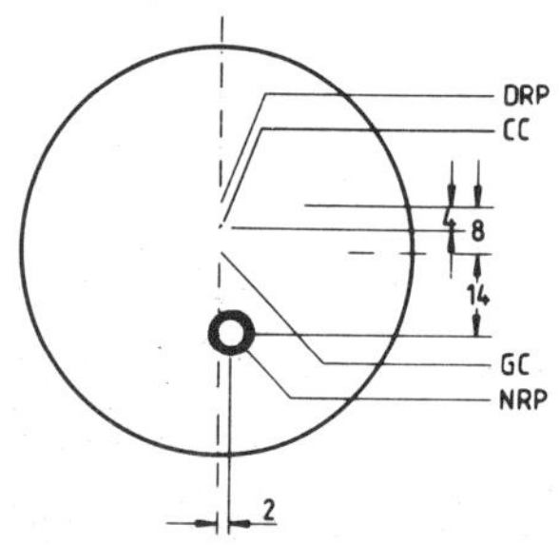

Progressiv R (Rodenstock)

Glass Clear and Photogray Extra (70 74mm blanks)

Base 9.00	+4.75 to +6.00 D
Base 7.00	+3.00 to +4.50 D
Base 5.00	Plano to + 2.75 D
Base 4.00	–0.25 to 4.00 D
Base 2.00	–4.25 to 8.00 D

Cylinder: –0.25 to 4.00 D
Additions: +0.50 to +3.50 D in 0.25 D steps

Hard Resin (plastic) and Hard Resin Duralux (scratch resistant coating) (74, 80mm blanks)

Base 7.00	+3.00 to +6.00 D
Base 5.00	Plano to +2.75 D
Base 4.00	0.25 to –4.00 D
Base 2.00	4.25 to –8.00 D

Cylinder - 0.25 to 4.00 D
Additions +0.50 to +3.50 D in 0.25 D steps (74mm blanks)
+0.50 to +3.00 D in 0.25 D steps (80 mm blanks)

Hard Resin (plastic)
*Photo-reactive Colormatic (brown to gray)
*Photocolor (Aquamarine = blue, Emerald = green, Amethyst = violet shades)

Base 7.00	+3.00 to +6.00 D
Base 5.00	+1.25 to +4.00 D
Base 4.00	+1.00 to –3.00 D
Base 2.00	–3.25 to –5.00 D

Cylinder: –0.25 to 4.00 D
Additions: +1.00 to +3.00 D in 0.25 D steps (74mm - 7 base/80mm - 2, 4, 5 bases)

High visual acuity for distance vision even in the periphery Progressive area that is soft and wide physiologically designed and proven by experience. Stabilized near portion that is extensive and clear. Unimpaired peripheral vision and orientation. Minimized distortion unsurpassed orthoscopy. Excellent adaptation and continuing success.
Cosmolit (Rodenstock)

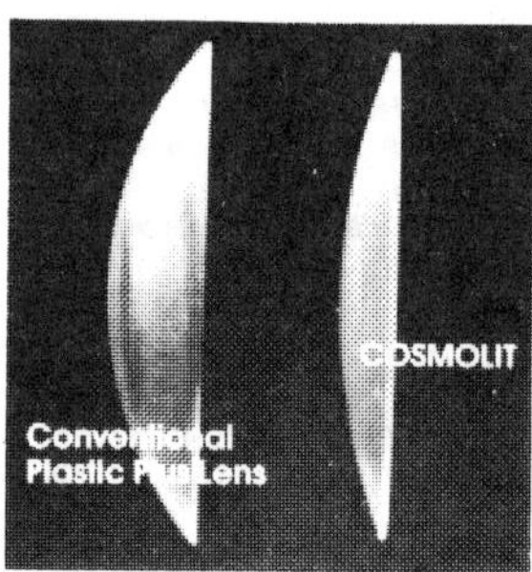

Hard Resin (plastic) Index 1.50
Aspheric single vision for low to moderate hyperopia.

Base 12.5	+11.25 to +12.00 D
Base 12.0	+10.25 to +11.00 D
Base 11.0	+9.25 to +10.00 D
Base 10.0	+8.25 to +9.00 D
Base 9.0	+7.25 to +8.00 D
Base 8.0	+6.25 to +7.00 D
Base 7.0	+5.25 to +6.00 D
Base 6.0	+4.25 to +5.00 D
Base 5.0	+2.25 to +4.00 D
Base 4.0	Plano to +2.00 D

Cylinder –0.25 to 4.00 D (Cylinders over 4.00 D but may limit eye size)

Fully aspheric base curvatures allow for flatter base curves reduced vertex heights reduced lens bulging, less magnification lower peripheral aberration thinner lighter less overall lens mass.

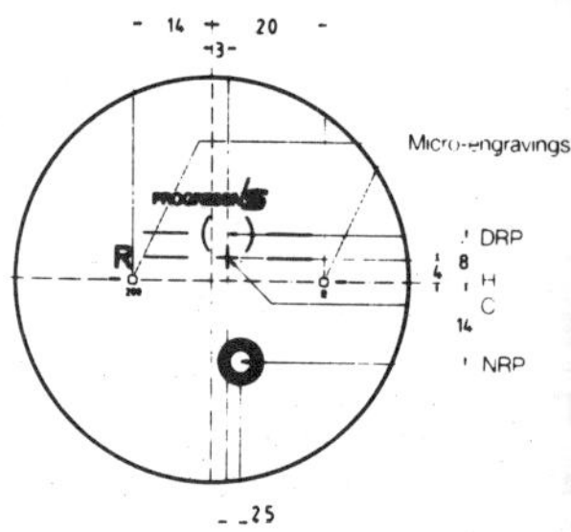

Progressiv S (Rodenstock)

Glass: White Index 1.60, Photogray Extra, Index 1.60

Base 8	+5.75 to +8.00 D	66/70 decentered blank
Base 6	+3.75 to +6.00 D	70/74 decentered blank
Base 5	+1.75 to +3.50 D	70/74 decentered blank
Base 4	–1.00 to +1.50 D	70/74 decentered blank
Base 3	–1.25 to –6.00 D	70/74 decentered blank
Base 2	–4.25 to –10.00 D	66/70 decentered blank

Cylinder: –0.25 to 4.00 D
Additions: +0.50 to 3.50 D in 0.25 D steps

Hard Resin (plastic) and Hard Resin Duralux (scratch resistant coating)

Base 8	+3.75 to +6.00 D	70/76 decentered blank
Base 6	+1.75 to +4.00 D	74/80 decentered blank
Base 5	-1.00 to +1.50 D	74/80 decentered blank
Base 4	-1.25 to -4.00 D	74/80 decentered blank
Base 3	-3.25 to -5.00 D	70/76 decentered blank
Base 2	-5.25 to -8.00 D	70/76 decentered blank

Cylinder: 0.25 to 4.00 D
Additions: +0.50 to 3.50 D in 0.25 D steps

Clear vision over the whole viewing field. Full size of the progressive corridor regardless which fitting method is chosen. Physiologically free of distortion. Unimpaired vision and spatial perception for both eyes. Thinner lighter flatter through built in prism thinning. Wider corridor and reading areas

4. FRESNEL LENSES AND PRISMS

TABLE 30

FRESNEL LENSES AND PRISMS

PRISMS	SEGMENT ADD	SPHERES (PLUS)	SPHERES (MINUS)
0.5Δ	+0.50	+0.50	
1.00Δ	+1.00	+1.00	
1.50Δ	+1.25 to +2.50(a)	+1.25 to +2.50(a)	
2Δ to 10Δ(c)	+3.00 to +4.00(b)	+3.00 to +4.00(b)	–1.00 to –14.00(c)
12Δ	+5.00 to +8.00(c)	+5.00 to +14.00(c)	
15Δ	segs above +3 have	+16.00	
20Δ	incorporated prism	+20.00	
25Δ			
30Δ			

Prism Bars: 1-40Δ Horizontal; 1-25Δ Vertical Prism Trial Set: 12, 15, 20, 25, 30, 35, 40ΔD.
Increments: (a) 0.25, (b) 0.50, (c) 1.00 steps in either prism diopters or lens.

5. SOFT CONTACT LENSES

TABLE 31

Soft contact lenses and lens materials approved by the F.D.A. as of Feb. 1991, as indicated by manufacturers. See **Table 32** for Gas Permeable Contact Lenses.

SPHERICAL DAILY WEAR HYDROGELS

RADE NAME	MANUFACTURER	MATERIAL	%H_2O	THICKNESS[1]	DIAMETERS	BASE CURVES[2]	POWERS
CCUGEL	Strieter	HEMA/PVP	47	.16	13.5,14.0	8.3, 8.6, 8.9	–10 to +10
				.07	13.5,14.0	7.8 to 9.2(.1)	–20 to +20
					13.0	7.6 to 8.6(.2)	+20 to +36
LGES	Miami C.L. Company	HEMA/NVP	45	.11	14.0	8.3, 8.6, 8.9	–20 to +20
L–47	Alden	HEMA	36	.12	12.5 to 14.0	7.7 to 8.9	–20 to +20
MSOF	Lombart Lenses	HEMA/BMA	43	.14	13.5	8.1, 8.4, 8.7	–10 to +5
				.06	13.8	8.3, 8.6, 8.9	–12 to –0.25
OSOFT	CIBA Vision	HEMA/NVP/MMA	42.5	.13	13.2	7.8 to 8.7(.3)[5]	–9.75 to PLANO
QUAFLEX	Wesley–Jessen	HEMA/NVP/MMA	43	.14	13.2	7.9 to 9.1(.3)[6]	–9.75 to PLANO
				.06	13.8	8.2 to 9.1(.3)[6]	–20 to –0.25
				.21	13.8	8.2 to 9.1(.3)[6]	+0.25 to +9.75
QUASIGHT	Lombart Lenses	HEMA/BMA	43	.14	13.5	8.1, 8.4, 8.7	–10 to +5
				.06	13.8	8.3, 8.6, 8.9	–12 to –0.25
ZTECH	Sola/Barnes–Hind	GMA/MMA	38	.05	14.0	8.2, 8.5	–6 to PLANO
IOCURVE	BioCurve Soft Lenses	HEMA	55	.11	14.0	8.4	
					14.5	8.4, 8.6, 8.8, 9.0	–20 to + 10
					15.0	8.9	
					14.0	8.4	+10.50 to +20
					14.5	8.8	
CELUSOFT	Fashion	HEMA	38	.06	14.0	8.4, 8.7, 8 .9	–20 to +20
CIBASOFT[3]	CIBA Vision	HEMA	37.5	.07(.14 for +)	13.8	8.3, 8.6, 8.9	–10 to +6
				.07(.14 for +)	14.5	8.6, 8.9, 9.2	–10 to PLANO
CONTINENTAL	Continental	HEMA	53	varies	13.5 to 15.0	8.2 to 9.8(.2)	–20 to +20
COOPER CLASSIC	CooperVision	HEMA/NVP/MMA	43	.03 to.13	14.0 14.4	8.6, 8.9 8.7	–10 to –0.25 –10 to –0.25
COOPERTHIN	CooperVision	HEMA	38	.06	14.0	8.4	–10 to –0.25
				.06	14.5	8.6	–6.50 to –0.25
CQ.4	Ocular Sciences	HEMA	38	.07	14.5	8.7	–8 to PLANO
CSI	Sola/Barnes–Hind	GMA/MMA	38	.05	13.8	8.0, 8.3, 8.6	–20 to +8
				.05	14.8	8.6, 8.9, 9.35	–20 to PLANO
CTL 38L CLEAR	Sola/Barnes–Hind	HEMA	38	.05	14.0	8.4, 8.7	—8 to +5
EDGE II	OcularSciences	HEMA	38	.10	14.0	8.6	–8 to PLANO
EDGE III	Ocular Sciences	HEMA	38	.10	14.0	8.3, 8.6, 8.9	–8 to PLANO
EDGE III THIN	Ocular Sciences	HEMA	38	.07	14.5	8.4, 8.7, 9.0	–8 to PLANO
EPCON SOFT[4]	Epcon	HEMA	38	.06	14.0	8.4, 8.7, 8.9	–20 to +20
FIRESOFT	FirestoneOptics	HEMA	55	.10 to.12	14.2	8.3, 8.6	–12 to +8
					15.0	8.6, 8.9, 9.2	–20 to +20

Reprinted from *Contact Lens Spectrum,* Feb. 1991, ED: White, P., and Scott, C.

Continued on next page

SPHERICAL DAILY WEAR HYDROGELS continued

TRADE NAME	MANUFACTURER	MATERIAL	%H_2O	THICKNESS[1]	DIAMETERS	BASE CURVES[2]	POWERS
FLEXLENS[4]	Flexlens	HEMA/NVP	45	.11	14.5, 15.0	8.5 to 9.25 (.25)	−10 to +10
				custom	12.5 to 16.5	6.0 to 11.0(.25)	−50 to +50
FRE–FLEX	Optech	HEMA	55	.04 to 1.0	10.0 to 17.5	6.0 to 11.0	−40 to +40
HYDRASOFT	CoastVision	HEMA	55	.12	15.0	8.6, 8.9, 9.2	−20 to +20
				.10	14.2	8.3, 8.6	−12 to +8
HYDROCURVE II	Sola/Barnes–Hind	HEMA/Acrylamide	45	.05	13.5	83, 8.6	−12 to +7
				.05	14.5	8.90	−12 to +7
HYDROMARC	Vistakon	HEMA/MA	43	.12	14.0, 14.5	8.15 to 9.05(.15)	−20 to +20
HYDRON Min	Allergan Optical	HEMA	38	.12 to.52	13.0	8.1 to 8.9(.2)	−20 to +20
Hydron Zero 6				.06(10 for +)	14.0	8.4, 8.7, 9.0	−10 to + 10
Hydron Zero 4				.04	13.8	Steep	−10 to PLANO
Hydron Zero 4 F2				.04	13.8	Flat	−5.25 to PLANO
Hydron Spincast				.07	14.5	Spin Cast	−8 to PLANO
IDEAL SOFT	Ideal Optics	HEMA	38	.08	14.0	8.3, 8.6, 8.9	−20 to +20
KONTUR 55	Kontur Kontact Lens	HEMA	55	.15	15.0	8.3, 8.6, 8.9	+20 to −20
LL-38	Lombart Lenses	HEMA	38	.07	14.5	8.4, 8.7, 9.0	PLANO to −8.00
LL–380	Lombart Lenses	HEMA	38	.10	14.0	8.3, 8.6, 8.9	PLANO to −8.00
LL–55	Lombart Lenses	HEMA	55	.09	14.5	8.4, 8.7	+5.00 to −10.00
LL–550	Lombart Lenses	HEMA	55		14.0	8.3, 8.6, 8.9	+5.00 to −10.00
METROSOFT II	Metro Optics	HEMA	38	.10	13.5	8.3, 8.6, 8.9	−20 to +20
				.06	14.0	8.70	−7 to PLANO
METROSOFT 55	Metro Optics	HEMA	55	.14	14.2	8.4, 8.7, 9.0	−10 to +10
N&N TRESOFT	N&N	HEMA/MA	46	.15	13.5,14.0,14.5	8.2, 8.4, 8.6, 8.8	−20 to +20
				.06	13.7	8.2, 8.5, 8.8	−20 to +20
OCU–FLEX–53	Ocu–Ease	HEMA/MA	53	.12	14.0, 14.5, 15.0	8.2, 8.4, 8.6, 8.8	−25 to +10
OPTIMA 38[3]	Bausch & Lomb	HEMA	38	.06 to.19	14.0	8.4, 8.7	−12 to +5
OTI–05	Ocu–Tec	HEMA	38	.05	14.0	8.4, 8.7	−8 to +5
PROFESSIONAL SERIES	CoastVision	HEMA	55	.10	14.2	8.3, 8.6	−12 to +8
				.12	15.0	8.6, 8.9	−12 to + 8
Q & E	Breger Mueller	HEMA/BMA	43	.06	13.8	8.3, 8.6, 8.9	−12 to PLANO
	Welt			.23	13.5	8.1, 8.4, 8.7	PLANO to +5
SOF–FORM II[4]	Salvatori	HEMA	38	.06	14.0	8.3, 8.5, 8.7, 8.9	−20 to +20
SOF–FORM 67	Salvatori	Xylofilcon A	67.5	0.5 to.08	13.8	8.3, 8.6	−7 to +4
					14.5	8.8	− 7 to + 5
SOFLENS	Bausch & Lomb	HEMA	38	.16	12.5	F	−0.25 to −9.50
				.52	13.5	F3	+6.50 to +20.00
				.26	12.5	N	+0.25 to +18.50
				.12(.55 for +)	13.5	B3	+6.00 to −20.00
				.12(.21 for +)	14.5	B4	+6.00 to −9.00
				.06	13.5	L3	−0.25 to −3.00
				.06	14.5	L4	−0.25 to −3.00
				.07(.12 for +)	13.5	U3	+6.00 to −9.00
				.07(.12 for +)	14.5	U4	+6.00 to −9.00
				.035	13.5	H03	−8.00 to −20.00
				.035	14.5	H04	−8.00 to −20.00
				.52	13.5	H3	+6.50 to +20.00
				.49 to .60	14.5	H4	+6.50 to +20.00

Reprinted from *Contact Lens Spectrum,* Feb. 1991, ED: White, P., and Scott, C.

Continued on next page

SPHERICAL DAILY WEAR HYDROGELS continued

TRADE NAME	MANUFACTURER	MATERIAL	%H_2O	THICKNESS[1]	DIAMETERS	BASE CURVES[2]	POWERS
SOFSPIN	Bausch & Lomb	HEMA	38	.05 to .09	14.0	Spin Cast	–6 to –0.25
SOFTACT II	C.L.Corp.of America	HEMA	38	.06	14.0	8.4, 8.7, 9.0	–20 to +20
SOFTCON	CIBA Vision	HEMA/PVP	55	.17–.32(–)	14.0	7.8, 8.7	–8 to +5
				.32–.64(+)	14.0	8.1, 8.4	–8 to +9.50
					14.5	8.1, 8.4, 8.7	–8 to +9.50
SOFTMATE B	Sola/Barnes–Hind	HEMA/Acryl	45	.07	14.3	8.7	–12 to +7
					14.8	9.0	–12 to +7
SEA VIEW[4]	Miami	HEMA/NVP	45	.10	14.0	8.3	–20 to +20
	C.L. Company				14.5	8.6, 8.9	–20 to +20
SPHEREX	GBF	HEMA	53	.06	13.5, 14.0, 14.5, 15.0	8.4, 8.6, 8.8, 9.2	–12 to + 12
SPORTMATE	Sola/Barnes–Hind	HEMA/Acryl	45	.05	15.5	9.5, 9.8	–12 to +6
				.05	15.5	9.2, 10.1	PLANO to –12
STD CLEAR	CIBA Vision	HEMA	37.5	.10(.17 for +)	13.8	8.3, 8.6, 8.9	–6 to +6
SUNFLEX	Sunsoft	HEMA	55	.10	14.0	8.3, 8.6, 8.9	10 to +5
					15.0	8.3, 8.6, 8.9	–20 to + 10
TECHNICON DW	Westcon	HEMA	55	.08 to.60	14.0,14.5	8.3	–20 to +20
					14.5, 15.0	8.6	
					15.0	8.9	
UCL 55%	United	HEMA	55	.12	14.0, 14.5	8.3	–20 to +20
					14.0, 14.5, 15.0	8.6	–20 to +20
					14.5, 15.0		–20 to +20
ULTRAFLEX	Ocular Sciences	HEMA	38	0.10	14.0	8.3, 8.6, 8.9	–8 to PLANO
ULTRAFLEX THIN	Ocular Sciences	HEMA	38	0.07	14.5	8.4, 8.7, 8.9	–8 to PLANO

(1) Center thickness for low minus power. (2) Increments in parentheses. (3) Available in blue visibility tint.
(4) Also can be custom designed. (5) Vaults 4 to 1. (6) Vaults 4 to 0. Editor's note: thickness. diameters, and base curves are in mm.

TINTED DAILY WEAR HYDROGELS

TRADE NAME	MANUFACTURER	MATERIAL	%H_2O	THICKNESS[1]	DIAMETERS	BASE CURVES[2]	POWERS
COMPLEMENTS	Wesley–Jessen	HEMA/MMA blue, brown, green, gray	55	.05	14.5	8.6	–4 to PLANO
COOPER CLASSIC	CooperVision	HEMA/NVP/MMA light blue visibility tint	43	.03 to.15	14.0	8.3, 8.6	PLANO to +6
					14.0	8.6, 8.9	–10 to –.25
					14.4	8.7	–10 to –.25
					14.7	8.7	PLANO to +6
CSI COLOURS	Sola/Barnes–Hind	GMA/MMA blue, green, violet, aqua	38.6	.05	13.8	8.3, 8.6	–6 to PLANO
CTL–M*	Sola/Barnes–Hind	HEMA blue, brown	38	.05	14.0	8.4, 8.7	
				.07	14.5	Spin Cast	
CTL 38L COSMETIC TINT	Sola/Barnes–Hind	HEMA aquamarine, cocoa, emerald, lavender, sapphire, topaz	38	.05	14.0	8.4, 8.7	–8 to +5

Reprinted from *Contact Lens Spectrum,* Feb. 1991, ED: White, P., and Scott, C.

Continued on next page

TINTED DAILY WEAR HYDROGELS continued

TRADE NAME	MANUFACTURER	MATERIAL	%H_2O	THICKNESS(1)	DIAMETERS	BASE CURVES(2)	POWERS
DURASOFT 2 COLORS	Wesley–Jessen	HEMA/MMA sky blue, jade green, aquamarine violet–blue	38	.05 .07	14.5 14.5	8.6 8.3 9.0	–8 to +4 –4 to PLANO
DURASOFT 2 LITE TINT (D2LT)	Wesley–Jessen	HEMA/MMA	38	.07 .07	13.8 14.5	8.0, 8.3,8 .6 8.3, 8.6, 9.0	–8 to +6 –8 to +6
DURASOFT 3 COLORS	Wesley–Jessen	HEMA/MMA baby blue opaque, aqua opaque, sapphire blue opaque, hazel opaque, jade green opaque, misty gray opaque, violet opaque, chestnut brown opaque, baby blue enhance	55	.05	14.5	8.3, 8.6 9.0 8.6 8.6	–8 to +6 –4 to PLANO –4 to PLANO –8 to + 6
EDGE II TINTS	Ocular Sciences	HEMA blue, green, aqua	38	.10	14.0	8.6	–6 to PLANO
HYDRON SOFBLUE	Allergan Optical	HEMA light blue visibility tint	38	.04 .06 .10	13.8 14.0 14.0 14.0	8.6 8.4, 8.7, 9.0 8.4, 9.0 8.7	–10 to PLANO –10 to PLANO PLANO to +6 PLANO to +10
METROLITE	Metro Optics	HEMA light blue	38	.10 .06	13.5 14.0	8.6 8.7	–20 to +20 –7 to PLANO
METROTINT	Metro Optics	HEMA blue, aqua, green	38	.06 .10	14.0 13.5	8.7 8.3, 8.6, 8.9	–7 to PLANO –20 to +20
MYSTIQUE OPAQUE	CooperVision	HEMA sapphire blue, crystal blue, jade green, willow green	38	.06	14.2	8.4, 8.7	–6 to PLANO
NARCISSUS	Narcissus Eye Research Foundation	Custom–Designed prosthetic masking lenses	ordering information upon request to manufacturer				
NATURAL TINT	Bausch & Lomb	HEMA aqua, blue, green, brown	38	.07	B3, U3, U4	Spin Cast	–6 to PLANO
OPTIMA	Bausch & Lomb	HEMA aqua, blue, green	38	.06	14.0	SAG I, SAG II	–9 to +5
PERMAFLEX THIN COLOR COLLECTION	CooperVision	HEMA/NVP/MMA sky blue, violet blue, spring green, turquoise	43	.035	13.8 14.4	8.4 8 9	–6 to PLANO – 6 to PLANO
SOFTCOLORS	CIBA Vision	HEMA aqua, blue, green, amber, royal blue, evergreen	37.5	.07(.14 for +)	13.8 14.5	8.3, 8.6, 8.9 8.6, 8.9, 9.2	–10 to +6 –10 to PLANO
			(Cibathin, TORISOFT, and STD parameters are available in tints)				
SOFTMATES LOCATOR TINT	Sola/Barnes–Hind	HEMA–light blue visibility tint	45	.07 .07	14.3 14.8	8.7 9.0	–4 to +4 –6 to +6
STD SOFTCOLORS	CIBA Vision	HEMA aqua, royal blue, evergreen	37.5	.10(.17 for +)	13.8	8.3, 8.6, 8.9	–6 to +6
STD VISITINT	CIBA Vision	HEMA light blue visibility tint	37.5	.10(.17 for +)	13.8	8.3, 8.6, 8.9	–6 to +6

Reprinted from *Contact Lens Spectrum*, Feb. 1991, ED: White, P., and Scott, C.

Continued on next page

TINTED DAILY WEAR HYDROGELS continued

TRADE NAME	MANUFACTURER	MATERIAL	%H_2O	THICKNESS[1]	DIAMETERS	BASE CURVES[2]	POWERS
*RESOFT LIGHT	N&N	HEMA/MA blue handling tint	46	.09	13.7	8.2, 8.5, 8.8	–6 to PLANO
*RESOFT COLORS	N&N	HEMA/MA–ice blue, Atlantic green, steel blue	46	.09	13.7	8.2, 8.5, 8.8	–6 to PLANO
*ANTAGE	CooperVision	HEMA/NVP/MMA light blue visibility tint	43	.03 to.15	14.0 14.4 14.0	8.3, 8.6, 8.9 8.7 8.3, 8.6	–10 to –0.25 –10 to +6 +.25 to +6
VANTAGE ACCENTS ENHANCEMENT TINTS	CooperVision	HEMA/NVP/MMA sky blue, violet blue, spring green, turquoise, auburn, misty brown	43	.035	14.0 14.7	8.3, 8.6, 8.9 8.7	–6.50 to PLANO – 6.50 to PLANO
VISITINT	CIBA Vision	HEMA - light blue visibility tint	37.5	.07(.14 for +)	13.8 14.5	8.3, 8.6, 8.9 8.6, 8.9, 9.2	–10 to +6 –10 to PLANO

*Ocular masking prosthetic tint.

(1) Center thickness for low minus power.

TORIC DAILY WEAR HYDROGELS

TRADE NAME	COMPANY	MATERIAL	%H_2O	DIAMETERS	BASE CURVES	SPHERES	CYLINDER[1]	AXIS	BALLAST
ACCUGEL TORIC[4]	Strieter	HEMA/PVP	47	14.0	7.8 to 9.9(.1)	–30 to +30	–.75 to –10.00[2]	Any; 5° Steps	Prism/ Slab–off
BIOCURVE TORIC[4]	BioCurve Soft Lenses	HEMA	55	14.0,14.5	8.4, 8.6, 8.8, 9.0	–20 to +10	–.75 to –5.00[2]	Any	Prism
CONTINENTAL TORIC	Continental	HEMA	53	13.5 to 15.0	8.2 to 9.8(.1)	–20 to +20	–.50 to –10.00[2]	Any	Prism
DURASOFT 2 OPTIFIT TORIC	Wesley–Jessen	HEMA/MMA	38	14.5	8.6	–12 to +4	–0.75 to –3.75[2]	Any	Pris Thin Zones
DURASOFT 3 OPTIFIT TORIC	Wesley–Jessen	HEMA/MMA	55	14.5	8.6	–8 to +4	–.75 to –2.25[3]	180° (±20°) 90° (±20°)	Prism/ Thin Zones
DURASOFT 3 TORIC	Wesley–Jessen	HEMA/MMA	55	14.5	8.3, 8.6	–8 to +4	–.75 to –2.00[3]	180° (±30°) 90° (±30°)	Periballast Truncation, Prism; Inf. Slab–off
DURASOFT 3 TORIC COLORS	Wesley–Jessen	HEMA/MMA opaques: baby blue, emerald green, aqua, hazel	55	14.5	8.6	PLANO to –4	–1.00 to –2.00[3]	180±20° 90 + 20°	Periballast, Truncation Prism; Inf. Slab–off
ECLIPSE	Sunsoft	HEMA	55	14.5		–6 to +2	–.75 to –2.00[2]	180° (±25°) 90° (±25°)	Prism Eccentric Lenticulation
FIRESOFT TORIC	Firestone Optics	HEMA	55	15.0	8.6, 8.9, 9.2	–12 to +6	–.75 to –10.00[2]	Any	Prism
FRE–FLEX TORIC	Optech	HEMA	55	10.0 to 17.5	6.0 to 11.0	–30 to +30	Up to –16.00[2]	Any	Prism Slab–off
HYDRASOFT[4)]	CoastVision	HEMA	55	14.2 15.0	8.3, 8.6 8.3, 8.6, 8.9, 9.2	+10 to –20	–.75 to –10.00[2]	Any	Prism, Eccentric Lenticulation
HYDRASOFT APHAKIC TORIC	CoastVision	HEMA	55	15.0	8.6, 8.9	+10 to +20	–.75 to –10.00[2]	Any	Prism, Eccentric Lenticulation

Reprinted from *Contact Lens Spectrum,* Feb. 1991, ED: White, P., and Scott, C.

Continued on next page

TORIC DAILY WEAR HYDROGELS continued

TRADE NAME	COMPANY	MATERIAL	%H_2O	DIAMETERS	BASE CURVES	SPHERES	CYLINDER[1]	AXIS	BALLAST
HYDROCURVE II TORIC	Sola/Barnes–Hind	HEMA/Acryl.	45	13.5	8.6	–6.25 to +3	–1.25, –2.00[2]	90°(±25°) 180°(±25°)	Prism
				14.5	8.9	–8 to +3	–1.25 to –2.00[2]	Full circle in 5° steps	
				14.5	8.9	– 6 to PLANO	– .75[2]	180°(±25°) 90°(±25°)	
HYDROMARC TORIC	Vistakon	HEMA/MA	43	14.5	8.4, 8.75, 9.05 (Series 1, 2, 3)	–5 to +4	–.75 to 2.00[3]	180°(+20°) 90°(+20°)	Prism; Slab–off
HYDRON CUSTOM TORIC[4]	Allergan Optical	HEMA	38	13.0, 13.5, 4.0, 14.5, 15.0	7.2–9.3	–20 to +20	–.50 to –6.00[3]	Any	Truncation Prism
HYDRON ULTRA T	Allergan Optical	HEMA	43	14.5	Spincast	–6 to PLANO	–1.00, –1.50, – 2.00[3]	Any; 10° steps	Prism
KONTUR 55 TORIC[4]	Kontur Kontact Lens	HEMA	55	15.0	8.6, 8.9	+10 to –20	–.75 to–5.00[2]	Any	Prism Eccentric Lenticulation
METROSOFT TORIC	Metro Optics	HEMA	38	14.0	8.7	–5 to –.25	–.75 to –3.00[3]	Any	Prism
OCU–FLEX–53	Ocu–Ease	HEMA/MA	53	13.5, 14.0, 14.5, 15.0	8.2 to 9.0(.2)	–20 to +20	Up to –4.50[2]	Any	Prism
OPTIMA TORIC	Bausch & Lomb	HEMA/NVP	45	14.0	8.3, 8.6, 8.9	–6 to +4	–.75, –1.25, –1.75[3]	Full circle in 10° steps	Prism
		Made–to–Order	45	14.0	8.3, 8.6, 8.9	+6.00 to – 7.00	–0.75,–1.25 – 1.75, – 2.25, – 2.75[3]	Full circle in 5° steps	Prism
PROFESSIONAL SERIES	CoastVision	HEMA	55	14.2	8.3, 8.6	–20 to +10	–.75 to –10.00	Any	Prism, Eccentric Lenticulation
				15.0	8.3, 8.6, 8.9, 9.2	– 20 to + 10	– .75 to –10.00	Any	
SIGNATURE	Sola/ Barnes–Hind	HEMA	55	14.5	8.9	–6 to PLANO	–1.00, –1.75	180°(±30°) 90°(± 30°)	Prism
SOF–FORM II TORIC	Salvatori	HEMA	55	14.0, 14.5, 15.0	8.6, 8.9. 9.2	–20 to +10	–.75 to –5[2]	Any	Prism
SUNSOFT[4] TORIC 15.0	Sunsoft	HEMA	55	15.0	8.3, 8.9	–20 to +10	– .75 to –7.00[2]	Any	Prism: Eccentric Lenticulation
TECHNICON TORIC	Westcon	HEMA	55	14.0, 14.5, 15.0	8.3, 8.6, 8.9	–10 to +10	– .75 to –5.00[2]	Any	Prism Eccentric Lenticulation
TOREX	GBF	HEMA	53	14.0 14.5 15.0	8.4, 8.6, 8.8, 9.2	–12 to +12	–.50 to –4.75[2]	Any; 5° Steps	Double Slab–off Periballast
TORISOFT CLEAR/ TORISOFT SOFTCOLORS (Special Order)	CIBA Vision	HEMA aqua, blue, royal blue, green, amber, evergreen	37.5	14.5	8.6, 8.9	–7 to +4	–1, –1.75[3]	0°±80°	Thin zones Double Slab–on
					9.2	–7 to PLANO	–1, –1.75[3]	180°±20° 90°±20° in 10° steps	Thin zones Double Slab–off
TRESOFT TORIC[4]	N&N	HEMA/MA	46	14.0, 14.5	8.8	–6 to +5	– .75 to – 3[2]	180°±20° 90° ± 20°	Prism Slab–off
UCL TORIC 55%[4]	United Contact Lens	HEMA	55	15.0	8.6, 8.9	+10 to –10	Any	Any	Prism Slab–off

Reprinted from *Contact Lens Spectrum,* Feb. 1991, ED: White, P., and Scott, C.

Continued on next page

TORIC DAILY WEAR HYDROGELS continued

TRADE NAME	COMPANY	MATERIAL	%H_2O	DIAMETERS	BASE CURVES	SPHERES	CYLINDER[1]	AXIS	BALLAST
ULTRA T	Allergan	HEMA	43	14.5	Varies with power	–6 to PLANO	1,1.50,2[3]	Any 10° steps	Prism Slab–off

(1) All lenses, whether manufactured with front surface toric or back surface toric, are listed in minus cylinder form, as that is how the lenses are ordered. However, we have also indicated by footnotes how they are manufactured.

(2) Manufactured with back toric.
(3) Manufactured with front toric.
(4) Custom designs available.

MULTI DAILY WEAR HYDROGELS

TRADE NAME	COMPANY	MATERIAL	%H_2O	DIAMETERS	BASE CURVES	POWERS	ADDS	DESIGN
ALGES BIFOCAL	Miami Contact Lens Company	HEMA/NVP	45	14.0	8.6, 8.9	–6 to +6	+1.50 to +3.50 (2.12, 2.35, 2.55, 3.00, 3.50 seg diameters)	concentric central near add
BI–TECH[1]	Bausch & Lomb	HEMA	38	14.5	SAG I, SAG II	–6 to +6	+2.00, +2.50 seg heights 4.75 and 5.25 mm	translating periballast
BI–SOFT	CIBAVision	HEMA	37.5	13.8	8.3, 8.6 8.9 only in +	–6 to +6	+1.50 to +3.00 in .50D steps	concentric simultaneous vision
FULFOCUS	CL Corp. of America	HEMA	38	14.2	8.7	–6 to +5	Progressive to +3.00	front aspheric[3]
HYDROCURVE II BIFOCAL	Sola/Barnes–Hind	HEMA/Acrylic Acid	45	14.8	9.0 Aspheric	–6 to +4	Progressive +1.50 to +3.00 at OZ Periphery	back aspheric central distance
HYDRON ECHELON BIFOCAL	Allergan Optical	HEMA	38	13.8	8.7	–6 to +4	+1.50, +2.00 +2.50	diffraction
PA–I[2]	Bausch & Lomb	HEMA	38	13.5	Aspheric (8.6, nominal)	–6 to +6	+1.50 (nominal)	back aspheric[3] central distanc
PS–45 MULTIFOCAL	Product Develop. Corp.	HEMA	38	14.0	8.7	–3 to +6	+2.00	front aspheric[3] central near
SOF•TOUCH MULTIFOCAL	N&N	HEMA	55	14.8	8.6, 8.9	–6 to +4	Progressive to +3.00	back aspheric[3] central distance
SYNSOFT	Salvatori/Vision–Ease	HEMA	38	13.5, 14.0	8.4, 8.7, 8.9	–6 to +4	+1.50 to +3.50	translating periballast
UNILENS	Unilens	HEMA/NVP	45	14.0, 14.5	8.7, 9.0, 9.3	–4 to +6	to +2.50	front aspheric[3] central near
V/X	GBF	HEMA	38	14.0, 14.3	8.2	±20	to +4.00	back aspheric central distance

(1) Available in blue visibility tint. (2) Available in blue, green, and aqua cosmetic tints. (3) With aspherics there is a progressive power change.

SPHERICAL COSMETIC EXTENDED WEAR HYDROGELS

TRADE NAME	MANUFACTURER	MATERIAL	%H_2O	DIAMETERS	BASE CURVES[2]	POWERS
B&L 70	Bausch & Lomb	MMA/NVP	70	14.3	8.4, 8.7, 9.0	–6 to +6
CIBATHIN	CIBA Vision	HEMA	37.5	13.8	8.6, 8.9	–6 to PLANO
CSI–T	Sola/Barnes–Hind	GMA/MMA	38	13.8	8.0 to 8.9(.3)	–10 to PLANO
				14.8	8.6, 8.9, 9.3	–7 to PLANO
DURASOFT 3	Wesley–Jessen	HEMA	55	13.5	8.2,.8.5	–6 to +6
				14.5	8.3, 8.6, 9.0	–20 to +20
EDGE III 55	Ocular Sciences	HEMA	55	14.0	8.3, 8.6, 8.9	–10 to + 5
				14.5	8.4, 8.7	–10 to +5

Reprinted from *Contact Lens Spectrum*, Feb. 1991, ED: White, P., and Scott, C.

Continued on next page

SPHERICAL COSMETIC EXTENDED WEAR HYDROGELS con tinued

TRADE NAME	MANUFACTURER	MATERIAL	%H_2O	DIAMETERS	BASE CURVES[2]	POWERS
FIRESOFT EW	Firestone Optics	HEMA	55	14.2	8.3, 8.6	–12 to +8
				15.0	8.6, 8.9, 9.2	–20 to +10
GENESIS 4	Lombart Lenses	MMA/NVP	70	14.3	8.4, 8.7, 9.0	–12 to +8
HYDRASOFT XW	CoastVision	HEMA	55	14.2	8.3, 8.6	–12 to +8
				15.0	8.6, 8.9, 9.2	–20 to +10
HYDROCURVE II 55	Sola/Barnes–Hind	HEMA/Acrylamide	55	14.0	8.50	–12 to +7
				14.5	8.8, 9.1	–12 to +7
HYDRON ZERO 4 SOFBLUE	Allergan Optical	HEMA	38	13.8	8.6	–10 to PLANO
HYDRON ZERO 4F	Allergan Optical	HEMA	38	13.8	8.8	–5.25 to PLANO
KONTUR 55 EW	Kontur Kontact Lens	HEMA	55	15.0	8.3, 8.6, 8.9	+10 to –20
N&N 70	N&N	MMA/NVP	70	14.3	8.4, 8.7, 9.0	–12 to +8
OPTIMA EW–FW	Bausch & Lomb	HEMA	38	14.0	8.7	–9 to +4
PERMALENS	CooperVision	HEMA/NVP/MMA	71	13.5	7.7, 8.0, 8.3	–20 to –0.25
				14.0	8.0, 8.3, 8.6	+8 to +0.25
				14.2	8.6	–10 to – 0.25
				14.5	8.3	–10 to–0.25
PERMAFLEX THIN	CooperVision	HEMA/NVP/MMA	43	13.8	8.4	–9.75 to PLANO
				14.4	8.9	
PERMAFLEX NATURALS	CooperVision	MMA/PVP	74	14.4	8.7	–10 to –0.25 + 6 to + 0.50
				14.4	8.9	–6 to –1
PERMAFLEX UV NATURALS	CooperVision	MMA/PVP	74	14.4	8.7	–10 to –0.25 +6 to + 0.50
PROFESSIONAL SERIES	CoastVision	HEMA	55	14.2	8.3, 8.6	–12 to +8
				15.0	8.6, 8.9	–12 to +8
Q&E 70	Breger Mueller Welt	MMA/NVP	70	14.3	8.4, 8.7, 9.0	–12 to +8
RYNCOSOFT	Rynco	MMA/NVP	70	14.3	8.4, 8.7, 9.0	– 6 to PLANO
SATIN SOFT	N&N	HEMA	55	14.0	8.4, 8.7, 9.0	–12 to +8
SOFFORM 55	Salvatori	HEMA	55	14.0	8.3, 8.6, 8.9	–20 to +20
				15.0	8.6, 8.9, 9.2	–20 to +20
SOFTCON EW	CIBAVision	HEMA/PVP	55	14.0	8.1, 8.4, 8.7	–8 to +9.5
				14.5	8.7	–8 to –0.25
SOFLENS O_3, O_4	Bausch & Lomb	HEMA	38	13.5	Spin Cast	–6 to–1
				14.5	(8.8, O_3) (8.5,O_4)	
SOFT MATE I	Sola/Barnes–Hind	HEMA/Acrylamide	45	14.3	8.7	– 6 to PLANO
				14.8	9.0	–6 to PLANO
SOFT MATE II	Sola/Barnes–Hind	HEMA/Acrylamide	55	14.3	8.7	–12 to +7
				14.8	9.0	–12 to +7
SPECTRUM SPHERICAL	CIBA Vision	HEMA/PVP light blue visibility tint	55	14.0	8.3, 8.6, 8.9	–8 to +9.50
				14.5	8.9, 9.2	–8 to PLANO
SUNFLEX	Sunsoft	HEMA	55	15.0	8.3, 8.6, 8.9	+10 to–20
				14.0	8.3, 8.6, 8.9	+ 5 to –10
ULTRAFLEX 55	Ocular Sciences	HEMA	55	14.0	8.3, 8.6, 8.9	–10 to +5
				14.5	8.4, 8.7	–10 to +5

Reprinted from *Contact Lens Spectrum,* Feb. 1991, ED: White, P., and Scott, C.

Continued on next page

SPHERICAL COSMETIC EXTENDED WEAR HYDROGELS continued

RADE NAME	MANUFACTURER	MATERIAL	%H_2O	DIAMETERS	BASE CURVES[(2)]	POWERS
ANTAGE HIN	CooperVision	HEMA/NVP/MMA	43	13.8	8.4	–10 to PLANO
				14.4	8.7	–10 to PLANO
ISTAMARC	Vistakon	HEMA/MA	58	14.0	8.0, 8.3, 8.6	–9 to +7
				14.5	8.7	–9 to + 7
T 70	Lombart Lenses	MMA/NVP	70	14.3	8.4, 8.7, 9.0	–12 to +8

TORIC EXTENDED WEAR HYDROGELS

RADE NAME	COMPANY	MATERIAL	%H_2O	DIAMETERS	BASE CURVES	SPHERES	CYLINDER[(1)]	AXIS	BALLAST
&L FW ORIC	Bausch & Lomb	MMA/NVP	70	14.0	8.7, 9.0	–6 to +4	–.75, –1.25, – 1.75[(3)]	Full circle 10° steps	Prism
URASOFT 3 ORIC	Wesley–Jessen	HEMA/MMA	55	14.5	8.3, 8.6	–8 to +4	–0.75 to –2.00[(3)]	180°±30° 90°±30°	Periballast truncation, Prism Inf Slab off
URASOFT 3 PTIFIT TORIC	Wesley–Jessen	HEMA/MMA	55	14.5	8.6	–8.00 to +4.00	–.75 to –2.25	180°±20° 90°±20°	Prism/ thin zones
URASOFT 3 ORIC COLORS	Wesley–Jessen	HEMA/MMA opaques: baby blue, emerald green, aqua, hazel	55	14.5	8.6	PLANO to –4	–1.00 to –2.00[(3)]	180±20 90 ± 20	Periballast truncation, Prism Inf. Slab off
IRESOFT ORIC FW	Firestone Optics	HEMA	55	15.0	8.6, 8.9	–12 to +8	–.75 to –5.00[(2)]	Any	Prism; Eccentric lenticulation
YDRASOFT[(4)] ORIC XW	CoastVision	HEMA	55	15.0	8.6, 8.9	–12 to +8	–.75 to –5.00[(2)]	Any	Prism; Eccentric lenticulation
YDROCURVE TORIC	Sola/Barnes–Hind	HEMA/Acryl.	55	14.5	8.5	–6 to PLANO	–1.25[(2)]	180°±25° 90°—25°	Prism
					8.8	–8 to +4	–.75,–1.25 – 2.00[(2)]	Any	
ROFESSIONAL ERIES	CoastVision	HEMA	55	15.0	8.6, 8.9	–12 to +8	–.75 to –5.00	Any	Prism– Eccentric lenticulation
PECTRUM ORIC	CIBAVision	HEMA/PVP	55	14.5	8.9, 9.2	–6 to +4	–1.00, –1.75[(2)]	Full circle in 10° steps	Prism; circumferentia comfort level
CLIPSE	Sunsoft	HEMA	55	14.5	N/A	–6 to +2	—.75 to –2.00[(2)]	180°±25° 90°±25°	Prism; Eccentric lenticulation
UNSOFT[(4)] ORIC 15.0	Sunsoft	HEMA	55	15.0	8.3, 8.9	–20 to +10	–.75 to –7.00[(2)]	Any	Prism
VISTAMARC ORIC	Vistakon	HEMA/MA	58	14.5	8.6	–6 to +5	–.75 to –2.50[(3)]	180°±20° 90°±20°	Prism Slab off

1) All lenses, whether manufactured with front surface toric or back surface toric, are sted in minus cylinder form, as that is how the lenses are ordered. However, we have lso indicated by footnotes how they are manufactured.

(2) Manufactured with back toric
(3) Manufactured with front toric.
(4) Custom designs available.

Reprinted from *Contact Lens Spectrum,* Feb. 1991, ED: White, P., and Scott, C.

TORIC EXTENDED WEAR HYDROGELS

TRADE NAME	COMPANY	MATERIAL	%H_2O	DIAMETERS	BASE CURVES[2]	POWERS
BANDAGE LENS	Breger Mueller Welt	HEMA/NVP	45	13.5	8.6	
				15.5	9.5, 9.8	PLANO
CSI–T	Sola/Barnes–Hind	GMA/MMA	38	13.8	8.0 to 8.9(.3)	
				14.8	8.6, 8.9, 9.35	—7 to PLANO
GENESIS 79	Lombart Lenses	MMA/NVP	79	14.4	8.1, 8.4, 8.7	+0.75 to +7.50 and PLANO
N&N PW	N&N	MMA/NVP	79	14.4	8.1, 8.4, 8.7	PLANO to +20
PERMALENS	CooperVision	HEMA/NVP/MMA	71	15.0	9.0	PLANO
				13.5	7.7, 8.0, 8.3	PLANO
				14.2	8.6	PLANO
SOFLENS	Bausch & Lomb	HEMA	38	12.5 13.5 14.5	U, T U_3 O_4, B_4,	-9 to PLANO
SOFTCON EW APHAKIC	CIBA Vision	HEMA/PVP	55	14.0	7.8 to 8.7(.3)	+10 to +18
				14.5	8.1, 8.4	+10 to +18
SEA VIEW BANDAGE	Miami Contact Lens Company	HEMA/NVP	45	14.0, 15.5	8.6, 9.5, 9.8	PLANO
SEA VIEW THERAPEUTIC	Miami Contact Lens Company	HEMA/NVP	45	14.5	8.6, 8.9	–20 to +20
VT 79	Lombart Lenses	MMA/NVP	79	14.4	8.1, 8.4, 8.7	PLANO to +7.50

TINTED EXTENDED WEAR HYDROGELS

TRADE NAME	COMPANY	MATERIAL	%H_2O	THICKNESS	DIAMETERS	BASE CURVES	POWERS
CIBATHIN SOFTCOLORS	CIBA Vision	HEMA aqua, royal blue, blue, green, amber	37.5	.035	13.8	8.6, 8.9	–6 to PLANO
DURASOFT 3 COLORS	Wesley–Jessen	HEMA/MMA baby blue opaque, emerald green opaque, aqua opaque, sapphire blue, hazel opaque, jade green opaque, misty gray opaque, violet opaque, chestnut opaque, baby blue enhance	55	.05	14.5	8.3, 8.6 9.0 8.6 8.6	–8 to +6 PLANO to – 4 – 4 to PLANO – 8 to + 6
DURASOFT 3 LITETINT (D3LT)	Wesley–Jessen	HEMA/MMA	55		14.5	8.3, 8.6, 9.0	–8 to +6
HYDRON ZERO 4 SOFBLUE	Allergan Optical	HEMA light blue visibility tint	38	.04	13.8	8.4	– 10 to PLANO
HYDRON ZERO 4•F	Allergan Optical	HEMA light blue visibility tint	38	.04	13.8	8.8	– 5.25 to PLANO
NATURAL TINT O_3, O_4	Bausch & Lomb	HEMA aqua, blue, green, brown	38	.035	13.5 14.5	Spin Cast 8.8 for O_3 8.5 for O_4	–6 to PLANO
OPTIMA EW–FW	Bausch & Lomb	HEMA	38	.06	14.0	8.7	–9 to PLANO

Reprinted from *Contact Lens Spectrum*, Feb. 1991, ED: White, P., and Scott, C.

Continued on next page

TINTED EXTENDED WEAR HYDROGELS continued

TRADE NAME	COMPANY	MATERIAL	%H_2O	THICKNESS	DIAMETERS	BASE CURVES	POWERS
PERMAFLEX THIN 43 COLOR COLLECTION	CooperVision	HEMA/NVP/MMA sky blue, violet blue, spring green, turquoise	43	.035	13.8	8.4	–6 to PLANO
					14 4	8.9	– 6 to PLANO
SOFTMATE CUSTOM EYES 55	Sola/Barnes–Hind	HEMA Acrylamide aqua, blue, green	55	.05	14.8	9.0	–6 to PLANO
					14.3	8.7	–6 to PLANO
SPECTRUM SPHERICAL	CIBA Vision	HEMA/PVP	55	.10	14.0	8.3, 8.6, 8.9	–8 to +9.50
		light blue visibility tint		(.15 for +)	14.5	8.9, 9.2	–8 to PLANO
VANTAGE THIN ACCENTS	CooperVision	HEMA/NVP/MMA sky blue, violet blue, spring green, turquoise, auburn, misty brown	43	.035	13.8	8.4	–6.50 to PLANO
					14.4	8.7	–6.50 to PLANO
VANTAGE THIN	CooperVision	HEMA/NVP/MMA light blue handling tint	43	.035	13.8	8.4	– 10 to PLANO
					14.4	8.7	– 10 to PLANO

MULTIFOCAL EXTENDED WEAR HYDROGELS

TRADE NAME	COMPANY	MATERIAL	%H_2O	DIAMETERS	BASE CURVES	DISTANCE POWERS	ADD POWERS	DESIGN
SPECTRUM BIFOCAL	CIBA Vision	HEMA/PVP	55	14.0	8.6, 8.9	–6 to +6	+1.50 to +3.00	Central near concentric

DISPOSABLE AND/OR FREQUENT REPLACEMENT COSMETIC EXTENDED AND/OR DAILY WEAR HYDROGELS

TRADE NAME	COMPANY	MATERIAL	%H_2O	DIAMETERS	BASE CURVES	POWERS
ACUVUE	Vistakon	HEMA/MA	58	14.0	8.8	–9 to –0.50
				14.4	9.1	+0.50 to +6
NEWVUES	CIBA Vision	HEMA/PVP	55	14.0	8.4, 8.8	–10 to +4
SEEQUENCE	Bausch & Lomb	HEMA	38	14.0	Spincast	–6 to –1

6. RIGID GAS PERMEABLE LENSES

TABLE 32

RGP DAILY WEAR STANDARD DESIGN LENSES

TRADE NAME	COMPANY	MATERIAL	DK[1]	COLOR	LENS DIAMETER	BASE CURVES	POWERS
ADVENT	Allergan Optical/3M	Fluoro Polymer	100	clear	10.1	7.2 to 8.4	–7 to –0.25
COOPER HGP	CooperVision	Siloxane Acrylale	14	clear	8.9	7.00 to 8.30	–20 to +20
				blue	9 3	7.00 to 8.50	
					9.7	7.00 to 8.70	
FLUOROFLEX	CooperVision	Fluoro–Siloxane Acrylate	70	blue	8.9	7.00 to 8.30	–20 to +12
					9,3	7.00 to 8.50	
					9.7	7.00 to 8.70	
FLUOROCON[3]	Sola/Barnes–Hind	Fluoro–Siloxane Acrylate	60	blue	9.0	7.10 to 8.45	–10 to +8
					9.0XT[2]	7.10 to 8.30	–8 to PLANO
					9.5	7.20 to 8.65	–10 to +8

Reprinted from *Contact Lens Spectrum*, Feb. 1991, ED: White, P., and Scott, C.

Continued on next page

RGP DAILY WEAR STANDARD DESIGN LENSES

TRADE NAME	COMPANY	MATERIAL	DK(1)	COLOR	LENS DIAMETER	BASE CURVES	POWERS
NOVALENS	Ocutec	Styrene/Silicone(5)	55	blue	9.3–10.0	7.47(6) to 8.22	–8 to PLANO
PERMAFLEX HGP	CooperVision	Siloxane Acrylate	28	clear	8.9	7.00 to 8.30	–20 to +20
				blue	9 3	7.00 to 8.50	
					9.7	7.00 to 8.70	
POLYCON II(3)	Sola/Barnes–Hind	Siloxane Acrylate	12	blue	8.5	7.10 to 8.30	–8 to PLANO
					9.0	7.10 to 8.30	– 8 to + 8
					9.0XT(2)	7.10 to 8.30	–8 to PLANO
					9.5	7.20 to 8.55	–8 to +8
POLYCON HDK(3)	Sola/Barnes–Hind	Siloxane Acrylate	40	blue	9.0	7.20 to 8.30	–6 to +1
					9.5	7.30 to 8.40	–6 to + 1
SOFTPERM	Sola/Barnes–Hind	t–Butyl Styrene/ Siloxane Acrylate HEMA Skirt	14 RGP 25% H_2O Skirt	clear	14.3	7.1 to 8.1	–13 to +6

(1) Company's published Dk values (2) Increased center thickness (3) Custom designs available
(5) hydrophilic surface (6) diameters are matched to base curves in 16 increments

RGP DAILY WEAR CUSTOM DESIGN LENSES

TRADE NAME	COMPANY	MATERIAL	COLOR	DK(1)
THE BOSTON II	Polymer Technology	Siloxane Acrylate	clear, blue	14
THE BOSTON IV		Siloxane Acrylate	clear, blue, green	28
THE BOSTON EOUALENS(4)		Fluoro–Siloxane Acrylate	clear, blue	60
THE BOSTON EOUALENS II(4,5)		Fluoro–Siloxane Acrylate	blue	127
THE BOSTON RXD(4)		Fluoro–Siloxane Acrylate	blue	45
THE BOSTON ENVISION(4,6)		Fluoro–Siloxane Acrylate	blue	45
FLUOREX 300	G.T. Laboratories	Fluoro–Silicate Acrylate	clear, blue, green, grey	30
FLUOREX 500		Fluoro–Silicate Acrylate	clear, blue, green, grey	50
FLUOREX 700		Fluoro–Silicate Acrylate	clear, blue, green, grey	70
FLUOROPERM 30(4)*	Paragon	Fluoro–Siloxane Acrylate	clear, blue, green, grey, majestic blue	30
FLUOROPERM 60(4)*		Fluoro–Siloxane Acrylale	clear, blue, green, grey	60
FLUOROPERM 92(4)*		Fluoro–Siloxane Acrylate	clear, blue, green, grey	92
NOVALENS	Ocutec	Styrene/Silicone(4)*	blue	55
OPTACRYL 60	Paragon	Siloxane Acrylate	blue	18
PARAPERM O_2	Paragon	Siloxane Acrylate	clear, blue, green	15.6
SGP	Permeable Contact	Siloxane Acrylate	clear, blue, green	19
SGP II	Lens	Siloxane Acrylate	clear, blue, green	43.5
SGP III		Fluoro–Siloxane Acrylate	blue	43.5

(4)* UV absorber/inhibitors available 5) not commercially available (6) Preformed bi–aspheric back surface.

Reprinted from *Contact Lens Spectrum*, Feb. 1991, ED: White, P., and Scott, C.

Continued on next page

RGP TORIC DAILY WEAR STANDARD DESIGN LENSES

RADE NAME	COMPANY	COLOR	MATERIAL	DK(1)	DIAMETERS	BASE CURVES	SPHERE	CYLINDER	AXIS
POLYCON II TORIC LENSES	Sola/Barnes-Hind	blue	Siloxane Acrylate	12					
Front toric prism ballast					8.0 to 10.0	7.00 to 8.65	–10 to + 10	to 3.00	0° to 180°
Back toric					8.0 to 10.0	7.00 to 8.65	–10 to + 10	to 5.00	N/A
Bitoric SPE and CPE					8.0 to 10.0	7.00 to 8.65	–10 to + 10	to 5.00	NIA

RGP TORIC DAILY WEAR CUSTOM DESIGN MATERIALS

TRADE NAME	COMPANY	COLOR	MATERIAL	DK(1)
THE BOSTON EQUALENS	Polymer Technology	clear, blue	Fluoro–Siloxane Acrylate	60
THE BOSTON RXD			Fluoro–Siloxane Acrylate	45

RGP EXTENDED WEAR STANDARD DESIGN MATERIALS

TRADE NAME	COMPANY	COLOR	MATERIAL	DK(1)	LENS DIAMETER	BASE CURVES	POWERS
ADVENT	Allergan Optical/3M	clear	Fluoropolymer	100	10.1	–7.2 to 8.4	–7 to PLANO

RGP EXTENDED WEAR CUSTOM DESIGN MATERIALS

TRADE NAME	COMPANY	COLOR	MATERIAL	DK
THE BOSTON EOUALENS	Polymer Technology	clear, blue	Fluoro–Siloxane Acrylate	60
THE BOSTON EOUALENS II		blue	Fluoro–Siloxane Acrylate	127
FLOROPERM 60	Paragon	clear, blue, green, gray	Fluoro–Siloxane Acrylate	60
FLUOROPERM 92			Fluoro–Siloxane Acrylate	92
PARAPERM EW	Paragon	clear, blue, green	Siloxane Acrylate	56

RGP MULTIFOCAL LENSES

TRADE NAME	COMPANY	COLOR	MATERIAL	DK	TYPE
VFL	Conforma	blue	Siloxane Acrylate Fluoro–Siloxane Acrylate	18–90	Aspheric back surface (simultaneous)
TANGENT STREAK	Fused Kontacts	clear, blue, green, grey	Fluoro–Silicate Acrylic	70	One–piece segmented, translating no–jump bifocal
V/X	GBF	clear, blue, green, grey	Siloxane Acrylate Fluoro–Siloxane Acrylate	18–90	Aspheric back surface (simultaneous)

Reprinted from *Contact Lens Spectrum*, Feb. 1991, ED: White, P., and Scott, C.

Continued on next page

TABLE 33

SOFT BIFOCAL CONTACT LENSES

COMPANY	ALLERGAN/ HYDRON	BAUSCH & LOMB	BAUSCH & LOMB	CIBA	CIBA	SOFTSITE (UNILENS)	SOFTSITE (UNILENS)	SOLA/ BARNES-HIND	PRODUCT DEVELOP-MENT	UNILENS
Trade Name	Echelon	BiTech	PA 1	BiSoft	Spectrum	Alges	True Bifocal	H/C II	PS-45	Unilens
Material	Polymacon	Polymacon	Polymacon	Tefilcon	Vifilcon A	Hefilcon A	Hefilcon A	Bufilcon A	Polymacon	Ocufilcon B
H_2O	38%	38%	38%	37.5%	58%	48%	48%	48%	38%	53%
CT	.07 (−) .14 (+)	.19 (−) .29 (+)	.15	.07 (−) .12 (+)		.16	.24 (−)	.05	.17 (+/−)	.16 (−) .24 (+)
dk x 10'	8.4	8.4	8.4	8.0		11.3	11.3	12.0	8.4	
BC	8.7	8.7 8.9	Back Aspheric	8.3(+/−) 8.6 (+/−) 8.9	8.6 8.9	8.6 8.9 Custom	8.6 8.9 9.2	Back Aspheric	8.7	8.7 9.0 9.3
Diameter	14.0	14.5	13.5	13.8	14.0	14.0	13.5, 14.0(+) 14.0, 14.5(−)	14.8	14.0	14.0 14.5
Distance power	+4 to −6	+/−6	+/−6	+/−6	+/−6	+/−6	+/−6	+4 to −6	+/−6	+6 to −4
Near add	+1.50 +2.00	+2.00 +2.50	Progressive to +1.25	+1.50, +2 +2.50, +3	+1.50, +2 +2.50, +3	+1.50, +2 +2.50, +3 + 3.50	+2.25	Progressive to +1.50	Progressive to +2.00	Progressive to +2.00
Segments	Annular Diffraction	4.75 high 5.25 high Translating	Progressive Center Far	Annular Center Far	Annular Center Near	Annular Center Near	Translating 1.8 mm below center	Progressive Center Far	Progressive Center Near	Progressive Center Near
Concept	Simultaneous	Alternating	Simultaneous	Simultaneous	Simultaneous	Simultaneous	Alternating	Simultaneous	Simultaneous	Simultaneous
Stability	None	Perl Ballast	None	None	None	None	Structural Vent	None	None	None
Cost	$89 Warr. $69	$59.90 Warr.	$57.50 Warr.	$60	$74 Warr.	$65 Warr. $52.50	$56	$65	$100 Warr. $70	$75 Warr.
Phone	800-645-7544	800-828-9030	800-828-9030	800-241-5999	800-241-5999	800-327-5761	800-327-5761	800-854-2790	800-222-7324	800-477-2020

Source: *Contact Lens Forum*, April 1991 © Gralla Publications

TABLE 34

DISPOSABLE CONTACT LENSES

NAME	MATERIAL	DIAM(mm)	BASE CURVE	POWER(D)	THICKNESS(mm)
Acuvue	Etafilcon A	14.0 14.4	8.8 9.1	+4.00 to −6.00	0.07 to 0.17
New Vues	Vifilcon A	14.0	8.4 and 8.8	+4.00 to −6.00	0.06 to 0.13
SeeQuence	Polymacon	13.8	3.6 (saggital depth)	−0.50 to −9.00	0.035
Medalist	HEMA	14.0	8.7	+0.25 to −9.00 +0.25 to +4.00	
SureVue	Etafilcon	14.0	8.8	−0.50 to −9.00	

Adapted from Ghormley, N.R., *Disposable Contact Lenses—A fresh Look* ICLC 17:61-62,1990.

7. Aphakia

A. Recent Methods of Correcting Aphakia

Aphkia generally requires optical correction for useful visual acuity. Spectacle correction has been the most common, safest, and generally most acceptable method of correcting aphakia. However, other useful methods have been developed in the past few decades, and these include daily wear contact lenses, both hard and soft, long-term wear soft lenses, and intraocular lenses. Long-term wear lenses with FDA approval are listed in **Table 34.**

Intraocular lenses were pioneered by Dr. Harold Ridly of England more than thirty years ago. Presently, in the United States more than 50% of patients undergoing cataract extraction will have placement of one or another type of intraocular lens. More than 300 intra-

Continued on next page

ocular lenses are available in various sizes, shapes, and intraocular powers and many are listed in **Table 35**. At the present time some intraocular lenses are considered investigational and implant surgeons must have investigator status from the various manufacturers in order to comply with FDA regulations. Proponents of the various lenses claim specific merits for their lenses. However, for many lenses there is insufficient data to support the advantage of one type of lens over another. Differences in manufacture or fabrication of intraocular lenses can be significant factors in the incidence of complications following lens implantation.

B. 4 Drop Aphakic Corrective Lenses

In contrast to aspheric aphakic lenses, the curves generated in the 4 drop lenses are spherical curves. Instead of a transition from maximum lens power centrally to lesser power peripherally, the 4 drop lens accomplishes this by 4 zones of diminishing spherical power. These powers can be measured by the Geneva lens measure type device. This optical design is claimed to minimize ring scotoma and distortions found in the aspheric lenses. The field of view is also increased.

Cosmesis is aided by elimination of the lenticular commonly used in the aspheric type lenses and by the provision of minimum effective diameter lens blanks permitting reduced thickness.

TABLE 35

APHAKIC EXTENDED WEAR HYDROGELS

Trade Name	Company	Material	%H_2O	Diameters	Base Curves	Powers
C.W.79	Bausch & Lomb	MMA/NVP	79	14.4	8.1, 8.4, 8.7	+10 to +20
NEW APHAKIC	Breger Mueller Welt	HEMA/NVP	45	14.0	8.6, 8.9	+9 to +20
GENESIS 79 APHAKIC	Lombart Lenses	MMA/NVP	79	14.4	8.1, 8.4, 8.7	+8 to +25
GENESIS 79 PEDIATRIC APHAKIC	Lombart Lenses	MMA/NVP	79	13.7	7.5, 7.8	+20 to +35
HYDROCURVE II 55	Sola/Barnes–Hind	HEMA/Acrylamide	55	14.0	8.5	+7.25 to +20
				14.5	8.8	+7.25 to +20
				15.5	9.5, 9.8	+7.25 to +20
				15.5	9.2	+12 to +16
N&N PW APHAKIC	N&N	MMA/NVP	79	14.4	8.1, 8.4, 8.7	+7 to +20
N&N PEDIATRIC			79	13.7	7.5, 7.8	+20 to +35
PERMALENS	CooperVision	HEMA/NVP/MMA	71	14.0	8.0, 8.3	+8.50 to +20
				14.5	8.3, 8.6, 8.9	+8.50 to +20
SILSOFT	Bausch & Lomb	Silicone	0	11.3, 12.5	7.5 to 8.3(.2)	+12 to +20
				11.3	7.5 to 7.9(.2)	+23 to +32
SOF–FORM 55	Salvatori	HEMA	55	14.0, 15.0	8.3, 8.6, 8.9, 9.2	+10 to +20
SOFTCON EW APHAKIC	CIBA Vision	HEMA/PVP	55	14.0	7.8 to 8.7(.3)	+10 to +18
			55	14.5	8.1, 8.4	+10 to +18
SEA VIEW APHAKIC	Miami Contact Lens Company	HEMA/NVP	45	14.5	8.6, 8.9	+9 to +20
				14.0	8.3	+9 to +20
SUNSOFT APHAKIC	Sunsoft	HEMA	55	15.0	8.3, 8.6, 8.9	+10.50 to +20
VT 79 APHAKIC	Lombart Lenses	MMA/NVP	79	14.4	8.1, 8.4, 8.7	+8 to +25
VT 79 PEDIATRIC APHAKIC				13.7	7.5, 7.8	+20 to +35

Reprinted from *Contact Lens Spectrum*, Feb. 1991, ED: White, P., and Scott, C.

TABLE 36

INTRAOCULAR LENSES AVAILABLE IN THE UNITED STATES[1]

COMPANY NAME	STYLES[2]	POWERS (DIOPTER)	HAPLIC MATERIAL[3]
Alcon Surgical	AC PC	+10.00 to +25.00 +10.00 to +25.00	PMMA/PCQ PPL
Allergan Medical Optics	AC PC	+10.00 to +24.00 +10.0 to +27.00	PCQ PPL
Colburn Optical	AC PC	+14.00 to +27.00 +14.00 to +30.00	PMMA PMMA
Cooper Vision CILCO	AC PC	+4.00 to +32.00 +4.00 to +30.00	PMMA PMMA
Domilens	PC	+8.00 to 28.00	Prol
Eye Technology Inc.	PC	+ 8.00 to +28.00	PMMA
Intraoptics	AC PC	+10.00 to +30 00 +10.00 to +30.00	PCQ
International Optics	PC	+8.00 to +35.00	Prol
IOLAB Corporation	AC PC	+4.00 to +25.00 +6.00 to +30.00	Prol Prol
IOPTEX, Inc	AC PC	+8.00 to +28.00 +8.00 to +28.00	PMMA PPL/Prol
Optical Radiation Corporation	AC PC	+6.00 to +28.00 +6.00 to +28.00	PMMA Prol
Pharmacia Ophthalmics	PC	+10.00 to +30.00	PMMA
Starr Surgical Co.	PC Foldable PC	+8.00 to +30.00 +14.00 to +24.00	PMMA Sil
Storz Intraocular Lens Co.	AC PC	+10.00 to +30.00 +10.00 to +30.00	PCQ/PMMA PMMA/Prol
Surgidev	AC PC	+10.00 to +27.00 +10.00 to +27.00	PMMA PMMA/Prol
3M Vision Care	PC	+9.00 to +28.00	PPL

1. Adapted from intraocular Lens Data, Colenbrander, A, Woods, LV and Stamper, RL in *Ophthalmology Instrument and Book Supplement*, 1989 pp 20–27.
2. AC = Anterior Chamber PC = Posterior Chamber

3. RELATIVE MAGNIFICATION, LENS EFFECTIVITY, INDEX OF REFRACTION, STOCK BASE CURVES AND CONVERSION TABLES

TABLE 37

THE RELATIVE MAGNIFICATION PRODUCED BY CONTACT & SPECTACLE LENSES

The percentage increase (or decrease) in the size of the retinal image afforded by contact lenses in comparison with orthodox spectacles fitted at 12 mm from the cornea. (after A.G. Bennett)

SPECTACLE REFRACTION	EQUIVALENT POWER OF CONTACT LENS SYSTEM	PERCENTAGE INCREASE AFFORDED BY CONTACT LENS	SPECTACLE REFRACTION	EQUIVALENT POWER OF CONTACT LENS SYSTEM	PERCENTAGE INCREASE AFFORDED BY CONTACT LENS	SPECTACLE REFRACTION	EQUIVALENT POWER OF CONTACT LENS SYSTEM	PERCENTAGE INCREASE AFFORDED BY CONTACT LENS
-20	–15.73	27.2	–8	–7.07	12.9	+6	+6.10	–4.7
-18	–14.41	24.8	–6	–5.42	10.5	+8	+8.29	–7.4
-16	–13.06	22.5	–4	–3.69	7.8	+10	+10.62	–10.3
-14	–11.65	20.1	–2	–1.88	5.4	+12	+13.07	–13.8
-12	–10.19	17.8	+2	+1.96	1.2	+14	+15.64	–17.3
-10	–8.66	15.3	+4	+3.99	–1.7			

TABLE 38

LENS EFFECTIVITY

The power of equivalent lens at reduced or increased vertex distance can be approximated by the formula:

$$> F = sD^2$$

Where: s = Change in vertex distance. in meters
D = Power of lens

Example: 10.00 D lens fitted at vertex distance 15mm.
1. Lens is refitted at 10mm. vertex distance
   $> F = .005\,(10)^2 = .005\,(100) = .0.50D$
2. Lens is fitted as a Contact Lens
   $> F = .015\,(10)^2 = .015\,(100) = 1.50D$

If lens is replaced by one closer to eye, plus power must be increased, minus power must be decreased by > F. If lens is replaced by one further from eye, plus power must be reduced. minus power must be increased by > F.

*Bennett, AG, *Optics of Contact Lenses.* 4th ed London Hatton Press, 1966.

TABLE 39

INDEX OF REFRACTION OF LENS MATERIAL

	CROWN GLASS	1.6 INDEX CROWNLITE GLASS	HILITE GLASS	INDEX 8 GLASS	CR-39 PLASTIC	HIRI PLASTIC	1.6 PLASTIC	POLYCAR-BONATE THIN-LITE PLASTIC
INDEX OF REFRACTION the higher the number, the thinner the material	1.523	1.601	1.701	1.805	1.498	1.56	1.6	1.586
SPECIFIC GRAVITY the higher the number, the heavier the material	2.5	2.67	2.99	3.37	1.32	1.216	1.34	1.20
DISPERSION the higher the number, the less chromatic aberration (ABBE value)	59	42.24	31	25	58	38	37	31
PERSONALITY	temperable, coatable, ease in handling, vast availability	chem. temperable, ease in handling, limited availability	chem. temperable, fairly easy to handle, SV & multi–focals, vacuum coatings cause lens to become highly sensitive to scratching	SV, difficult to temper, highly reflective so A/R coatings recommended, but has same problems as hilite: Mfrs. suggest having patient sign liability waiver when ground thin. Multifocal available in laminate.	strong, tintable, coatable, ease in handling, vast availability	SV & bifocal, tints well before SRC, edges well, must be SRC, extremely brittle	SV only, tints well before SRC, edges well must be SRC	SV & multifocal, strongest lens material available, limited tintability, must be SPC, no fast fabrication, special edging equipment needed, must for children and athletes

SRC–scratch resistant coating

TABLE 40

AVAILABLE STOCK BASE CURVES

POWER OF LENS (DIOPTERS)	NEAREST STANDARD BASE CURVE
0.0 to + 7.0	– 6.0 (back surface)
– 0.12 to – 5.0	+ 6.0 (front surface)
– 5.0 to – 9.0	+ 3.0 (front surface)
– 10.0 to – 15.0	+ 1.25 (front surface)
– 15.0 to – 20.0	plano (front surface)

TABLE 41

CYLINDER POWER IN OFF-AXIS MERIDIAN

DEGREES FROM CYLINDER AXIS

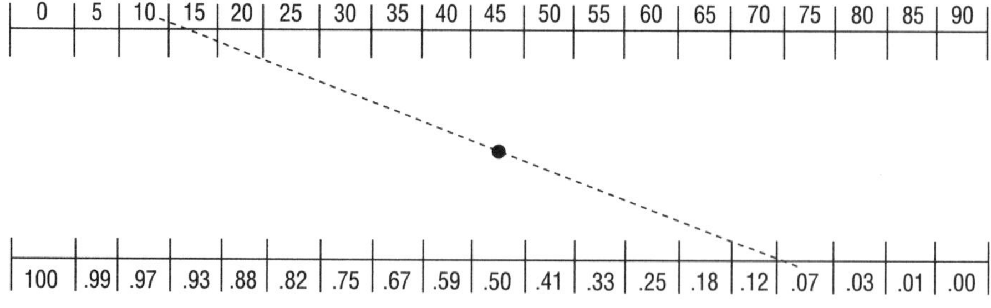

PERCENTAGE OF CYLINDER POWER IN OFF-AXIS MERIDIAN

To determine cylinder power in an off–axis meridian, place straight–edge on diagram below so that it intersects center dot and upper scale position for number of degrees that the meridian sought is off–axis. Percentage of cylinder power in the meridian sought is indicated on lower scale at point of intersection with straight–edge.

Example: 2 00D. Cyl x 75° What is the power at 90° which is 15° off axis?
Reading on lower scale is .07, therefore, power in 90th meridian is .14D

TABLE 42

CORNEAL RADIUS EQUIVALENCE DIOPTERS/MILLIMETERS

DIOPTERS	MM.	DIOPTERS	MM.	DIOPTERS	MM.	DIOPTERS	MM.	DIOPTERS	MM.	DIOPTERS	MM.	DIOPTERS	MM.	DIOPTERS	MM.
20.00	16.875	36.00	9.375	39.00	8.653	42.00	8.035	45.00	7.500	48.00	7.031	51.00	6.617	54.00	6.250
22.00	15.340	36.12	9.343	39.12	8.627	42.12	8.012	45.12	7.480	48.12	7.013	51.12	6.602	54.12	6.236
24.00	14.062	36.25	9.310	39.25	8.598	42.25	7.988	45.25	7.458	48.25	6.994	51.25	6.585	54.25	6.221
26.00	12.980	36.37	9.279	39.37	8.572	42.37	7.965	45.37	7.438	48.37	6.977	51.37	6.569	54.37	6.207
27.00	12.500	36.50	9.246	39.50	8.544	42.50	7.941	45.50	7.417	48.50	6.958	51.50	6.553	54.50	6.192
28.00	12.053	36.62	9.216	39.62	8.518	42.62	7.918	45.62	7.398	48.62	6.941	51.62	6.538	54.62	6.179
29.00	11.638	36.75	9.183	39.75	8.490	42.75	7.894	45.75	7.377	48.75	6.923	51.75	6.521	54.75	6.164
29.50	11.441	36.87	9.153	39.87	8.465	42.87	7.872	45.87	7.357	48.87	6.906	51.87	6.506	54.87	6.150
30.00	11.250	37.00	9.121	40.00	8.437	43.00	7.848	46.00	7.336	49.00	6.887	52.00	6.490	55.00	6.136
30.50	11.065	37.12	9.092	40.12	8.412	43.12	7.826	46.12	7.317	49.12	6.870	52.12	6.475	55.12	6.123
31.00	10.887	37.25	9.060	40.25	8.385	43.25	7.803	46.25	7.297	49.25	6.852	52.25	6.459	55.25	6.108
31.50	10.714	37.37	9.031	40.37	8.360	43.37	7.781	46.37	7.278	49.37	6.836	52.37	6.444	55.37	6.095
32.00	10.547	37.50	9.000	40.50	8.333	43.50	7.758	46.50	7.258	49.50	6.818	52.50	6.428	55.50	6.081
32.50	10.385	37.62	8.971	40.62	8.308	43.62	7.737	46.62	7.239	49.62	6.801	52.62	6.413	55.62	6.068
33.00	10.227	37.75	8.940	40.75	8.282	43.75	7.714	46.75	7.219	49.75	6.783	52.75	6.398	55.75	6.054
33.50	10.075	37.87	8.912	40.87	8.257	43.87	7.693	46.87	7.200	49.87	6.767	52.87	6.383	55.87	6.041
34.00	9.926	38.00	8.881	41.00	8.231	44.00	7.670	47.00	7.180	50.00	6.750	53.00	6.367	56.00	6.027
34.25	9.854	38.12	8.853	41.12	8.207	44.12	7.649	47.12	7.162	50.12	6.733	53.12	6.353	56.50	5.973
34.50	9.783	38.25	8.823	41.25	8.181	44.25	7.627	47.25	7.142	50.25	6.716	53.25	6.338	57.00	5.921
34.75	9.712	38.37	8.795	41.37	8.158	44.37	7.606	47.37	7.124	50.37	6.700	53.37	6.323	57.50	5.869
35.00	9.643	38.50	8.766	41.50	8.132	44.50	7.584	47.50	7.105	50.50	6.683	53.50	6.308	58.00	5.819
35.25	9.574	38.62	8.738	41.62	8.109	44.62	7.563	47.62	7.087	50.62	6.667	53.62	6.294	58.50	5.769
35.50	9.507	38.75	8.708	41.75	8.083	44.75	7.541	47.75	7.068	50.75	6.650	53.75	6.279	59.00	5.720
35.75	9.440	38.87	8.682	41.87	8.060	44.87	7.521	47.87	7.050	50.87	6.634	53.87	6.265	60.00	5.625

TABLE 43

VERTEX DISTANCE CONVERSION SCALE

SPECTACLE LENS POWER	PLUS LENSES				VERTEX DISTANCE/MILLIMETERS								MINUS LENSES			
	8	9	10	11	12	13	14	15	8	9	10	11	12	13	14	15
4.00	4.12	4.12	4.12	4.12	4.25	4.25	4.25	4.25	3.87	3.87	3.87	3.87	3.87	3.75	3.75	3.75
4.50	4.62	4.75	4.75	4.75	4.75	4.75	4.75	4.87	4.37	4.37	4.25	4.25	4.25	4.25	4.25	4.25
5.00	5.25	5.25	5.25	5.25	5.25	5.37	5.37	5.37	4.75	4.75	4.75	4.75	4.75	4.75	4.62	4.62
5.50	5.75	5.75	5.75	5.87	5.87	5.87	6.00	6.00	5.25	5.25	5.25	5.12	5.12	5.12	5.12	5.12
6.00	6.25	6.37	6.37	6.37	6.50	6.50	6.50	6.62	5.75	5.62	5.62	5.62	5.62	5.50	5.50	5.50
6.50	6.87	6.87	7.00	7.00	7.00	7.12	7.12	7.25	6.12	6.12	6.12	6.00	6.00	6.00	6.00	5.87
7.00	7.37	7.50	7.50	7.62	7.62	7.75	7.75	7.75	6.62	6.62	6.50	6.50	6.50	6.37	6.37	6.37
7.50	8.00	8.00	8.12	8.12	8.25	8.25	8.37	8.50	7.12	7.00	7.00	6.87	6.87	6.87	6.75	6.75
8.00	8.50	8.62	8.75	8.75	8.87	8.87	9.00	9.12	7.50	7.50	7.37	7.37	7.25	7.25	7.25	7.25
8.50	9.12	9.25	9.25	9.37	9.50	9.50	9.62	9.75	8.00	7.87	7.87	7.75	7.75	7.62	7.62	7.50
9.00	9.75	9.75	9.87	10.00	10.12	10.25	10.37	10.37	8.37	8.37	8.25	8.25	8.12	8.00	8.00	8.00
9.50	10.25	10.37	10.50	10.62	10.75	10.87	11.00	11.12	8.87	8.75	8.62	8.62	8.50	8.50	8.37	8.37
10.00	10.87	11.00	11.12	11.25	11.37	11.50	11.62	11.75	9.25	9.12	9.12	9.00	8.87	8.87	8.75	8.75
10.50	11.50	11.62	11.75	11.87	12.00	12.12	12.25	12.50	9.62	9.62	9.50	9.37	9.37	9.25	9.12	9.12
11.00	12.00	12.25	12.37	12.50	12.75	12.87	13.00	13.12	10.12	10.00	9.87	9.75	9.75	9.62	9.50	9.50
11.50	12.62	12.87	13.00	13.12	13.37	13.50	13.75	13.87	10.50	10.37	10.37	10.25	10.12	10.00	9.87	9.87
12.00	13.25	13.50	13.62	13.87	14.00	14.25	14.50	14.62	11.00	10.87	10.75	10.62	10.50	10.37	10.25	10.12
12.50	13.87	14.12	14.25	14.50	14.75	15.00	15.25	15.37	11.37	11.25	11.12	11.00	10.87	10.75	10.62	10.50
13.00	14.50	14.75	15.00	15.25	15.50	15.62	16.00	16.12	11.75	11.62	11.50	11.37	11.25	11.12	11.00	10.87
13.50	15.12	15.37	15.62	15.87	16.12	16.37	16.62	16.87	12.25	12.00	11.87	11.75	11.62	11.50	11.37	11.25
14.00	15.75	16.00	16.25	16.50	16.75	17.12	17.50	17.75	12.62	12.50	12.25	12.12	12.00	11.87	11.75	11.50
14.50	16.50	16.75	17.00	17.25	17.50	17.87	18.25	18.50	13.00	12.75	12.62	12.50	12.37	12.25	12.00	11.87
15.00	17.00	17.37	17.75	18.00	18.25	18.62	19.00	19.37	13.37	13.25	13.00	12.87	12.75	12.50	12.37	12.25
15.50	17.75	18.00	18.25	18.75	19.00	19.37	19.75	20.25	13.75	13.62	13.50	13.25	13.00	12.87	12.75	12.62
16.00	18.25	18.75	19.00	19.37	19.75	20.25	20.50	21.00	14.25	14.00	13.75	13.62	13.50	13.25	13.00	12.87
16.50	19.00	19.37	19.75	20.25	20.50	21.00	21.50	21.87	14.50	14.37	14.12	14.00	13.75	13.62	13.50	13.25
17.00	19.75	20.25	20.50	21.00	21.50	22.00	22.25	22.87	15.00	14.75	14.50	14.25	14.12	14.00	13.75	13.50
17.50	20.50	20.75	21.25	21.75	22.25	22.75	23.25	23.75	15.37	15.12	14.87	14.75	14.50	14.25	14.00	13.87
18.00	21.00	21.50	22.00	22.50	23.00	23.50	24.00	24.62	15.75	15.50	15.25	15.00	14.75	14.62	14.37	14.12
18.50	21.75	22.25	22.75	23.25	23.75	24.50	25.00	25.62	16.12	15.87	15.62	15.37	15.12	14.87	14.75	14.50
19.00	22.50	23.00	23.50	24.00	24.75	25.25	26.00	26.50	16.50	16.25	16.00	15.75	15.50	15.25	15.00	14.75

TABLE 44

MJK SPHERO-CYLINDRICAL VERTEX CHART

VERTEX DISTANCE = 13.00 MM | CYLINDER INCREMENT = 0.25 DIOPTERS | SPHERE INCREMENTS = 0.125 DIOPTERS

SR	SRV	−0.25	−0.50	−0.75	−1.00	−1.25	−1.50	-1.75	-2.00	-2.25	-2.50	-2.75	−3.00
−3.00	−2.87	−0.25	−0.50	−0.75	−1.00	−1.25	−1.25	−1.50	−1.75	−2.00	−2.25	−2.50	−2.75
−3.25	−3.12	−0.25	−0.50	−0.75	−1.00	−1.25	−1.25	−1.50	−1.75	−2.00	−2.25	−2.50	−2.75
−3.50	−3.37	−0.25	−0.50	−0.75	−1.00	−1.25	−1.25	−1.50	−1.75	−2.00	−2.25	−2.50	−2.75
−3.75	−3.62	−0.25	−0.50	−0.75	−1.00	−1.00	−1.25	−1.50	−1.75	−2.00	−2.25	−2.50	−2.75
−4.00	−3.75	−0.25	−0.50	−0.75	−1.00	−1.00	−1.25	−1.50	−1.75	−2.00	−2.25	−2.50	−2.50
−4.25	−4.00	−0.25	−0.50	−0.75	−1.00	−1.00	−1.25	−1.50	−1.75	−2.00	−2.25	−2.50	−2.50
−4.50	−4.25	−0.25	−0.50	−0.75	−1.00	−1.00	−1.25	−1.50	−1.75	−2.00	−2.25	−2.25	−2.50
−4.75	−4.50	−0.25	−0.50	−0.75	−1.00	−1.00	−1.25	−1.50	−1.75	−2.00	−2.25	−2.25	−2.50
−5.00	−4.75	−0.25	−0.50	−0.75	−0.75	−1.00	−1.25	−1.50	−1.75	−2.00	−2.25	−2.25	−2.50
−5.25	−4.87	−0.25	−0.50	−0.75	−0.75	−1.00	−1.25	−1.50	−1.75	−2.00	−2.25	−2.25	−2.50
−5.50	−5.12	−0.25	−0.50	−0.75	−0.75	−1.00	−1.25	−1.50	−1.75	−2.00	−2.00	−2.25	−2.50
−5.75	−5.37	−0.25	−0.50	−0.75	−0.75	−1.00	−1.25	−1.50	−1.75	−2.00	−2.00	−2.25	−2.50
−6.00	−5.62	−0.25	−0.50	−0.75	−0.75	−1.00	−1.25	−1.50	−1.75	−2.00	−2.00	−2.25	−2.50
−6.25	−5.75	−0.25	−0.50	−0.75	−0.75	−1.00	−1.25	−1.50	−1.75	−1.75	−2.00	−2.25	−2.50
−6.50	−6.00	−0.25	−0.50	−0.75	−0.75	−1.00	−1.25	−1.50	−1.75	−1.75	−2.00	−2.25	−2.50
−6.75	−6.25	−0.25	−0.50	−0.75	−0.75	−1.00	−1.25	−1.50	−1.75	−1.75	−2.00	−2.25	−2.50
−7.00	−6.37	−0.25	−0.50	−0.50	−0.75	−1.00	−1.25	−1.50	−1.75	−1.75	−2.00	−2.25	−2.50
−7.25	−6.62	−0.25	−0.50	−0.50	−0.75	−1.00	−1.25	−1.50	−1.75	−1.75	−2.00	−2.25	−2.50
−7.50	−6.87	−0.25	−0.50	−0.50	−0.75	−1.00	−1.25	−1.50	−1.50	−1.75	−2.00	−2.25	−2.50
−7.75	−7.00	−0.25	−0.50	−0.50	−0.75	−1.00	−1.25	−1.50	−1.50	−1.75	−2.00	−2.25	−2.50
−8.00	−7.25	−0.25	−0.50	−0.50	−0.75	−1.00	−1.25	−1.50	−1.50	−1.75	−2.00	−2.25	−2.50
−8.25	−7.50	−0.25	−0.50	−0.50	−0.75	−1.00	−1.25	−1.50	−1.50	−1.75	−2.00	−2.25	−2.25
−8.50	−7.62	−0.25	−0.50	−0.50	−0.75	−1.00	−1.25	−1.50	−1.50	−1.75	−2.00	−2.25	−2.25
−8.75	−7.87	−0.25	−0.50	−0.50	−0.75	−1.00	−1.25	−1.50	−1.50	−1.75	−2.00	−2.25	−2.25
−9.00	−8.00	−0.25	−0.50	−0.50	−0.75	−1.00	−1.25	−1.25	−1.50	−1.75	−2.00	−2.25	−2.25
−9.25	−8.25	−0.25	−0.50	−0.50	−0.75	−1.00	−1.25	−1.25	−1.50	−1.75	−2.00	−2.00	−2.25
−9.50	−8.50	−0.25	−0.50	−0.50	−0.75	−1.00	−1.25	−1.25	−1.50	−1.75	−2.00	−2.00	−2.25
−9.75	−8.62	−0.25	−0.50	−0.50	−0.75	−1.00	−1.25	−1.25	−1.50	−1.75	−2.00	−2.00	−2.25
−10.00	−8.87	−0.25	−0.50	−0.50	−0.75	−1.00	−1.25	−1.25	−1.50	−1.75	−2.00	−2.00	−2.25
−10.25	−9.00	−0.25	−0.50	−0.50	−0.75	−1.00	−1.25	−1.25	−1.50	−1.75	−2.00	−2.00	−2.25
−10.50	−9.25	−0.25	−0.50	−0.50	−0.75	−1.00	−1.25	−1.25	−1.50	−1.75	−2.00	−2.00	−2.25
−10.75	−9.37	−0.25	−0.50	−0.50	−0.75	−1.00	−1.25	−1.25	−1.50	−1.75	−1.75	−2.00	−2.25
+4.00	+4.25	−0.25	−0.50	−0.75	−1.00	−1.25	−1.75	−2.00	−2.25	−2.50	−2.75	−3 00	−3.25
+4.25	+4.50	−0.25	−0.50	−0.75	−1.00	−1 .50	−1.75	−2.00	−2.25	−2.50	−2.75	−3.00	−3.25
+4.50	+4.75	−0.25	−0.50	−0.75	−1.00	−1.50	−1.75	−2.00	−2.25	−2.50	−2.75	−3.00	−3.25
+4.75	+5.12	−0.25	−0.50	−0.75	−1.00	−1.50	−1.75	−2.00	−2.25	−2.50	−2.75	−3.00	−3.25
+5.00	+5.37	−0.25	−0.50	−0.75	−1.00	−1.50	−1.75	−2.00	−2.25	−2.50	−2.75	−3.00	−3.25
+5.25	+5.62	−0.25	−0.50	−0.75	−1.00	−1.50	−1.75	−2.00	−2.25	−2.50	−2.75	−3.00	−3.25
+5.50	+5.87	−0.25	−0.50	−0.75	−1.25	−1.50	−1.75	−2.00	−2.25	−2.50	−2.75	−3.00	−3.25
+5.75	+6.25	−0.25	−0.50	−0.75	−1.00	−1.50	−1.75	−2.00	−2.25	−2.50	−2.75	−3.00	−3.25
+6.00	+6.50	−0.25	−0.50	−0.75	−1.00	−1.50	−1.75	−2.00	−2.25	−2.50	−2.75	−3.00	−3.50
+6.25	+6.75	−0.25	−0.50	−1.00	−1.00	−1.50	−1.75	−2.00	−2.25	−2.50	−2.75	−3.25	−3.50
+6.50	+7.12	−0.25	−0.50	−1.00	−1.00	−1.50	−1.75	−2.00	−2.25	−2.50	−3.00	−3.25	−3.50
+6.75	+7.37	−0.25	−0.50	−1.00	−1.00	−1.50	−1.75	−2.00	−2.25	−2.50	−3.00	−3.25	−3.50
+7.00	+7.75	−0.25	−0.50	−1.00	−1.00	−1.50	−1.75	−2.00	−2.25	−2.75	−3.00	−3.25	−3.50
+7.25	+8 00	−0.25	−0.50	−1.00	−1.00	−1.50	−1.75	−2.00	−2.25	−2.75	−3.00	−3.25	−3.50
+7.50	+8.25	−0.25	−0.50	−1.00	−1.00	−1.50	−1.75	−5.00	−2.50	−2.75	−3.00	−3.25	−3.50
+7.75	+8.62	−0.25	−0.50	−1.00	−1.00	−1.50	−1.75	−2.00	−2.50	−2.75	−3.00	−3 25	−3.50
+8.00	+8.87	−0.25	−0.50	−1.00	−1.00	−1.50	−1.75	−2.25	−2.50	−2.75	−3.00	−3.25	−3.50
+8.25	+9.25	−0.25	−0.50	−1.00	−1.00	−1.50	−1.75	−2.25	−2.50	−2.75	−3.00	−3.25	−3.50
+8.50	+9 25	−0.25	−0.75	−1.00	−1.25	−1.50	−1.75	−2.25	−2.50	−2.75	−3.00	−3.25	−3.75
+8.75	+9.87	−0.25	−0.75	−1.00	−1.25	−1.50	−1.75	−2.25	−2.50	−2.75	−3.00	−3.25	−3.75
+9.00	+10.25	−0.25	−0.75	−1.00	−1.25	−1.50	−2.00	−2.25	−2.50	−2.75	−3.00	−3.50	−3.75
+9.25	+10.50	−0.25	−0.75	−1.00	−1.25	−1.50	−2.00	−2.25	−2.50	−2.75	−3.00	−3.50	−3.75
+9.50	+10.87	−0.25	−0.75	−1.00	−1.25	−1.50	−2.00	−2.25	−2.50	−2.75	−3.25	−3.50	−3.75
+9.75	+11.12	−0.25	−0.75	−1.00	−1.25	−1.50	−2.00	−2.25	−2.50	−2.75	−3.25	−3.50	−3.75
+10.00	+11.50	−0.25	−0.75	−1.00	−1.25	−1.50	−2.00	−2.25	−2.50	−3.00	−3.25	−3.50	−3.75
+10.25	+11.87	−0.25	−0.75	−1.00	−1.25	−1.75	−2.00	−2.25	−2.50	−3.00	−3.25	−3.50	−3.75
+10 50	+12.12	−0.25	−0.75	−1.00	−1.25	−1.75	−2.00	−2.25	−2.50	−3.00	−3 25	−3.50	−3.75
+10.75	+12.50	−0.25	−0.75	−1.00	−1.25	−1.75	−2.00	−2.25	−2.50	−3.00	−3.25	−3.50	−4.00
+11.00	+12.87	−0.25	−0.75	−1.00	−1.25	−1.75	−2.00	−2.25	−2.75	−3.00	−3.25	−3.50	−4.00
+11.25	+13.12	−0.25	−0.75	−1.00	−1.25	−1.75	−2.00	−2.25	−2.75	−3.00	−3.25	−3.50	−4.00
+11.50	+13.50	−0.25	−0.75	−1.00	−1.25	−1.75	−2.00	−2.25	−2.75	−3.00	−3.25	−3.75	−4.00
+11.75	+13.87	−0.25	−0.75	−1.00	−1.25	−1.75	−2.00	−2.25	−2.75	−3.00	−3.25	−3.75	−4.00

Example: Spectacle Refraction at 13 mm = 1)-5.75 −2 50 × 180
Matching up 3)-5.75 on the left, gives effective spherical power of −5.37.
Following underlined values to the right and reading in the 2)-2.50 cylinder column gives a cylinder value of 4)-2.00.

Corneal Plane Refraction = -5.37 −2.00 × 180

Legend: In this chart of sphero-cylindrical corneal plane refractions, the spherical value is calculated and rounded off to the nearest 0.12 diopter, while the cylinder value is rounded off to the nearest 0.25 diopter.

SECTION 5

VISION STANDARDS AND LOW VISION

Vision standards for interstate commercial drivers and pilots as well as state motor vehicle standards are included in the first part of this section.

A discussion of low vision and a directory of state service facilities follows.

1. VISION STANDARDS

TABLE 45

VISION STANDARDS FOR INTERSTATE COMMERCIAL DRIVERS

1. Distant visual acuity of at least 20/40 (Snellen) in each eye with or without corrective lenses.
2. Distant binocular acuity of at least 20/40 (Snellen) in both eyes with or without corrective lenses.
3. A field of vision of at least 120° in the horizontal Meridian in each eye.
4. Ability to recognize the colors of traffic signals and devices showing standard red, green, and amber.

Note: Contact lenses are permissible if there is sufficient evidence that the driver has good tolerance and is well adapted to their use.
Section 391.41 (b) (10) U.S. Department of Transportation, Federal Highway Administration

TABLE 46

VISION STANDARDS FOR PILOTS

	WITHOUT RX[1]	REQUIRING RX[1] CORRECTED TO	NEAR VISION WITH/WITHOUT RX	PHORIAS[2]	FIELDS	COLOR	PATHOLOGY
1st Class	20/20	20/100 to 20/20	20/40 (J_3)	6D Eso/Exo 1Δ Hyper	Normal	Normal	4
2nd Class	20/20	20/100 to 20/20	20/40 (J_3)	6D Eso/Exo 1Δ Hyper	Normal	3	5
3rd Class	20/50	To 20/30	20/60 (J_6)	....	....	3	5

1. Each eye.
2. If exceeded, further evaluation required to determine if bifoveal fixation and adequate vergence phoria relationship.
3. Able to distinguish aviation signal red, aviation signal green, and white.
4. No acute or chronic pathological condition of either eye of adnexae that might interfere with its proper function, might progress to that degree, or be aggravated by flying.
5. No serious pathology.

Note: By amendment regulations (12/21/76) correction may be by spectacles or contact lenses.

TABLE 47

VISION STANDARDS FOR ADMISSION TO SERVICE ACADEMIES*

Coast Guard Academy	Minimum Uncorrected 20/200 each eye Correctible to 20/20 each eye Refractive error: Not more than ±5.50D. any meridian. Astigmatism not over 3.00D. Anisometropia not exceeding 3.50D. Full visual fields Normal color vision No chronic, disfiguring, disabling, ocular pathology.
U.S. Merchant Marine Academy	Minimum uncorrected 20/100 each eye. Correctible to 20/20 each eye. Refractive error: As Coast Guard Academy Color Vision, normal by Farnsworth Lantern Test or Pseudoisochromatic plates. Certain pathologies may disqualify.
U.S. Naval Academy	Uncorrected vision 20/20 each eye. Limited waivers if correctable to 20/20 each eye and to Refraction Standards, Coast Guard Academy. ColorVision, normal. No waivers. No chronic, disfiguring, disabling ocular pathology.
U.S. Military Academy	Distance vision correctable to 20/20 each eye Refractive error: As Coast Guard Academy Able to distinguish vivid red and green. ET less than 15 prism diopters XT less than 10 prism diopters Hypertropia less than 2 prism diopters Certain pathologies may disqualify.
U.S. Air Force Academy	*Pilot:* Uncorrected vision 20/20 or better each eye, far and near. Refractive error: Hyperopia no greater than +1.75 diopters and nearsightedness less than plano in any one meridian, the astigmatic error must not exceed 0.75 diopters. *Navigator:* Uncorrected vision 20/70 or better correctable with ordinary glasses to 20/20 each eye. Near Acuity 20/20 or better each eye, uncorrected. Hyperopia not greater than +3.00 diopters and Myopia not greater than –1.50 diopters any meridian. Astigmatism not to exceed 2.00 diopters. *Commission:* Distant acuity correctable 20/40 one eye and 20/70 in other, or 20/30 one eye and 20/100 in other. Near acuity correctable to 20/20 (J_1) one eye and 20/30 (J_2) in other. Refractive error of equivalent sphere of not more than ±8.00 D. No chronic, disfiguring, disabling ocular pathology

*Based on information as of 17 May, 1983 Medical Examination Review Board, Department of Defense

TABLE 48

VISION STANDARDS FOR MOTOR VEHICLE OPERATION*

	WITHOUT GLASSES 2 EYES	WITHOUT GLASSES 1 BLIND EYE	WITH GLASSES 2 EYES	WITH GLASSES 1 BLIND EYE	DEPTH PERCEPTION	COLOR BLINDNESS	VISUAL FIELDS
AL	20/40	20/30	20/70	20/60	S	S	X
AK	20/40	20/40	20/40	20/40	S	X	X—T
AZ	20/40	20/40	20/40	20/40	S	S	X
AR	20/40	20/30	20/50	20/40	X	S	110°
CA	20/40	20/40	20/40	20/40	X	X	X—T
CO	20/40	20/40	20/40	20/40	S	S	X
CT	20/40	20/30	20/40	20/30	S	S	120°
DE	20/40	20/40	20/40	20/40	S	S	X-T
DC	20/40	20/40	20/40	20/40	SC	S	130°
FL	20/70	20/40	20/70	20/40	X	X	X
GA	20/60	20/60	20/60	20/60	S	S	140°
HI	20/40	20/40	20/40	20/40	S	S	140°
ID	20/40	20/40	20/40	20/40	S	S	S—T
IL	20/40	20/40	20/40	20/40	X	S	X—T
IN	20/40	20/30	20/50	20/40	S	S	S—T
IA	20/40	20/40	20/40	20/40	S	SC	X
KS	20/40	20/30	20/70	20/30	X	X	X—T
KY	20/45	20/33	20/60	20/45	S	X	X
LA	20/40	20/40	20/40	20/40	S	S	SC—T
ME	20/40	20/40	20/40	20/40	S	S	S—T
MD	20/40	20/40	20/40	20/40	S	S	140°
MA	20/40	20/40	20/40	20/40	X	S	120°-T
MI	20/40	20/40	20/40	20/40	X	X	140°
MN	20/40	20/30	20/40	20/30	S	S	S-T
MS	20/40	20/30	20/30	20/30	S	S	120°
MO	20/40	20/40	20/70	20/70	S	S	140°—T
MT	20/40	20/40	20/40	20/40	S	S	X
NB	20/40	20/30	20/40	20/30	S	S	120°
NV	20/40	20/30	20/40	20/50	S	S	X—T
NH	20/40	20/30	20/40	20/30	S	S	120°
NJ	20/50	20/50	20/50	20/50	X	S	X
NM	20/40	20/40	20/40	20/40	X	S	X
NY	20/40	20/40	20/40	20/40	X	S	X**—T
NC	20/40	20/29	20/50	20/40	X	S	X
ND	20/40	20/30	20/40	20/30	OP	OP	OP
OH	20/40	20/30	20/70	20/60	S	S	X
OK	20/40	20/30	20/40	20/30	S	S	140°
OR	20/40	20/40	20/40	20/40	S	S	100°
PA	20/40	20/40	20/40	20/40	SC	SC	SC
RI	20/40	20/40	20/40	20/40	S	S	S
SC	20/40	20/20	20/40	20/40	X	S	X
SD	20/40	20/40	20/40	20/40	S	S	X—T
TN	20/70	20/40	20/70	20/40	X	X	X
TX	20/40	20/25	20/70	20/70	X	S	X—T
UT	20/40	20/40	20/40	20/40	X	X	X
VT	20/40	20/40	20/40	20/40	S	S	120°
VA	20/40	20/40	20/40	20/40	X	S	100°
WA	20/40	20/40	20/40	20/40	FU	S	X
WV	20/40	20/40	20/40	20/40	S	S	X
WI	20/40	20/40	20/40	20/40	S	S	X
WY	20/40	20/40	20/40	20/40	S	S	X-T

T License Bioptic Drivers
X Not required
S Standard Practice
SC Special Cases
OP Optional with examiner, or hearing officer
FU Fusion Test
** 20/70 with 140° field

*Adapted from "1977 Survey of State Standards for Motor Vehicle Operators." American Optometric Assn., St. Louis. MO

2. LOW VISION

Federal regulation establishes legal blindness when the best vision obtained, in the better, is 20/200 or less, or when, despite the acuity attained, the field of vision of the better eye is 20° or less. While most states have adopted these standards, individual variations may exist at the local level.

Patients having reduced or subnormal vision for their visual tasks, whose best corrected vision ranges from 20/50 downwards toward the 20/200 level can frequently be aided by the same techniques and devices used for the legally blind and visually rehabilitated.

Many of the legally blind can be helped to work, travel, enjoy social and educational activities. Rehabilitation training programs, in addition to optical and non-optical aids, can help restore and maintain independence and mobility, make them productive individuals.

Increased vision is obtained for those patients, considered partially sighted rather than partially blind, by magnification or approximation. This is accomplished by low vision procedures, aids, and devices. At distance this may be accomplished by telescopic devices. Although these devices are difficult to use while moving about, they may be quite effective to momentarily see a street sign, house or bus number, etc. Seated, they are effective aids in the theatre, at sporting events, or in the classroom to view the blackboard. They are obtainable in magnifications of 2.2, 2.5, 3.0, 3.5, 4.0, 6.0, 8.0 10x. (Designs for Vision, Keeler, Nikon, Selsi. Walters, Zeiss). Some are fixed focus, others may be refocused for view of closer material. Minimum magnification to secure desired acuity is used because of the diminishing field as the power is increased. Individual design and construction may result in a slight variance between the fields produced with each magnification by different manufacturers. An estimate may be drawn from the devices produced by Designs for Vision:

MAGNIFICATION	FIELD AT 20 FT.
2.2 Standard	12°
2.2 Wide angle	17°
3.0 Standard	8°
	12°
4.0 Standard	6°

Telescopes, fitted with reading cap lenses permit reading at further distances than high plus aids. A familiar example of this system is the surgical loupe.

Near vision is augmented by higher adds, high plus "Micro' lenses (American Optical Corp, Lucerne Optical), binocular loupes, hand-held or stand magnifiers. The higher plus values permit approximation to increase the angle subtended with lesser or no demand on the accommodation. The add to obtain J5 can be estimated by the inverse of the best distance vision obtained. For example, best distance vision 20/200, therefore 200/20 or 10D. Further detail may be obtained through increased add power or supplementary hand-held or stand magnifiers. If the patient will not read at extremely close range, lower adds may be used in combination with hand-held or stand magnifiers, or a telemicroscope system used to provide required magnification and desired working distance by use of a reading cap or objective lens power modification, as in a surgical loupe. When binocular function is present, prism base-in may be required in the near Rx (about 1 prism diopter per diopter of add). Plastic lens half-eye spectacles of 6, 8 or 10D, with incorporated prism are available. (American Optical Company, Lucerne Optical). Hand-held magnifiers range from 2x to 8x (Bausch & Lomb, Coburn, Coil, Eschenbach, McLeod, Selsi). Once again, the higher powers have increasingly diminished fields of view. Patients with physical infirmities can use stand magnifiers which rest on the material and remain in focus as they are moved across the page.

Non-optical aids include reading masks, large print books, newspapers, and periodicals, heavy ruled stationery, check-writing guides, large playing cards, easy threading needles. There are also fixed magnification opaque projection magnifiers (Nesbit Co.) and closed circuit television devices (CCTV) with variable magnification. The closed circuit television permits a greater range of magnification and can, by reversal of polarity, provide a white on black image rather than a black on white. This for many, is an additional aid in seeing the material (Telesensory Systems, Visualtek). Advances in electronics have made possible talking clocks, calculators, and many business machines whose "voices" open the way to gainful employment for the visually impaired. A "Catalogue of Optical Aids" is available from the New York Association for the Blind, 111 East 59th Street, New York, N.Y. 10022.

The American Foundation for the Blind, 15 West 16 St., NY, NY 10011, has "Aids for the 80's", "Products for People with Visual Handicaps" and a "Catalogue of Publications" . All of these can serve to be of further help to the low-visioned patient.

The Talking Books Program may be joined by application to the National Library Science for the Blind and Physically Handicapped, Library of Congress, Washington, DC, 20542.

Absorptive lenses provide glare protection and can also help to improve acuity when the media are clouded. 5% to 15% transmission neutral grey lenses are specifically recommended for achromatopes who may also require the protection of wide side-shield frames. Albinotic patients are aided by the brown tints. 75% transmission indoors and 25% transmission outdoors. Retinitis Pigmentosa patients generally require daytime outdoor protection with the darker sunglass tints and many are aided in night vision by the Kalichrome (Bausch & Lomb) and Hazemaster (American Optical Company) lenses.

TABLE 49

DIRECTORY OF STATE SERVICES FOR THE VISUALLY HANDICAPPED*

AL	Voc. Rehab., 2129 E. South Blvd. POB 11586, Montgomery 36111
AK	Office of Voc. Rehab., Pouch F. Mail Sta. 0581, Juneau 99811
AZ	Rehab. Svcs. Bureau, Dept. Econ. Sec., 1535 West Jefferson, Suite 155, Phoenix 85007
AR	Dept. of Soc. & Rehab. Svcs., 1801 Rebsamen Pk. Rd., POB 3781, Little Rock 72203
CA	Dept. of Rehab., Health & Welf. Agency, 722 Capitol Mall, Sacramento 95814
CO	Div. of Rehab., Dept. Soc. Svcs., 1575 Sherman St., Denver 80203
CT	Bd. of Ed. & Svcs. for Blind, 170 Ridge Rd., Wethersfield 06109
DE	Del. Bureau for Vis. Impaired, Dept Health & S.S., 305 W 8th St., Wilmington 19801
DC	Soc. & Rehab. Adm., Dept. Human Res., 122 C St., N.W., 8 Fl., Washington 20001
FL	Bureau Blind Services, Dept. of Ed., 1309 Winewood Blvd., Tallahassee 32301
GA	Dept. Human Res., Div. Voc. Rehab., 47 Trinity Ave., Atlanta 30334
GU	Div. Voc. Rehab., Bd. of Control Voc. Rehab., Dept of Ed. POB IO-C, Agana 96910
HI	Div. Voc. Rehab., Dept. Soc. Svcs. Queen Liliuokalani Bldg., POB 339 Honolulu 96809
ID	Idaho Comm. for Blind, Statehouse, Boise 83720
IL	Bd. Voc. Ed. & Rehab., Div Voc. Rehab., 623 E. Adams St., Springfield 62706
IN	Indiana Rehab. Svcs, 1028 Illinois Bldg, 17 W. Market St., Indianapolis 46204
IA	Comm. for the Blind, 4th & Keosauqua, Des Moines 50309
KS	Svcs. for Blind & Vis. Handicapped, Soc. & Rehab. Svce. 2700 W. 6th St., Topeka 66606
KY	Bur. of Rehab. Svcs., Capital Plaza Office Tower, Frankfort 40601
LA	La. Health & Human Res., Family Svce., 755 Riverside N. Box 44065, Baton Rouge 70804
ME	Bureau of Rehab., 32 Winthrop St., Augusta 04330
MD	Div. Voc. Rehab., State Dept. Ed., Bx 8717, Balt./Wash. Intnl. Airport Baltimore 21240
MA	Mass. Commission for Blind, 39 Boylston St., Boston 02116
MI	Dept. Soc. Svcs., Div, Svcs. for Blind, 300 S. Capitol Ave, Lansing 48926
MN	State Svcs. for Blind & Vis. Handicapped, 1745 University Ave, St. Paul 55104
MS	Vocational Rehab. for Blind, POB 4872, Jackson 39216
MO	Bur. for Blind, Dept. Soc. Svcs, B'way State Office Bldg, Jefferson City 65101
MT	Visual Svce. Div., Dept. Soc & Rehab. Svcs, POB 1723, Helena 59601
NB	Svce. for the Visually Impaired, 1047 South St., Lincoln 68502
NV	Bureau of Svcs. for Blind, Dept. Human Res., 308 N. Curry St., Rm. 200, Carson City 89701
NH	State Dept. Ed., Div Voc. Rehab., 105 Loudon Rd., Bldg 3, Concord 03301
NJ	Comm. for Blind & Vis. Impaired; 1100 Raymond Blvd., Newark 07102
NM	Dept. of Ed., 231 Washington Ave., POB 1830, Sante Fe 87503
NY	State Dept. Soc. Svcs., Comm. for Visually Handicapped, 40 No. Pearl St., Albany 12243
NC	Div. Svcs. for Blind, N.C. Dept. Human Res., 410 N. Boylan Ave., Box 2658 Raleigh 27602
ND	Div. Voc. Rehab., 1025 N. 3rd St., Box 1037, Bismarck 58501
OH	Rehab. Svcs. Comm., 4656 Heaton Rd., Columbus 43229
OK	Dept. of Instit., Rehab. Svcs, Div. Rehab & Vis. Svcs., POB 25352, Oklahoma City 73125
OR	Comm. for Blind, 535 S.E. 12th Ave, Portland 97214
PA	Dept. Public Welfare, Bureau for Vis. Handicapped, Capital Assn. Bldg, POB 2675 Harrisburg 17120
PR	Asst. Secy. Voc. Rehab., Dept. Soc. Svcs., POB 1118, Hato Rey 00919
RI	Dept. of Soc. & Rehab. Svce, Svcs. for Blind, 46 Aborn St., Providence 02903
SC	Comm. for Blind, POB 11638, Capital Sta., Columbia 29211
SD	Dept. Soc. Svcs., Div. Rehab. Svcs, State Office Bldg, Illinois St., Pierre 57501
TN	Div. Svcs. for the Blind, Dept. Human Svcs, 303 State Office Bldg, Nashville 37219
TX	State Comm for the Blind, POB 12866, Capital Sta., 800 City Natn'l. Bank Bldg., Austin 78711
UT	Div. of Rehab. Svcs. 250 E. 5th Utah St. Bd. of Ed., Salt Lake City 84111
VT	Div. for the Blind & Vis. Handicapped, Dept. Soc. & Rehab. Svcs. 81 River St., Montpelier 05602
VA	Virginia Comm. for Visually ,Handicapped, 3003 Parkwood Ave, Richmond 23221
VI	Dept. Soc. Welf., Div. Voc. Rehab., POB 539, St Thomas 00801
WA	Off. Svcs for Blind, Dept. Soc. & Health Svcs., 3411 So Alaska St., Seattle 98118
WV	Div. Voc. Rehab., State Bd. Voc. Ed., State Capital, P&G Bldg, Washington St., Charleston 25305
WIS	Div. Voc. Rehab., Dept. Health & Soc. Svcs., 1 W. Wilson St., Rm 720, Madison 53702
WY	Div. Voc. Rehab., Hathaway Bldg., West, Cheyenne 82002

*Compiled by Massachusetts Eye & Ear Infirmary from AFB Directory of agencies serving the visually handicapped.

SECTION 6

EVALUATION OF PERMANENT VISUAL IMPAIRMENT

The purpose of this chapter is to provide criteria for use in evaluating permanent impairment resulting from dysfunction of the visual system, which consists of the eyes, ocular adnexa and the visual pathways. A simplified method is provided for quantitating visual impairment, which can then be translated into impairment of the whole person.

Visual impairment in varying degrees occurs in the presence of a deviation from normal in one or more functions of the eye, including (1.) corrected visual acuity for objects at distance and near; (2.) visual fields; and (3.) ocular motility with diplopia. Evaluation of visual impairment is based on these three functions. Although they are not equally important, vision is imperfect without the coordinated function of all three.

Other ocular functions and disturbances are considered to the extent that they are reflected in one or more of the three coordinated functions. These other functions include color perception, adaptation to light and dark, contrast sensitivity, accommodation, metamorphopsia, and stereoscopic vision. Ocular disturbances include paresis of accommodation, iridoplegia, entropion, ectropion, epiphora, lagophthalmos and scarring. To the extent that any ocular disturbance causes impairment not reflected in visual acuity, visual fields, or ocular motility with diplopia, the impairment must be evaluated by the physician and be added to the impairment of the visual system.

One or more other ocular impairments, such as vitreous opacities, a nonreactive pupil, and light scattering disturbances of the cornea or other media, may be calculated as an additional 5% to 10% impairment of the involved eye. Permanent deformities of the orbit, scars, and cosmetic defects that may not alter ocular function should be considered individually as an additional factor that can cause up to 10% impairment of the whole person. If facial disfigurement due to scarring above the upper lip is evaluated, then any overlapping percentage of impairment due to ocular scarring should be subtracted from the larger percentage.

The following equipment is necessary to test the functions of the eyes:

1. Visual acuity test charts for distance and near vision. For distance vision, the Snellen test chart with nonserif block letters* or numbers, or the illiterate E chart, or Landolt's broken-ring chart is desirable. For near vision, many charts are available, such as those with print similar to that of the Snellen chart, with Revised Jaeger Standard print, or with American point-type notation for use at 35 cm or 14 inches.

2. An arc, bowl, or other validated perimeter with standard radius of 30 cm to 33 cm, or with a larger radius, if an appropriately larger target is used.

3. Refraction equipment.

Before using the information in this chapter, the reader is urged to consult the Preface to the Guides, which provides a general discussion of the purpose of the Guides, and of the situations in which they are useful; and discusses techniques for the evaluation of the patient and for report preparation .

The report should include the information found in the following outline.

A. *Medical Evaluation*

1. Narrative history of medical conditions
2. Results of the most recent clinical evaluation
3. Assessment of current clinical status and state ment of future plans
4. Diagnoses and clinical impressions
5. Expected date of full or partial recovery

B. *Analysis of Findings*

1. Impact of medical condition(s) on life activities
2. Explanation for concluding that the medical condition(s) has or has not become.static or well-stabilized
3. Explanation for concluding that the individual is or is not likely to suffer from sudden or subtle incapacitation
4. Explanation for concluding that the individual is or is not likely to suffer injury or further impairment by engaging in life activities or by attempting to meet personal, social and occupational demands
5. Explanation for concluding that accommodations and/or restrictions are or are not warranted

C. *Comparison of Results of Analysis with Impairment Criteria*

1. Description of clinical findings, and how these findings relate to specific criteria in the chapter
2.. Explanation of each percent of impairment rating
3. Summary list of all impairment ratings
4. Overall rating of impairment of the whole person

---

*The 10 equally difficult letters (D, K, R, H, V, C, N, Z, S, O) of Louise L. Sloan are recommended for uniformity. Each letter subtends a visual angle of 5 minutes and a stroke width of I minute.

1. CRITERIA AND METHODS FOR EVALUATING PERMANENT IMPAIRMENT

Central Visual Acuity

Test chart illumination of at least 5 foot-candles is recommended to attain a distinct contrast of .85 or greater and a comfortable luminance of approximately 85 ± 5 candelas per square meter. The chart or reflecting surface should not be dirty or discolored. The far test distance simulates infinity at 6 m (20 ft) or at no less than 4 m (13 ft 1 in). The near test distance should be fixed at 35 cm (14 in) in keeping with the Revised Jaeger Standard. Adequate and comfortable illumination must be diffused onto the test card at a level about three times greater than that of usual room illumination. Measurements of visual acuity at near have less interest reproducibility than those made of visual acuity at distance. Many occupational needs depend disproportionately on acuity of near vision.

Central vision should be measured and recorded for distance and for near objects, with and without wearing conventional spectacles. The use of contact lenses may further improve vision reduced by irregular astigmatism due to corneal injury or disease. However, practical problems related to fitting, expense, development of tolerance, and the fact that contact lenses are at times medically contraindicated, are sufficient at present to justify the recommendation that conventional ophthalmic lenses be used to obtain best corrected vision. In the absence of contraindications, if the patient is well adapted to contact lenses and wishes to wear them, correction by contact lenses is acceptable.

Visual acuity for distance should be recorded in the Snellen notation, using a fraction in which the numerator is the test distance in feet or meters, and the denominator is the distance at which the smallest letter discriminated by the patient would subtend 5 minutes of arc, that is, the distance at which an eye with 20/20 vision would see that letter. The fraction notation is one of convenience that does not imply percentage of visual acuity. A similar Snellen notation using centimeters or inches, or a comparable Revised Jaeger Standard or American point-type notation, may be used in designating near visual acuity.

The notations for acuity of distance and near vision that appear in **Table 50**, with corresponding percentages of loss of central vision, are included only to indicate the basic values used in developing **Table 51.** Simply adding two percentages of loss, corresponding to appropriate notations for distance and near vision, does not provide the true percentage of loss of central vision. Rather, the functional loss of central vision is the mean of the two percentages.

Monocular aphakia or monocular pseudophakia is considered to be an additional visual impairment, and if it is present, it is weighted by an additional 50% decrease in the value for remaining corrected central vision, as noted in **Table 51.**

TABLE 50

VISUAL ACUITY NOTATIONS WITH CORRESPONDING PERCENTAGES OF LOSS OF CENTRAL VISION

FOR DISTANCE			
	SNELLEN NOTATIONS		
ENGLISH	METRIC 6	METRIC 4	% LOSS
20/15	6/5	4/3	0
20/20	6/6	4/4	0
20/25	6/75	4/5	5
20/30	6/10	4/6	10
20/40	6/12	4/8	15
20/50	6/15	4/10	25
20/60	6/20	4/12	35
20/70	6/22	4/14	40
20/80	6/24	4/16	45
20/100	6/30	4/20	50
20/125	6/38	4/25	60
20/150	6/50	4/30	70
20/200	6/60	4/40	80
20/3 00	6/90	4/60	85
20/400	6/120	4/80	90
20/800	6/240	4/160	95

		FOR NEAR		
INCHES	NEAR SNELLEN CM.	REVISED JAEGER STANDARD	AMERICAN POINT-TYPE	%LOSS
14/14	35/35	1	3	0
14/18	35/45	2	4	0
14/21	35/53	3	5	5
14/24	35/60	4	6	7
14/28	35/70	5	7	10
14/35	35/88	6	8	50
14/40	35/100	7	9	55
14/45	35/113	8	10	60
14/60	35/150	9	11	80
14/70	35/175	10	12	85
14/80	35/200	11	13	87
14/88	35/220	12	14	90
14/112	35/280	13	21	95
14/140	35/350	14	23	98

The procedure for determining loss of central vision in one eye is us follows:

1. Measure and record best central visual acuity for distance and for near, with and without conventional corrective spectacles or contact lenses.

2. Consult **Table 51** to derive the percentage loss by combining best connected near and distance acuities, and to calculate the additional loss of central vision that results from the presence of aphakia or pseudophakia.

Example: Without allowance for monocular aphakia. 14/70 for near vision and 20/200 for distance produce 83% loss of central vision. With allowance for monocular aphakia, which is applicable to corrected vision only, 14/70 for near vision and 20/200 for distance produce 91% loss of central vision.

continued on next page

TABLE 51

LOSS OF CENTRAL VISION* IN PERCENTAGE

SNELLEN RATING FOR DISTANCE IN FEET	APPROXIMATE SNELLING RATING FOR NEAR IN INCHES													
	14/14	14/18	14/21	14/24	14/28	14/35	14/40	14/45	14/60	14/70	14/80	14/88	14/112	14/140
20/15	0	0	3	4	5	25	27	30	40	43	44	45	48	49
	50	50	52	52	53	63	64	65	70	72	72	73	74	75
20/20	0	0	3	4	5	25	27	30	40	43	44	46	48	49
	50	50	52	52	53	63	64	65	70	72	72	73	74	75
20/25	3	3	5	6	8	28	30	33	43	45	46	48	50	52
	52	52	53	53	54	64	65	67	72	73	73	74	75	76
20/30	5	5	8	9	10	30	32	35	45	48	49	50	53	54
	53	53	54	54	55	65	66	68	73	74	74	75	76	77
20/40	8	8	10	11	13	33	35	38	48	50	51	53	55	57
	54	54	55	56	57	67	68	69	74	75	76	77	78	79
20/50	13	13	15	16	18	38	40	43	53	55	56	58	60	62
	57	57	58	58	59	69	70	72	77	78	78	79	80	81
20/60	16	16	18	20	22	41	44	46	56	59	60	61	64	65
	58	58	59	60	61	70	72	73	78	79	80	81	82	83
20/80	20	20	23	24	25	45	47	50	60	63	64	65	68	69
	60	60	62	62	63	73	74	75	80	82	82	83	84	85
20/100	25	25	28	29	30	50	52	55	65	68	69	70	73	74
	63	63	64	64	65	75	76	78	83	84	84	85	87	87
20/125	30	30	33	34	35	55	57	60	70	73	74	75	78	79
	65	65	67	67	68	78	79	80	85	87	87	88	89	90
20/150	34	34	37	38	39	59	61	64	74	77	78	79	82	83
	67	67	68	69	70	80	81	82	87	88	89	90	91	92
20/200	40	40	43	44	45	65	67	70	80	83	84	85	88	89
	70	70	72	72	73	83	84	85	90	91	92	93	94	95
20/300	43	43	45	46	48	68	70	73	83	85	86	88	90	92
	72	72	73	73	74	84	85	87	91	93	93	94	95	96
20/400	45	45	48	49	50	70	72	75	85	88	89	90	93	94
	73	73	74	74	75	85	86	88	93	94	94	95	97	97
20/800	48	48	50	51	53	73	75	78	88	90	91	93	95	97
	74	74	75	76	77	87	88	89	94	95	96	97	98	99

*Upper figure = % loss of central vision without allowance for monocular aphakia or monocular pseudophakia; low figure = % loss of central vision with allowance for monocular aphakia or monocular pseudophakia.

Visual Fields

For the purposes of these *Guides*, one level suprathreshold screening is acceptable. The standard reference for visual field measurement is the Goldmann kinetic outer isopter of the III/4e stimulus. This is approximately equivalent to the arc perimeter examination using a 3 mm white test target at a radius of 330 mm which is also acceptable under these *Guides*. Automated programs cannot be used to quantify visual field impairments between the outer limit of their radii (usually 30° or 60° and, less frequently, 70° or 80° from fixation) and the normal outer extent of the functional visual field.

Current and widely available automated perimeters, such as the Allergan-Humphrey 635 or the Techna Vision, Inc. (formerly Coopervision) Dicon, can test only those points of the visual field that are within the radius or the bowl or radius of the specific programmed test sequence used. Thus, the Allergan-Humphrey Field Analyzer with its 30-1 or 30-2 program tests only within a field radius of 30°. At the 10 decibel level this provides an equivalent stimulus to the Goldmann III/4e but no direct test of the visual field between 30° from fixation and the outer limit or normal extent of the visual field. The Humphrey "full field 81-point program" tests only within the radius of 60° from fixation: however, threshold peripheral tests from 30° to 60° from fixation are available. The Squid (Synemed, Inc.) provides a peripheral field program covering the outer ring from 30° to 70° from fixation. Techna Vision offers a 30-2 program with two peripheral isopters at 30° and 80° plus Esterman monocular and binocular grid programs at a suitable target intensity of 2500 apostilbs. Software packages are available to deliver Esterman monocular and binocular scores.

If the ocular history and examination are essentially normal and suggest no lesions involving the outer extent of the visual fields, then normal central visual fields produced by automated programs within 30° or 60° may be submitted to confirm a report of normal visual fields. Alternatively, if the history and examination indicate circumferential impairment of the peripheral fields extending within the programmed test radius of 30° or 60° from fixation, then automated programs may be used to report visual field loss of such a greater extent. This will be based on findings transferred to an Esterman Grid or plotted as loss from the normal extent of visual field from point of fixation (Figure 1).

Figure 1.—Example of Perimetric Charts Used to Plot Extent or Outline of Visual Field Along the Eight Principal Meridians that are Separated by 45° Intervals.

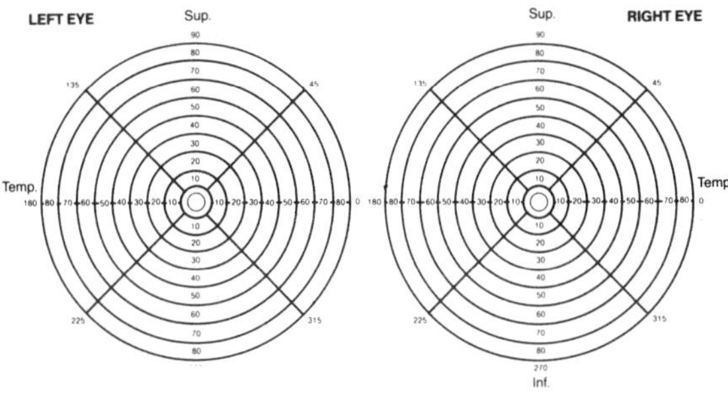

The examiner should use preferentially a binocular test of the functional visual field in distinction to the monocular visual field test, which is done for diagnostic purposes and may be assessed with a wide range of instruments. For binocular field testing the patient should have two eyes, proper alignment of the eyes, and no diplopia. If the patient has only one eye, if there is deviation (heterotropia) of either eye, or diplopia, then monocular visual field testing must be done. The binocular or functional field is derived from the usual use of the two eyes together and involves an overlapping area in the nasal portion of each field. This produces some enhancement of object awareness in the overlapping areas, although apparently not in the patient with advanced glaucoma. The chin rest must be positioned in the midline for suitable candidates so that the two eyes are evenly to the right and to the left of the central fixation target. Both eyes are kept open and the seeing field outline (isopter) is recorded on an Esterman Grid or similar chart (Figure 2A). A normal or standard outer isopter for the binocular field has been validated in studies of more than 2,000 individuals.

Accordingly, an outer limit (isopter) of functional awareness must be established from examination by arc perimeter, bowl perimeter, or other validated instrument and transferred as a line to the Esterman 120 unit binocular grid. A simple count of all the printed dots seen to be entirely outside of or falling on the line (isopter) marking the extent of the visual field provides for the scoring of functional loss to a maximum of 120 units. This is multiplied by 5/6 to yield the percentage loss of the binocular functional field.

For the one-eyed patient or the individual with diplopia or with apparent deviation of either eye (heterotropia), the Esterman 100 unit monocular field is preferably used (Figure 2B). A simple count of all the printed dots seen to be entirely outside of or falling on the line (isopter) marking the extent of the visual field provides an immediate percentage of field loss. (Conversely, a simple count of the printed dots within each grid square which fall within or do not touch the contour line gives the percentage of visual field retention for that eye.)

For an examination with an arc perimeter, the examiner should use a white disc that is 6 mm in diameter, at a distance of 33 cm, to test an aphakic patient whose eye is uncorrected, that is, not adapted to a contact lens or to an intraocular (pseudophake) implant, or whose eye is fitted with aphakic spectacles. If in these instances a Goldmann bowl perimeter is used, the target should be IV/4e in the kinetic mode. If the aphakic patient is well adapted to a contact lens or an intraocular lens, then the examiner should use the 3 mm diameter white target at 33 cm, or the Goldmann III/4e target, or equivalent.

In kinetic testing, the object is brought from the periphery to the seeing area. At least two peripheral fields

Figure 2A.—Esterman 120-unit Binocular Scoring Grid for Use with Both Eyes Open.

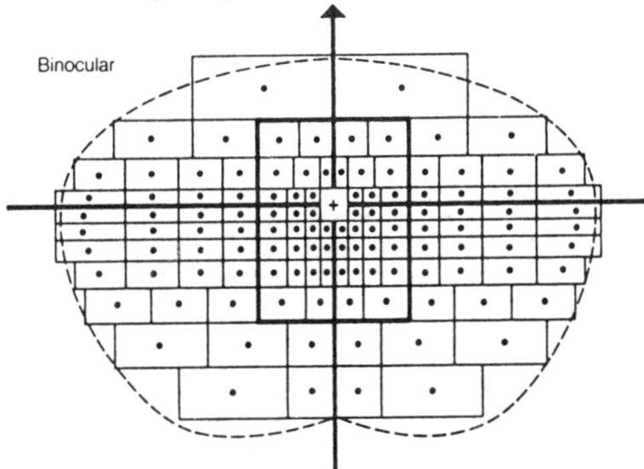

Figure 2B.—Esterman 100-unit Monocular Scoring Grid for Arc or Bowl Perimeter or Similar Automated Instrument Providing Full Monocular Field Analysis.

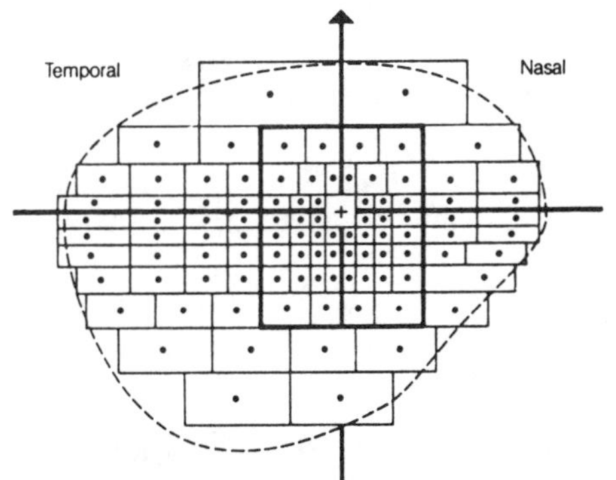

(Grids may be obtained from the Manhattan Eye Ear and Throat Hospital, 210 East 64th Street, NY, NY 10021)

continued on next page

should be obtained that agree within 15° in each meridian. The reliability of the patient's responses should be noted. The result is plotted on a visual field chart for each of the eight principal meridians that are separated by 45° intervals (Figure 1). The minimal normal extent of the visual field from the point of fixation is indicated in **Table 51** on page 54. The figures represent somewhat less than average normal performance, which allows for poor or delayed subjective responses or for unusual prominence of brow or nose.

The percentage of retained visual field in one eye is obtained by adding to the number of degrees remaining along the eight principal meridians given in **Table 51** for the 3/330 white isopter; which normally sum to 500 degrees, and dividing the total by 5. Conversely, the percentage loss of visual field is obtained by adding the number of degrees lost along each of the eight meridians, and dividing the total by 5. Where there is loss of a quadrant or of half a field, one-half of the value of each of the two boundary meridians should be added to the calculated loss. Visual field losses of other amounts and from other conditions can be calculated in a similar manner.

Although the extent of loss of visual fields cannot be determined accurately for a scotoma, an approximation can be obtained by subtracting the width of the scotoma from the peripheral visual field value at the same meridians. A similar estimation of visual field loss can be applied to enlargement of the blind spot with the use of a 2 mm test object at a distance of 1 m from the tangent screen while the patient is wearing corrective lenses. For example, a general enlargement of the blind spot of 5° would result in a visual field loss of 8 × 5 ÷ 5 = 8% loss. Because a central scotoma directly affects central visual acuity, which is evaluated first, such visual field loss is not used again in the final calculation of visual loss.

Determining Loss of Monocular Visual Fields

The following steps are taken to determine the loss of monocular visual fields in each eye.

1. The nontested eye is occluded, and the patient is positioned on the chin rest so that the tested eye is centered on the fixation target.

2. Plot the extent of the visual fields on each of the eight principal meridians of a visual field chart (See Figure 1).

3. (a) Determine the degrees lost by adding the degrees of visual field lost in each of the principal meridians (See **Table 53**).

(b) If half of a field is lost, include the two boundary meridians at a value equal to one half their total degrees value (**Table 53**).

4. Consult **Table 54** to ascertain corresponding percentage of visual field loss.

5. Because the inferior visual field is occupationally more significant than the superior visual field, lower quadrant defects are weighted by an additional 5% loss of the visual field. Correspondingly, an inferior hemianopic loss is weighted by an additional 10% loss of the visual field.

6. When the monocular Esterman scale (Figure 2B) is used, count all the printed dots seen to be entirely outside of or falling on the line (isopter) marking the extent of the visual field. This number is the final percent of visual field loss for that eye and automatically takes into account the additional weighting for lower field defects.

Abnormal Ocular Motility and Binocular Diplopia

Unless a patient has diplopia within 30° of the center of fixation, the diplopia rarely causes significant visual

TABLE 52

MINIMAL NORMAL EXTENT OF VISUAL FIELD FROM POINT OF FIXATION

	DEGREES
Temporally	85
Down temporally	85
Down	65
Down nasally	50
Nasally	60
Up nasally	55
Up	45
Up temporally	55
Total	500

TABLE 53

LOSS OF VISUAL FIELD

Example 1: A patient has a concentric contraction to 30 degrees:

LOSS	DEGREES
Temporally	55
Down temporally	55
Direct down	35
Down nasally	20
Nasally	30
Up nasally	25
Direct up	15
Up temporally	25
Total loss	260

The loss of 260 degrees is equivalent to 52% loss of visual field.

Example 2. A patient has an entire temporal field loss.

LOSS	DEGREES
Up temporally	55
Temporally	85
Down temporally	85
Half of direct up and direct down (45 & 65)	55
Total loss	280

The loss of 280 degrees is equivalent to 56% loss of visual field.

TABLE 54

LOSS OF MONOCULAR VISUAL FIELD

Total Degrees Lost	Total Degrees Retained	% of Loss	Total Degrees Lost	Total Degrees Retained	% of Loss	Total Degrees Lost	Total Degrees Retained	% of Loss
0	500*	0	170	330	34	340	160	68
5	495	1	175	325	35	345	155	69
10	490	2	180	320	36	350	150	70
15	485	3	185	315	37	355	145	71
20	480	4	190	310	38	360	140	72
25	475	5	195	305	39	365	135	73
30	470	6	200	300	40	370	130	74
35	465	7	205	295	41	375	125	75
40	460	8	210	290	42	380	120	76
45	455	9	215	285	43	385	115	77
50	450	10	220	280	44	390	110	78
55	445	11	225	275	45	395	105	79
60	440	12	230	270	46	400	100	80
65	435	13	235	265	47	405	95	81
70	430	14	240	260	48	410	90	82
75	425	15	245	255	49	415	85	83
80	420	16	250	250	50	420	80	84
85	415	17	255	245	51	425	75	85
90	410	18	260	240	52	430	70	86
95	405	19	265	235	53	435	65	87
100	400	20	270	230	54	440	60	88
105	395	21	275	225	55	445	55	89
110	390	22	280	220	56	450	50	90
115	385	23	285	215	57	455	45	91
120	380	24	290	210	58	460	40	92
125	375	25	295	205	59	465	35	93
130	370	26	300	200	60	470	30	94
135	365	27	305	195	61	475	25	95
140	360	28	310	190	62	480	20	96
145	355	29	315	185	63	485	15	97
150	350	30	320	180	64	490	10	98
155	345	31	325	175	65	495	5	99
160	340	32	330	170	66	500	0	100
165	335	33	335	165	67			

*Or more

impairment. An exception is diplopia upon looking downward. The extent of diplopia in the various directions of gaze is determined on an arc perimeter at 33 cm, or at an equivalent bowl perimeter radius, from the patient's eyes. Examination is made in each of the eight major meridians by using a small test light, or the projected light of approximately Goldmann III/4e without adding colored lenses or correcting prisms.

To determine the impairment of ocular motility the patient is seated with both eyes open and the chin resting in the chin rest, approximately centered so that the eyes are equidistant to either side of the central fixation target.

1. Plot the presence of diplopia along the meridians of a suitable visual field chart.

2. Add the percentages for loss of ocular motility due to diplopia in the meridian of maximum impairment as indicated in Figure 3.

3. In the patient with one eye, with profound amblyopia or with profound loss of vision, individual evaluation of motility will be made by the examiner.

Example: Diplopia within the central 20° is equivalent to 100% impairment of ocular motility.

Example: Diplopia on looking horizontally off center from 20° to 30° is equivalent to 20% loss of ocular motility; 30° to 40° is equivalent to 10% loss of ocular motility; for a total of 30% loss of ocular motility.

Steps to Determine Impairment of the Visual System and of the Whole Person Contributed by the Visual System

Calculate and record:

- percentage loss of central vision (CV) for each eye separately,
- percentage loss of visual field (VF) for each eye separately,

and

- percentage loss of ocular motility (OM).

continued on next page

A. If the percentage loss of VF is calculated for each eye separately (monocular), using the Combined Values Chart, combine the percentage loss of central vision with the percentage loss of visual field in each eye and record these values.

Example:

Right eye—

loss of central vision
(both near and distance)..............................56%
loss of visual field 32%
56% combined with 32%..............................70%

Left eye—

loss of central vision
(both near and distance)..............................46%
loss of visual field 32%
46% combined with 32%..............................63%

Again using the Combined Values Chart, combine the percentage loss of ocular motility with the combined value for central vision and visual field in the eye manifesting greater impairment. Disregard loss of ocular motility in other eye.

Example:

Right eye—

combined value of CV and VF 70%
loss of ocular motility 25%
70% combined with 25% 78%

Consult **Table 56** to ascertain impairment of the visual system.

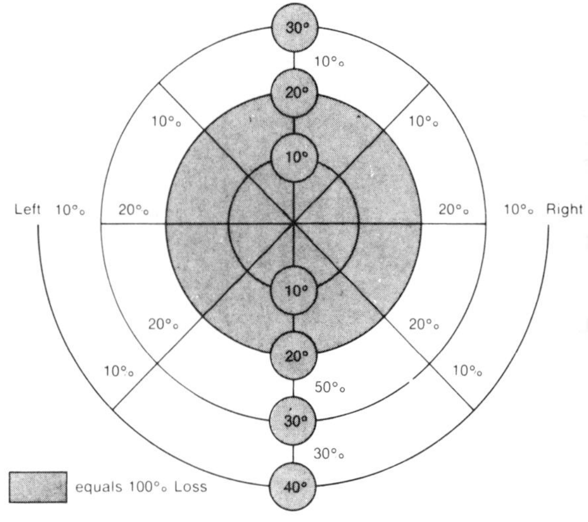

Figure 3—Percentage loss of ocular motility of one eye in diplopia fields.

Example:

Impairment of right (worse) eye 78%
Impairment of left (better) eye 63%
Impairment of visual system 67%

Consult **Table 55** to ascertain the impairment of the whole person that is contributed by impairment of the visual system.

TABLE 55

IMPAIRMENT OF THE VISUAL SYSTEM AS IT RELATES TO IMPAIRMENT OF THE WHOLE PERSON

% IMPAIRMENT OF		% IMPAIRMENT OF		% IMPAIRMENT OF		% IMPAIRMENT OF		% IMPAIRMENT OF		% IMPAIRMENT OF	
VISUAL SYSTEM	WHOLE PERSON	VISUAL SYSTEM	WHOLE PERSON	VISUAL SYSTEM	WHOLE PERSON	VISUAL SYSTEM	WHOLE PERSON	VISUAL SYSTEM	WHOLE PERSON	VISUAL SYSTEM	WHOLE PERSON
0	0	15	14	30	28	45	42	60	57	75	71
1	1	16	15	31	29	46	43	61	58	76	72
2	2	17	16	32	30	47	44	62	59	77	73
3	3	18	17	33	31	48	45	63	59	78	74
4	4	19	18	34	32	49	46	64	60	79	75
5	5	20	19	35	33	50	47	65	61	80	76
6	6	21	20	36	34	51	48	66	62	81	76
7	7	22	21	37	35	52	49	67	63	82	77
8	8	23	22	38	36	53	50	68	64	83	78
9	8	24	23	39	37	54	51	69	65	84	79
10	9	25	24	40	38	55	52	70	66	85	80
11	10	26	25	41	39	56	53	71	67	86	81
12	11	27	25	42	40	57	54	72	68	87	82
13	12	28	26	43	41	58	55	73	69	88	83
14	13	29	27	44	42	59	56	74	70	89	84
										90-100	85

	% IMPAIRMENT VISUAL SYSTEM	% IMPAIRMENT WHOLE PERSON
Total loss of vision one eye	25	24
Total loss of vision both eyes	100	85

Example: 67% impairment of the visual system is equivalent to 63% impairment of the whole person.

3. If the percentage loss of VF is calculated for both eyes together (using the Esterman binocular grid), consult **Table 56** to ascertain impairment of the visual system due to loss of central vision .

Using a similar example:

Right eye

loss of CV (both near and distance)...............56%

Left eye

loss of CV (both near and distance)...............46%
impairment due to loss of CV of both eyes ...49%

Using the Combined Values Chart combine the impairment due to loss of CV with the impairment due to binocular visual field loss. *Note:* No value for loss of ocular motility is provided since binocular VF testing is not recommended when loss of ocular motility is present.

Example:

impairment due to loss of CV of both eyes....49%
impairment due to binocular VF loss 20%
impairment of visual system...........................59%

Consult Table 55 to ascertain the impairment of the whole person that is contributed by the visual system.

Example:

59% impairment of the visual system is equivalent to 56% impairment of the whole person.

Other Conditions

Up to an additional 10% impairment may be combined with the impairment of the whole person caused by the visual system for such conditions as permanent deformities of the orbit, scars, and other cosmetic deformities that do not otherwise alter ocular function.

REFERENCES

1. Sloan LL: New test charts for the measurement of visual acuity. *Am J Opthalmol* 1959;48:807-813 .
2. Report of Working Group 39, Committee on Vision, National Academy of Sciences: Recommended Standard Procedures for the Clinical Measurement and Specification of Visual Acuity. *Adv Ophthalmol* 1980;41; 103-143.
3. Esterman B: Grids for scoring visual fields, II perimeter. *Arch Ophthalmol* 1968;79:400-406.
4. Keeney AH. Duerson HL, Jr: Collated near-vision test card. *Am J Opthalmol* 1958; 469(4):592-594.
5. Keeney AH: *Ocular Examination: Basis and Technique* (ed 2). St Louis, CV Mosby Co., 1976.
6. Newell FW: *Ophthalmology: Principles and Concepts* (ed 5). St Louis, CV Mosby Co., 1982.
7. Esterman B: Functional scoring of the binocular visual field. *Ophthalmol* 1982;89;1226-1234.
8. Esterman B, Blanche E, Wallach M, Bonelli A: Computerized scoring of the functional field: Preliminary report. *Doc Ophthalmol Proc Ser* 1985; 42:333-339.
9. Keltner JC, Johnson CA: Comparative materials on automated and semi-automated perimeters in 1985. *Ophthalmol* 1985;92:34-37.
10. Anderson DR: *Perimetry: With and Without Automation* (ed 2). St Louis, CV Mosby Co., 1987.

TABLE 56

VISUAL SYSTEM

The values in this table are based on the following formula:

$$\frac{3 \times \text{impairment value of better eye} + \text{impairment value of worse eye}}{4} = \text{impairment of visual system}$$

The guides to the table are percentage impairment values for each eye. The percentage for the worse eye is read at the side of the table. The percentage for the better eye is read at the bottom of the table. At the intersection of the column for the worse eye and the column for the better eye is the impairment of visual system value.

For example, when there is 60% impairment of one eye and 30% impairment of the other eye, read down the side of the table until you come to the larger value (60%). Then follow across the row until it is intersected by the column headed by 30% at the bottom of the page. At the intersection of these two columns is printed the number 38. This number (38) represents the percentage impairment of the visual system when there is 60% impairment of one eye and 30% impairment of the other eye.

If bilateral aphakia is present and corrected central vision has been used in evaluation, impairment of the visual system is weighted by an additional 25% decrease in the value of the remaining corrected vision. For example, a 38% impairment (62% remaining) would be increased to 38% + (25%) (62%) = 54%.

% IMPAIRMENT WORSE EYE																																																		
0	0																																																	
1	0	1																																																
2	1	1	2																																														
3	1	2	2	3																																												
4	1	2	3	3	4																																										
5	1	2	3	4	4	5																																									
6	2	2	3	4	5	5	6																																								
7	2	3	3	4	5	6	6	7																																							
8	2	3	4	4	5	6	7	7	8																																						
9	2	3	4	5	5	6	7	8	8	9																																					
10	3	3	4	5	6	6	7	8	9	9	10																																				
11	3	4	4	5	6	7	7	8	9	10	10	11																																			
12	3	4	5	5	6	7	8	8	9	10	11	11	12																																		
13	3	4	5	6	6	7	8	9	9	10	11	12	12	13																																	
14	4	4	5	6	7	7	8	9	10	10	11	12	13	13	14																																
15	4	5	5	6	7	8	8	9	10	11	11	12	13	14	14	15																															
16	4	5	6	6	7	8	9	9	10	11	12	12	13	14	15	15	16																														
17	4	5	6	7	7	8	9	10	10	11	12	13	13	14	15	16	16	17																													
18	5	5	6	7	8	8	9	10	11	11	12	13	14	14	15	16	17	17	18																												
19	5	6	6	7	8	9	9	10	11	12	12	13	14	15	15	16	17	18	18	19																											
20	5	6	7	7	8	9	10	10	11	12	13	13	14	15	16	16	17	18	19	19	20																										
21	5	6	7	8	8	9	10	11	11	12	13	14	14	15	16	17	17	18	19	20	20	21																									
22	6	6	7	8	9	9	10	11	12	12	13	14	15	15	16	17	18	18	19	20	21	21	22																								
23	6	7	7	8	9	10	10	11	12	13	13	14	15	16	16	17	18	19	19	20	21	22	22	23																							
24	6	7	8	8	9	10	11	11	12	13	14	14	15	16	17	17	18	19	20	20	21	22	23	23	24																						
25	6	7	8	9	9	10	11	12	12	13	14	15	15	16	17	18	18	19	20	21	21	22	23	24	24	25																					
26	7	7	8	9	10	10	11	12	13	13	14	15	16	16	17	18	19	19	20	21	22	22	23	24	25	25	26																				
27	7	8	8	9	10	11	11	12	13	14	14	15	16	17	17	18	19	20	20	21	22	23	23	24	25	26	26	27																			
28	7	8	9	9	10	11	12	12	13	14	15	15	16	17	18	18	19	20	21	21	22	23	24	24	25	26	27	27	28																		
29	7	8	9	10	10	11	12	13	13	14	15	16	16	17	18	19	19	20	21	22	22	23	24	25	25	26	27	28	28	29																	
30	8	8	9	10	11	11	12	13	14	14	15	16	17	17	18	19	20	20	21	22	23	23	24	25	26	26	27	28	29	29	30																
31	8	9	9	10	11	12	12	13	14	15	15	16	17	18	18	19	20	21	21	22	23	24	24	25	26	27	27	28	29	30	30	31															
32	8	9	10	10	11	12	13	13	14	15	16	16	17	18	19	19	20	21	22	22	23	24	25	25	26	27	28	28	29	30	31	31	32														
33	8	9	10	11	11	12	13	14	14	15	16	17	17	18	19	20	20	21	22	23	23	24	25	26	26	27	28	29	29	30	31	32	32	33													
34	9	9	10	11	12	12	13	14	15	15	16	17	18	18	19	20	21	21	22	23	24	24	25	26	27	27	28	29	30	30	31	32	33	33	34												
35	9	10	10	11	12	13	13	14	15	16	16	17	18	19	19	20	21	22	22	23	24	25	25	26	27	28	28	29	30	31	31	32	33	34	34	35											
36	9	10	11	11	12	13	14	14	15	16	17	17	18	19	20	20	21	22	23	23	24	25	26	26	27	28	29	29	30	31	32	32	33	34	35	35	36										
37	9	10	11	12	12	13	14	15	15	16	17	18	18	19	20	21	21	22	23	24	24	25	26	27	27	28	29	30	30	31	32	33	33	34	35	36	36	37									
38	10	10	11	12	13	13	14	15	16	16	17	18	19	19	20	21	22	22	23	24	25	25	26	27	28	28	29	30	31	31	32	33	34	34	35	36	37	37	38								
39	10	11	11	12	13	14	14	15	16	17	17	18	19	20	20	21	22	23	23	24	25	26	26	27	28	29	29	30	31	32	32	33	34	35	35	36	37	38	38	39							
40	10	11	12	12	13	14	15	15	16	17	18	18	19	20	21	21	22	23	24	24	25	26	27	27	28	29	30	30	31	32	33	33	34	35	36	36	37	38	39	39	40									
41	10	11	12	13	13	14	15	16	16	17	18	19	19	20	21	22	22	23	24	25	25	26	27	28	28	29	30	31	31	32	33	34	34	35	36	37	37	38	39	40	40	41								
42	11	11	12	13	14	14	15	16	17	17	18	19	20	20	21	22	23	23	24	25	26	26	27	28	29	29	30	31	32	32	33	34	35	35	36	37	38	38	39	40	41	41	42							
43	11	12	12	13	14	15	15	16	17	18	18	19	20	21	21	22	23	24	24	25	26	27	27	28	29	30	30	31	32	33	33	34	35	36	36	37	38	39	39	40	41	42	42	43						
44	11	12	13	13	14	15	16	16	17	18	19	19	20	21	22	22	23	24	25	25	26	27	28	28	29	30	31	31	32	33	34	34	35	36	37	37	38	39	40	40	41	42	43	43	44					
45	11	12	13	14	14	15	16	17	17	18	19	20	20	21	22	23	23	24	25	26	26	27	28	29	29	30	31	32	32	33	34	35	35	36	37	38	38	39	40	41	41	42	43	44	44	45				
46	12	12	13	14	15	15	16	17	18	18	19	20	21	21	22	23	24	24	25	26	27	27	28	29	30	30	31	32	33	33	34	35	36	36	37	38	39	39	40	41	42	42	43	44	45	45	46			
47	12	13	13	14	15	16	16	17	18	19	19	20	21	22	22	23	24	25	25	26	27	28	28	29	30	31	31	32	33	34	34	35	36	37	37	38	39	40	40	41	42	43	43	44	45	46	46	47		
48	12	13	14	14	15	16	17	17	18	19	20	20	21	22	23	23	24	25	26	26	27	28	29	29	30	31	32	32	33	34	35	35	36	37	38	38	39	40	41	41	42	43	44	44	45	46	47	47	48	
49	12	13	14	15	15	16	17	18	18	19	20	21	21	22	23	24	24	25	26	27	27	28	29	30	30	31	32	33	33	34	35	36	36	37	38	39	39	40	41	42	42	43	44	45	45	46	47	48	48	49
	0	**1**	**2**	**3**	**4**	**5**	**6**	**7**	**8**	**9**	**10**	**11**	**12**	**13**	**14**	**15**	**16**	**17**	**18**	**19**	**20**	**21**	**22**	**23**	**24**	**25**	**26**	**27**	**28**	**29**	**30**	**31**	**32**	**33**	**34**	**35**	**36**	**37**	**38**	**39**	**40**	**41**	**42**	**43**	**44**	**45**	**46**	**47**	**48**	**49**

% IMPAIRMENT BETTER EYE

% IMPAIRMENT WORSE EYE

	0	1	2	3	4	5	6	7	8	9	10	11	12	13	14	15	16	17	18	19	20	21	22	23	24	25	26	27	28	29	30	31	32	33	34	35	36	37	38	39	40	41	42	43	44	45	46	47	48	49	
50	13	13	14	15	16	16	17	18	19	19	20	21	22	22	23	24	25	25	26	27	28	28	29	30	31	31	32	33	34	34	35	36	37	37	38	39	40	40	41	42	43	43	44	45	46	46	47	48	49	49	50
51	13	14	14	15	16	17	17	18	19	20	20	21	22	23	23	24	25	26	26	27	28	29	29	30	31	32	32	33	34	35	35	36	37	38	38	39	40	41	41	42	43	44	44	45	46	47	47	48	49	50	51
52	13	14	15	15	16	17	18	18	19	20	21	21	22	23	24	24	25	26	27	27	28	29	30	30	31	32	33	33	34	35	36	36	37	38	39	39	40	41	42	42	43	44	45	45	46	47	48	48	49	50	52
53	13	14	15	16	16	17	18	19	19	20	21	22	22	23	24	25	25	26	27	28	28	29	30	31	31	32	33	34	34	35	36	37	37	38	39	40	40	41	42	43	43	44	45	46	46	47	48	49	49	50	53
54	14	14	15	16	17	17	18	19	20	20	21	22	23	23	24	25	26	26	27	28	29	29	30	31	32	32	33	34	35	35	36	37	38	38	39	40	41	41	42	43	44	44	45	46	47	47	48	49	50	50	54
55	14	15	15	16	17	18	18	19	20	21	21	22	23	24	24	25	26	27	27	28	29	30	30	31	32	33	33	34	35	36	36	37	38	39	39	40	41	42	42	43	44	45	45	46	47	48	48	49	50	51	55
56	14	15	16	16	17	18	19	19	20	21	22	22	23	24	25	25	26	27	28	28	29	30	31	31	32	33	34	34	35	36	37	37	38	39	40	40	41	42	43	43	44	45	46	46	47	48	49	49	50	51	56
57	14	15	16	17	17	18	19	20	20	21	22	23	23	24	25	26	26	27	28	29	29	30	31	32	32	33	34	35	35	36	37	38	38	39	40	41	41	42	43	44	44	45	46	47	47	48	49	50	50	51	57
58	15	15	16	17	18	18	19	20	21	21	22	23	24	24	25	26	27	27	28	29	30	30	31	32	33	33	34	35	36	36	37	38	39	39	40	41	42	42	43	44	45	45	46	47	48	48	49	50	51	51	58
59	15	16	16	17	18	19	19	20	21	22	22	23	24	25	25	26	27	28	28	29	30	31	31	32	33	34	34	35	36	37	37	38	39	40	40	41	42	43	43	44	45	46	46	47	48	49	49	50	51	52	59
60	15	16	17	17	18	19	20	20	21	22	23	23	24	25	26	26	27	28	29	29	30	31	32	32	33	34	35	35	36	37	38	38	39	40	41	41	42	43	44	44	45	46	47	47	48	49	50	50	51	52	60
61	15	16	17	18	18	19	20	21	21	22	23	24	24	25	26	27	27	28	29	30	30	31	32	33	33	34	35	36	36	37	38	39	39	40	41	42	42	43	44	45	45	46	47	48	48	49	50	51	51	52	61
62	16	16	17	18	19	19	20	21	22	22	23	24	25	25	26	27	28	28	29	30	31	31	32	33	34	34	35	36	37	37	38	39	40	40	41	42	43	43	44	45	46	46	47	48	49	49	50	51	52	52	62
63	16	17	17	18	19	20	20	21	22	23	23	24	25	26	26	27	28	29	29	30	31	32	32	33	34	35	35	36	37	38	38	39	40	41	41	42	43	44	44	45	46	47	47	48	49	50	50	51	52	53	63
64	16	17	18	18	19	20	21	21	22	23	24	24	25	26	27	27	28	29	30	30	31	32	33	33	34	35	36	36	37	38	39	39	40	41	42	42	43	44	45	45	46	47	48	48	49	50	51	51	52	53	64
65	16	17	18	19	19	20	21	22	22	23	24	25	25	26	27	28	28	29	30	31	31	32	33	34	34	35	36	37	37	38	39	40	40	41	42	43	43	44	45	46	46	47	48	49	49	50	51	52	52	53	65
66	17	17	18	19	20	20	21	22	23	23	24	25	26	26	27	28	29	29	30	31	32	32	33	34	35	35	36	37	38	38	39	40	41	41	42	43	44	44	45	46	47	47	48	49	50	50	51	52	53	53	66
67	17	18	18	19	20	21	21	22	23	24	24	25	26	27	27	28	29	30	30	31	32	33	33	34	35	36	36	37	38	39	39	40	41	42	42	43	44	45	45	46	47	48	48	49	50	51	51	52	53	54	67
68	17	18	19	19	20	21	22	22	23	24	25	25	26	27	28	28	29	30	31	31	32	33	34	34	35	36	37	37	38	39	40	40	41	42	43	43	44	45	46	46	47	48	49	49	50	51	52	52	53	54	68
69	17	18	19	20	20	21	22	23	23	24	25	26	26	27	28	29	29	30	31	32	32	33	34	35	35	36	37	38	38	39	40	41	41	42	43	44	44	45	46	47	47	48	49	50	50	51	52	53	53	54	69
70	18	18	19	20	21	21	22	23	24	24	25	26	27	27	28	29	30	30	31	32	33	33	34	35	36	36	37	38	39	39	40	41	42	42	43	44	45	45	46	47	48	48	49	50	51	51	52	53	54	54	70
71	18	19	19	20	21	22	22	23	24	25	25	26	27	28	28	29	30	31	31	32	33	34	34	35	36	37	37	38	39	40	40	41	42	43	43	44	45	46	46	47	48	49	49	50	51	52	52	53	54	55	71
72	18	19	20	20	21	22	23	23	24	25	26	26	27	28	29	29	30	31	32	32	33	34	35	35	36	37	38	38	39	40	41	41	42	43	44	44	45	46	47	47	48	49	50	50	51	52	53	53	54	55	72
73	18	19	20	21	21	22	23	24	24	25	26	27	27	28	29	30	30	31	32	33	33	34	35	36	36	37	38	39	39	40	41	42	42	43	44	45	45	46	47	48	48	49	50	51	51	52	53	54	54	55	73
74	19	19	20	21	22	22	23	24	25	25	26	27	28	28	29	30	31	31	32	33	34	34	35	36	37	37	38	39	40	40	41	42	43	43	44	45	46	46	47	48	49	49	50	51	52	52	53	54	55	55	74
75	19	20	20	21	22	23	23	24	25	26	26	27	28	29	29	30	31	32	32	33	34	35	35	36	37	38	38	39	40	41	41	42	43	44	44	45	46	47	47	48	49	50	50	51	52	53	53	54	55	56	75
76	19	20	21	21	22	23	24	24	25	26	27	27	28	29	30	30	31	32	33	33	34	35	36	36	37	38	39	39	40	41	42	42	43	44	45	45	46	47	48	48	49	50	51	51	52	53	54	54	55	56	76
77	19	20	21	22	22	23	24	25	25	26	27	28	28	29	30	31	31	32	33	34	34	35	36	37	37	38	39	40	40	41	42	43	43	44	45	46	46	47	48	49	49	50	51	52	52	53	54	55	55	56	77
78	20	20	21	22	23	23	24	25	26	26	27	28	29	29	30	31	32	32	33	34	35	35	36	37	38	38	39	40	41	41	42	43	44	44	45	46	47	47	48	49	50	50	51	52	53	53	54	55	56	56	78
79	20	21	21	22	23	24	24	25	26	27	27	28	29	30	30	31	32	33	33	34	35	36	36	37	38	39	39	40	41	42	42	43	44	45	45	46	47	48	48	49	50	51	51	52	53	54	54	55	56	57	79
80	20	21	22	22	23	24	25	25	26	27	28	28	29	30	31	31	32	33	34	34	35	36	37	37	38	39	40	40	41	42	43	43	44	45	46	46	47	48	49	49	50	51	52	52	53	54	55	55	56	57	80
81	20	21	22	23	23	24	25	26	26	27	28	29	29	30	31	32	32	33	34	35	35	36	37	38	38	39	40	41	41	42	43	44	44	45	46	47	47	48	49	50	50	51	52	53	53	54	55	56	56	57	81
82	21	21	22	23	24	24	25	26	27	27	28	29	30	30	31	32	33	33	34	35	36	36	37	38	39	39	40	41	42	42	43	44	45	45	46	47	48	48	49	50	51	51	52	53	54	54	55	56	57	57	82
83	21	22	22	23	24	25	25	26	27	28	28	29	30	31	31	32	33	34	34	35	36	37	37	38	39	40	40	41	42	43	43	44	45	46	46	47	48	49	49	50	51	52	52	53	54	55	55	56	57	58	83
84	21	22	23	23	24	25	26	26	27	28	29	29	30	31	32	32	33	34	35	35	36	37	38	38	39	40	41	41	42	43	44	44	45	46	47	47	48	49	50	50	51	52	53	53	54	55	56	56	57	58	84
85	21	22	23	24	24	25	26	27	27	28	29	30	30	31	32	33	33	34	35	36	36	37	38	39	39	40	41	42	42	43	44	45	45	46	47	48	48	49	50	51	51	52	53	54	54	55	56	57	57	58	85
86	22	22	23	24	25	25	26	27	28	28	29	30	31	31	32	33	34	34	35	36	37	37	38	39	40	40	41	42	43	43	44	45	46	46	47	48	49	49	50	51	52	52	53	54	55	55	56	57	58	58	86
87	22	23	23	24	25	26	26	27	28	29	29	30	31	32	32	33	34	35	35	36	37	38	38	39	40	41	41	42	43	44	44	45	46	47	47	48	49	50	50	51	52	53	53	54	55	56	56	57	58	59	87
88	22	23	24	24	25	26	27	27	28	29	30	30	31	32	33	33	34	35	36	36	37	38	39	39	40	41	42	42	43	44	45	45	46	47	48	48	49	50	51	51	52	53	54	54	55	56	57	57	58	59	88
89	22	23	24	25	25	26	27	28	28	29	30	31	31	32	33	34	34	35	36	37	37	38	39	40	40	41	42	43	43	44	45	46	46	47	48	49	49	50	51	52	52	53	54	55	55	56	57	58	58	59	89
90	23	23	24	25	26	26	27	28	29	29	30	31	32	32	33	34	35	35	36	37	38	38	39	40	41	41	42	43	44	44	45	46	47	47	48	49	50	50	51	52	53	53	54	55	56	56	57	58	59	59	90
91	23	24	24	25	26	27	27	28	29	30	30	31	32	33	33	34	35	36	36	37	38	39	39	40	41	42	42	43	44	45	45	46	47	48	48	49	50	51	51	52	53	54	54	55	56	57	57	58	59	60	91
92	23	24	25	25	26	27	28	28	29	30	31	31	32	33	34	34	35	36	37	37	38	39	40	40	41	42	43	43	44	45	46	46	47	48	49	49	50	51	52	52	53	54	55	55	56	57	58	58	59	60	92
93	23	24	25	26	26	27	28	29	29	30	31	32	32	33	34	35	35	36	37	38	38	39	40	41	41	42	43	44	44	45	46	47	47	48	49	50	50	51	52	53	53	54	55	56	56	57	58	59	59	60	93
94	24	24	25	26	27	27	28	29	30	30	31	32	33	33	34	35	36	36	37	38	39	39	40	41	42	42	43	44	45	45	46	47	48	48	49	50	51	51	52	53	54	54	55	56	57	57	58	59	60	60	94
95	24	25	25	26	27	28	28	29	30	31	31	32	33	34	34	35	36	37	37	38	39	40	40	41	42	43	43	44	45	46	46	47	48	49	49	50	51	52	52	53	54	55	55	56	57	58	58	59	60	61	95
96	24	25	26	26	27	28	29	29	30	31	32	32	33	34	35	35	36	37	38	38	39	40	41	41	42	43	44	44	45	46	47	47	48	49	50	50	51	52	53	53	54	55	56	56	57	58	59	59	60	61	96
97	24	25	26	27	27	28	29	30	30	31	32	33	33	34	35	36	36	37	38	39	39	40	41	42	42	43	44	45	45	46	47	48	48	49	50	51	51	52	53	54	54	55	56	57	57	58	59	60	60	61	97
98	25	25	26	27	28	28	29	30	31	31	32	33	34	34	35	36	37	37	38	39	40	40	41	42	43	43	44	45	46	46	47	48	49	49	50	51	52	52	53	54	55	55	56	57	58	58	59	60	61	61	98
99	25	26	26	27	28	29	29	30	31	32	32	33	34	35	35	36	37	38	38	39	40	41	41	42	43	44	44	45	46	47	47	48	49	50	50	51	52	53	53	54	55	56	56	57	58	59	59	60	61	62	99
100	25	26	27	27	28	29	30	30	31	32	33	33	34	35	36	36	37	38	39	39	40	41	42	42	43	44	45	45	46	47	48	48	49	50	51	51	52	53	54	54	55	56	57	57	58	59	60	60	61	62	100
	0	1	2	3	4	5	6	7	8	9	10	11	12	13	14	15	16	17	18	19	20	21	22	23	24	25	26	27	28	29	30	31	32	33	34	35	36	37	38	39	40	41	42	43	44	45	46	47	48	49	

% IMPAIRMENT BETTER EYE

% IMPAIRMENT WORSE EYE

Worse eye	50	51	52	53	54	55	56	57	58	59	60	61	62	63	64	65	66	67	68	69	70	71	72	73	74	75	76	77	78	79	80	81	82	83	84	85	86	87	88	89	90	91	92	93	94	95	96	97	98	99	100
50	50																																																		
51	50	51																																																	
52	51	51	52																																															
53	51	52	52	53																																													
54	51	52	53	53	54																																											
55	51	52	53	54	54	55																																									
56	52	52	53	54	55	55	56																																								
57	52	53	53	54	55	56	56	57																																							
58	52	53	54	54	55	56	57	57	58																																						
59	52	53	54	55	55	56	57	58	58	59																																					
60	53	53	54	55	56	56	57	58	59	59	60																																				
61	53	54	54	55	56	57	57	58	59	60	60	61																																			
62	53	54	55	55	56	57	58	58	59	60	61	61	62																																		
63	53	54	55	56	56	57	58	59	59	60	61	62	62	63																																	
64	54	54	55	56	57	57	58	59	60	60	61	62	63	63	64																																
65	54	55	55	56	57	58	58	59	60	61	61	62	63	64	64	65																															
66	54	55	56	56	57	58	59	59	60	61	62	62	63	64	65	65	66																														
67	54	55	56	57	57	58	59	60	60	61	62	63	63	64	65	66	66	67																													
68	55	55	56	57	58	58	59	60	61	61	62	63	64	64	65	66	67	67	68																												
69	55	56	56	57	58	59	59	60	61	62	62	63	64	65	65	66	67	68	68	69																											
70	55	56	57	57	58	59	60	60	61	62	63	63	64	65	66	66	67	68	69	69	70																										
71	55	56	57	58	58	59	60	61	61	62	63	64	64	65	66	67	67	68	69	70	70	71																									
72	56	56	57	58	59	59	60	61	62	62	63	64	65	65	66	67	68	68	69	70	71	71	72																								
73	56	57	57	58	59	60	60	61	62	63	63	64	65	66	66	67	68	69	69	70	71	72	72	73																							
74	56	57	58	58	59	60	61	61	62	63	64	64	65	66	67	67	68	69	70	70	71	72	73	73	74																						
75	56	57	58	59	59	60	61	62	62	63	64	65	65	66	67	68	68	69	70	71	71	72	73	74	74	75																					
76	57	57	58	59	60	60	61	62	63	63	64	65	66	66	67	68	69	69	70	71	72	72	73	74	75	75	76																				
77	57	58	58	59	60	61	61	62	63	64	64	65	66	67	67	68	69	70	70	71	72	73	73	74	75	76	76	77																			
78	57	58	59	59	60	61	62	62	63	64	65	65	66	67	68	68	69	70	71	71	72	73	74	74	75	76	77	77	78																		
79	57	58	59	60	60	61	62	63	63	64	65	66	66	67	68	69	69	70	71	72	72	73	74	75	75	76	77	78	78	79																	
80	58	58	59	60	61	61	62	63	64	64	65	66	67	67	68	69	70	70	71	72	73	73	74	75	76	76	77	78	79	79	80																
81	58	59	59	60	61	62	62	63	64	65	65	66	67	68	68	69	70	71	71	72	73	74	74	75	76	77	77	78	79	80	80	81															
82	58	59	60	60	61	62	63	63	64	65	66	66	67	68	69	69	70	71	72	72	73	74	75	75	76	77	78	78	79	80	81	81	82														
83	58	59	60	61	61	62	63	64	64	65	66	67	67	68	69	70	70	71	72	73	73	74	75	76	76	77	78	79	79	80	81	82	82	83													
84	59	59	60	61	62	62	63	64	65	65	66	67	68	68	69	70	71	71	72	73	74	74	75	76	77	77	78	79	80	80	81	82	83	83	84												
85	59	60	60	61	62	63	63	64	65	66	66	67	68	69	69	70	71	72	72	73	74	75	75	76	77	78	78	79	80	81	81	82	83	84	84	85											
86	59	60	61	61	62	63	64	64	65	66	67	67	68	69	70	70	71	72	73	73	74	75	76	76	77	78	79	79	80	81	82	82	83	84	85	85	86										
87	59	60	61	62	62	63	64	65	65	66	67	68	68	69	70	71	71	72	73	74	74	75	76	77	77	78	79	80	80	81	82	83	83	84	85	86	86	87									
88	60	60	61	62	63	63	64	65	66	66	67	68	69	69	70	71	72	72	73	74	75	75	76	77	78	78	79	80	81	81	82	83	84	84	85	86	87	87	88								
89	60	61	61	62	63	64	64	65	66	67	67	68	69	70	70	71	72	73	73	74	75	76	76	77	78	79	79	80	81	82	82	83	84	85	85	86	87	88	88	89							
90	60	61	62	62	63	64	65	65	66	67	68	68	69	70	71	71	72	73	74	74	75	76	77	77	78	79	80	80	81	82	83	83	84	85	86	86	87	88	89	89	90										
91	60	61	62	63	63	64	65	66	66	67	68	69	69	70	71	72	72	73	74	75	75	76	77	78	78	79	80	81	81	82	83	84	84	85	86	87	87	88	89	90	90	91									
92	61	61	62	63	64	64	65	66	67	67	68	69	70	70	71	72	73	73	74	75	76	76	77	78	79	79	80	81	82	82	83	84	85	85	86	87	88	88	89	90	91	91	92								
93	61	62	62	63	64	65	65	66	67	68	68	69	70	71	71	72	73	74	74	75	76	77	77	78	79	80	80	81	82	83	83	84	85	86	86	87	88	89	89	90	91	92	92	93							
94	61	62	63	63	64	65	66	66	67	68	69	69	70	71	72	72	73	74	75	75	76	77	78	78	79	80	81	81	82	83	84	84	85	86	87	87	88	89	90	90	91	92	93	93	94						
95	61	62	63	64	64	65	66	67	67	68	69	70	70	71	72	73	73	74	75	76	76	77	78	79	79	80	81	82	82	83	84	85	85	86	87	88	88	89	90	91	91	92	93	94	94	95					
96	62	62	63	64	65	65	66	67	68	68	69	70	71	71	72	73	74	74	75	76	77	77	78	79	80	80	81	82	83	83	84	85	86	86	87	88	89	89	90	91	92	92	93	94	95	95	96				
97	62	63	63	64	65	66	66	67	68	69	69	70	71	72	72	73	74	75	75	76	77	78	78	79	80	81	81	82	83	84	84	85	86	87	87	88	89	90	90	91	92	93	93	94	95	96	96	97			
98	62	63	64	64	65	66	67	67	68	69	70	70	71	72	73	73	74	75	76	76	77	78	79	79	80	81	82	82	83	84	85	85	86	87	88	88	89	90	91	91	92	93	94	94	95	96	97	97	98		
99	62	63	64	65	65	66	67	68	68	69	70	71	71	72	73	74	74	75	76	77	77	78	79	80	80	81	82	83	83	84	85	86	86	87	88	89	89	90	91	92	92	93	94	95	95	96	97	98	98	99	
100	63	63	64	65	66	66	67	68	69	69	70	71	72	72	73	74	75	75	76	77	78	78	79	80	81	81	82	83	84	84	85	86	87	87	88	89	90	90	91	92	93	93	94	95	96	96	97	98	99	99	100

% IMPAIRMENT BETTER EYE

SECTION 7

Product Identification Section

This section is designed to help you identify ophthalmic products and their packaging.

Participating manufacturers have included selected products in full color. Where capsules and tablets are included they are shown in actual size. Solutions, tubes and so forth are reduced in size to fit available space.

For more information on products included, refer to the description in the PRODUCT INFORMATION SECTION EIGHT or check directly with the manufacturer.

On page 106 of the Product Identification Section there is a Color Vision Screening Chart which can be used to test your patients for color blindness.

While every effort has been made to reproduce products faithfully, this section should be considered only as a quick-reference identification aid.

INDEX OF MANUFACTURERS

Akorn, Inc. **103**
Bausch & Lomb **103**
IOLAB Corporation **103**
Merck Sharp & Dohme **103**
Parke-Davis **104**
Pfizer Consumer Health Care **104**
Polymer Technology Corporation **104**
Roche Laboratories **105**
Ross Laboratories **105**
Storz Ophthalmic Pharmaceuticals **105**
Wyeth-Ayerst **105**

PRODUCT INDEX

Achromycin Ophthalmic Suspension 1% (Storz) 105
AK-Pred (Akorn) 103
AK-Sulf (Akorn) 103
Bio-Cor (Bausch & Lomb) 103
Boston Advance Care System (Polymer) 104
Chibroxin (Merck Sharp & Dohme) 103
Chloromycetin Ophthalmic Solution (Parke-Davis) 104
Chloromycetin Ophthalmic Ointment 1% (Parke-Davis) 104
Chloromycetin Hydrocortisone Ophthalmic (Parke-Davis) 104
Clear Eyes (Ross) 105
Collyrium Fresh (Wyeth-Ayerst) 105
Collyrium For Fresh Eyes (Wyeth-Ayerst) 105
Daranide (Merck Sharp & Dohme) 103
Decadron Phosphate Sterile Ophthalmic Ointment (Merck Sharp & Dohme) 103
Decadron Phosphate Sterile Ophthalmic Solution (Merck Sharp & Dohme) 103
Diamox Tablets & Sequels (Storz) 105
Floropryl (Merck Sharp & Dohme) 103
Fluor-I-Strip (Wyeth-Ayerst) 105
Fluor-I-Strip A.T. For Applanation Tonometry (Wyeth-Ayerst) 105
Gantrisin Ophthalmic Solution (Roche) 105
Humorsol Sterile Ophthalmic Solution (Merck Sharp & Dohme) 104
Lacrisert Sterile Ophthalmic Insert (Merck Sharp & Dohme) 104
Miochol With IOCARE Steri-Tags (IOLAB) 103
Miochol System Pak (IOLAB) 103
Miochol System Pak Plus IOCARE Balanced Salt Solution (IOLAB) 103
Muro 128 (Bausch & Lomb) 103
NeoDecadron Sterile Ophthalmic Ointment (Merck Sharp & Dohme) 104
NeoDecadron Sterile Ophthalmic Solution (Merck Sharp & Dohme) 104
Neptazane (Storz) 105
Occucoat (Storz) 105
Ophthalgan (Wyeth-Ayerst) 105
Ophthocort (Parke-Davis) 104
Ophthochlor (Parke-Davis) 104
OptiPranolol (Bausch & Lomb) 103
Phospholine Iodide (Wyeth-Ayerst) 105
Pilocar Ophthalmic Solution (IOLAB) 103
Timoptic Sterile Ophthalmic Solution (Merck Sharp & Dohme) 104
Timoptic Ophthalmic Solution in Ocudose (Merck Sharp & Dohme) 104
Vira-A (Parke-Davis) 104
Visine (Pfizer Consumer) 104
Voltaren Ophthalmic (CIBA Vision) 103

AKORN, INC.

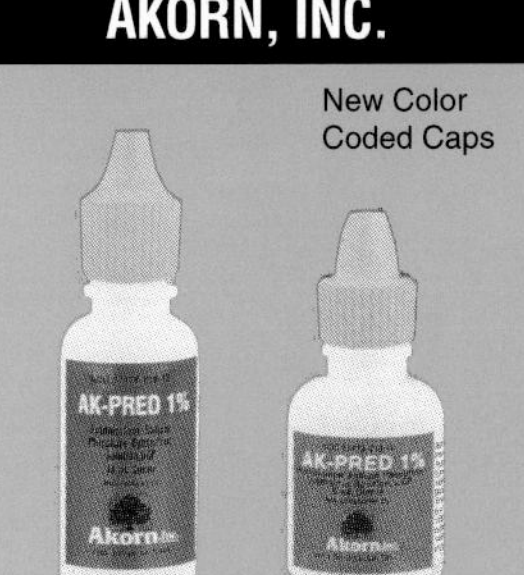

New Color Coded Caps

15 mL 5 mL

AK-PRED 1%
(prednisolone sodium phosphate)

Also available in 0.125% 5 mL

Akorn, Inc.

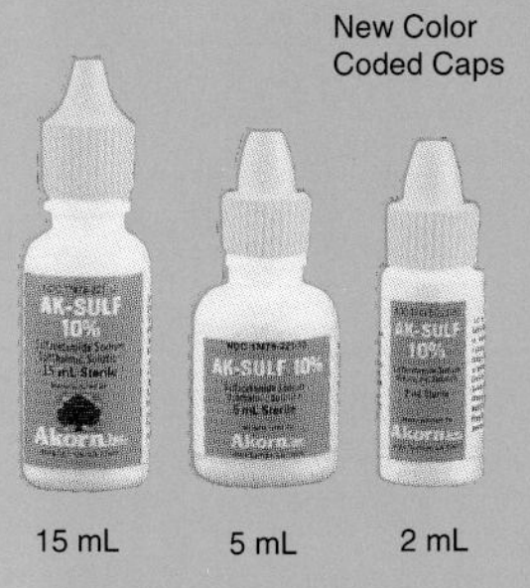

New Color Coded Caps

15 mL 5 mL 2 mL

AK-SULF 10%
(sulfacetamide sodium 10%)

Also available in 3.5 gm ointment

BAUSCH & LOMB

Pharmaceutical Division

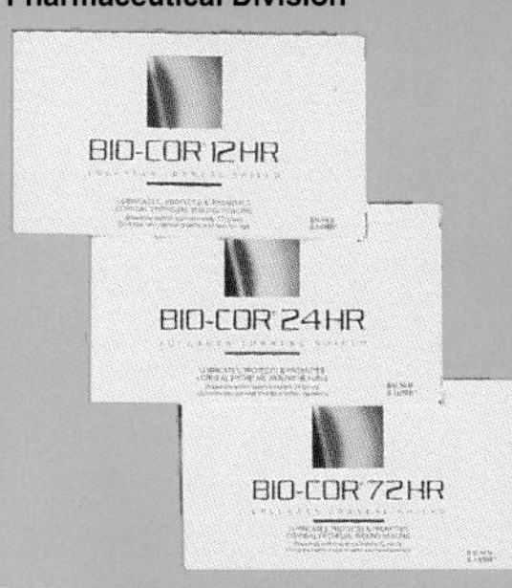

BIO-COR
Collagen Corneal Shield
12 HR, 24 HR, 72 HR

Bausch & Lomb

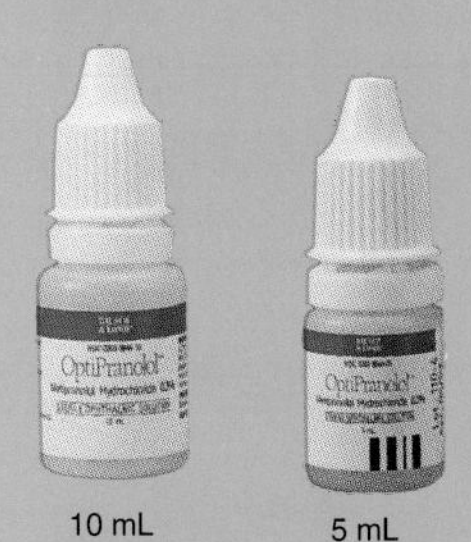

10 mL 5 mL

OptiPranolol
Sterile Ophthalmic Solution

(metipranolol HCl 0.3%)

Bausch & Lomb

2% 15 mL 5% 15 mL

5% Ointment 3.5 g

MURO 128
Hypertonicity Solutions & Ointment
(sodium chloride 2%, 5%)

CIBA Vision Ophthalmics

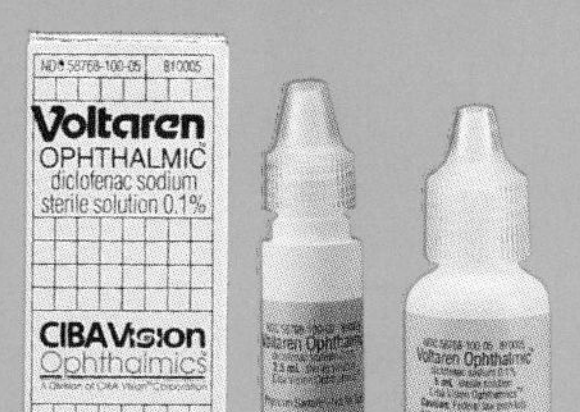

2.5 mL 5 mL

VOLTAREN OPHTHALMIC
(diclofenac sodium
sterile solution 0.1%)

IOLAB

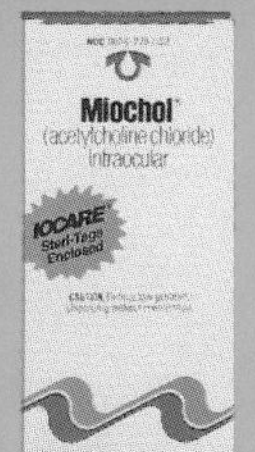

Pack contains:
Miochol 2ml univial,
IOCARE Steri-Tags
(sterile syringe labels for drug identification)

MIOCHOL
with IOCARE Steri-Tags
(acetylcholine chloride intraocular)

IOLAB

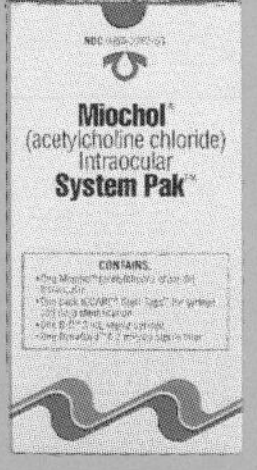

Pack contains:
Miochol 2ml univial,
IOCARE Steri-Tags sterile labels,
B-D 3ml sterile syringe, DynaGard
0.2 micron sterile filter

MIOCHOL
System Pak
(acetylcholine chloride intraocular)

IOLAB

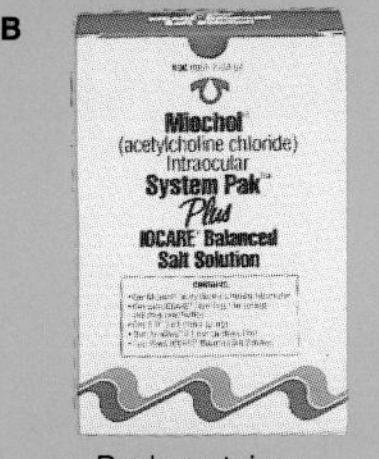

Pack contains:
Miochol 2ml univial, IOCARE
Steri-Tags sterile labels, B-D 3ml
sterile syringe, DynaGard 0.2 micron
sterile filter, 2x15ml IOCARE
Balanced Salt Solution

MIOCHOL
System Pak Plus
IOCARE Balanced Salt Solution
(acetylcholine chloride intraocular)

IOLAB

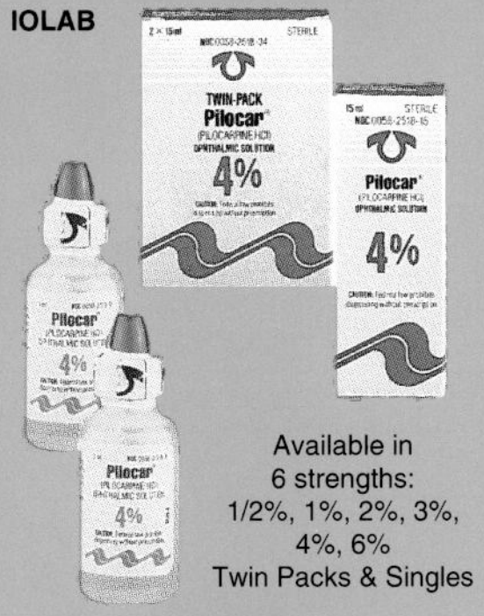

Available in
6 strengths:
1/2%, 1%, 2%, 3%,
4%, 6%
Twin Packs & Singles

PILOCAR
Ophthalmic Solution
(pilocarpine HCl)

MERCK SHARP & DOHME

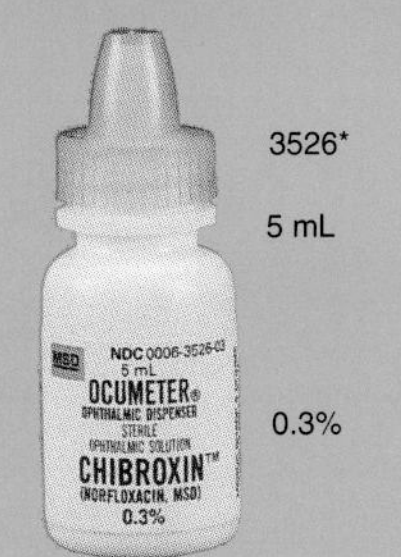

3526*
5 mL
0.3%

CHIBROXIN
Sterile Ophthalmic Solution
(Norfloxacin | MSD)
OCUMETER Ophthalmic Dispenser

Merck Sharp & Dohme

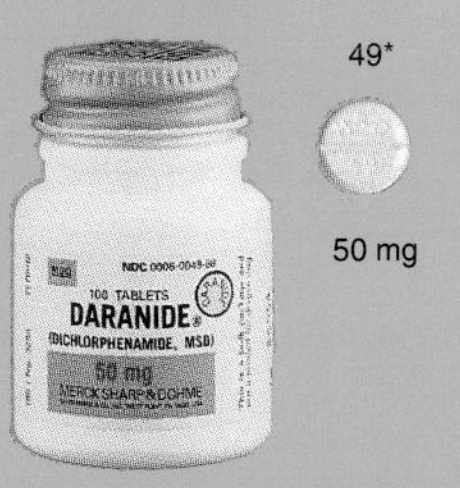

49*
50 mg

Bottle of 100

DARANIDE
(Dichlorphenamide | MSD)

Merck Sharp & Dohme

7615*
3.5-g tube

DECADRON
Phosphate Sterile
Ophthalmic Ointment
(Dexamethasone Sodium Phosphate | MSD)

Merck Sharp & Dohme

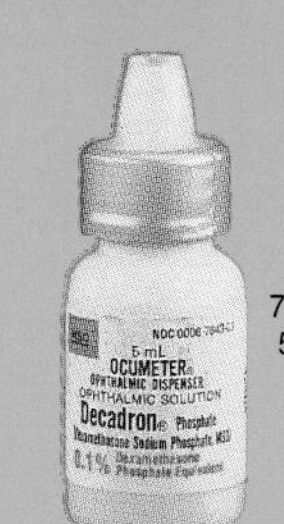

7643*
5 mL

DECADRON
Phosphate Sterile
Ophthalmic Solution
(Dexamethasone Sodium
Phosphate | MSD)
OCUMETER Ophthalmic Dispenser

Merck Sharp & Dohme

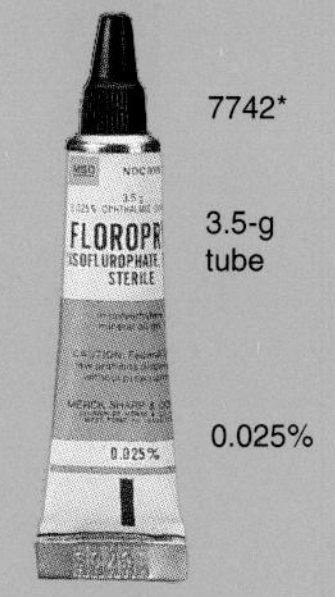

7742*
3.5-g tube
0.025%

FLOROPRYL
Sterile Ophthalmic Ointment
(Isoflurophate | MSD)

Merck Sharp & Dohme

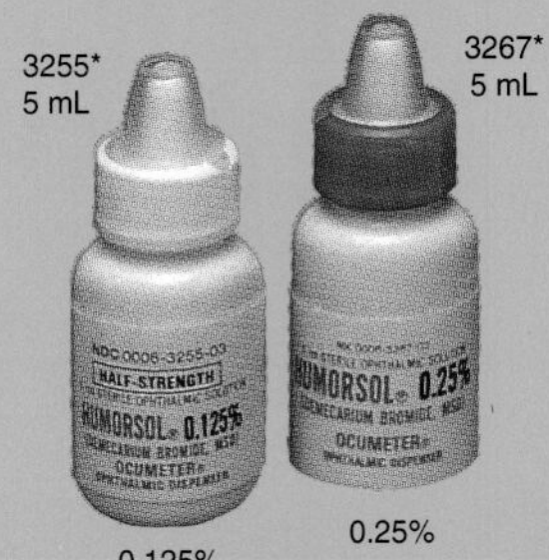

3255*
5 mL
3267*
5 mL

0.125% 0.25%

HUMORSOL
Sterile Ophthalmic Solution
(Demecarium Bromide | MSD)
OCUMETER Ophthalmic Dispenser

*Manufacturer's identification code

Merck Sharp & Dohme

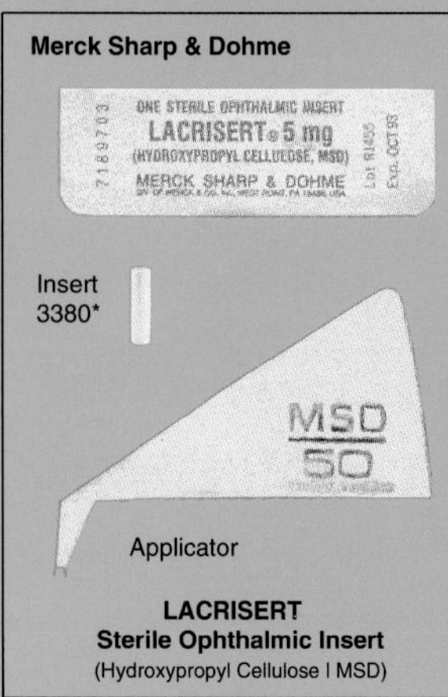

Insert 3380*

Applicator

LACRISERT
Sterile Ophthalmic Insert
(Hydroxypropyl Cellulose | MSD)

Merck Sharp & Dohme

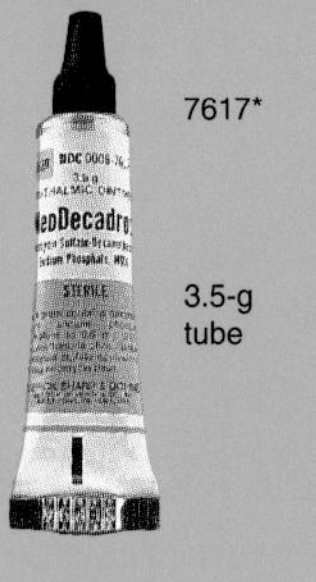

7617*

3.5-g tube

NEODECADRON
Sterile Ophthalmic Ointment
(Neomycin Sulfate-Dexamethasone Sodium Phosphate | MSD)

Merck Sharp & Dohme

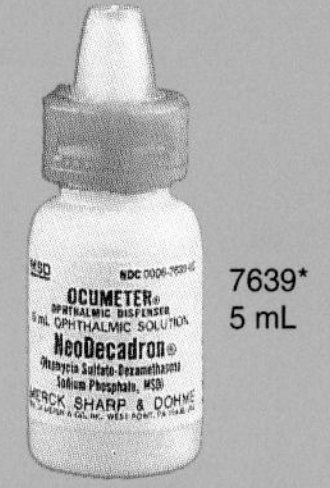

7639*
5 mL

NEODECADRON
Sterile Ophthalmic Solution
(Neomycin Sulfate-Dexamethasone Sodium Phosphate | MSD)
OCUMETER Ophthalmic Dispenser

Merck Sharp & Dohme

3542*

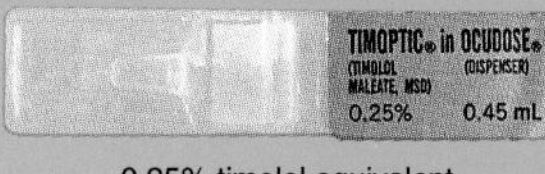

0.25% timolol equivalent

3543*

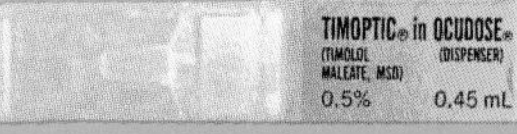

0.5% timolol equivalent

TIMOPTIC
Preservative-Free
Sterile Ophthalmic Solution
(Timolol Maleate | MSD)
in OCUDOSE (Dispenser)

Merck Sharp & Dohme

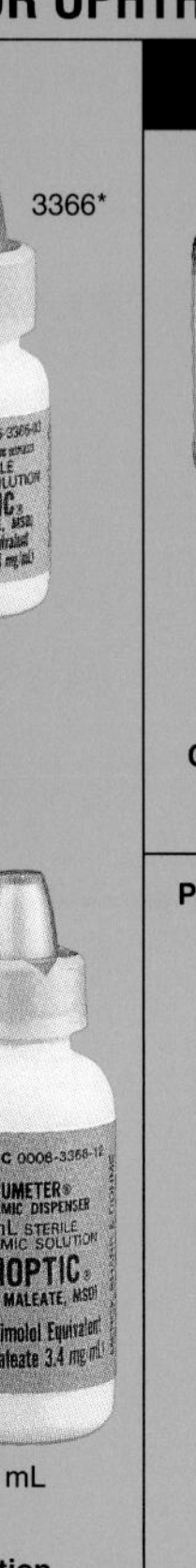

3366*

2.5 mL

5 mL

10 mL

0.25% timolol equivalent

15 mL

TIMOPTIC
Sterile Ophthalmic Solution
(Timolol Maleate | MSD)
OCUMETER Ophthalmic Dispenser

Merck Sharp & Dohme

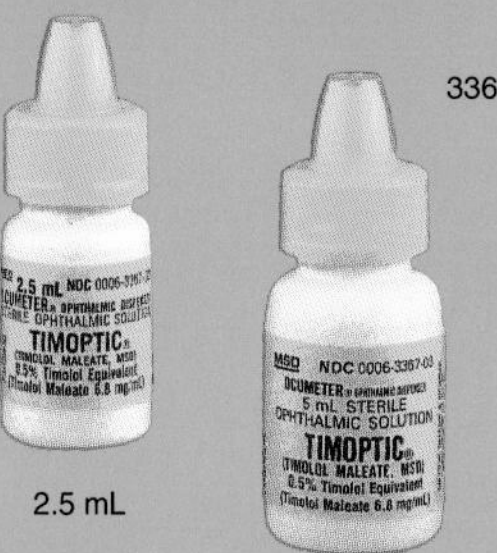

3367*

2.5 mL

5 mL

10 mL

0.5% timolol equivalent

15 mL

TIMOPTIC
Sterile Ophthalmic Solution
(Timolol Maleate | MSD)
OCUMETER Ophthalmic Dispenser

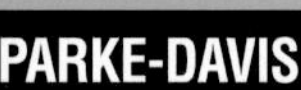

PARKE-DAVIS

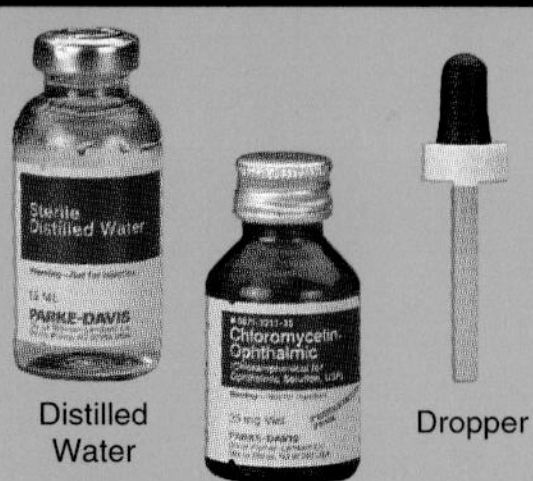

Distilled Water

Dropper

25 mg
Sterile Powder

Preservative Free
CHLOROMYCETIN OPHTHALMIC
(chloramphenicol for ophthalmic solution, USP)

Parke-Davis

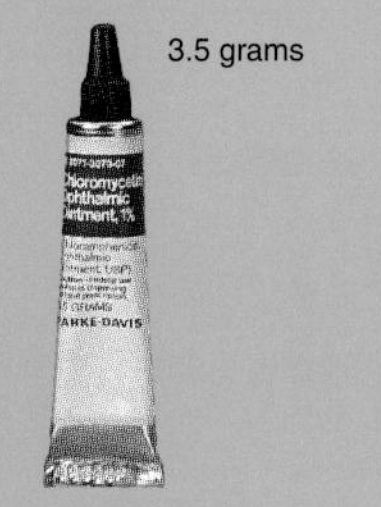

3.5 grams

Preservative Free
CHLOROMYCETIN
OPHTHALMIC OINTMENT 1%
(chloramphenicol ophthalmic ointment, USP)

Parke-Davis

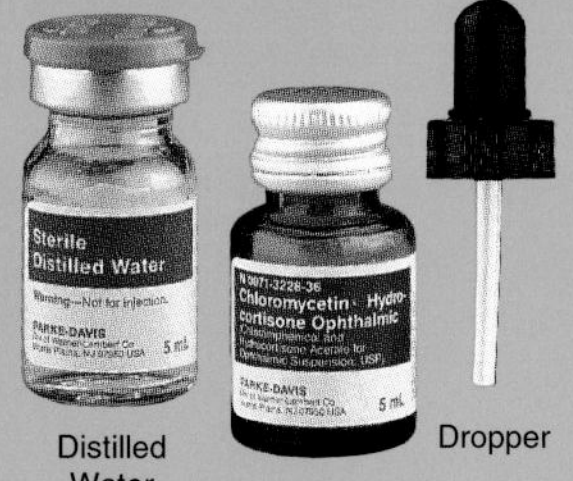

Distilled Water

Dropper

5 mL
Sterile Powder

CHLOROMYCETIN
HYDROCORTISONE OPHTHALMIC
(chloramphenicol and hydrocortisone acetate for ophthalmic suspension, USP)

Parke-Davis

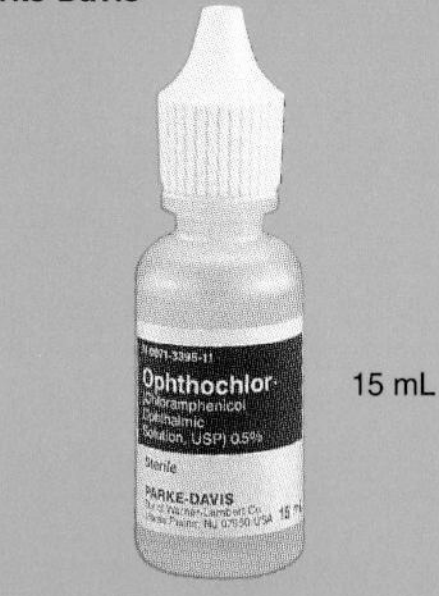

15 mL

Preservative Free

OPHTHOCHLOR
(chloramphenicol ophthalmic solution, USP) 0.5%

Parke-Davis

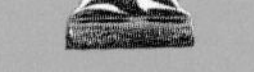

3.5 grams

Preservative Free

OPHTHOCORT
(chloramphenicol, polymyxin B sulfate, and hydrocortisone acetate ophthalmic ointment, USP)

Parke-Davis

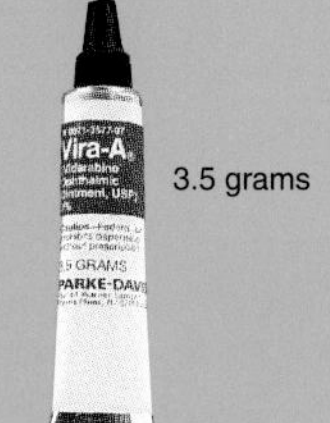

3.5 grams

Preservative Free

VIRA-A
(vidarabine ophthalmic ointment, USP) 3%

PFIZER Health Care

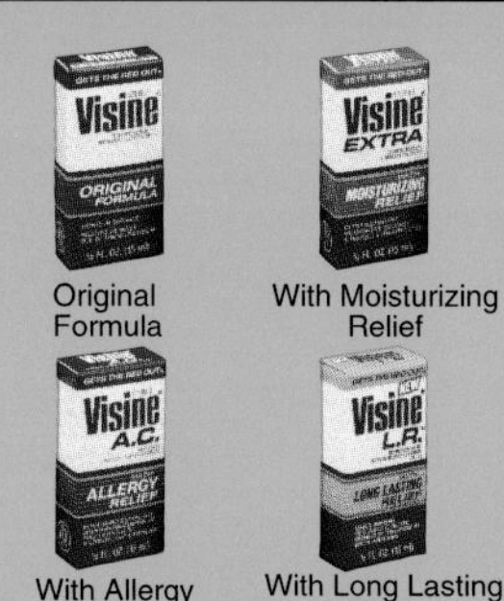

Original Formula

With Moisturizing Relief

With Allergy Relief

With Long Lasting Relief

VISINE Redness Reliever Eye Drops

POLYMER TECHNOLOGY

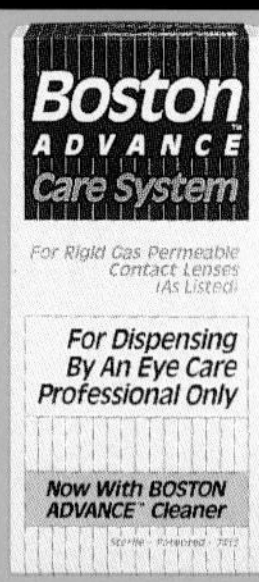

BOSTON ADVANCE
Care System
Also Available: Deluxe Care System (with travel pouch) and Starter Kit

*Manufacturer's identification code

ROCHE

15 mL

GANTRISIN
4% (40 mg/mL)
(sulfisoxazole diolamine/Roche)

Ophthalmic Solution

ROSS

0.5 Fl. Oz.

Also available in 1.0 Fl. Oz.
CLEAR EYES ACR
Astringent/Lubricating Eye Redness Reliever Drops

STORZ OPHTHALMICS

(Shown smaller than actual size)

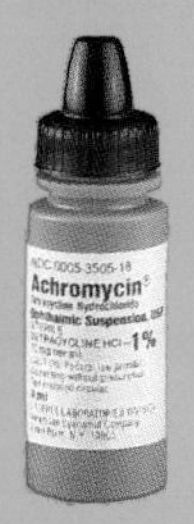

ACHROMYCIN
Ophthalmic Suspension 1.0%
(tetracycline HCl)

Storz Ophthalmics

D1** 125 mg.

D2** 250 mg.

†DIAMOX Tablets

D3** 500 mg.

†DIAMOX Sequels
(acetazolamide)

Storz Ophthalmics

N2** 25 mg.

N1** 50 mg.

NEPTAZANE
(methazolamide)

Storz Ophthalmics

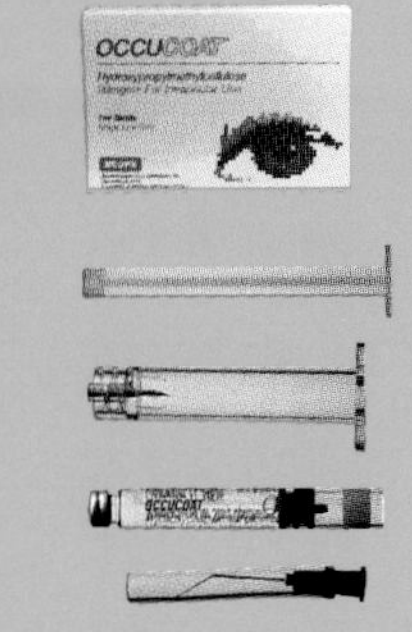
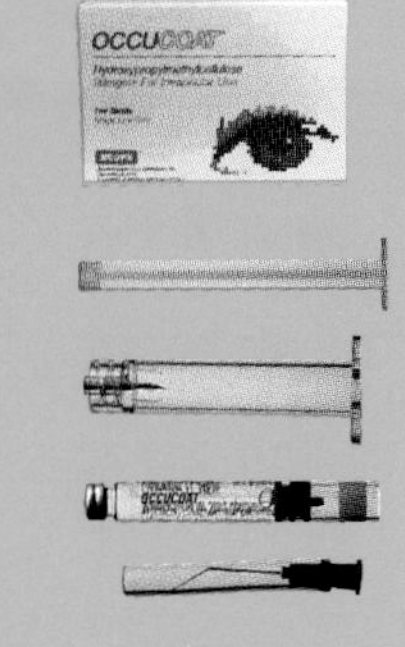
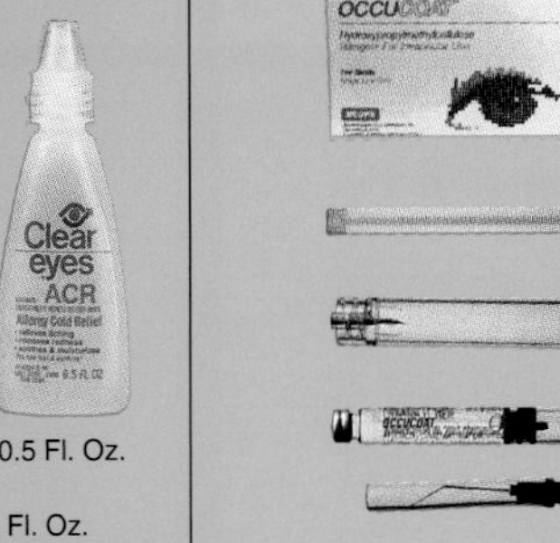

OCCUCOAT
2% Hydroxypropylmethylcellulose

For more detailed information on products illustrated in this section, consult the Product Information Section or manufacturers may be contacted directly.

The Indices are divided into 5 parts–

Part I	**Manufacturers' Index**
Part II	**Product Name Index**
Part III	**Product Category Index**
Part IV	**Active Ingredients Index**
Part V	**Instrumentation Index and**

WYETH-AYERST

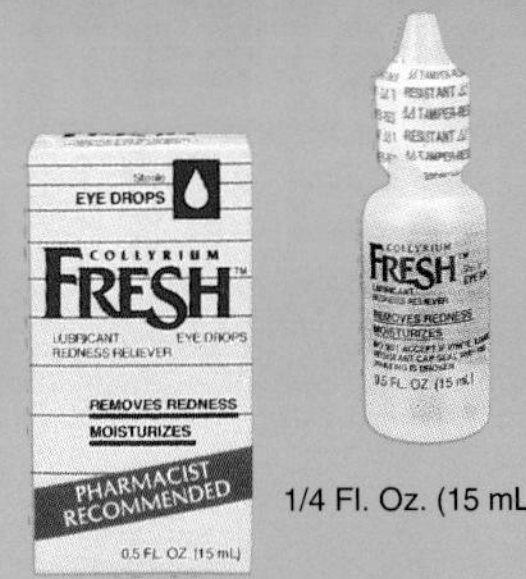

1/4 Fl. Oz. (15 mL)

COLLYRIUM FRESH

Eye drops with tetrahydrozoline HCl plus glycerin

Wyeth-Ayerst

Lotion 4 Fl. Oz. (118 mL)
with separate eyecup bottle cap

COLLYRIUM for FRESH EYES
Eye Wash

Wyeth-Ayerst

Box of 300 strips

Each strip contains
9 mg fluorescein sodium

FLUOR-I-STRIP
(fluorescein sodium ophthalmic strips)

Wyeth-Ayerst

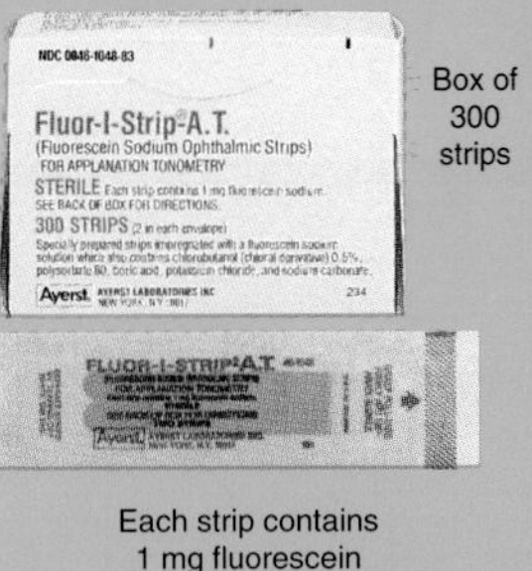

Box of 300 strips

Each strip contains
1 mg fluorescein sodium

FLUOR-I-STRIP -A.T.
(fluorescein sodium ophthalmic strips)
For Applanation Tonometry

Wyeth-Ayerst

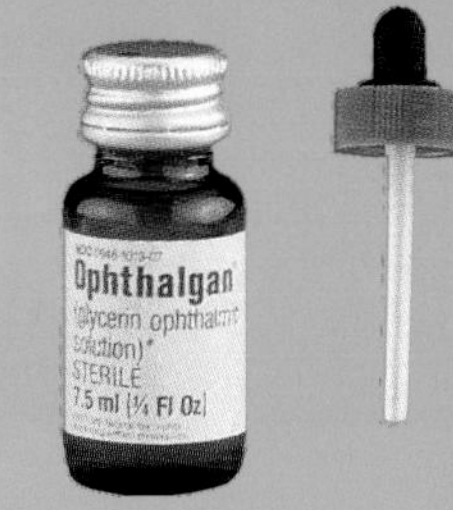

7.5 mL
(1/4 Fl. Oz.)

OPHTHALGAN
(glycerin ophthalmic solution)

Sterile

Wyeth-Ayerst

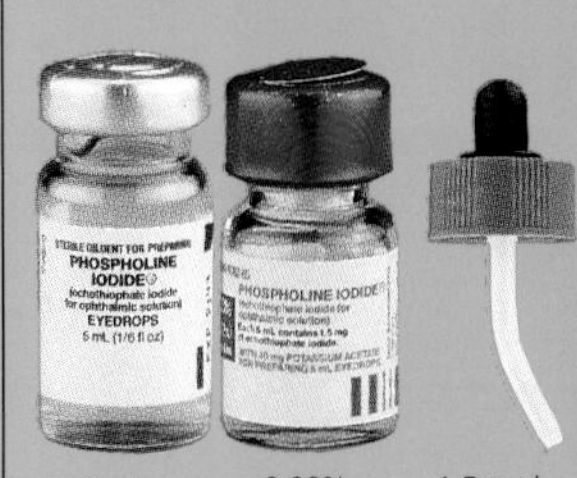

Sterile diluent | 0.03% (1/32%) sterile powder | 1.5 mg/5 mL

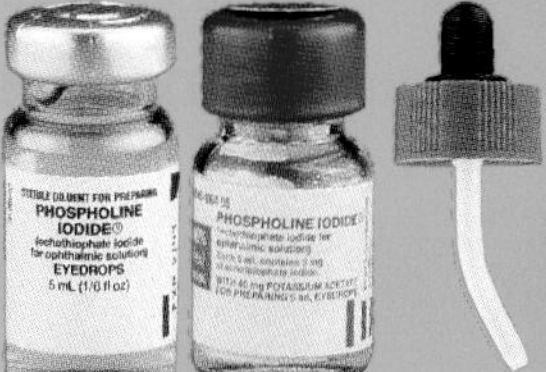

Sterile diluent | 0.06% (1/16%) sterile powder | 3 mg/5 mL

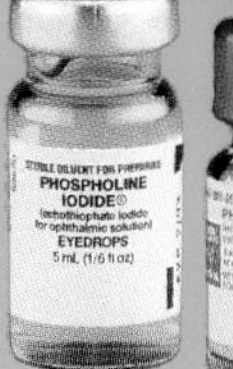

Sterile diluent | 0.125% (1/8%) sterile powder | 6.25 mg/5 mL

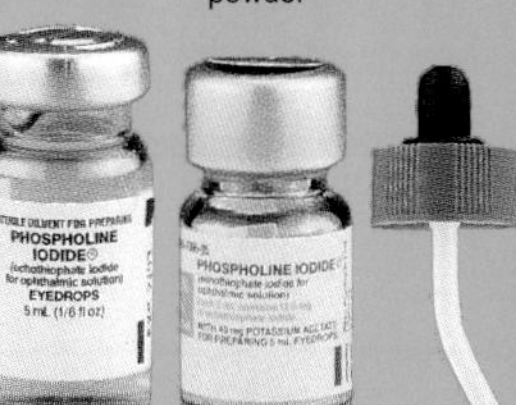

Sterile diluent | 0.25% (1/4%) sterile powder | 12.5 mg/5 mL

PHOSPHOLINE IODIDE
(echothiophate iodide for ophthalmic solution)

**Ledermark Product Identification Codes.

COLOR VISION SCREENING CHART

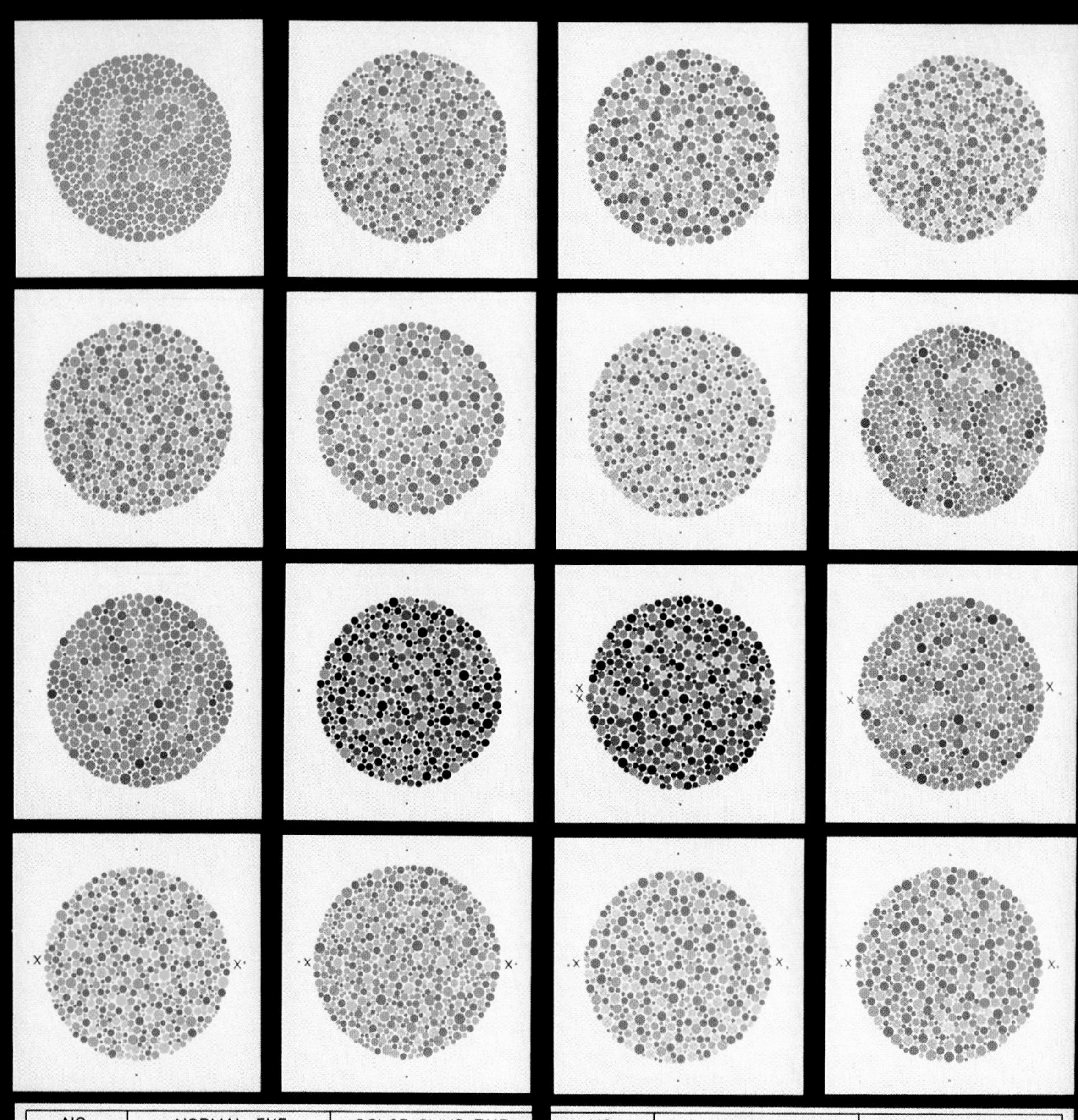

NO.	NORMAL EYE	COLOR BLIND EYE
1	12	12
2	8	3
3	29	70
4	5	2
5	74	21
6	45	NOTHING
7	5	NOTHING
8	NOTHING	5

NO.	NORMAL EYE	COLOR BLIND EYE
9	NOTHING	45
10	26	2 OR 6
11	2 LINES X TO X	LINE X TO X
12	NOTHING	LINE X TO X
13	LINE X TO X	NOTHING
14	LINE X TO X	NOTHING
15	LINE X TO X	NOTHING
16	LINE X TO X	LINE X TO X

COVER ANSWERS BEFORE TESTING PATIENT

SECTION 8

Pharmaceutical Product Information

This book is made possible through the courtesy of the manufacturers whose products appear on the following pages. The information concerning each product has been prepared by the manufacturer, and edited and approved by the medical department, medical director, or medical counsel of each manufacturer.

In presenting the following material to the medical profession, the publisher is not necessarily advocating the use of any product listed.

Akorn, Inc.
100 AKORN DRIVE
ABITA SPRINGS, LA 70420

AKARPINE ℞
[-kar'pēn]
(pilocarpine hydrochloride)
Sterile Ophthalmic Solution

Description: An aqueous solution containing Pilocarpine Hydrochloride, hydroxypropyl methylcellulose (4000 centipoise), sodium phosphate, purified water. Preservatives: Benzalkonium Chloride 0.01% and EDTA disodium.

Action: Constricts the pupil by direct action on the myoneural junction of the sphincter muscle. Constriction of the pupil moves the iris away from the narrow filtration angle facilitating the outflow of aqueous.

Indications and Uses: As a myotic, especially in the management of open angle glaucoma; in the control of pre- and post-operative intraocular tension; and as an antidote for mydriasis after use of mydriatic or cycloplegic drugs.

Precautions: Keep container tightly closed. Do not touch dropper tip to any surface since this may contaminate solution. Store in a cool place protected from light.

If accidentally swallowed, evacuate stomach and treat promptly with atropine.

Side Effects: Occasional sensitization of the lids and conjuctiva may occur. Reduce concentration or discontinue if condition persists.

Administration: Frequency and concentration of dosage must be determined by the Ophthalmologist based on the effective response of each patient. Usual dose: 1 drop 3 times daily. Acute narrow-angle glaucoma: 1 drop every 5 to 15 minutes for 1 or 2 hours until miosis occurs and ocular tension is reduced.

How Supplied: 15 ml Plastic Dropper Bottles

1%—NDC 17478-223-12
2%—NDC 17478-224-12
4%—NDC 17478-226-12

AK-CHLOR ℞
(chloramphenicol)
Sterile Ophthalmic Solution
Sterile Ophthalmic Ointment

Description: This product is a sterile ophthalmic antibacterial prepared as a solution and ointment. The active ingredient is Chloramphenicol.

Each ml of the solution contains:
Chloramphenicol 0.5%
in a base containing Polyoxyl 40 Stearate, Polyethyene Glycol & Water. Preserved with Chlorobutanol 0.5%. pH adjusted with Sodium Hydroxide or Hydrochloric Acid.

Each ml of the ointment contains:
Chloramphenicol 1.0%
in a base containing the inactive ingredients: Mineral Oil, White Petrolatum and Polysorbate 60

Clinical Pharmacology: Chloramphenicol is a broad-spectrum antibiotic originally isolated from Streptomyces venezuelae. It is primarily bacteriostatic and acts by inhibition of protein synthesis by interfering with the transfer of activated amino acids from soluble RNA to ribosomes. It has been noted that chloramphenicol is found in measurable amounts in the aqueous humor following local application to the eye. Development of resistance to chloramphenicol can be regarded as minimal for staphlococci and many other species of bacteria.

Indications and Usage: Chloramphenicol should be used only in those serious infections for which less potentially dangerous drugs are ineffective or contraindicated. Bacteriological studies should be performed to determine the causative organisms and their sensitivity to chloramphenicol ***(See Box Warning).***

AK-CHLOR is indicated for the treatment of superficial ocular infections involving the conjuctiva and/or cornea caused by chloramphenicol-susceptible organisms. Bacteriological studies should be performed to determine the causative organisms and their sensitivity to chloramphenicol.

Contraindications: This product is contraindicated in persons sensitive to any of its components.

Warnings:

Bone marrow hypoplasia, including aplastic anemia and death has been reported following local application of chloramphenicol. Chloramphenicol should not be used when less potentially dangerous agents would be expected to provide effective treatment.

Precautions: The prolonged use of antibiotics may occasionally result in overgrowth of nonsusceptible organisms, including fungi. If the new infections appear during medication, the drug should be discontinued and appropriate measures should be taken. In all except very superficial infections the topical use of chloramphenicol should be supplemented by appropriate systemic medication.

Continued on next page

Akorn—Cont.

Adverse Reactions: Blood dyscrasias have been reported in association with the use of chloramphenicol (See WARNINGS).
Dosage and Administration: Solution: Two drops applied to the affected eye every three hours or more frequently if deemed advisable by the prescribing physician. Administration should be continued day and night for the first 48 hours, after which the interval between applications may be increased. Treatment should be continued for at least 48 hours after the eye appears normal.
Ointment: Apply a small amount to the lower conjunctival sac(s) at bedtime as a supplement to the drops.
Storage: Solution:
Refrigerate at 36°–46°F (2°–8°C). Protect from light. Remove from refrigerator for dispensing; discard 21 days thereafter. Ointment: Store at controlled room temperature 15°–30°C (59°–86°F)
How Supplied: Plastic Dropper Bottles containing: 7.5 and 15 ml.; 3.5 gm ointment.
7.5 mL NDC 17478-281-09
15 mL NDC 17478-281-12
3.5 gm NDC 17478-280-35

AK-CIDE ℞
(prednisolone acetate, USP and sulfacetamide sodium, USP)
Sterile Ophthalmic Suspension
Sterile Ophthalmic Ointment

Description: AK-Cide Ophthalmic Suspension (Sterile) is a steroid/anti-infective sterile preparation having a pH range of 6.6 - 7.4. Each ml contains: 5 mg. prednisolone acetate, USP; 100 mg. sulfacetamide sodium, USP; sodium phosphate (monobasic and dibasic), anhydrous polysorbate 80, hydroxypropyl methylcellulose 2906 (viscosity type 4000), benzalkonium chloride 0.01%, sodium thiosulfate pentahydrate and purified water.
Description: AK-Cide Ophthalmic Ointment (Sterile) is a steroid/anti-infective sterile preparation containing in each gram 5 mg. prednisolone acetate, USP and 100 mg. sulfacetamide sodium, USP; 0.5 mg. methylparaben and 0.1 mg. propylparaben as preservatives in a bland unctuous base of mineral oil, white petrolatum and lanolin.
Clinical Pharmacology: Corticosteroids suppress the inflammatory response to a variety of agents and they probably delay or slow healing. Since corticoids may inhibit the body's defense mechanism against infection, a concomitant antimicrobial drug may be used when this inhibition is considered to be clinically significant in a particular case.
The anti-infective component in the combination is included to provide action against specific organisms susceptible to it. Sulfacetamide sodium is considered active against the following microorganisms: **Escherichia coli, Staphylococcus aureus, Streptococcus pneumoniae, Streptococcus (viridans group), Pseudomonas** species, **Haemophilus influenzae, Klebsiella** species, and **Enterobacter** species.
Does not provide adequate coverage against **Hemophilus influenzae, Klebsiella/Enterobacter** species, **Neisseria species** and **Serratia marcescens.**
When a decision is made to administer both a corticoid and an antimicrobial, the administration of such drugs in combination has the advantages of greater patient compliance and convenience and added assurance that the appropriate dosage of both drugs is administered. There is also assured compatibility of ingredients when both types of drug are in the same formulation and, particularly, that the correct volume of drug is delivered and retained.
The relative potency of corticosteroids depends on the molecular structure, concentration, and release from the vehicle.
Indications and Usage: AK-Cide Ophthalmic Suspension or Ointment is indicated for ocular inflammation when concurrent use of an antimicrobial and a steroid is judged necessary.
Contraindications: AK-Cide Ophthalmic Suspension and Ophthalmic Ointment are contraindicated in: epithelial herpes simplex keratitis (dendritic keratitis), vaccinia, varicella, and many other viral diseases of the cornea or conjunctiva; mycobacterial infection of the eye; and fungal diseases of ocular structures. AK-Cide Ophthalmic Suspension and AK-Cide Ophthalmic Ointment are contraindicated in individuals with known or suspected hypersensitivity to any of the ingredients of the preparation, or to other sulfonamides, or other corticosteroids. (Hypersensitivity to the antibacterial components.) The use of these combinations is always contraindicated after uncomplicated removal of a corneal foreign body.
Warnings: Prolonged use may result in glaucoma, with damage to the optic nerve, defects in visual acuity and fields of vision, and in posterior subcapsular cataract formation. Prolonged use may suppress the host response and thus increase the hazard of secondary ocular infections. In those diseases causing thinning of the cornea or sclera, perforations have been known to occur with the use of topical steroids. In acute purulent conditions of the eye, steroids may mask infection or enhance existing infection. If these products are used for 10 days or longer, intraocular pressure should be routinely monitored even though this may be difficult in children and uncooperative patients. Employment of steroid medication in the treatment of herpes simplex requires great caution. A significant percentage of staphylococcal isolates are completely resistant to sulfonamides.
Precautions: The initial prescription and renewal of the medication order beyond 20 ml of AK-Cide Ophthalmic Suspension or beyond 8 gm of the Ointment should be made by a physician only after examination of the patient with the aid of magnification such as slitlamp biomicroscopy and where appropriate, fluorescein staining.
The possibility of fungal infections of the cornea should be considered after prolonged steroid dosing.
Sensitization may recur when a sulfonamide is readministered irrespective of the route of administration and cross-sensitivity among different sulfonamides may occur. (See ADVERSE REACTIONS.) Cross-allergenicity among corticosteroids has been demonstrated. If signs of hypersensitivity or other untoward reactions occur, discontinue use of the preparation.
Adverse Reactions: Adverse reactions have occurred which can be attributed to the steroid component, the anti-infective component, or the combination. Exact incidence figures are not available since no denominator of treated patients is available.
Instances of Stevens-Johnson syndrome and systemic lupus erythematosus (in one case producing a fatal outcome) have been reported following the use of ophthalmic sulfonamide-containing preparations.
The reactions due to the steroid component in decreasing order of frequency are: elevation of intraocular pressure (IOP) with possible development of glaucoma, and infrequent optic nerve damage; posterior subcapsular cataract formation; and delayed wound healing.
Corticosteroid-containing preparations can also cause acute anterior uveitis or perforation of the globe. Mydriasis, loss of accommodation, and ptosis have occasionally been reported following local use of corticosteroids.
Secondary Infection: The development of secondary infection has occurred after use of combinations containing steroids and antimicrobials. Fungal infections of the cornea are particularly prone to develop coincidentally with long term applications of the steroid. The possibility of fungal invasion must be considered in any persistent corneal ulceration where steroid treatment has been used.
Secondary bacterial ocular infection following suppression of host responses also occurs.
Dosage and Administration: AK-Cide Ophthalmic Suspension: One or two drops should be instilled into the conjunctival sac every one to two hours during the day and at bedtime until a favorable response is obtained.
AK-Cide Ophthalmic Ointment: A thin film should be applied three or four times daily and once at bedtime until a favorable response is obtained.
The initial prescription of AK-Cide Ophthalmic should **not** be more than 20 ml of the Suspension or 8g of the Ointment and the prescription should not be refilled without further evaluation as outlined in the PRECAUTIONS Section.
Dosage should be adjusted according to the specific needs of the patient. AK-Cide Ophthalmic Suspension or Ointment dosage may be reduced, but care should be taken not to discontinue therapy prematurely. In chronic conditions, withdrawal of treatment should be carried out by gradually decreasing the frequency of application.
Storage: Store between 2° and 30° C (36° and 86° F). Protect from light. Clumping may occur on long standing at high temperatures. Shake well before using.
How Supplied: Ophthalmic Suspension, 5 ml and 15 ml dropper bottle. Ophthalmic Ointment, 3.5 gm applicator tube.
5 mL NDC 17478-275-10
15 mL NDC 17478-275-12
3.5 gm NDC 17478-275-35

AK-CON ℞
(naphazoline hydrochloride 0.1%)
Sterile Ophthalmic Solution

Description: An ocular vasoconstrictor ophthalmic containing: Naphazoline Hydrochloride 0.1% in a Boric Acid-Sodium Carbonate buffered isotonic saline solution preserved with Benzalkonium Chloride 0.01%, and Disodium Edetate 0.01%.
Actions: Constricts the vascular system of the conjunctiva. It is presumed this effect is due to the direct action of the drug upon the alpha (excitatory) receptors of the vascular smooth muscle.
Indications: For use as a topical ocular vasoconstrictor.
Contraindications: Hypersensitivity to a component of this medication. Narrow-Angle glaucoma.
Warnings: A severe hypertensive crisis may ensue in patients under MAO inhibitor medication from use of a sympathomimetic drug.
Precautions: Use only with caution in the presence of hypertension, cardiac irregularities, hyperglycemia (diabetes), hyperthyroidism.
Adverse Reactions: Pupillary dilation with increase in intraocular pressure, systemic effects due to absorption (hypertension, cardiac irregularities, hyperglycemia). Accidental ingestion (especially in children) may cause marked sedation requiring emergency treatment.
Dosage and Administration: 1–2 drops every 3–4 hours.
Supply: 15 ml. Plastic Dropper Bottles.
NDC 17478-216-12

AK-CON-A ℞
(Naphazoline Hydrochloride and Pheniramine Maleate)
Sterile Ophthalmic Solution

Description: AK-CON-A is a combination of a decongestant and an antihistamine prepared as a sterile topical ophthalmic solution.
Each ml contains: Active: Naphazoline Hydrochloride 0.025% Pheniramine Maleate 0.3%. Preservative: Benzalkonium Chloride 0.01%. Inactive: Boric Acid, Sodium Borate, Edetate Disodium, Sodium Chloride, Sodium Hydroxide and/or Hydrochloric Acid (to adjust pH), and Purified Water.
Clinical Pharmacology: AK-CON-A combines the effects of the antihistamine, pheniramine maleate, and the decongestant, naphazoline.

Indications and Usage: Based on a review of a related combination of drugs by the National Academy of Sciences—National Research Council and/or other information, FDA has classified the indications as follows: "Possibly" effective: For relief of ocular irritation and/or congestion or for the treatment of allergic or inflammatory ocular conditions. Final classification of the less-than-effective indication requires further investigation.

Contraindications: Hypersensitivity to one or more of the components of this preparation.
Warnings: Do not use in the presence of narrow angle glaucoma. Patients under MAO inhibitors may experience a severe hypertensive crisis if given a sympathomimetic drug. Use in infants and children may result in CNS depression leading to coma and marked reduction in body temperature.
Precautions: This preparation should be used with caution in elderly patients with severe cardiovascular disease including cardiac arrhythmias; patients with poorly controlled hypertension; patients with diabetes, especially those with a tendency toward diabetic ketoacidosis. To prevent contaminating the dropper tip and solution, care should be taken not to touch the eyelids or surrounding area with the dropper tip of the bottle.
Adverse Reactions: The following adverse reactions may occur: Pupillary dilation, increase in intraocular pressure, systemic effects due to absorption (i.e., hypertension, cardiac irregularities, hyperglycemia).
Dosage and Administration: One or two drops instilled in each eye every 3 to 4 hours or less frequently, as required to relieve symptoms.
Storage: Store at 36° to 80°F. Keep bottle tightly closed when not in use. Protect from light and excessive heat.
How Supplied: 15ml plastic dropper bottle.
NDC 17478-215-12

AK-DEX ℞
(dexamethasone sodium phosphate)
Sterile Ophthalmic/Otic Solution
Sterile Ophthalmic Ointment

Description: AK-Dex Solution is a water soluble form of the synthetic anti-inflammatory steroid dexamethasone.
Each ml. of solution contains:
Dexamethasone Sodium Phosphate (Equivalent to Dexamethasone Phosphate) 0.1%
Benzalkonium Chloride (Preservative) 0.01%
In an isotonic, phosphate buffered saline solution containing Sodium Edetate and Hydroxyethyl cellulose.
Description: AK-Dex Ointment is an adrenocortical steroid prepared as a sterile ophthalmic ointment containing Dexamethasone Sodium Phosphate equivalent to 0.5 mg (0.05%). Dexamethasone Phosphate in each gram. Inactive ingredients: Mineral Oil, White Petrolatum, Lanolin Anhydrous, Propylparaben, Methylparaben, Polyethylene Glycol 400 and Purified Water.
Dexamethasone Sodium Phosphate is an inorganic ester of dexamethasone.
Actions: This drug causes inhibition of inflammatory response to inciting agents of mechanical, chemical, or immunological nature. No generally accepted explanation of this steroid property has been advanced.
Indications: For the treatment of the following conditions:
Ophthalmic:
Steroid responsive inflammatory conditions of the palpebral and bulbar conjunctiva, cornea, and anterior segment of the globe, such as allergic conjunctivitis, acne rosacea, superficial punctate keratitis, herpes zoster keratitis, iritis, cyclitis, selected infective conjunctivitis when the inherent hazard of steroid use is accepted to obtain an advisable diminution in edema and inflammation; corneal injury from chemical, radiation, or thermal burns, or penetration of foreign bodies.
Contraindications:
1. Acute superficial herpes simplex keratitis
2. Fungal diseases of ocular structures
3. Taccinia, varicella and most other viral diseases of the cornea and conjunctiva
4. Tuberculosis of the eye
5. Hypersensitivity to a component of this medication.

Warnings:
1. Steroid medication in the treatment of herpes simplex keratitis involving the stroma requires great caution; frequent slit-lamp microscopy is mandatory.
2. Prolonged use may result in glaucoma, damage to the optic nerve, defect in visual acuity and fields of vision, posterior subcapsular cataract formation, or may aid in the establishment of secondary ocular infections from pathogens liberated from ocular tissues.
3. In those diseases causing thinning of the cornea or sclera, perforation has been known to occur with the use of topical steroids.
4. Acute purulent untreated infection of the eye may be masked or activity enhanced by presence of steroid medication.
5. Usage in pregnancy: Safety of intensive or protracted use of topical steroids during pregnancy has not been established.

Precautions: As fungal infection of the cornea are particularly prone to develop coincidentally with long-term steroid applications, fungus invasion must be suspected in any persistent corneal ulceration where a steroid has been used or is in use.
Intraocular pressure should be checked frequently.
The use of this drug should be discontinued if improvement in the condition being treated does not occur within several days.
Care should be exercised to avoid contamination of the material during its use.
Store in a cool place.
Protect from light.
Adverse Reactions: Glaucoma with optic nerve damage, visual acuity and field defects, posterior subcapsular cataract formation, secondary ocular infections from pathogens liberated from ocular tissues, perforation of the globe
Dosage:
Solution: Initially, 1 or 2 drops placed in the conjunctival sac every hour until improvement occurs. Thereafter, gradually reduce to 1 or 2 drops every 3 or 4 hours.
Ointment: Apply a thin coating of ointment three or four times a day. When a favorable response is observed, reduce the number of daily applications to two, and later to one a day as a maintenance dose if this is sufficient to control symptoms. AK-Dex Ophthalmic Ointment, is particularly convenient when an eye pad is used. It may also be the preparation of choice for patients in whom therapeutic benefit depends on prolonged contact of the active ingredients with ocular tissues.
Advise: Occasional stinging or burning of the eye may occur after application. Notify physician if eye pain or infection occurs.
Caution: Federal law prohibits dispensing without prescription.
How Supplied: Solution: 5 ml plastic squeeze bottles with dropper tip.
Ointment: 3.5 gram (1/8 ounce) tube with applicator tip.
5 mL NDC 17478-279-10
3.5 gm NDC 17478-278-35

AK-DILATE ℞
(phenylephrine hydrochloride)
Sterile Ophthalmic Solution

Description: AK-DILATE is a sterile ophthalmic solution. Each ml. contains phenylephrine hydrochloride 2.5%, or 10% with boric acid, sodium borate, edetate disodium, and sodium bisulfite. Preserved with benzalkonium chloride 0.01%. AK-DILATE contains a sympathomimetic agent producing both vasoconstricting and mydriatic effects. Phenylephrine hydrochloride is a synthetic sympathomimetic compound structurally similar to epinephrine and ephedrine. A prompt, short acting mydriatic, it causes little or no cycloplegia or irritation.
Actions: Phenylephrine hydrochloride is presumed to have a direct effect upon the alpha-adrenergic receptor stimulator producing pupil dilation and vasoconstriction.
Indications: As an ophthalmic decongestant and vasoconstrictor and for pupil dilation in uveitis (posterior synechiae), wide angle glaucoma, surgery, refraction, ophthalmoscopic examination and diagnostic procedures.
Contraindications: Narrow-angle glaucoma, hypertension, and in persons with a known hypersensitivity to any component.
Warning: For topical ophthalmic use only. As with all other adrenergic drugs, when administered simultaneously with, or up to 21 days after, administration of monoamine oxidase (MAO) inhibitors, careful supervision and adjustment of dosages are required since exaggerated adrenergic effects may result. The pressor response of adrenergic agents may also be potentiated by tricyclic antidepressants.
Precautions: AK-DILATE should be used with caution in patients with advanced arteriosclerotic conditions or severe hypertension. Phenylephrine may be used in patients with glaucoma when temporary dilation of the pupil may free adhesions or when vasoconstriction of intrinsic vessels may lower intraocular tension: these advantages may temporarily outweigh the danger from coincident dilation of the pupil.
Do not use if solution is discolored or contains a precipitate.
Do not touch dropper tip to any surface, since this may contaminate the solution.
Adverse Reactions: It is well to bear in mind that phenylephrine is, in fact, a sympathomimetic drug related to epinephrine and ephedrine, and that although the incidence is rare, it may produce such reactions as tremor, pallor, perspiration, palpitation or collapse.
Dosage and Administration: Topically, 1 or 2 drops into the conjunctiva of each eye for refraction, in conjunction with the cycloplegic of choice, and ophthalmoscopic examination. AK-DILATE may be applied topically from 30 to 60 minutes prior to surgery.
Storage: Keep container tightly closed. Store in a cool place, protected from light.

Continued on next page

Akorn—Cont.

How Supplied:
2.5%—2 mL NDC 17478-200-20
2.5%—15mL NDC 17478-200-12
10%—2mL NDC 17478-205-20
10%—5mL NDC 17478-205-10

AK-FLUOR Injection ℞
(fluorescein injection, U.S.P.)

Description: AK-FLUOR is a sterile, aqueous solution of Fluorescein Sodium in Water for Injection. pH is adjusted with Sodium Hydroxide, and/or Hydrochloric Acid.
See "How Supplied" for potencies available.
Actions: Fluorescein will create a yellowish-green fluorescence which delineates the vascular area under study from adjacent areas.
Indications: Indicated for angiography of retinal vessels. To detect occlusion or obliteration of retinal vessels, vascular malformations, neovascularization, changes in vascular permeability, ocular tumors, and defects in the retinal pigment epithelium.
Contraindications: Known hypersensitivity to any of the components.
Precautions: Patients with a history of either allergy or bronchial asthma should be evaluated and caution exercised.
Use in Pregnancy: Avoid angiography on patients who are pregnant, especially those in first trimester. There have been no reports of fetal complications for fluorescein injection during pregnancy.
Adverse Reactions: Nausea, vomiting, headache, gastrointestinal distress, syncope, hypotension, and other symptoms and signs of hypersensitivity have occurred. Immediate hypersensitivity reactions have occurred only rarely, but there should be facilities to treat these reactions available. Cardiac arrest, basilar artery ischemia, severe shock, convulsions, and thrombophlebitis at the injected site have been reported. Following systemic absorption, this dye causes transient fluorescence of the skin and appears in the urine. Discoloration of the skin fades in 6 to 12 hours, urine fluorescence in approximately 24 to 36 hours.
Dosage and Administration:
AK-FLUOR 10% (Fluorescein Injection 10%, USP—Sterile)
Adults: 5mL (500mg) injected rapidly in the antecubital vein.
Children: 0.035mL (3.5mg) for each pound of body weight, injected rapidly in the antecubital vein.
AK-FLUOR 25% (Fluorescein Injection 25%, USP—Sterile)
Adults: 2 mL (500mg) (3 mL = 750mg) injected rapidly in the antecubital vein.
Children: 0.02mL (5mg) for each pound of body weight, injected rapidly in the antecubital vein.
Fluorescence of the retinal vessels should occur within 12–30 seconds.
IN CASE OF EMERGENCY, INTRAVENOUS EPINEPHRINE 1:1000 SHOULD BE AVAILABLE AT THE TIME OF DRUG ADMINISTRATION. AN ANTIHISTAMINE SHOULD ALSO BE AVAILABLE.
Inject rapidly into the antecubital vein. The dye should appear in the central retinal artery in 9 to 15 seconds. This may be observed with standard viewing equipment. At the time of administration, an emergency tray including such items as 0.1% epinephrine for intravenous or intramuscular use, an antihistamine, soluble steroid, aminophylline for intravenous use, and oxygen should be available in the event of possible reaction to fluorescein injection.
In patients with inaccessible veins where early phases of an angiogram are not necessary, such as cystoid macular edema, one gram of **AK-FLUOR** has been administered orally. Ten to fifteen minutes is usually required before evidence of dye appears in the fundus.
Parenteral drug products should be inspected visually for particulate matter and discoloration, whenever solution and container permit.
How Supplied:
AK-FLUOR 10%
NDC 17478-253-10 12 × 5mL Single Dose Vials
NDC 17478-254-10 25 × 5mL Ampules
AK-FLUOR 25%
NDC 17478-250-20 12 × 2mL Single Dose Vials
NDC 17478-251-20 12 × 2mL Ampules

AK-MYCIN Ointment ℞
(erythromycin U.S.P.)

AK-Mycin is a wide-range antibiotic prepared in a sterile ophthalmic ointment.
Contents: Each gram of the sterile ointment contains:
ACTIVE: Erythromycin base 5 mg.
INACTIVE: White Petrolatum and Mineral Oil. Contains no preservatives.
Indications and Usage: For the treatment of superficial ocular infections involving the conjunctiva and/or cornea caused by organisms susceptible to erythromycin.
For prophylaxis of ophthalmia neonatorium due to *Neisseria gonorrhoeae* or *Chlamydia trachomatis.* The Center for Disease Control and the Committee on Drugs, the Committee on Fetus and Newborn, and the Committee on Infectious Diseases of the American Academy of Pediatrics recommend 1% silver nitrate solution in single-use tubes of an ophthalmic ointment containing 0.5% erythromycin or 1% tetracycline as "effective and acceptable regimens for prophylaxis of gonococcal ophthalmia neonatorum". (For infants born to mothers with clinically apparent gonorrhea, intravenous or intramuscular injections of aqueous crystalline penicillin G should be given: a single dose of 50,000 units for term infants or 20,000 units for infants of low birth weight. Topical prophylaxis alone is inadequate for these infants. AK-Mycin ointment also has been effective for prevention of neonatal conjunctivitis due to C. trachomatis, a condition that may develop 1 to several weeks after delivery in infants of mothers whose birth canals harbor the organism.
Contraindications: This drug is contraindicated in patients with a history of hypersensitivity to erythromycin.
Precautions: The use of antimicrobial agents may be associated with the overgrowth of antibiotic-resistant organisms, in such a case antibiotic administration should be stopped and appropriate measures taken.
Adverse Reactions: As with any other medication intended for topical use, there is always the possibility that sensitivity reactions will occur in certain individuals. If such reactions develop, the medication should be discontinued.
Dosage and Administration: In the treatment of external ocular infections, AK-Mycin Ointment should be applied directly to the infected structure one or more times daily, depending on the severity of the infection. For prophylaxis of neonatal gonococcal or chlamydial conjuctivitis, a ribbon of ointment approximately 0.5 to 1 cm in length should be instilled into each conjuctival sac. The ointment should not be flushed from the eye following instillation.
A new tube should be used for each infant. Infants born by cesarean section as well as those delivered by the vaginal route should receive prophylaxis.
How Supplied: 3.5 gm (1/8oz.) applicator tube
NDC 17478-801-35

AK-NaCl 5% Ointment & Solution OTC
(sodium chloride 5%)

Description: A sterile ophthalmic hypertonic ointment containing Sodium Chloride 5% in a base of Anhydrous Lanolin, Mineral Oil, White Petrolatum and Purified Water.
Description: A sterile ophthalmic hypertonic solution of Sodium Chloride 5% with Hydroxypropyl Methylcellulose. Also contains Propylene Glycol and Purified Water, buffered with Sodium Borate and Boric Acid. Preservatives are Methylparaben and Propylparaben.
Indications: For the temporary relief of corneal edema.
Contraindications: Hypersensitivity to any ingredient in the preparation.
Warnings: Do not use this product except under the supervision of a physician. If you experience severe pain, headache, rapid change in vision (side and straight ahead), sudden appearance of floating spots, acute redness of the eyes, pain on exposure to light, or double vision, consult a physician at once. To avoid contamination of this product, do not touch the tip of the container to any surface. Replace cap after using. This product may cause temporary burning and irritation on being instilled into the eye.
Directions: Apply one or more times a day or as directed by a physician.
How Supplied:
15 mL Solution NDC 17478-621-12
3.5 gm Ointment NDC 17478-620-35

AK-PENTOLATE ℞
(cyclopentolate hydrochloride)
Sterile Ophthalmic Solution

Description:
Each ml contains:
Active:
Cyclopentolate Hydrochloride 1.0%
Inactive:
Benzalkonium Chloride 0.01%
Potassium Chloride 0.2%
Disodium Edetate 0.01%
Boric Acid 1.0%
Sodium Carbonate ....to adjust pH
Purified Water ....q.s.
Actions: This anticholinergic preparation blocks the responses of the sphincter muscle of the iris and the accommodative muscle of the ciliary body to cholinergic stimulation, producing pupillary dilation (mydriasis) and paralysis of accommodation (cycloplegia). It acts rapidly, but has a shorter duration than atropine.
Indications: For mydriasis and cycloplegia for diagnostic purposes.
Contraindications: Should not be used where narrow-angle glaucoma is present.
Precautions: In the elderly and others where increased intraocular pressure may be encountered, mydriatics and cycloplegics should be used cautiously. Tonometric examination prior to drop instillation is advisable. Systemic absorption may be minimized by compressing the lacrimal sac for a minute or two during the following instillation of the drops. Sac compression blocks passage of the drops to the wide absorption area of the nasal and pharyngeal mucosa. This is advisable especially in children.
Adverse Reactions: Increased intraocular pressure. Use of Cyclopentolate has been associated with psychotic reactions and behavioral disturbances in children especially in higher concentrations. Ataxia, incoherent speech, restlessness, hallucinations, disorientation as to time and place, failure to recognize people, and tachycardia, have been reported.

Dosage and Administration: Adults: One drop is instilled in each eye at the time of retraction, followed 10 minutes later by a second application if necessary. Although complete recovery usually occurs in 24 hours, 1 or 2 drops of 1% or 2% pilocarpine reduces recovery time to 3 to 6 hours in most eyes.

How Supplied:
15 mL NDC 17478-100-12
2 mL NDC 17478-100-20

Storage: Store at 59°–86°F. (15°–30°C.)

AK-POLY-BAC Ointment ℞
(bacitracin zinc, polymyxin B sulfate)

Description: AK-Poly-Bac Ophthalmic Ointment is a sterile anti-microbial ointment formulated for ophthalmic use to contain bacitracin zinc and polymyxin B sulfate in a special white petrolatum-mineral oil base. Contains no preservatives.

Each gram contains 500 units of bacitracin zinc and 10,000 units of polymyxin B sulfate.

Bacitracin zinc is the zinc salt of bacitracin, a mixture of related cyclic polypeptides (mainly bacitracin A) produced by the growth of an organism of the *licheniformis* group of *Bacillus subtilis* (Fam. Bacillaceae). It has a potency of not less than 40 bacitracin units per milligram. The precise formula is not known.

Polymixin B Sulfate is the sulfate salt of polymyxin B_1 and B_2 which are produced by the growth of *Bacillus polymyxa* (Prazmowski) Migula (Fam. Bacillaceae). It has a potency of not less than 6,000 polymyxin B units per milligram, calculated on an anhydrous basis.

Indications and Usage: For the treatment of superficial ocular infections involving the conjunctive and/or cornea caused by organisms susceptible to Polymyxin B Sulfate and Bacitracin Zinc.

Contraindications: This product is contraindicated in those individuals who have shown hypersensitivity to any of its components.

Warnings: Ophthalmic Ointments may retard corneal healing.

Precautions: As with other antibiotic preparations, prolonged use may result in overgrowth of non-susceptible organisms, including fungi. Appropriate measures should be taken if this occurs.

Information for Patients: If redness, irritation, swelling or pain persists or increases, discontinue use and contact your physician.

Avoid contaminating the applicator tip with material from the eye, fingers, or other source. This caution is necessary if the sterility of the ointment is to be preserved.

Adverse Reactions: The most frequent adverse reactions are localized hypersensitivity including itching, swelling and conjunctival erythema.

Dosage and Administration: Apply every 3 or 4 hours, depending on the severity of the infection.

How Supplied:
3.5 gm (⅛oz.) NDC 17478-238-35

AK–PRED ℞
(prednisolone sodium phosphate) Sterile Ophthalmic Solution

Description: AK-PRED is a water soluble form of the synthetic anti-inflammatory steroid prednisolone.

Available in two strengths as follows:

Contents:
Each ml contains:

	Ak-Pred 0.125%	Ak-Pred-1%
Prednisolone Sodium Phosphate	0.125%	1.0%
Equivalent to Prednisolone)	0.1%	0.8%
Benzalkonium Chloride (Preservative)	0.01%	0.01%

In an isotonic, phosphate buffered saline solution containing Sodium Bisulfite, Sodium Edetate and Hydroxypropyl Methylcellulose.

Actions: This drug causes inhibition of inflammatory response to inciting agents of mechanical, chemical, or immunological nature. No generally accepted explanation of this steroid property has been advanced.

Indications: For the treatment of: Steroid responsive inflammatory conditions of the palpebral and bulbar conjuctiva, cornea and anterior segment of the globe, such as allergic conjunctivitis, acne rosacea, superficial punctate keratitis, herpes zoster keratitis, iritis, cyclitis, selected infective conjunctivitis when the inherent hazard of steroid use is accepted to obtain an advisable diminution in edema and inflammation: corneal injury from chemical, radiation, or thermal burns, or penetration of foreign bodies.

Contraindications:
1. Acute superficial herpes simplex keratitis
2. Fungal diseases of ocular structures
3. Vaccinia, varicella and most other viral diseases of the cornea and conjunctiva
4. Tuberculosis of the eye
5. Hypersensitivity to a component of this medication.

Warnings:
1. Steroid medication in the treatment of herpes simplex keratitis involving the stroma requires great caution; frequent slit-lamp microscopy is mandatory.
2. Prolonged use may result in glaucoma, damage to the optic nerve, defect in visual acuity and fields of vision, posterior subcapsular cataract formation, or may aid in the establishment of secondary ocular infections from pathogens liberated from ocular tissues.
3. In those diseases causing thinning of the cornea or sclera, perforation has been known to occur with the use of topical steroids.
4. Acute purulent untreated infection of the eye may be masked or activity enhanced by presence of steroid medication.
5. Usage in pregnancy: Safety of intensive or protracted use of topical steroids during pregnancy has not been established.

Precautions: As fungal infections of the cornea are particularly prone to develop coincidentally with long-term steroid applications, fungus invasion must be suspected in any persistent corneal ulceration where a steroid has been used or is in use.

Introacular pressure should be checked frequently.

The use of AK-PRED should be discontinued if improvement in the condition being treated does not occur within several days.

Care should be exercised to avoid contamination of the material during its use.

Store in a cool place. Protect from light.

Adverse Reactions: Glaucoma with optic nerve damage, visual acuity and field defects, posterior subcapsular cataract formation, secondary ocular infections from pathogens liberated from ocular tissues, perforation of the globe.

Dosage: Initially, 1 or 2 drops placed in the conjunctival sac every hour until improvement occurs. Thereafter, gradually reduce to 1 or 2 drops every 3 or 4 hours.

Supply:
0.125%—5 mL NDC 17478-218-10
1%—5 mL NDC 17478-219-10
1%—5 mL NDC 17478-219-12

Shown in Product Identification Section, page 103

AK–SPORE ℞
(neomycin sulfate-polymyxin B sulfate-gramicidin) Sterile Ophthalmic Solution (neomycin sulfate-polymyxin B sulfate-bacitracin zinc) Sterile Ophthalmic Ointment

Description: Solution—AK-SPORE Solution is a sterile aqueous solution formulated for ophthalmic use in the treatment of superficial external ocular infections. Each ml contains Polymyxin B Sulfate 10,000 units, Neomycin Sulfate (equivalent to 1.75 mg Neomycin base), Gramicidin 0.025 mg. The vehicle contains Alcohol 0.5%, Thimerosal (preservative) 0.001%, Propylene glycol, Polyoxyethylene-polyoxypropylene compound, Sodium chloride and Purified Water.

Ointment—AK-SPORE ointment is a sterile antimicrobial ointment formulated for ophthalmic use to contain bacitracin zinc, neomycin sulfate, and polymyxin B sulfate in a special white petrolatum-mineral oil base. Each gram contains 400 units of bacitracin, 3.5 milligrams of neomycin, and 10,000 units of Polymyxin B. Contains no preservatives.

Clinical Pharmacology: The anti-infective components in AK-SPORE Solution and Ointment are included to provide action against specific organisms susceptible to them. Neomycin Sulfate is considered effective against a wide range of gram-negative and gram-positive organisms, including many strains of **Proteus, Klebsiella, Staphylococcus aureus, Escherichia coli,** and **Haemophilus influenzae.** Polymyxin B Sulfate's effectiveness is sharply restricted to gram-negative bacteria, including many strains of **Escherichia coli, Haemophilus influenzae,** and **Pseudomonas aeruginosa.** Gramicidin is effective against gram-positive organisms including **Pneumococci, Staphylococci, Streptococci, Diphtheria bacilli,** and certain **anaerobic bacilli.**

Bacitracin is bactericidal for a variety of gram-positive and gram-negative organisms. It interferes with bacterial cell wall synthesis by inhibition of the regeneration of phospholipid receptors involved in peptidoglycan synthesis.

Indications and Usage: This product is indicated in the short-term treatment of superficial external ocular infections. The particular anti-infective drug(s) in this product are active against the following common bacterial eye pathogens:

Staphylococcus aureus
Streptococci, including **Streptococcus pneumoniae**
Escherichia coli
Haemophilus influenzae
Klebsiella/Enterobacter species
Nelsseria species
Pseudomonas aeruginosa

The product does not provide adequate coverage against:

Serratia marcescens

Contraindications: This product is contraindicated in those persons who have shown sensitivity to any of its components.

Warnings: Neomycin sulfate may cause cutaneous sensitization. A precise incidence of hypersensitivity reactions (primarily skin rash) due to topical neomycin is now known. The ophthalmic manifestations of sensitization to neomycin are usually itching, reddening and edema of the conjunctiva and eyelid. It may be manifest simply as a failure to heal. During long-term use of neomycin-containing products, periodic examination for such signs is advisable, and the patient should be told to discontinue the product if they are observed. These symptoms subside quickly on withdrawing the medication. Neomycin-containing applications should be avoided for the patient thereafter.

Continued on next page

Akorn—Cont.

Precautions: General: As with other antibiotic preparations, prolonged use may result in overgrowth of nonsusceptible organisms including fungi. Appropriate measures should be taken if this occurs.
Culture and susceptibility testing should be performed during treatment.
Allergic cross-reactions may occur which could prevent the use of any or all of the following antibiotics for the treatment of future infections; kanamycin, paromomycin, streptomycin, and possibly gentamicin.
Information for Patients: If redness, irritation, swelling or pain persists or increases, discontinue use and contact your physician.
Avoid contaminating the applicator tip with material from the eye, fingers, or other source. This caution is necessary if the sterility of the solution is to be preserved.
Adverse Reactions: The most frequent adverse reactions are localized hypersensitivity, including itching, swelling, and conjunctival erythema. Local irritation on instillation has also been reported. Exact incidence figures are not available since no denominator of treated patients is available.
Dosage and Administration: The suggested dosage is one or two drops in the affected eye, two to four times daily or more frequently, as required. In acute infection, initiate therapy with one or two drops every 15 to 30 minutes, reducing the frequency of instillation gradually as the infection is controlled. The patient should be instructed to avoid contaminating the applicator tip with material from an infected eye or other source. This is best done by preventing the tip from touching the eyelid or surrounding area. This caution is necessary in order to keep the sterile solution as free from contaminating organisms as possible. Apply the ointment every 3 or 4 hours for 7 to 10 days, depending on the severity of the infection.
How Supplied:
2 mL NDC 17478-790-20
10 mL NDC 17478-790-11
3.5 gm (1/8oz.) NDC 17478-235-35

AK-SPORE H.C. ℞

(neomycin sulfate-polymyxin B sulfate, hydrocortisone) Sterile Ophthalmic Suspension-
(neomycin sulfate-bacitracin zinc-polymyxin B sulfate-hydrocortisone) Sterile Ophthalmic Ointment

Description: Suspension—AK-Spore H.C. is a sterile antimicrobial and anti-inflammatory suspension intended for ophthalmic use.
Each ml contains: Polymyxin B Sulfate 10,000 units, Neomycin Sulfate equivalent to 3.5 mg Neomycin base and Hydrocortisone 10 mg (1%) in a vehicle containing 0.01% Benzalkonium Chloride (added as a preservative) and the inactive ingredients Cetyl Alcohol, Glyceryl Monostearate, Mineral Oil, Polyoxyl 40 Stearate, Propylene Glycol, Boric Acid, Sodium Borate and Purified Water.
Description: Ointment—A sterile antimicrobial/anti-inflammatory ointment formulated for ophthalmic use to contain bacitracin zinc, neomycin sulfate, and polymyxin B sulfate in a special white petrolatum-mineral oil base. Each gram contains 400 units of bacitracin, 3.5 milligrams of neomycin, 10,000 units of polymyxin B, 10 milligrams (1%) of Hydrocortisone in a white petrolatum base.
Bacitracin zinc is the zinc salt of bacitracin, a mixture of related cyclic polypeptides (mainly bacitracin A) produced by the growth of an organism of the **licheniformis** group of **Bacillus subtillis** (Fam. Bacillaceae). It has a potency of not less than 40 bacitracin units per milligram.
Clinical Pharmacology: Corticoids suppress the inflammatory response to a variety of agents and they may delay healing. Since corticoids may inhibit the body's defense mechanism against infection, a concomitant antimicrobial drug may be used when this inhibition is considered to be clinically significant in a particular case.
The anti-infective components in the combination are included to provide action against specific organisms susceptible to them. Polymyxin B Sulfate and Neomycin Sulfate together are considered active against the following microorganisms: *Staphylococcus aureus, Escherichia coli, Haemophilus influenzae, Klebsiella-Enterobacter* species, *Niesseria* species and *Pseudomonas aeruginosa.*
When a decision to administer both a corticoid and antimicrobials is made, the administration of such drugs in combination has the advantage of greater patient compliance and convenience, with the added assurance that the intended dosage of both drugs is administered, plus assured compatibility of ingredients when both types of drug are in the same formulation and, particularly, that the intended volume of drug is delivered simultaneously, thereby avoiding dilution of either medication by successive instillations.
The relative potency of corticosteroids depends on the molecular structure, concentration, and release from the vehicle.
Indications and Usage: For steroid-response inflammatory ocular conditions for which a corticosteroid is indicated and where bacterial infection or risk of bacterial ocular infection exists.
Ocular steroids are indicated in inflammatory conditions of the palpebral and bulbar conjunctiva, cornea and anterior segment of the globe where the inherent risk of steroid use in certain infective conjunctivitides is accepted to obtain a diminution in edema and inflammation. They are also indicated in chronic anterior uveitis and corneal injury from chemical, radiation, or thermal burns, or penetration of foreign bodies.
The use of a combination drug with an anti-infective component is indicated where the risk of infection is high or where there is an expectation that potentially dangerous numbers of bacteria will be present in the eye.
The particular anti-infective drugs in this product are active against the following common bacterial eye pathogens: *Staphyloccus aureus, Escherichia coli, Haemophilus influenzae, Klebsiella-Enterobacter* species, *Niesseria* species, and *Pseudomonas aeruginosa.*
The product does not provide adequate coverage against *Serratia marcescens* and streptococci, including *Streptoccus pneumoniae.*
Contraindications: Epithelial herpes simplex keratitis (dendritic keratitis), vaccinia, vancella, and many other viral diseases of the cornea and conjunctiva. Myobacterial infection of the eye. Fungal diseases of ocular structures. Hypersensitivity to a component of the medication. (Hypersensitivity to the antibiotic component occurs at a higher rate than for other components.)
The use of these combinations is contraindicated after uncomplicated removal of a cornea foreign body.
Warnings: Prolonged use may result in glaucoma, with damage to the optic nerve, defects in visual acuity and fields of vision, and posterior subcapsular cataract formation. Prolonged use may suppress the host response and thus increase the hazard of secondary ocular infections. In those diseases causing thinning of the cornea or sclera, perforations have been known to occur with the use of topical steroids. In acute purulent conditions of the eye, steroids may mask infections or enhance existing infection. If these products are used for 10 days or longer, intraocular pressure should be routinely monitored even though it may be difficult in children and uncooperative patients. Employment of steroid medication in the treatment of herpes simplex requires great caution. Neomycin sulfate may cause cutaneous sensitization. A precise incidence of hypersensitivity reactions (primarily skin rash) due to topical neomycin is not known.
The manifestations of sensitization to neomycin are usually itching, reddening and edema of the conjunctiva and eyelid. It may be manifest simply as a failure to heal. During long-term use of neomycin-containing products periodic examination for such signs is advisable, and the patient should be told to discontinue the product if they are observed. These symptoms subside quickly on withdrawing the medication. Neomycin-containing applications should be avoided for the patient thereafter.
Precautions: General: The initial prescription and renewal of the medication order beyond 20 milliliters should be made by a physician only after examination of the patient with the aid of magnification, such as slit lamp biomicroscopy and, where appropriate, fluorescein staining.
The possibility of persistent fungal infections of the cornea should be considered after prolonged steroid dosing.
Allergic-cross-reactions may occur which could prevent the use of any or all of the following antibiotics for the treatment of future infections: kanamycin, paramomycin, streptomycin, and possibly gentamicin.
Carcinogenesis, Mutageneisis, Impairment Of Fertility: Long-term studies in animals (rats, rabbits, mice) showed no evidence of carcinogenicity attributable to oral administration of corticosteroids.
Pregnancy: Teratogenic Effects: Pregnancy Category C. Corticosteroids have been shown to be teratogenic in rabbits when applied topically at concentrations of 0.5% on days 6–18 of gestation and in mice when applied topically at a concentration of 15% on days 10–13 of gestation. There are no adequate and well-controlled studies in pregnant women. Corticosteroids should be used during pregnancy only if the potential benefit justifies the potential risk to the fetus.
Nursing Mothers: Hydrocortisone appears in human milk following oral administration of the drug. Since systemic absorption of hydrocortisone may occur when applied topically caution should be exercised when Neomycin Sulfate-Polymixin B Sulfate-Hydrocortisone Ophthalmic Suspension is used by a nursing woman.
Adverse Reactions: Adverse reactions have occurred with steroid/anti-infective combination drugs which can be attributed to the steroid component, the anti-infective component, or the combination. Reactions occurring most often from the presence of the anti-infective ingredient are localized hypersensitivity, including itching, swelling and conjunctival erythema. Local irritation on instillation has also been reported. Exact incidence figures are not available since no denominator of treated patients is available.
The reactions due to the steroid component in decreasing order of frequency are elevation of intraocular pressure (IOP) with possible development of glaucoma, and infrequent optic nerve damage; posterior subcapsular cataract formation; and delayed wound healing.
Secondary Infection: The development of secondary infection has occurred after use of combinations containing steroids and antimicrobials. Fungal infections of the cornea are particularly prone to develop coincidentally with long-term applications of steroid. The possibility of fungal invasion must be considered in any persistent corneal ulceration where steroid treatment has been used.

Secondary bacterial ocular infection following suppression of host responses also occurs.

Dosage and Administration: One or two drops in the affected eye every three or four hours, depending on the severity of the condition. The suspension may be used more frequently if necessary.

Not more than 20 milliliters should be prescribed initially and the prescription should not be refilled without further evaluation as outlined in **PRECAUTIONS** above. SHAKE WELL BEFORE USING.

How Supplied: 7.5 mL Suspension in plastic squeeze bottle. 3.5 gm (1/8oz.) Ointment with ophthalmic applicator tip.

7.5 mL NDC 17478-231-09
3.5 gm (1/8oz.) NDC 17478-232-35

AK-SULF ℞

(sodium sulfacetamide 10%)
Sterile Ophthalmic Solution
Sterile Ophthalmic Ointment

Description: Aqueous solution containing Sodium Sulfacetamide 10%, with Hydroxyethyl Cellulose 0.35%, Sodium Borate and Boric Acid as buffers; Sodium Thiosulfate 2.0mg; Chlorobutanol 2.0mg Methylparaben 0.15 mg and Propylparaben 0.15 mg as preservatives.

Sulfacetamide Sodium 10% Ophthalmic Ointment (sterile) contains in each gram of sterile ointment 100 mg. Sulfacetamide Sodium, 0.5 mg. Methylparaben, 0.1 mg. Propylparaben in a bland, special petrolatum base.

Action: Sulfonamides exert a bacteriostatic effect against a wide range of gram-positive and gram-negative micro-organisms by restricting through competition with para-aminobenzoic acid, the synthesis of folic acid which bacteria require for growth.

Indications: For the treatment of conjunctivitis; corneal ulcer and other superficial ocular infections due to susceptible micro-organisms; and as an adjunct in the systemic sulfonamide therapy of trachoma.

Contraindications: Hypersensitivity to sulfonamide preparations.

Precautions: Sulfacetamide solutions are incompatible with silver preparations. Nonsusceptible organisms, including fungi, may proliferate with the use of this preparation. Sulfonamides are inactivated by the para-aminobenzoic acid present in purulent exudates.

Dosage: Instill 1-2 drops into lower conjunctival sac every 2-3 hours during the day, less often at night. The ointment may be used adjunctively with any of the solution forms.

Storage: Store in cool place. Protect from light. Dark or precipitated solutions should be discarded.

Supply:
2 mL NDC 17478-221-20
5 mL NDC 17478-221-10
15 mL NDC 17478-221-12
3.5 gm NDC 17478-227-35

Shown in Product Identification Section, page 103

AK-TAINE ℞

(proparacaine HCl)
Sterile Ophthalmic Solution

Description:
Proparacaine HCl 0.5%
Benzalkonium Chloride 0.01%
In a glycerine/purified water base with hydrochloric acid and/or sodium hydroxide to adjust pH.

Actions: A rapidly acting topical anesthetic with induced anethesia lasting 15 minutes or longer.

Indications: For procedures in which a topical ophthalmic anesthetic is indicated: corneal anesthesia of short duration, e.g., tonometry, gonioscopy, removal of corneal foreign bodies, and for short corneal and conjunctival procedures.

Contraindications: Known hypersensitivity to any component of this drug.

Warnings: Prolonged use of a topical ocular anesthetic is not recommended. It may produce permanent corneal opacification with accompanying visual loss.

Precautions: Proparacaine should be used cautiously and sparingly in patients with known allergies, cardiac disease, or hyperthyroidism. The long-term toxicity of proparacaine is unknown; prolonged use may possibly delay wound healing. Although exceedingly rare with ophthalmic application of local anesthetics, it should be borne in mind that systemic toxicity (manifested by central nervous system stimulation followed by depression) may occur.

Protection of the eye from irritating chemicals, foreign bodies and rubbing during the period of anesthesia is very important. Tonometers soaked in sterilizing or detergent solutions should be thoroughly rinsed with sterile distilled water prior to use. Patients should be advised to avoid touching the eye until the anesthesia has worn off.

Adverse Reactions: Occasional temporary stinging, burning, and conjunctival redness have been reported after use of proparacaine, as well as a rare, severe, immediate-type, apparently hyperallergic corneal reaction, with acute, intense and diffuse epithelial keratitis, a gray, ground glass appearance, sloughing of large areas of necrotic epithelium, corneal filaments and sometimes, iritis with descemetitis. Allergic contact dermatitis from proparacaine with drying and fissuring of the fingertips has been reported.

Dosage and Administraiton:

Usual Dosage: Removal of foreign bodies and sutures, and for tonometry; 1 to 2 drops (in single instillations) in each eye before operating.

Deep Ophthalmic Anesthesia: 1 drop in each eye every 5 to 10 minutes for 5-7 doses.

Note: Do not use if solution is discolored (amber).

Storage: Unopened bottles may be stored at room temperature. After bottles are opened, refrigeration is recommended as it will retard discoloration of the solution. Solutions which have become discolored should not be used.

Supply: 15 mL and 2 mL Plastic squeeze bottles with dropper tip.

15 mL NDC 17478-240-12
2 mL NDC 17478-240-20

AK-TROL ℞

(neomycin sulfate–polymyxin B sulfate–dexamethasone 0.1%)
Sterile Ophthalmic Suspension
Sterile Ophthalmic Ointment

Description: AK-Trol Ophthalmic Ointment and Suspension are anti-infective steroid combinations in a sterile suspension form and sterile ointment form for topical application.

Contents: Each ml of the suspension and each gram of the ointment contains:

Neomycin Sulfate ... Equivalent to 3.5 mg Neomycin base
Polymyxin B Sulfate 10,000 units
Dexamethasone 0.1%

In a solution containing Benzalkonium Chloride 0.01% (preservative) with Polysorbate 20, Sodium Chloride, Hydroxpropyl Methylcellulose, Hydrochloric Acid and/or Sodium Hydroxide to adjust the pH and Purified Water or in an ointment base containing Methylparaben 0.05%, Propylparaben 0.01% (as preservatives) with White Petrolatum, Anhydrous Liquid Lanolin and Mineral Oil as inactive ingredients.

Clinical Pharmacology: Corticoids suppress the inflammatory response to a variety of agents and they probably delay or slow healing. Since corticoids may inhibit the body's defense mechanism against infection, a concomitant antimicrobial drug may be used when this inhibition is considered to be clinically significant in a particular case.

The anti-infective component in the combination is included to provide action against specific organisms susceptible to it. Neomycin Sulfate and Polymyxin B Sulfate are considered active against the following microrganisms:

Staphylococcus aureus
Escherichia coli
Haemophilus influenzae
Klebsiella/Enterobacter species
Neisseria species
Pseudomonas aeruginosa

When a decision to administer both a corticoid and an antimicrobial is made, the administration of such drugs in combination has the advantage of greater patient compliance and convenience, with the added assurance that the appropriate dosage of both drugs is administered, plus assured compatibility of ingredients when both types of drug are in the same formulation and, particularly, that the correct volume of drug is delivered and retained.

The relative potency of corticosteroids depends on the molecular structure, concentration, and release from the vehicle.

Indications and Usage: For steroid-responsive inflammatory ocular conditions for which a corticosteroid is indicated and where bacterial infection or a risk of bacterial ocular infection exists.

Ocular steroids are indicated in inflammatory conditions of the palpebral and bulbar conjunctiva, cornea, and anterior segment of the globe where the inherent risk of steroid use in certain infective conjunctivitides is accepted to obtain a diminution in edema and inflammation. They are also indicated in chronic anterior uveitis and corneal injury from chemical, radiation or thermal burns, or penetration of foreign bodies.

The use of a combination drug with an anti-infective component is indicated where the risk of infection is high or where there is an expectation that potentially dangerous numbers of bacteria will be present in the eye.

The particular anti-infective drugs in this product are active against the following common bacterial eye pathogens:

Staphylococcus aureus
Escherichia coli
Haemophilus influenzae
Klebsiella/Enterobacter species
Neisseria species
Pseudomonas aerugenosa

The product does not provide adequate coverage against:

Serratia marcescens
Streptococci, including *Streptococcus pneumoniae*

Contraindications: Epithelial herpes simplex keratitis (dendritic keratitis), vaccinia, varicella and many other viral diseases of the cornea and conjunctiva. Mycobacterial infection of the eye. Fungal diseases of ocular structures. Hypersensitivity to a component of the medication. (Hypersensitivity to the antibiotic component occurs at a higher rate than for other components.)

The use of these combinations is always contraindicated after uncomplicated removal of a corneal foreign body.

Warnings: Prolonged use may result in glaucoma, with damage to the optic nerve, defects in visual acuity and fields of vision, and posterior subcapsular cataract formation. Prolonged use may suppress the host response and thus increase the hazard of secondary ocular infections. In those diseases causing thinning of the cornea of sclera, perforations have been

Continued on next page

Akorn—Cont.

known to occur with the use of topical steroids. In acute purulent conditions of the eye, steroids may mask infection or enhance existing infection. If these products are used for 10 days or longer, intraocular pressure should be routinely monitored even though it may be difficult in children and uncooperative patients.
Employment of steroid medication in the treatment of herpes simplex requires great caution.
Neomycin Sulfate cause cutaneous sensitization. A precise incidence of hypersensitivity reactions (primarily skin rash) due to topical neomycin is not known.
Precautions: The initial prescription and renewal of the medication beyond 20 milliliters should be made by a physician only after examination of the patient with the aid of magnification, such as slit lamp biomicroscopy and where appropriate, flourescein staining. The possibility of persistent fungal infections of the cornea should be considered after prolonged steroid dosing.
Adverse Reactions: Adverse reactions have occurred with steroid/anti-infective combination drugs which can be attributed to the steroid component, the anti-infective component, or the combination. Exact incidence figures are not available since no denominator of treated patients is available. Reactions occurring most often from the presence of the anti-infective ingredients are allergic sensitizations. The reactions due to the steroid component in decreasing order of frequency are; elevation of intraocular pressure (OP) with possible development of glaucoma and infrequent optic nerve damage; posterior subcapsular cataract formation; and delayed wound healing.
Secondary Infection:
The development of secondary infection has occurred after use of combinations containing steroids and antimicrobials. Fungal infections of the cornea are particularly prone to develop coincidentally with long-term applications of steroids. The possibility of fungal invasion must be considered in any persistent corneal ulceration where steroid treatment has been used. Secondary bacterial ocular infection following suppression of host responses also occurs.
Dosage and Administration: AK-Trol Ophthalmic Suspension: One to two drops topically in the conjunctival sac(s). In severe disease, drops may be used hourly, being tapered to discontinuation as the inflammation subsides. In mild disease, drops may be used up to four to six times daily. Not more than 20 milliliters should be prescribed initially and the prescription should not be refilled without further evaluation as outlined in PRECAUTIONS above.
SHAKE WELL BEFORE USING.
AK-Trol Ophthalmic Ointment: Apply a small amount into the conjunctival sac(s) up to three or four times daily. Not more than 8 grams should be prescribed initially and the prescription should not be refilled without further evaluation as outlined in PRECAUTIONS above.
How Supplied: Ophthalmic Suspension is supplied in 5 ml (plastic drop container). Ointment is supplied in 3.5 gram (1/8oz.) ophthalmic tube.
5 mL NDC 17478-239-10
3.5 gm NDC 17478-240-35

AKWA TEARS Ointment — OTC

Description: An ocular emollient containing white petrolatum, mineral oil and lanolin. Contains no preservatives.
Indications: For use as a protectant or lubricant to prevent further irritation or to relieve dryness of the eye.
Dosage: Apply a thin film of ointment to affected eye(s) one or more times daily or as directed by physician.
How Supplied: 3.5 gm (1/8 oz.) ophthalmic tube.
NDC 17478-062-35

AKWA TEARS Solution — OTC
(polyvinyl alcohol)

Description: AKWA TEARS from Akorn, Inc. is a sterile buffered, isotonic solution formulated to provide soothing, cooling lubrication for various ocular irritations including dry eye. AKWA TEARS also enhances lens (hard) wearing comfort by providing lubrication and rewetting the lenses while being worn. AKWA TEARS provides temporary relief from such non-specific patient complaints as dry, itchy eyes.
Contains: Polyvinyl Alcohol in an isotonic phosphate buffered sodium chloride solution preserved with Disodium Edetate and Benzalkonium Chloride 0.01%.
Directions: Instill one or two drops as necessary or as directed by your doctor. In hard contact lens use, if the lenses begin to feel uncomfortable, apply one or two drops directly in the eyes. If irritation persists or increases, discontinue use.
Precaution: Avoid contamination. Always replace the cap securely and avoid touching the dropper tip.
How Supplied: Economical 15 ml plastic bottle.
NDC 17478-060-12

FLUORACAINE — ℞
(fluorescein sodium—proparacaine HCl)
Ophthalmic Solution
Sterile

Description: This product is a sterile ophthalmic solution combining the disclosing action of Fluorescein with the anesthetic action of Proparacaine HCl.
Each ml. contains:
Fluorescein Sodium 0.25%
Proparacaine Hydrochloride 0.5%
with Povidone and glycerin in purified water. Preserved with 0.01% Thimerosal.
Actions: This product is the combination of a disclosing agent with a rapidly acting anesthetic of short duration.
Indications: For procedures requiring a disclosing agent in combination with an anesthetic agent such as tonometry, gonioscopy, removal of corneal foreign bodies and other short corneal or conjunctival procedures.
Contraindications: Known hypersensitivity to any component of this product.
Warning: Prolonged use of a topical ocular anesthetic is not recommended. It may produce corneal opacification with accompanying visual loss.
Precautions: This product should be used cautiously and sparingly in patients with known allergies, cardiac disease, or hyperthyroidism. The long-term toxicity is unknown; prolonged use may possibly delay wound healing. Although exceedingly rare with ophthalmic application of local anesthetics, it should be borne in mind that systemic toxicity (manifested by central nervous system stimulation followed by depression) may occur.
Protection of the eye from irritating chemicals, foreign bodies and rubbing during the period of anesthesia is very important. Tonometers soaked in sterilizing or detergent solutions should be thoroughly rinsed with sterile distilled water prior to use. Patients should be advised to avoid touching the eye until the anesthesia has worn off.
Adverse Reactions: Occasional temporary stinging, burning, and conjunctival redness have been reported after use of ocular anesthetics, as well as a rare, severe, immediate-type, apparently hyperallergic corneal reaction, with acute, intense and diffuse epithelial keratitis, a gray, ground glass appearance, sloughing of large areas of necrotic epithelium, corneal filaments and sometimes, iritis with descemetitis.
Allergic contact dermatitis with drying and fissuring of the fingertips has been reported.
Dosage and Administration:
Usual Dosage: Removal of foreign bodies and sutures, and for tonometry; 1 to 2 drops (in single instillations) in each eye before operating.
Deep Ophthalmic Anesthesia: 1 drop in each eye every 5 to 10 minutes or 5–7 doses.
NOTE: The use of an eye patch is recommended.
Storage: Protect from light.
How Supplied: 5 ml. Plastic bottles with dropper tip or 5 ml glass bottle with dropper.
Glass NDC 17478-311-10
Plastic NDC 17478-310-10

FLUORETS™ — ℞
(Fluorescein Sodium Ophthalmic Strips)
Diagnostic Agent

Description: Fluorets are sterile, individually wrapped paper strips each impregnated with 1 mg. of fluorescein sodium.
Usage: Fluorescein is a corneal stain and can be used in diagnostic examinations, including Goldman tonometry and contact lens fitting.
Contraindications: Known hypersensitivity to fluorescein sodium.
Directions For Use: Pull tabs apart at right-hand end of envelope and withdraw Fluoret. Moisten tip with tear fluid from lower fornix, sterile water or sterile ophthalmic solution. Then gently stroke the Fluoret across the conjunctiva. For the best results the patient should blink several times.
The applicator should be used once and then discarded. Care should be taken to handle the strip by the non-impregnated end only.
How Supplied: Gravity-delivery cartons of 100 individually wrapped Fluorets.
NDC 17478-400-01

GENTAK — ℞
(gentamicin sulfate, U.S.P.)
Sterile Ophthalmic Solution
Sterile Ophthalmic Ointment

Description: Gentak Ophthalmic Solution is a sterile, aqueous solution buffered to approximately pH 7.0 and formulated for ophthalmic use against a wide variety of pathogenic gram-negative and gram-positive bacteria.
Each ml Contains:
ACTIVE: Gentamicin sulfate (equivalent to 3.0 mg gentamicin base)
INACTIVES: Sodium phosphate anhydrous mono. and dibasic, sodium chloride and purified water.
PRESERVATIVE: Benzalkonium chloride 0.1%
Gentak Ophthalmic Ointment is a sterile ointment formulated for ophthalmic use against a wide variety of pathogenic gram-negative and gram-positive bacteria.
Each gram contains:
ACTIVE: Gentamicin sulfate (equivalent to 3.0 mg gentamicin base)
INACTIVES: Liquid lanolin (anhydrous), white petrolatum and mineral oil.
PRESERVATIVES: Methylparaben and propylparaben.
Gentamicin is an aminoglyoside antibiotic obtained from cultures of *Micromonospora purpurea.* It is a mixture of the sulfate salts of gentamicin C_1, C_2, and C_{1a}; all 3 components appear to have similar antimicrobial activity. Gentamicin sulfate occurs as a white powder and is soluble in water and insoluble in alcohol.

Indications and Usage: Gentak Solution and Ointment are indicated in the topical treatment of infections of the external eye and its adnexa caused by susceptible bacteria. Such infections embrace conjunctivitis, keratitis and keratoconjunctivitis, corneal ulcers, blepharitis and blepharoconjunctivitis, acute meibomianitis, and dacryocystitis.
Contraindications: This product is contraindicated in patients with known hypersensitivity to any of the components.
Warnings: Gentak Ophthalmic Solution is not for injection. It should never be injected subconjunctivally, nor should it be directly introduced into the anterior chamber of the eye.
Precautions: Prolonged use of topical antibiotics may give rise to overgrowth of nonsusceptible organisms, such as fungi. Should this occur, or if irritation or hypersensitivity to any component of the drug develops, discontinue use of the preparation and institute appropriate therapy.
Ophthalmic ointments may retard corneal healing.
Adverse Reactions: Occasional burning or stinging may occur with the use of Gentamicin Sulfate Ophthalmic Ointment.
Transient irritation has been reported with the use of Gentamicin Sulfate Ophthalmic Solution.
Dosage and Administration: Gentak Ophthalmic Ointment, USP-Sterile: Apply a small amount to the affected eye 2 to 3 times a day.
Gentak Ophthalmic Solution, USP-Sterile: Instill (1) one or (2) two drops into the affected eye(s) every (4) four hours. In the case of a severe infection, dosage may be increases to as much as (2) two drops once every hour.
How Supplied:
5 mL and 15 mL Solution;
3.5 gm (1/8oz.) Ointment
3.5 gm NDC 17478-384-35
5 mL NDC 17478-283-10
15 mL NDC 17478-283-12

GONAK OTC
Hydroxypropyl Methylcellulose 2.5%
Ophthalmic Demulcent Solution

Indications: For professional use in gonioscopic examinations.
Directions: Fill gonioscopic prism with solution necessary.
Warnings: Do not touch dropper tip to any other surface. Replace cap after use. If solution changes color or becomes cloudy, do not use. Solution clouding may occur.
Note: If this solution dries on optical surfaces, let them stand in cool water before cleansing.
Contents: Hydroxypropyl Methylcelllulose 2.5% in an isotonic, buffered, sterile aqueous solution of Boric Acid, Potassium Chloride, Sodium Borate and Edetate Disodium; preserved with BenzalkoniumChloride 0.01%.
How Supplied: 15 ml dropper bottles.
NDC 17478-070-12

ROSE BENGAL 1% ℞
Sterile Ophthalmic Solution
Sterile Ophthalmic Strips

A fluorescein derivative (4,5,6,7 Tetrachloro 2′, 4′, 5′, 7′, Tetra-Iodofluorescein Sodium).
A Specific diagnostic stain for dead and degenerated corneal and conjunctival epithelial cells and mucus.
Composition: Rose Bengal 1% in a base containing Polyvinylpyrrolidone, Sodium Borate, Polyethylene Glycol p-Isooctylphenol 10 $(CH_2)_2O$, made isotonic with Sodium Chloride.
Preservative: Thimerosal 0.01%.
Staining Properties
Rose Bengal
1. Stains dead and degenerated epithelial cells-corneal and conjunctival.
2. Stains mucus.
3. Does not stain epithelial defects.
4. Doesn't pass into intercellular spaces.
5. Normally stains line behind meibomian gland outlets.

Uses: Dry eyes-stains dead cells and filaments as well as mucus. Ulcers-delineated margins. Any corneal or conjunctival erosion. Aids in diagnosis of squamous cell carcinoma.
Caution: This solution may be irritating.
Supply: 5 ml plastic squeeze bottle with dropper tip and individually wrapped sterile strips. 100 per box.
5 mL NDC 17478-261-10
Strips NDC 17478-402-01

SNO® STRIPS OTC
(Sterile Tear Flow Test Strips)
Diagnostic Agent
For Professional Use Only

Description: Sno Strips are sterile, individually wrapped paper strips for testing tear flow.

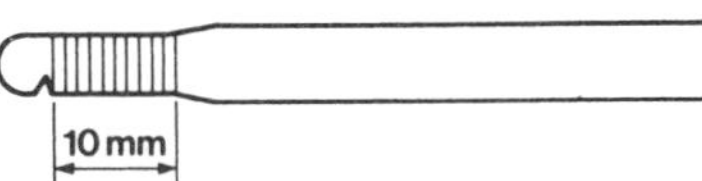

Directions For Use: The Sno strip tear test should be performed on the eye before any topical medication (especially local anaesthetic) is administered or other procedures carried out, such as manipulation of the eyelids.
The patient should be seated with the head supported by a headrest.
1 Hold the sterile unopened Sno strip up to the light, locate the strip and through the overwrap, make a bend in the strip in line with the notch in the thin end of the strip.
2 Open the overwrap towards the broad end of the Sno strip. Remove the strip by holding the broad end.
3 Each strip should be applied to the lower temporal lid margin of the eye under investigation, so that the strip fits snugly. The patient should be gazing up and in.
4 Commence timing. The distance between the notch and the shoulder of the strip is 10 mm. This should be wetted in about 3 minutes. If the time is in excess of 5 minutes, a further test should be carried out after a suitable interval. A time of greater than 10 minutes indicates a reduced tear secretion.

How Supplied: Gravity-delivery cartons of 100 individually wrapped Sno Strips.
NDC 17478-401-01

TEARS RENEWED OTC
(dextran 70, hydroxypropyl methylcellulose)

Tears Renewed is a sterile solution for use as an artificial tear and lubricant in the relief of ocular irritations due to Dry Eye Syndrome.
Dosage: Instill one or two drops as frequently as required to relieve irritation or as directed by your doctor.
Caution: If irritation persists, discontinue use and consult physician. To avoid contamination, do not touch dropper tip to any surface.
Contains: Dextran 70, Hydroxypropyl Methylcellulose, Sodium Chloride, Potassium Chloride and Purified Water with Benzalkonium Chloride 0.01% and Edetate Disodium 0.05% as preservatives.
How Supplied: Economical 15 ml plastic bottle.
NDC 17478-061-12

TEARS RENEWED OINTMENT OTC
Preservative Free and Lanolin-Free
Sterile Ophthalmic Lubricating Ointment

Description: An ocular emollient containing white petrolatum and light mineral oil. Contains no preservatives and no lanolin.
Indications: For use as a lubricant or protectant to prevent further irritation or to relieve dryness of the eye.
Directions: Pull down lower lid of the affected eye and apply a small amount (1/4 inch) of ointment to the inside of the eyelid.
How Supplied: 3.5 gm (1/8 oz.) ophthalmic tube with applicator tip. NDC 17478-063-35

TROPICACYL ℞
(tropicamide)
Sterile Ophthalmic Solution

Description: Tropicamide Ophthalmic Solution USP Sterile is an anticholingeric prepared as a sterile topical ophthalmic solution in two strengths.
Each ml of the solution contains:
Active: Tropicamide 0.5% or 1.0%
Inactives: Boric Acid, Edetate Disodium, Hydrochloric Acid and/or Sodium Hydroxide (to adjust pH) and Purified Water.
Preservative: Benzalkonium Chloride 0.1%
Clinical Pharmacology: This anticholinergic preparation blocks the responses of the sphincter muscle of the iris and the cillary muscle to cholinergic stimulation, dilating the pupil (mydriasis). The 1.0% solution also paralyzes accommodation. This preparation acts rapidly and the duration of activity is relatively short.
Indications and Usage: For mydriasis and cycloplegia in diagnostic procedures. When a short acting mydriatic is needed for some pre and post-operative states.
Contraindications: This product is contraindicated in narrow-angle glaucoma, and in persons showing hypersensitivity to any component of the preparation.
Warnings: For topical use only - not for injection. Reproductive studies have not been performed in animals. There is not adequate information on whether this drug may affect fertility in human males or females or have a teratogenic potential or other adverse effect on the fetus. This preparation may cause CNS disturbances which may be dangerous in infants and children. Possibility of occurrence of psychotic reaction and behavioral disturbance due to hypersensitivity to anti cholinergic drugs should be borne in mind.
Precautions: In the elderly and others where increased intraocular pressure may be encountered, mydriatics and cycloplegics should be used cautiously. To avoid inducing angle closure glaucoma, an estimation of the depth of the angle of the anterior chamber should be made. The lacrimal sac should be compressed by digital pressure for one minute after instillation to avoid excessive systemic absorption.
Patient Warning: Patient should be advised not to drive or engage in other hazardous activities while pupils are dilated. Patient may experience sensitivity to light and should protect eyes in bright illumination during dilation. Parents should be warned not to get this preparation in their child's mouth and to wash their hands and the child's hands following administration.
Adverse Reactions: Increased intraocular pressure. Psychotic reactions, behavioral disturbances, and cardiorespiratory collapse in children with this class of drugs have been reported. Transient stinging, dryness of the mouth, blurred vision, photophobia with or without corneal staining, tachycardia, headache, parasympathetic stimulation, or allergic reaction may occur.
Dosage and administration: For refraction, one or two drops of 1.0% solution in the eye(s), repeated in five minutes. If patient is not seen within 20 to 30 minutes, an additional drop may be instilled to prolong mydriatic ef-

Continued on next page

Akorn—Cont.

fect. For examination of fundus, one or two drops of 0.5% solution 15 or 20 minutes prior to examination.

How Supplied:
1% - 2 ml and 15 ml plastic drop container
0.5% - 15 ml plastic drop container

1% 2 mL NDC 17478-102-20
1% 15 mL NDC 17478-102-12
½% 15 mL NDC 17478-101-12

Storage: Store at 46° to 75°F. Do not refrigerate or store at high temperatures.
Keep containers tightly closed.

Alcon Laboratories, Inc.
and its affiliates
CORPORATE HEADQUARTERS:
6201 SOUTH FREEWAY
FORT WORTH, TX 76134

ADSORBONAC®* 2% and 5% OTC
(Sodium Chloride Ophthalmic Solution)
Hypertonicity Eye Drops

Ingredients: Each mL contains: **Active:** Sodium chloride 2% or 5%. **Preservative:** Thimerosal 0.004%, added. **Inactive:** ADSORBOBASE®* polymers (Povidone, PEG-90M, Hydroxyethyl Cellulose and Poloxamer 188), Edetate Disodium, Dibasic Sodium Phosphate, Hydrochloric Acid and/or Sodium Hydroxide to adjust pH, Purified Water.

Indications:

FDA APPROVED USE
For the temporary relief of corneal edema.

Directions: Instill 1 or 2 drops in the affected eye(s) every 3 or 4 hours, or as directed by a doctor.

Warnings: This product contains thimerosal 0.004% added as a preservative. Do not use this product if you are sensitive to thimerosal or any other ingredient containing mercury. Do not use this product except under the advice and supervision of a doctor. If you experience eye pain, changes in vision, continued redness or irritation of the eye, or if the condition worsens or persists, consult a doctor. This product may cause temporary burning and irritation on being instilled into the eye. If solution changes color or becomes cloudy, do not use. To avoid contamination, do not touch tip of container to any surface. Replace cap after using. Keep this and all drugs out of the reach of children. In case of accidental ingestion, seek professional assistance or contact a Poison Control Center immediately.

How Supplied: 15mL sterile control dropper dispensers—2% and 5% strengths.
Protect from light—Store container in original carton at 46°-80°F.
2% NDC 0998-0504-15
5% NDC 0998-0505-15
*U.S. Patent No. 3,767,788

ADSORBOTEAR® OTC
Artificial Tear

Indications: ADSORBOTEAR® is a sterile, tear-like lubricant (and ocular wetting agent) which provides temporary relief for dry eye conditions.

ADSORBOTEAR® contains ADSORBOBASE®* (povidone 1.67% with water soluble polymers) and hydroxyethylcellulose, as a viscosity agent, in a buffered isotonic solution. Thimerosal 0.004% and edetate disodium 0.1% are added as preservatives.

FOR TOPICAL EYE USE ONLY.

ADSORBOTEAR® provides relief of dry eye symptoms for a prolonged period. It substitutes for both the aqueous and the mucin layers of the tear film.

ADSORBOTEAR® contains a mucin-like substance which mimics the action of the conjunctival mucus to render the surface of the eye more wettable. Its special polymeric formulation helps keep the eye moist and assures that the tear film can spread easily and evenly over the surface of the eye.

Directions for Use: Apply one or two drops of ADSORBOTEAR® to the eye(s) three times a day or as needed.

Warning: This product contains thimerosal 0.004% added as a preservative. Do not use this product if you are sensitive to thimerosal or any other ingredient containing mercury.
If you experience eye pain, changes in vision, continued redness or irritation of the eye, or if the condition worsens or persists for more than 72 hours, discontinue use and consult a doctor. If solution changes color or becomes cloudy, do not use.
To avoid contamination, do not touch tip of container to any surface. Replace cap after using. Keep this and all drugs out of the reach of children. In case of accidental ingestion, seek professional assistance or contact a Poison Control Center immediately.

How Supplied: 15mL sterile control dropper dispensers. Protect from light. Store container in original carton at 46°–80°F.
NDC 0998-0410-15
*U.S. Patent No. 3,767,788

ALCAINE® ℞
(proparacaine hydrochloride)
Sterile Ophthalmic Solution, 0.5%

Description: ALCAINE® (Proparacaine Hydrochloride) is a topical anesthetic prepared as a sterile aqueous ophthalmic solution. The active ingredient is represented by the chemical structure:

$CH_3CH_2CH_2O-C_6H_3(NH_2)-COOCH_2CH_2N(C_2H_5)_2 \cdot HCl$

Established name:
Proparacaine Hydrochloride

Chemical name:
Benzoic acid, 3-amino-4-propoxy-, 2-(diethylamino) ethyl ester, monohydrochloride.

Each mL contains: Active: Proparacaine Hydrochloride 0.5% (5mg). Preservative: Benzalkonium Chloride 0.01%. Inactive: Glycerin, Hydrochloric Acid and/or Sodium Hydroxide (to adjust pH), Purified Water.

Clinical Pharmacology: ALCAINE Solution is a rapid acting local anesthetic suitable for ophthalmic use. The onset of anesthesia usually begins within 30 seconds and persists for 15 minutes or longer.
The main site of anesthetic action is the nerve cell membrane where proparacaine interferes with the large transient increase in the membrane permeability to sodium ions that is normally produced by a slight depolarization of the membrane. As the anesthetic action progressively develops in a nerve, the threshold for electrical stimulation gradually increases and the safety factor for conduction decreases; when this action is sufficiently well developed, block of conduction is produced.
The exact mechanism whereby proparacaine and other local anesthetics influence the permeability of the cell membrane is unknown; however, several studies indicate that local anesthetics may limit sodium ion permeability through the lipid layer of the nerve cell membrane. This limitation prevents the fundamental change necessary for the generation of the action potential.

Indications and Usage: ALCAINE (Proparacaine Hydrochloride) Ophthalmic Solution is indicated for topical anesthesia in ophthalmic practice. Representative ophthalmic procedures in which the preparation provides good local anesthesia include measurement of intraocular pressure (tonometry), removal of foreign bodies and sutures from the cornea, conjunctival scraping in diagnosis and gonioscopic examination; it is also indicated for use as a topical anesthetic prior to surgical operations such as cataract extraction.

Contraindications: This preparation is contraindicated in patients with known hypersensitivity to any component of the solution. This product should never be prescribed for the patient's own use.

Warnings: For topical ophthalmic use only. Prolonged use of a topical ocular anesthetic may produce permanent corneal opacification with accompanying loss of vision.

Precautions:
General. Proparacaine hydrochloride should be used cautiously and sparingly in patients with known allergies, cardiac disease, or hyperthyroidism. The long-term toxicity of proparacaine is unknown; prolonged use may possibly delay wound healing. Although exceedingly rare with ophthalmic application of local anesthetics, it should be borne in mind that systemic toxicity (manifested by central nervous system stimulation followed by depression) may occur.
Protection of the eye from irritating chemicals, foreign bodies and rubbing during the period of anesthesia is very important. Tonometers soaked in sterilizing or detergent solutions should be thoroughly rinsed with sterile distilled water prior to use. Patients should be advised to avoid touching the eye until the anesthesia has worn off. Do not touch dropper tip to any surface as this may contaminate the solution.
Carcinogenesis, Mutagenesis, Impairment of Fertility. Long-term studies in animals have not been performed to evaluate carcinogenic potential, mutagenicity, or possible impairment of fertility in males or females.
Pregnancy Category C. Animal reproduction studies have not been conducted with ALCAINE (Proparacaine Hydrochloride) Ophthalmic Solution. It is also not known whether proparacaine hydrochloride can cause fetal harm when administered to a pregnant woman or can affect reproduction capacity. Proparacaine hydrochloride should be administered to a pregnant woman only if clearly needed.
Nursing Mothers. It is not known whether this drug is excreted in human milk. Because many drugs are excreted in human milk, caution should be exercised when proparacaine hydrochloride is administered to a nursing woman.
Pediatric Use. Controlled clinical studies have not been performed with ALCAINE (Proparacaine Hydrochloride) Ophthalmic Solution to establish safety and effectiveness in children; however, the literature cites the use of proparacaine hydrochloride as a topical ophthalmic anesthetic agent in children.

Adverse Reactions: Pupillary dilation or cycloplegic effects have rarely been observed with proparacaine hydrochloride. The drug appears to be safe for use in patients sensitive to other local anesthetics, but local or systemic sensitivity occasionally occurs. Instillation of proparacaine in the eye at recommended concentration and dosage usually produces little or no initial irritation, stinging, burning, conjunctival redness, lacrimation or increased winking. However, some local irritation and stinging may occur several hours after the instillation.

Rarely, a severe, immediate-type, apparently hyperallergic corneal reaction may occur which includes acute, intense and diffuse epithelial keratitis; a gray, ground-glass appearance; sloughing of large areas of necrotic epithelium; corneal filaments and, sometimes, iritis with descemetitis.

Allergic contact dermatitis with drying and fissuring of the fingertips has been reported. Softening and erosion of the corneal epithelium and conjunctival congestion and hemorrhage have been reported.

Dosage and Administration:

Deep anesthesia as in cataract extraction: Instill 1 drop every 5 to 10 minutes for 5 to 7 doses.

Remove of sutures: Instill 1 or 2 drops 2 or 3 minutes before removal of stitches.

Removal of foreign bodies: Instill 1 or 2 drops prior to operating.

Tonometry: Instill 1 or 2 drops immediately before measurement.

How Supplied: ALCAINE (Proparacaine Hydrochloride) Ophthalmic Solution, 0.5% is supplied in 15 mL DROP-TAINER® dispensers.

NDC 0998-0016-15

Storage: Store at 46° to 75°F before opening. Store at 35° to 46°F after opening to retard discoloration of solution. Do not use a discolored solution.

Caution: Federal (USA) law prohibits dispensing without prescription.

BETOPTIC® ℞
(betaxolol hydrochloride)
0.5% as base
Sterile Ophthalmic Solution

Description: BETOPTIC® Sterile Ophthalmic Solution contains betaxolol hydrochloride, a cardioselective beta-adrenergic receptor blocking agent, in a sterile isotonic solution. Betaxolol hydrochloride is a white, crystalline powder, soluble in water, with a molecular weight of 343.89. The chemical structure is presented below:

$(CH_3)_2CHNHCH_2CHCH_2O-C_6H_4-CH_2CH_2OCH_2-C_3H_5 \cdot HCl$ (OH on the CH)

Empirical Formula:
$C_{18}H_{29}NO_3 \cdot HCl$

Chemical Name:
(±)-1-[p-[2-(Cyclopropylmethoxy)ethyl] phenoxy]-3-(isopropylamino)-2-propanol hydrochloride.

Each mL of BETOPTIC Ophthalmic Solution (0.5%) contains: Active: 5.6 mg betaxolol hydrochloride equivalent to betaxolol base 5 mg. Preservative: Benzalkonium Chloride 0.01%. Inactive: Edetate Disodium, Sodium Chloride, Hydrochloric Acid and/or Sodium Hydroxide (to adjust pH), and Purified Water.

Clinical Pharmacology: Betaxolol HCl, a cardioselective (beta-1-adrenergic) receptor blocking agent, does not have significant membrane-stabilizing (local anesthetic) activity and is devoid of intrinsic sympathomimetic action. Orally administered beta-adrenergic blocking agents reduce cardiac output in healthy subjects and patients with heart disease. In patients with severe impairment of myocardial function beta-adrenergic receptor antagonists may inhibit the sympathetic stimulatory effect necessary to maintain adequate cardiac function.

When instilled in the eye, BETOPTIC Ophthalmic Solution has the action of reducing elevated as well as normal intraocular pressure, whether or not accompanied by glaucoma. Ophthalmic betaxolol has minimal effect on pulmonary and cardiovascular parameters.

Ophthalmic betaxolol (one drop in each eye) was compared to timolol and placebo in a three-way crossover study challenging nine patients with reactive airway disease who were selected on the basis of having at least a 15% reduction in the forced expiratory volume in one second (FEV_1) after administration of ophthalmic timolol. Betaxolol HCl had no significant effect on pulmonary function as measured by FEV_1, Forced Vital Capacity (FVC) and FEV_1/VC. Additionally, the action of isoproterenol, a beta stimulant, administered at the end of the study was not inhibited by ophthalmic betaxolol. In contrast, ophthalmic timolol signficantly decreased these pulmonary functions.

[See table above.]

FEV_1 —Percent Change from Baseline[1]

	Means		
	Betaxolol 1.0%[a]	Timolol 0.5%	Placebo
Baseline	1.6	1.4	1.4
60 Minutes	2.3	−25.7*	5.8
120 Minutes	1.6	−27.4*	7.5
240 Minutes	−6.4	−26.9*	6.9
Isoproterenol[b]	36.1	−12.4*	42.8

[1] Schoene, R. B., *et al.* Am. J. Ophthal. 97:86, 1984.
[a] Twice the clinical concentration.
[b] Inhaled at 240 minutes; measurement at 270 minutes.
*Timolol statistically different from betaxolol and placebo ($p < 0.05$).

No evidence of cardiovascular beta-adrenergic blockade during exercise was observed with betaxolol in a double masked, three-way crossover study in 24 normal subjects comparing ophthalmic betaxolol, timolol and placebo for effect on blood pressure and heart rate. Mean arterial blood pressure was not affected by any treatment; however, ophthalmic timolol produced a significant decrease in the mean heart rate.

[See table below.]

Mean Heart Rates[1]

Bruce Stress Exercise Test	TREATMENT		
Minutes	Betaxolol 1%[a]	Timolol 0.5%	Placebo
0	79.2	79.3	81.2
2	130.2	126.0	130.4
4	133.4	128.0*	134.3
6	136.4	129.2*	137.9
8	139.8	131.8*	139.4
10	140.8	131.8*	141.3

[1] Atkins, J. M., *et al.* Am. J. Oph. 99:173–175, Feb., 1985.
[a] Twice the clinical concentration.
*Mean pulse rate significantly lower for timolol than betaxolol or placebo ($p < 0.05$).

Clinical Studies: Optic nerve head damage and visual field loss are the result of a sustained elevated intraocular pressure and poor ocular perfusion. BETOPTIC Ophthalmic Solution has the action of reducing elevated as well as normal intraocular pressure, and the mechanism of ocular hypotensive action appears to be a reduction of aqueous production as demonstrated by tonography and aqueous fluorophotometry. The onset of action with BETOPTIC Ophthalmic Solution can generally be noted within 30 minutes and the maximal effect can usually be detected 2 hours after topical administration. A single dose provides a 12-hour reduction in intraocular pressure. Clinical observation of glaucoma patients treated with BETOPTIC Ophthalmic Solution for up to three years shows that the intraocular pressure lowering effect is well maintained. Clinical studies show that topical BETOPTIC Ophthalmic Solution reduces mean intraocular pressure 25% from baseline. In trials using 22 mmHg as a generally accepted index of intraocular pressure control, BETOPTIC Ophthalmic Solution was effective in more than 94% of the population studied, of which 73% were treated with the beta blocker alone. In controlled, double-masked studies, the magnitude and duration of the ocular hypotensive effect of BETOPTIC Ophthalmic Solution and ophthalmic timolol solution were clinically equivalent.

BETOPTIC Ophthalmic Solution has also been used successfully in glaucoma patients who have undergone a laser trabeculoplasty and have needed additional long-term ocular hypotensive therapy.

BETOPTIC Ophthalmic Solution has been well-tolerated in glaucoma patients wearing hard or soft contact lenses and in aphakic patients.

BETOPTIC Ophthalmic Solution does not produce miosis or accommodative spasm which are frequently seen with miotic agents. The blurred vision and night blindness often associated with standard miotic therapy are not associated with BETOPTIC Ophthalmic Solution. Thus, patients with central lenticular opacities

Continued on next page

Alcon—Cont.

avoid the visual impairment caused by a constricted pupil.

Indications and Usage: BETOPTIC® Ophthalmic Solution has been shown to be effective in lowering intraocular pressure and is indicated in the treatment of ocular hypertension and chronic open-angle glaucoma. It may be used alone or in combination with other anti-glaucoma drugs.

In clinical studies BETOPTIC® safely controlled the intraocular pressure of 47 patients with glaucoma and reactive airway disease followed for a mean period of 15 months. However, caution should be used in treating patients with severe reactive airway disease.

Contraindications: Hypersensitivity to any component of this product.

BETOPTIC Ophthalmic Solution is contraindicated in patients with sinus bradycardia, greater than a first degree atrioventricular block, cardiogenic shock, or patients with overt cardiac failure.

Warning: Although BETOPTIC Ophthalmic Solution has had little or no effect on heart rate or blood pressure in clinical studies, caution should be observed in treating patients with a history of cardiac failure. Treatment with BETOPTIC Ophthalmic Solution should be discontinued at the first signs of cardiac failure.

Precautions: General. Patients who are receiving a beta-adrenergic blocking agent orally and BETOPTIC Ophthalmic Solution should be observed for a potential additive effect either on the intraocular pressure or on the known systemic effects of beta blockade.

While BETOPTIC Ophthalmic Solution has demonstrated a low potential for systemic effect, it should be used with caution in patients with diabetes (especially labile diabetes) because of possible masking of signs and symptoms of acute hypoglycemia. Beta-adrenergic blocking agents may mask certain signs and symptoms of hyperthyroidism and their abrupt withdrawal might precipitate a thyroid storm.

Consideration should be given to the gradual withdrawal of beta-adrenergic blocking agents prior to general anesthesia because of the reduced ability of the heart to respond to beta-adrenergically mediated sympathetic reflex stimuli.

Information for Patients: Do not touch dropper tip to any surface as this may contaminate the solution.

Pulmonary: Caution should be exercised in the treatment of glaucoma patients with excessive restriction of pulmonary function. Ophthalmic betaxolol has minimal systemic effects and has been used by over 100,000 patients with glaucoma or ocular hypertension and coexisting reactive airway disease. Nonetheless, there have been reports of asthmatic attacks and pulmonary distress during betaxolol treatment. Although rechallenges of such patients with ophthalmic betaxolol have not adversely affected pulmonary function test results, the possibility of adverse pulmonary effects in patients unusually sensitive to beta blockers cannot be ruled out.

Drug Interactions: Although BETOPTIC Ophthalmic Solution used alone has little or no effect on pupil size, mydriasis resulting from concomitant therapy with BETOPTIC Ophthalmic Solution and epinephrine has been reported occasionally. Close observation of the patient is recommended when a beta-blocker is administered to patients receiving catecholamine-depleting drugs such as reserpine, because of possible additive effects and the production of hypotension and/or bradycardia. Caution should be exercised in patients using concomitant adrenergic psychotropic drugs.

Ocular: In patients with angle-closure glaucoma, the immediate treatment objective is to re-open the angle by constriction of the pupil with a miotic agent. Betaxolol has no effect on the pupil; therefore, BETOPTIC Ophthalmic Solution should be used with a miotic to reduce elevated intraocular pressure in angle-closure glaucoma.

As with the use of other antiglaucoma drugs, diminished responsiveness to BETOPTIC Ophthalmic Solution after prolonged therapy has been reported in some patients. However in one long-term study in which 250 patients have been followed for a mean period of two years, no significant difference in mean intraocular pressure has been observed after initial stabilization.

Animal Studies: No adverse ocular effects were observed following topical ocular administration of BETOPTIC Ophthalmic Solution to rabbits for one year.

Carcinogenesis, Mutagenesis, Impairment of Fertility: Lifetime studies with betaxolol HCl have been completed in mice at oral doses of 6, 20 or 60 mg/kg/day and in rats at 3, 12 or 48 mg/kg/day; betaxolol HCl demonstrated no carcinogenic effect. Higher dose levels were not tested. In a variety of *in vitro* and *in vivo* bacterial and mammalian cell assays, betaxolol HCl was nonmutagenic.

Pregnancy Category C: Reproduction, teratology, and peri- and post-natal studies have been conducted with orally administered betaxolol HCl in rats and rabbits. There was evidence of drug related post-implantation loss in rabbits and rats at dose levels above 12 mg/kg and 128 mg/kg, respectively. Betaxolol HCl was not shown to be teratogenic, however, and there were no other adverse effects on reproduction at subtoxic dose levels. There are, however, no adequate and well-controlled studies in pregnant women. Because animal reproductive studies are not always predictive of human response, this drug should be used during pregnancy only if clearly indicated.

Nursing Mothers: It is not known whether BETOPTIC Ophthalmic Solution is excreted in human milk. Because many drugs are excreted in human milk, caution should be exercised when BETOPTIC Ophthalmic Solution is administered to nursing women.

Usage in Children: Clinical studies to establish the safety and efficacy in children have not been performed.

Adverse Reactions: The following adverse reactions have been reported in clinical trials with BETOPTIC Ophthalmic Solution.

Ocular: BETOPTIC Ophthalmic Solution has been well tolerated. Discomfort of short duration was experienced by one in four patients, but none discontinued therapy; occasional tearing has been reported. Rare instances of decreased corneal sensitivity, erythema, itching sensation, corneal punctate staining, keratitis, anisocoria and photophobia have been reported.

Systemic: Systemic reactions following administration of ophthalmic betaxolol have been reported rarely. These include: insomnia, depression, headache, hives, toxic epidermal necrolysis, bradycardia, asthma, and dyspnea (see Pulmonary Precautions section).

Overdosage: No information is available on overdosage of humans. The oral LD_{50} of the drug ranged from 350–920 mg/kg in mice and 860–1050 mg/kg in rats. The symptoms which might be expected with an overdose of a systemically administered beta-1-adrenergic receptor blocker agent are bradycardia, hypotension and acute cardiac failure.

A topical overdose of BETOPTIC Ophthalmic Solution may be flushed from the eye(s) with warm tap water.

Dosage and Administration: The usual dose is one drop of BETOPTIC Ophthalmic Solution in the affected eye(s) twice daily. In some patients, the intraocular pressure lowering response to BETOPTIC Ophthalmic Solution may require a few weeks to stabilize. Clinical follow-up should include a determination of the intraocular pressure during the first month of treatment with BETOPTIC Ophthalmic Solution. Thereafter, intraocular pressures should be determined on an individual basis at the judgment of the physician.

When a patient is transferred from a single anti-glaucoma agent, continue the agent already used and add one drop of BETOPTIC Ophthalmic Solution in the affected eye(s) twice a day. On the following day, discontinue the previous anti-glaucoma agent completely and continue with BETOPTIC Ophthalmic Solution.

Because of diurnal variations of intraocular pressure in individual patients, satisfactory response to twice a day therapy is best determined by measuring intraocular pressure at different times during the day. Intraocular pressures ≤22 mmHg may not be optimal for control of glaucoma in each patient; therefore therapy should be individualized.

If the intraocular pressure of the patient is not adequately controlled on this regimen, concomitant therapy with pilocarpine, other miotics, epinephrine or systemically administered carbonic anhydrase inhibitors can be instituted.

When a patient is transferred from several concomitantly administered anti-glaucoma agents, individualization is required. Adjustment should involve one agent at a time made at intervals of not less than one week. A recommended approach is to continue the agents being used and add one drop of BETOPTIC Ophthalmic Solution in the affected eye(s) twice a day. On the following day, discontinue one of the other anti-glaucoma agents. The remaining anti-glaucoma agents may be decreased or discontinued according to the patient's response to treatment. The physician may be able to discontinue some or all of the other anti-glaucoma agents.

How Supplied: BETOPTIC Ophthalmic Solution is a sterile, isotonic, aqueous solution of betaxolol hydrochloride. Supplied as follows: 2.5, 5, 10 and 15 mL in plastic ophthalmic DROP-TAINER® dispensers.

2.5 mL: NDC 0065-0245-20
5 mL: NDC 0065-0245-05
10 mL: NDC 0065-0245-10
15 mL: NDC 0065-0245-15

U.S. Patent Nos. 4,252,984; 4,311,708; 4,342,783

Caution: Federal (USA) law prohibits dispensing without prescription.

Storage: Store at room temperature.

BETOPTIC® S ℞
(betaxolol HCl)
0.25% as base
Sterile Ophthalmic Suspension

Description: BETOPTIC S Ophthalmic Suspension 0.25% contains betaxolol hydrochloride, a cardioselective beta-adrenergic receptor blocking agent, in a sterile resin suspension formulation. Betaxolol hydrochloride is a white, crystalline powder, with a molecular weight of 343.89. The chemical structure is presented below:

$(CH_3)_2CHNHCH_2CHCH_2O$—[benzene ring]—$CH_2CH_2OCH_2$—[cyclopropyl] •HCl (OH on CH)

Empirical Formula:
$C_{18}H_{29}NO_3 \cdot HCl$

Chemical Name:
(±)-1-[p-[2-(cyclopropylmethoxy)ethyl]phenoxy]-3-(isopropylamino)-2-propanol hydrochloride.

Each mL of BETOPTIC S Ophthalmic Suspension contains: Active: betaxolol HCl 2.8 mg equivalent to 2.5 mg of betaxolol base. Preservative: benzalkonium chloride 0.01%. Inactive: Mannitol, Poly(Styrene-Divinyl Benzene) sulfonic acid, Carbomer 934P, edetate disodium, hydrochloric acid or sodium hydroxide (to adjust pH) and purified water.

Clinical Pharmacology: Betaxolol HCl, a cardioselective (beta-1-adrenergic) receptor blocking agent, does not have significant membrane-stabilizing (local anesthetic) activity and is devoid of intrinsic sympathomimetic action. Orally administered beta-adrenergic blocking agents reduce cardiac output in healthy subjects and patients with heart disease. In patients with severe impairment of myocardial function, beta-adrenergic receptor antagonists may inhibit the sympathetic stimulatory effect necessary to maintain adequate cardiac function.

When instilled in the eye, BETOPTIC S Ophthalmic Suspension 0.25% has the action of reducing elevated intraocular pressure, whether or not accompanied by glaucoma. Ophthalmic betaxolol has minimal effect on pulmonary and cardiovascular parameters.

Elevated IOP presents a major risk factor in glaucomatous field loss. The higher the level of IOP, the greater the likelihood of optic nerve damage and visual field loss. Betaxolol has the action of reducing elevated as well as normal intraocular pressure and the mechanism of ocular hypotensive action appears to be a reduction of aqueous production as demonstrated by tonography and aqueous fluorophotometry. The onset of action with betaxolol can generally be noted within 30 minutes and the maximal effect can usually be detected 2 hours after topical administration. A single dose provides a 12-hour reduction in intraocular pressure.

In controlled, double-masked studies, the magnitude and duration of the ocular hypotensive effect of BETOPTIC S Ophthalmic Suspension 0.25% and BETOPTIC Ophthalmic Solution 0.5% were clinically equivalent. BETOPTIC S Suspension was significantly more comfortable than BETOPTIC Solution.

Ophthalmic betaxolol solution at 1% (one drop in each eye) was compared to placebo in a crossover study challenging nine patients with reactive airway disease. Betaxolol HCl had no significant effect on pulmonary function as measured by FEV_1, Forced Vital Capacity (FVC), FEV_1/FVC and was not significantly different from placebo. The action of isoproterenol, a beta stimulant, administered at the end of the study was not inhibited by ophthalmic betaxolol.

No evidence of cardiovascular beta adrenergic-blockade during exercise was observed with betaxolol in a double-masked, crossover study in 24 normal subjects comparing ophthalmic betaxolol and placebo for effects on blood pressure and heart rate.

Indications and Usage: BETOPTIC S Ophthalmic Suspension 0.25% has been shown to be effective in lowering intraocular pressure and may be used in patients with chronic open-angle glaucoma and ocular hypertension. It may be used alone or in combination with other intraocular pressure lowering medications.

Contraindications: Hypersensitivity to any component of this product. BETOPTIC S Ophthalmic Suspension 0.25% is contraindicated in patients with sinus bradycardia, greater than a first degree atrioventricular block, cardiogenic shock, or patients with overt cardiac failure.

Warning: Topically applied beta-adrenergic blocking agents may be absorbed systemically. The same adverse reactions found with systemic administration of beta-adrenergic blocking agents may occur with topical administration. For example, severe respiratory reactions and cardiac reactions, including death due to bronchospasm in patients with asthma, and rarely death in association with cardiac failure, have been reported with topical application of beta-adrenergic blocking agents.

BETOPTIC S Ophthalmic Suspension 0.25% has been shown to have a minor effect on heart rate and blood pressure in clinical studies. Caution should be used in treating patients with a history of cardiac failure or heart block. Treatment with BETOPTIC S Ophthalmic Suspension 0.25% should be discontinued at the first signs of cardiac failure.

Precautions:

General:

Diabetes Mellitus. Beta-adrenergic blocking agents should be administered with caution in patients subject to spontaneous hypoglycemia or to diabetic patients (especially those with labile diabetes) who are receiving insulin or oral hypoglycemic agents. Beta-adrenergic receptor blocking agents may mask the signs and symptoms of acute hypoglycemia.

Thyrotoxicosis. Beta-adrenergic blocking agents may mask certain clinical signs (e.g., tachycardia) of hyperthyroidism. Patients suspected of developing thyrotoxicosis should be managed carefully to avoid abrupt withdrawal of beta-adrenergic blocking agents, which might precipitate a thyroid storm.

Muscle Weakness. Beta-adrenergic blockade has been reported to potentiate muscle weakness consistent with certain myasthenic symptoms (e.g., diplopia, ptosis and generalized weakness).

Major Surgery. Consideration should be given to the gradual withdrawal of beta-adrenergic blocking agents prior to general anesthesia because of the reduced ability of the heart to respond to beta-adrenergically mediated sympathetic reflex stimuli.

Pulmonary. Caution should be exercised in the treatment of glaucoma patients with excessive restriction of pulmonary function. There have been reports of asthmatic attacks and pulmonary distress during betaxolol treatment. Although rechallenges of some such patients with ophthalmic betaxolol has not adversely affected pulmonary function test results, the possibility of adverse pulmonary effects in patients sensitive to beta blockers cannot be ruled out.

Drug Interactions: Patients who are receiving a beta-adrenergic blocking agent orally and BETOPTIC S Ophthalmic Suspension 0.25% should be observed for a potential additive effect either on the intraocular pressure or on the known systemic effects of beta blockade. Close observation of the patient is recommended when a beta blocker is administered to patients receiving catecholamine-depleting drugs such as reserpine, because of possible additive effects and the production of hypotension and/or bradycardia.

Betaxolol is an adrenergic blocking agent; therefore, caution should be exercised in patients using concomitant adrenergic psychotropic drugs.

Ocular: In patients with angle-closure glaucoma, the immediate treatment objective is to reopen the angle by constriction of the pupil with a miotic agent. Betaxolol has little or no effect on the pupil. When BETOPTIC S Ophthalmic Suspension 0.25% is used to reduce elevated intraocular pressure in angle-closure glaucoma, it should be used with a miotic and not alone.

Carcinogenesis, Mutagenesis, Impairment of Fertility: Lifetime studies with betaxolol HCl have been completed in mice at oral doses of 6, 20 or 60 mg/kg/day and in rats at 3, 12 or 48 mg/kg/day; betaxolol HCl demonstrated no carcinogenic effect. Higher dose levels were not tested.

In a variety of *in vitro* and *in vivo* bacterial and mammalian cell assays, betaxolol HCl was nonmutagenic.

Pregnancy:

Pregnancy Category C. Reproduction, teratology, and peri- and postnatal studies have been conducted with orally administered betaxolol HCl in rats and rabbits. There was evidence of drug related postimplantation loss in rabbits and rats at dose levels above 12 mg/kg and 128 mg/kg, respectively. Betaxolol HCl was not shown to be teratogenic, however, and there were no other adverse effects on reproduction at subtoxic dose levels. There are no adequate and well-controlled studies in pregnant women. BETOPTIC S should be used during pregnancy only if the potential benefit justifies the potential risk to the fetus.

Nursing Mothers: It is not known whether betaxolol HCl is excreted in human milk. Because many drugs are excreted in human milk, caution should be exercised when BETOPTIC S Ophthalmic Suspension 0.25% is administered to nursing women.

Pediatric Use: Safety and effectiveness in children have not been established.

Adverse Reactions:

Ocular: In clinical trials, the most frequent event associated with the use of BETOPTIC S Ophthalmic Suspension 0.25% has been transient ocular discomfort. The following other conditions have been reported in small numbers of patients: blurred vision, corneal punctate keratitis, foreign body sensation, photophobia, tearing, itching, dryness of eyes, erythema, inflammation, discharge, ocular pain, decreased visual acuity and crusty lashes.

Additional medical events reported with other formulations of betaxolol include allergic reactions, decreased corneal sensitivity, edema and anisocoria.

Systemic: Systemic reactions following administration of BETOPTIC S Ophthalmic Suspension 0.25% or BETOPTIC Ophthalmic Solution 0.5% have been rarely reported. These include:

Cardiovascular: Bradycardia, heart block and congestive failure.

Pulmonary: Pulmonary distress characterized by dyspnea, bronchospasm, thickened bronchial secretions, asthma and respiratory failure.

Central Nervous System: Insomnia, dizziness, vertigo, headaches, depression, and lethargy.

Other: Hives, toxic epidermal necrolysis, hair loss, and glossitis.

Overdosage: No information is available on overdosage of humans. The oral LD50 of the drug ranged from 350–920 mg/kg in mice and 860–1050 mg/kg in rats. The symptoms which might be expected with an overdose of a systemically administered beta-1-adrenergic receptor blocking agent are bradycardia, hypotension and acute cardiac failure.

A topical overdose of BETOPTIC S Ophthalmic Suspension 0.25% may be flushed from the eye(s) with warm tap water.

Dosage and Administration: The recommended dose is one to two drops of BETOPTIC S Ophthalmic Suspension 0.25% in the affected eye(s) twice daily. In some patients, the intraocular pressure lowering responses to BETOPTIC S may require a few weeks to stabilize. As with any new medication, careful monitoring of patients is advised.

If the intraocular pressure of the patient is not adequately controlled on this regimen, concomitant therapy with pilocarpine and other miotics, and/or epinephrine and/or carbonic anhydrase inhibitors can be instituted.

How Supplied: BETOPTIC S Ophthalmic Suspension 0.25% is supplied as follows: 2.5, 5

Continued on next page

Alcon—Cont.

and 15 mL in plastic ophthalmic DROP-TAINER® dispensers.

2.5 mL: **NDC** 0065-0246-20
5.0 mL: **NDC** 0065-0246-05
15.0 mL: **NDC** 0065-0246-15

Storage: Store at room temperature. Shake well before using.

Caution: Federal (USA) Law Prohibits Dispensing Without a Prescription.

U.S. Patent Nos. 4,252,984; 4,311,708; 4,342,783; 4,911,920.

CILOXAN™ ℞
(Ciprofloxacin HCl)
0.3% as base
Sterile Ophthalmic Solution

Description: CILOXAN™ (Ciprofloxacin HCl) Ophthalmic Solution is a synthetic, sterile, multiple dose, antimicrobial for topical ophthalmic use. Ciprofloxacin is a fluoroquinolone antibacterial active against a broad spectrum of gram-positive and gram-negative ocular pathogens. It is available as the monohydrochloride monohydrate salt of 1-cyclopropyl-6-fluoro-1,4-dihydro-4-oxo-7- (1-piperazinyl)-3-quinoline-carboxylic acid. It is a faint to light yellow crystalline powder with a molecular weight of 385.8. Its empirical formula is $C_{17}H_{18}FN_3O_3 \cdot HCl \cdot C_2O$ and its chemical structure is as follows:

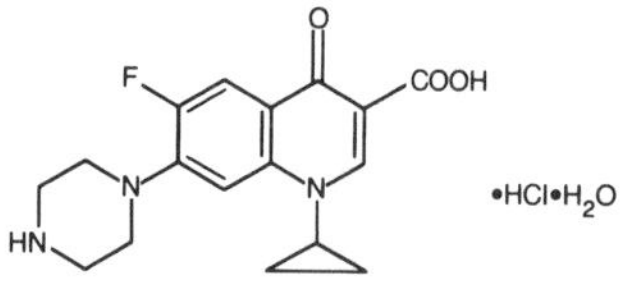

Ciprofloxacin differs from other quinolones in that it has a fluorine atom at the 6-position, a piperazine moiety at the 7-position, and a cyclopropyl ring at the 1-position.

Each mL of CILOXAN Ophthalmic Solution contains: Active: Ciprofloxacin HCl 3.5 mg equivalent to 3 mg base. Preservative: Benzalkonium Chloride 0.006%. Inactive: Sodium Acetate, Acetic Acid, Mannitol 4.6%, Edetate Disodium 0.05%, Hydrochloric Acid and/or Sodium Hydroxide (to adjust pH) and Purified Water. The pH is approximately 4.5 and the osmolality is approximately 300 mOsm.

Clinical Pharmacology:

Systemic Absorption: A systemic absorbtion study was performed in which CILOXAN Ophthalmic Solution was administered in each eye every two hours while awake for two days followed by every four hours while awake for an additional 5 days. The maximum reported plasma concentration of ciprofloxacin was less than 5 ng/mL. The mean concentration was usually less than 2.5 ng/mL.

Microbiology: Ciprofloxacin has *in vitro* activity against a wide range of gram-negative and gram-positive organisms. The bactericidal action of ciprofloxacin results from interference with the enzyme DNA gyrase which is needed for the synthesis of bacterial DNA.

Ciprofloxacin has been shown to be active against most strains of the following organisms both *in vitro* and in clinical infections. (See *Indications and Usage* section).

Gram-Positive:
Staphylococcus aureus (including methicillin-susceptible and methicillin-resistant strains)
Staphylococcus epidermidis
Streptococcus pneumoniae
Streptococcus (Viridans Group)

Gram-Negative:
Pseudomonas aeruginosa
Serratia marcescens

Ciprofloxacin has been shown to be active *in vitro* against most strains of the following organisms, however, *the clinical significance of these data is unknown:*

Gram-Positive:
Enterococcus faecalis (Many strains are only moderately susceptible)
Staphylococcus haemolyticus
Staphylococcus hominis
Staphylococcus saprophyticus
Streptococcus pyogenes

Gram-Negative:
Acinetobacter calcoaceticus subsp. anitratus
Aeromonas caviae
Aeromonas hydrophila
Brucella melitensis
Campylobacter coli
Campylobacter jujuni
Citrobacter diversus
Citrobacter freundii
Edwardsiella tarda
Enterobacter aerogenes
Enterobacter cloacae
Escherichia coli
Haemophilus ducreyi
Haemophilus influenzae
Haemophilus parainfluenzae
Klebsiella pneumoniae
Klebsiella oxytoca
Legionella pneumophila
Moraxella (Branhamella) catarrhalis
Morganella morganii
Neisseria gonorrhoeae
Neisseria meningitidis
Pasteurella multocida
Proteus mirabilis
Proteus vulgaris
Providencia rettgeri
Providencia stuartii
Salmonella enteritidis
Salmonella typhi
Shigella sonneii
Shigella flexneri
Vibrio cholerae
Vibrio parahaemolyticus
Vibrio vulnificus
Yersinia enterocolitica

Other Organisms: *Chlamydia trachomatis* (only moderately susceptible) and *Mycobacterium tuberculosis* (only moderately susceptible).

Most strains of *Pseudomonas cepacia* and some strains of *Pseudomonas maltophilia* are resistant to ciprofloxacin as are most anaerobic bacteria, including *Bacteroides fragilis* and *Clostridium difficile.*

The minimal bactericidal concentration (MBC) generally does not exceed the minimal inhibitory concentration (MIC) by more than a factor of 2. Resistance to ciprofloxacin *in vitro* usually develops slowly (multiple-step mutation).

Ciprofloxacin does not cross-react with other antimicrobial agents such as beta-lactams or aminoglycosides; therefore, organisms resistant to these drugs may be susceptible to ciprofloxacin.

Clinical Studies:
Following therapy with CILOXAN Ophthalmic Solution, 76% of the patients with corneal ulcers and positive bacterial cultures were clinically cured and complete re-epithelialization occurred in about 92% of the ulcers.

In 3 and 7 day multicenter clinical trials, 52% of the patients with conjunctivitis and positive conjunctival cultures were clinically cured and 70–80% had all causative pathogens eradicated by the end of treatment.

Indications and Usage: CILOXAN Ophthalmic Solution is indicated for the treatment of infections caused by susceptible strains of the designated microorganisms in the conditions listed below:

Corneal Ulcers:	*Pseudomonas aeruginosa*
	*Serratia marcescens**
	Staphylococcus aureus
	Staphylococcus epidermidis
	Streptococcus pneumoniae
	Streptococcus (Viridans Group)*
Conjunctivitis:	*Staphylococcus aureus*
	Staphylococcus epidermidis
	*Streptococcus pneumoniae**

*Efficacy for this organism was studied in fewer than 10 infections.

Contraindications: A history of hypersensitivity to ciprofloxacin or any other component of the medication is a contraindication to its use. A history of hypersensitivity to other quinolones may also contraindicate the use of ciprofloxacin.

Warnings: NOT FOR INJECTION INTO THE EYE.

Serious and occasionally fatal hypersensitivity (anaphylactic) reactions, some following the first dose, have been reported in patients receiving systemic quinolone therapy. Some reactions were accompanied by cardiovascular collapse, loss of consciousness, tingling, pharyngeal or facial edema, dyspnea, urticaria, and itching. Only a few patients had a history of hypersensitivity reactions. Serious anaphylactic reactions require immediate emergency treatment with epinephrine and other resuscitation measures, including oxygen, intravenous fluids, intravenous antihistamines, corticosteroids, pressor amines and airway management, as clinically indicated.

Precautions

General: As with other antibacterial preparations, prolonged use of ciprofloxacin may result in overgrowth of nonsusceptible organisms, including fungi. If superinfection occurs, appropriate therapy should be initiated. Whenever clinical judgment dictates, the patient should be examined with the aid of magnification, such as slit lamp biomicroscopy and, where appropriate, fluorescein staining.

Ciprofloxacin should be discontinued at the first appearance of a skin rash or any other sign of hypersensitivity reaction.

In clinical studies of patients with bacterial corneal ulcer, a white crystalline precipitate located in the superficial portion of the corneal defect was observed in 35 (16.6%) of 210 patients. The onset of the precipitate was within 24 hours to 7 days after starting therapy. In one patient, the precipitate was immediately irrigated out upon its appearance. In 17 patients, resolution of the precipitate was seen in 1 to 8 days (seven within the first 24–72 hours); in five patients, resolution was noted in 10–13 days. In nine patients, exact resolution days were unavailable; however, at follow-up examinations, 18–44 days after onset of the event, complete resolution of the precipitate was noted. In three patients, outcome information was unavailable. The precipitate did not preclude continued use of ciprofloxacin, nor did it adversely affect the clinical course of the ulcer or visual outcome (SEE ADVERSE REACTIONS).

Drug Interactions: Specific drug interaction studies have not been conducted with ophthalmic ciprofloxacin. However, the systemic administration of some quinolones has been shown to elevate plasma concentrations of theophylline, interfere with the metabolism of caffeine, enhance the effects of the oral anticoagulant, warfarin, and its derivatives and have been associated with transient elevations in serum creatinine in patients receiving cyclosporine concomitantly.

Carcinogenesis, Mutagenesis, Impairment of Fertility: Eight *in vitro* mutagenicity tests have been conducted with ciprofloxacin and the test results are listed below:

Salmonella/Microsome Test (Negative)
E. coli DNA Repair Assay (Negative)
Mouse Lymphoma Cell Forward Mutation Assay (Positive)
Chinese Hamster V_{79} Cell HGPRT Test (Negative)
Syrian Hamster Embryo Cell Transformation Assay (Negative)
Saccharomyces cerevisiae Point Mutation Assay (Negative)
Saccharomyces cerevisiae Mitotic Crossover and Gene Conversion Assay (Negative)
Rat Hepatocyte DNA Repair Assay (Positive)

Thus, two of the eight tests were positive, but the results of the following three *in vivo* test systems gave negative results:
Rat Hepatocyte DNA Repair Assay
Micronucleus Test (Mice)
Dominant Lethal Test (Mice)

Long term carcinogenicity studies in mice and rats have been completed. After daily oral dosing for up to two years, there is no evidence that ciprofloxacin had any carcinogenic or tumorigenic effects in these species.

Pregnancy—Pregnancy Category C: Reproduction studies have been performed in rats and mice at doses up to six times the usual daily human oral dose and have revealed no evidence of impaired fertility or harm to the fetus due to ciprofloxacin. In rabbits, as with most antimicrobial agents, ciprofloxacin (30 and 100 mg/kg orally) produced gastrointestinal disturbances resulting in maternal weight loss and an increased incidence of abortion. No teratogenicity was observed at either dose. After intravenous administration, at doses up to 20 mg/kg, no maternal toxicity was produced and no embryotoxicity or teratogenicity was observed. There are no adequate and well controlled studies in pregnant women. CILOXAN Ophthalmic Solution should be used during pregnancy only if the potential benefit justifies the potential risk to the fetus.

Nursing Mothers: It is not known whether topically applied ciprofloxacin is excreted in human milk; however, it is known that orally administered ciprofloxacin is excreted in the milk of lactating rats and oral ciprofloxacin has been reported in human breast milk after a single 500 mg dose. Caution should be exercised when CILOXAN Ophthalmic Solution is administered to a nursing mother.

Pediatric Use: Safety and effectiveness in children below the age of 12 have not been established.

Although ciprofloxacin and other quinolones cause arthropathy in immature animals after oral administration, topical ocular administration of ciprofloxacin to immature animals did not cause any arthropathy and there is no evidence that the ophthalmic dosage form has any effect on the weight bearing joints.

Adverse Reactions: The most frequently reported drug related adverse reaction was local burning or discomfort. In corneal ulcer studies with frequent administration of the drug, white crystalline precipitates were seen in approximately 17% of patients (SEE PRECAUTIONS). Other reactions occurring in less than 10% of patients included lid margin crusting, crystals/scales, foreign body sensation, itching, conjunctival hyperemia and a bad taste following instillation. Additional events occurring in less than 1% of patients included corneal staining, keratopathy/keratitis, allergic reactions, lid edema, tearing, photophobia, corneal infiltrates, nausea and decreased vision.

Overdosage: A topical overdose of CILOXAN Ophthalmic Solution may be flushed from the eye(s) with warm tap water.

Dosage and Administration: The recommended dosage regimen for the treatment of **corneal ulcers** is: Two drops into the affected eye every 15 minutes for the first six hours and then two drops into the affected eye every 30 minutes for the remainder of the first day. On the second day, instill two drops in the affected eye hourly. On the third through the fourteenth day, place two drops in the affected eye every four hours. Treatment may be continued after 14 days if corneal re-epithelialization has not occurred.

The recommended dosage regimen for the treatment of **bacterial conjunctivitis** is: One or two drops instilled into the conjunctival sac(s) every two hours while awake for two days and one or two drops every four hours while awake for the next five days.

How Supplied: As a sterile ophthalmic solution: 2.5 mL and 5 mL in plastic DROP-TAINER® dispensers.
2.5 mL—NDC 0065-0656-25
5 mL —NDC 0065-0656-05

Storage: Store at 2° to 30°C (36° to 86°F). Protect from light.

Animal Pharmacology: Ciprofloxacin and related drugs have been shown to cause arthropathy in immature animals of most species tested following oral administration. However, a one-month topical ocular study using immature Beagle dogs did not demonstrate any articular lesions.

Caution: Federal (USA) law prohibits dispensing without prescription.
U.S. Patent No. 4,670,444

CYCLOGYL® ℞
(cyclopentolate hydrochloride ophthalmic solution)

Description: CYCLOGYL® (cyclopentolate hydrochloride ophthalmic solution) is an anticholinergic prepared as a sterile, borate buffered solution for topical ocular use. It is supplied in three strengths. The active ingredient is represented by the chemical structure:

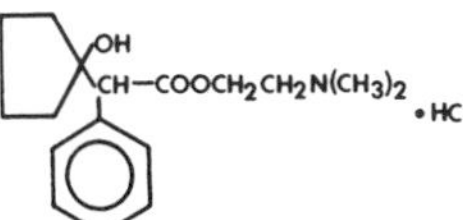

Established name:
Cyclopentolate Hydrochloride

Chemical name:
2-(Dimethylamino)ethyl 1-hydroxy-α-phenylcyclopentaneacetate hydrochloride

Each mL contains: Active: Cyclopentolate Hydrochloride 0.5%, 1% or 2%. **Preservative:** Benzalkonium Chloride 0.01%. **Inactive:** Boric Acid, Edetate Disodium, Potassium Chloride (except 2% strength), Sodium Carbonate and/or Hydrochloric Acid (to adjust pH), Purified Water.

Clinical Pharmacology: This anticholinergic preparation blocks the responses of the sphincter muscle of the iris and the accommodative muscle of the ciliary body to cholinergic stimulation, producing pupillary dilation (mydriasis) and paralysis of accommodation (cycloplegia). It acts rapidly, but has a shorter duration than atropine. Maximal cycloplegia occurs within 25 to 75 minutes after instillation. Complete recovery of accommodation usually takes 6 to 24 hours. Complete recovery from mydriasis in some individuals may require several days.

Indications and Usage: Cyclopentolate hydrochloride is used to produce mydriasis and cycloplegia.

Contraindications: Should not be used when narrow-angle glaucoma or anatomical narrow angles are present, or where there is hypersensitivity to any component of this preparation.

Warnings: Do not touch dropper tip to any surface as this may contaminate the solution. For topical use only—not for injection. This preparation may cause CNS disturbances. This is especially true in younger age groups, but may occur at any age, especially with the stronger solutions. Premature and small infants are especially prone to CNS and cardiopulmonary side effects from systemic absorption of cyclopentolate. To minimize absorption, use only 1 drop of 0.5% CYCLOGYL solution per eye, followed by pressure applied over the nasolacrimal sac for two to three minutes. Observe infants closely for at least 30 minutes following instillation.

Precautions:

General: To avoid inducing angle closure glaucoma, an estimation of the depth of the angle of the anterior chamber should be made. The lacrimal sac should be compressed by digital pressure for two to three minutes after instillation to avoid excessive systemic absorption. Caution should be observed when considering use of this medication in the presence of Down's syndrome or mongolism, and in those predisposed to angle-closure glaucoma.

Patient Information: A transient burning sensation may occur upon instillation. Patients should be advised not to drive or engage in other hazardous activities while pupils are dilated. Patients may experience sensitivity to light and should protect eyes in bright illumination during dilation. Parents should be warned not to get this preparation in their child's mouth and to wash their own hands and the child's hands following administration.

Drug Interactions: Cyclopentolate may interfere with the anti-glaucoma action of carbachol or pilocarpine; also, concurrent use of these medications may antagonize the anti-glaucoma and miotic actions of ophthalmic cholinesterase inhibitors.

Carcinogenesis, Mutagenesis, and Impairment of Fertility: Studies in animals or humans have not been conducted to evaluate the potential of these effects.

Pregnancy Category C: Animal reproduction studies have not been conducted with cyclopentolate. It is also not known whether cyclopentolate can cause fetal harm when administered to a pregnant woman or can affect reproduction capacity. Cyclopentolate should be administered to a pregnant woman only if clearly needed.

Nursing Mothers: It is not known whether this drug is excreted in human milk. Because many drugs are excreted in human milk, caution should be exercised when cyclopentolate hydrochloride is administered to a nursing woman.

Pediatrics: Increased susceptibility to cyclopentolate has been reported in infants, young children, and in children with spastic paralysis or brain damage. Therefore, cyclopentolate should be used with great caution in these patients. Feeding intolerance may follow ophthalmic use of this product in neonates. It is recommended that feeding be withheld for four (4) hours after examination. Do not use in concentrations higher than 0.5% in small infants (see WARNINGS).

Geriatrics: In the elderly and others where increased intraocular pressure may be encountered, mydriatics and cycloplegics should be used cautiously.

Adverse Reactions:

Ocular: Increased intraocular pressure, burning, photophobia, blurred vision, irritation, hyperemia, conjunctivitis, blepharoconjunctivitis, punctate keratitis, synechiae.

Systemic: Use of cyclopentolate has been associated with psychotic reactions and behavioral disturbances, usually in children, especially with 2% concentration. These disturbances include ataxia, incoherent speech, restlessness, hallucinations, hyperactivity, seizures, disorientation as to time and place, and failure to recognize people. This drug produces

Continued on next page

Alcon—Cont.

reactions similar to those of other anticholinergic drugs, but the central nervous system manifestations as noted above are more common. Other toxic manifestations of anticholinergic drugs are skin rash, abdominal distention in infants, unusual drowsiness, tachycardia, hyperpyrexia, vasodilation, urinary retention, diminished gastrointestinal motility and decreased secretion in salivary and sweat glands, pharynx, bronchii and nasal passages. Severe manifestations of toxicity include coma, medullary paralysis and death.

Overdosage: Excessive dosage may produce exaggerated symptoms as noted in ADVERSE REACTIONS. When administration of the drug product is discontinued, the patient usually recovers spontaneously. In case of severe manifestations of toxicity the antidote of choice is physostigmine salicylate.

Pediatric Dose: As an antidote, slowly inject intravenously 0.5 mg physostigmine salicylate. If toxic symptoms persist and no cholinergic symptoms are produced, repeat at five minute intervals to a maximum cumulative dose of 2 mg.

Adolescent and Adult: As an antidote, slowly inject 2 mg physostigmine salicylate intravenously. A second dose of 1 to 2 mg may be given after 20 minutes if no reversal of toxic manifestations has occurred.[1,2,3]

Dosage and Administration: Adults: One or two drops of 0.5%, 1% or 2% solution in the eye which may be repeated in five to ten minutes if necessary. Complete recovery usually occurs in 24 hours. **Children:** One or two drops of 0.5%, 1% or 2% solution in the eye which may be repeated five to ten minutes later by a second application of 0.5% or 1% solution if necessary. **Small Infants:** A single instillation of one drop of 0.5% CYCLOGYL in the eye. To minimize absorption, apply pressure over the nasolacrimal sac for two to three minutes. Observe infant closely for at least 30 minutes following instillation. Individuals with heavily pigmented irides may require higher strengths.

How Supplied:
In multiple-dose plastic DROP-TAINER® dispensers:

0.5% CYCLOGYL
- 2mL NDC 0065-0395-02
- 5mL NDC 0065-0395-05
- 15mL NDC 0065-0395-15

1% CYCLOGYL
- 2mL NDC 0065-0396-02
- 5mL NDC 0065-0396-05
- 15mL NDC 0065-0396-15

2% CYCLOGYL
- 2mL NDC 0065-0397-02
- 5mL NDC 0065-0397-05
- 15mL NDC 0065-0397-15

Storage: Store at 46°–80°F.

References:

1. Rumack, B. H.: Anticholinergic Poisoning: Treatment with Physostigmine. **Pediatrics** 52(6):449–51, 1973.
2. Duvoisin, R. C. and Katz, R.: Reversal of Central Anticholinergic Syndromes in Man by Physostigmine, **J. Am. Med. Assn.** 206(9): 1963–65, 1968.
3. Grant, W. M.: *Toxicology of the Eye.* Second Edition, Volume 1. Springfield, Illinois, Charles C. Thomas: 1974.

Caution: Federal (USA) law prohibits dispensing without prescription.

CYCLOMYDRIL® ℞
(cyclopentolate hydrochloride, phenylephrine hydrochloride)
STERILE OPHTHALMIC SOLUTION

Description: CYCLOMYDRIL® (Cyclopentolate Hydrochloride, Phenylephrine Hydrochloride) is a mydriatic prepared as a sterile topical ophthalmic solution. The active ingredients are represented by the chemical structures:

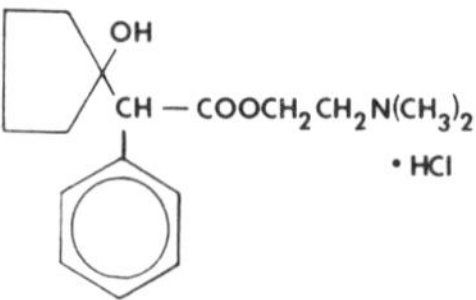

Established name:
Cyclopentolate Hydrochloride

Chemical name:
2-(Dimethylamino)ethyl 1-hydroxy-α-phenylcyclopentaneacetate hydrochloride

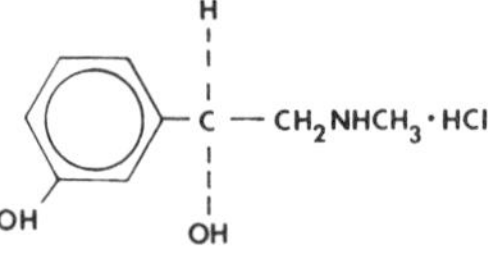

Established name:
Phenylephrine Hydrochloride

Chemical name:
3-hydroxy- α[(methylamino)-methyl]-, Benzenemethanol, hydrochloride (*R*)-.

Each mL contains: Active: Cyclopentolate Hydrochloride 0.2%, Phenylephrine Hydrochloride 1%. Preservative: Benzalkonium Chloride 0.01%. Inactive: Edetate Disodium, Boric Acid, Hydrochloric Acid and/or Sodium Carbonate (to adjust pH), Purified Water.

Clinical Pharmacology: Cyclopentolate Hydrochloride is an anticholinergic drug and Phenylephrine Hydrochloride is an adrenergic drug. This combination induces mydriasis that is considerably greater than that of either drug alone. The concentrations of Cyclopentolate Hydrochloride and of Phenylephrine Hydrochloride have been selected to induce safe and rapid mydriasis with little or no accompanying cycloplegia.

Indications and Usage: For the production of mydriasis.

Contraindications: Do not use in patients with narrow-angle glaucoma or with anatomically narrow angles or where there is hypersensitivity to any component of this preparation.

Warnings: Do not touch dropper tip to any surface, as this may contaminate the solution. For topical use only—not for injection. The use of this combination may have an adverse effect on individuals suffering from cardiovascular disease, hypertension, and hyperthyroidism, and it may cause CNS disturbances. Small infants are especially prone to CNS and cardiopulmonary side effects from systemic absorption of cyclopentolate.

Precautions: To avoid inducing angle closure glaucoma, an estimation of the depth of the angle of the anterior chamber should be made. The lacrimal sac should be compressed by digital pressure for two to three minutes after instillation to avoid excessive systemic absorption. The effect of long-term use of this preparation has not been established, therefore it should be restricted to short-term use.

Patient Warning: Patient should be advised not to drive or engage in other hazardous activities while pupils are dilated. Patient may experience sensitivity to light and should protect eyes in bright illumination during dilation. Parents should be warned not to get this preparation in their child's mouth and to wash their own hands and the child's hands following administration. Feeding intolerance may follow ophthalmic use of this product in neonates. It is recommended that feeding be withheld for four (4) hours after examination.

Adverse Reactions: Increased intraocular pressure. Use of Cyclopentolate has been associated with psychotic reactions and behavioral disturbances in children, especially with 2% concentration. These disturbances include ataxia, incoherent speech, restlessness, hallucinations, hyperactivity, seizures, disorientation as to time and place, and failure to recognize people. This drug produces reactions similar to those of other anticholinergic drugs; however, the central nervous system manifestations as noted above are more common. Other toxic manifestations of anticholinergic drugs are tachycardia, hyperpyrexia, vasodilation, urinary retention, diminished gastrointestinal motility and decreased secretion in salivary and sweat glands, pharynx, bronchii and nasal passages. Severe manifestations of toxicity include coma, medullary paralysis and death.

Overdosage: When administration of the drug product is discontinued, the patient usually recovers spontaneously. In case of severe manifestations of toxicity, the antidote of choice is physostigmine salicylate.

Pediatric Dose: As an antidote, slowly inject intravenously 0.5 mg of physostigmine salicylate. If toxic symptoms persist and no cholinergic symptoms are produced repeat at five minute intervals to a maximum dose of 2.0 mg.

Adolescent and Adult Dose: As an antidote, slowly inject intravenously 2.0 mg of physostigmine salicylate. A second dose of 1–2 mg may be given after 20 minutes if no reversal of toxic manifestations has occurred.[1,2,3]

Dosage and Administration: For funduscopy, instill one drop in each eye every five to ten minutes, not to exceed three times, to produce rapid mydriasis, permitting ready visual access to the fundus. Heavily pigmented irides may require larger doses. To minimize absorption in premature and small infants, apply pressure over the nasolacrimal sac for two to three minutes following instillation. Observe infants closely for at least 30 minutes.

How Supplied: In 2 mL and 5 mL plastic DROP-TAINER® dispensers.
- 2mL NDC 0065-0359-02
- 5mL NDC 0065-0359-05

Storage: Store at 46° to 80°F.

References:

1. Rumack, B. H.: Anticholinergic Poisoning: Treatment with Physostigmine. PEDIATRICS 52(6):449-51, 1973.
2. Duvoisin, R. C. and Katz, R.: Reversal of Central Anticholinergic Syndromes in Man by Physostigmine. J. AM. MED. ASSN. 206(9): 1963-65, 1968.
3. Grant, W. M.: *Toxicology of the Eye.* Second Edition, Volume 1. Springfield, Illinois. Charles C. Thomas: 1974.

DURATEARS NATURALE® OTC
Lubricant Eye Ointment

Description: A sterile bland, non-medicated unpreserved ointment.

Ingredients: Each gram contains: **Active:** White Petrolatum and Mineral Oil. **Inactive:** Anhydrous Liquid Lanolin.

Indications: For nighttime use as a lubricant to relieve dryness of the eye. For topical eye use only.

Warnings: If you experience eye pain, changes in vision, continued redness or irritation of the eye, or if the condition worsens or persists for more than 72 hours, discontinue use and consult a doctor.
To avoid contamination, do not touch tip of container to any surface. Replace cap after using. Keep this and all drugs out of the reach of children. In case of accidental ingestion,

seek professional assistance or contact a Poison Control Center immediately.
Directions: Pull down the lower lid of the affected eye and apply a small amount (one-fourth inch) of ointment to the inside of the eyelid.
Storage: Store at 46°–80°F.
Supplied: As a sterile ophthalmic ointment in 3.5 g tubes.
NDC 0065-0414-35

⅛ % ECONOPRED® ℞
and
1% ECONOPRED® Plus ℞
(prednisolone acetate)
Ophthalmic Suspension

Description: ECONOPRED® (prednisolone acetate) is an adrenocortical steroid prepared as a sterile ophthalmic suspension. The active ingredient is represented by the chemical structure:

[Chemical structure of prednisolone acetate]

Established name:
Prednisolone Acetate

Chemical name:
Pregna-1,4-diene-3,20-dione, 21-(acetyloxy)-11,17-dihydroxy-, (11β)-.

Each mL contains: Active: Prednisolone Acetate 0.125% or 1.0%. Preservative: Benzalkonium Chloride 0.01%. Vehicle: Hydroxypropyl Methylcellulose. Inactive: Dried Sodium Phosphate, Polysorbate 80, Edetate Disodium, Glycerin, Citric Acid and/or Sodium Hydroxide (to adust pH), Purified Water.
Clinical Pharmacology: This drug causes inhibition of the inflammatory response to inciting agents of a mechanical, chemical, or immunological nature. No generally accepted explanation of this steroid property has been advanced.
Indications and Usage: Steroid responsive inflammatory conditions of the palpebral and bulbar conjunctiva, cornea, and anterior segment of the globe. These include allergic conjunctivitis, acne rosacea, superficial punctate keratitis, herpes zoster keratitis, iritis, cyclitis, selected infective conjunctivitises, corneal injury from chemical, radiation, or thermal burns, or penetration of foreign bodies, when the inherent hazard of steroid use is accepted to obtain an advisable diminution in edema and inflammation. 1% may be used to suppress graft reaction after keratoplasty. ⅛% may be used for superficial inflammation and 1% for deeper inflammations.
Contraindications: Contraindicated in epithelial herpes simplex keratitis (dendritic keratitis), vaccinia, varicella, and most other viral diseases of the cornea and conjunctiva; tuberculosis; fungal diseases; acute purulent untreated infections which, like other diseases caused by microorganisms, may be masked or enhanced by the presence of the steroid; hypersensitivity to any component of the medication. Steroids should not be used after the uncomplicated removal of a superficial foreign body.
Warnings: Do not touch dropper tip to any surface, as this may contaminate the suspension. Employment of steroid medication in the treatment of stromal herpes simplex requires great caution; frequent slit-lamp microscopy is mandatory. Prolonged use may result in glaucoma, damage to the optic nerve, defects in visual acuity and visual field, posterior subcapsular cataract formation, or may aid in the establishment of secondary ocular infection from pathogens liberated from ocular tissue. In those diseases causing thinning of the cornea or sclera, perforation has been known to occur with the use of topical steroids. Steroid use may potentiate viral infections (herpes). This drug is not effective in the treatment of Sjögren's Keratoconjunctivitis. Rarely, filtering blebs have been reported when topical steroids have been used following cataract surgery.
Precautions: During the course of the therapy, if the inflammatory reaction does not respond within a reasonable period, other forms of therapy should be instituted. As fungal infections of the cornea are particularly prone to develop coincidentally with long-term local steroid application, fungus invasion must be considered in any persistent corneal ulceration where a steroid has been used or is in use. Intraocular pressure should be checked frequently. Steroids should be used with caution in the presence of glaucoma. This product should not be used without continuing medical supervision. The initial prescription and renewal of the medication order should be made by a physician only after examination of the patient with the aid of magnification, such as slit lamp biomicroscopy, and, where appropriate, fluorescein staining.
Usage in Pregnancy: Safety of intensive or protracted use of topical steroids during pregnancy has not been substantiated.
Adverse Reactions: Glaucoma with optic nerve damage, visual acuity and field defects, posterior subcapsular cataract formation, secondary ocular infections from pathogens including herpes simplex liberated from ocular tissues, perforation of the globe. Viral and fungal infections of the cornea may be exacerbated by the application of steroids.
Dosage and Administration: Shake well before using. Two drops topically in the eye(s) four times daily. In cases of bacterial infections, concomitant use of antibiotics or chemotherapeutic agents is mandatory.
How Supplied: In 5mL and 15mL (10mL fill) plastic DROP-TAINER® dispensers.
⅛% ECONOPRED®:
5 mL NDC 0998-0635-05
10 mL NDC 0998-0635-10
1% ECONOPRED® Plus:
5 mL NDC 0998-0637-05
10 mL NDC 0998-0637-10
Storage: Store at 46°–75°F in an upright position.

EYE-STREAM® OTC
Sterile Eye Irrigating Solution

EYE-STREAM® is a sterile and stable irrigating solution that is specially designed and packaged for use in the eye(s). Formulated as a balanced salt solution, it closely approximates normal human tear fluid.
Indications:

FDA APPROVED USES
For irrigating the eye to help relieve irritation, discomfort and burning by removing loose foreign material, air pollutants (smog or pollen), or chlorinated water.

Ingredients: Each mL contains: **Tonicity Agents:** Sodium Chloride 0.64%, Potassium Chloride 0.075%, Calcium Chloride Dihydrate 0.048%, Magnesium Chloride Hexahydrate 0.03%. **Buffering Agents:** Sodium Acetate Trihydrate 0.39%, Sodium Citrate Dihydrate 0.17%. **pH Adjusters:** Sodium Hydroxide and/or Hydrochloric Acid. **Preservative:** Benzalkonium Chloride 0.013%. **Purified Water.** The pH of the solution is in the physiologic range.
Directions: Flush the affected eye as needed, controlling the rate of flow of solution by pressure on the bottle.
Warnings: If you experience eye pain, changes in vision, continued redness or irritation of the eye, or if the condition worsens or persists, consult a doctor. Obtain immediate medical treatment for all open wounds in or near the eyes. If solution changes color or becomes cloudy, do not use. To avoid contamination, do not touch tip of container to any surface. Replace cap after using. Keep this and all drugs out of the reach of children. In case of accidental ingestion, seek professional assistance or contact a Poison Control Center immediately. Not to be used as a saline solution for rinsing and soaking soft contact lenses. Not for injection or intraocular surgery.
How Supplied: In 1 fluid ounce and 4 fluid ounce plastic squeeze bottles.
1 fl. oz: NDC 0065-0530-01
4 fl. oz.: NDC 0065-0530-04
Storage: Store at 46°–80°F.

FLUORESCITE® INJECTION ℞
(fluorescein injection)
Sterile

Description: FLUORESCITE® INJECTION is a sterile aqueous solution in two strengths for use intravenously as a diagnostic aid. The active ingredient is represented by the chemical structure:

[Chemical structure of fluorescein sodium]

Established name:
Fluorescein Sodium
Chemical name:
Spiro[isobenzofuran-1(3*H*),9'-[9*H*] xanthene]-3-one, 3'6'dihydroxy, disodium salt.

The solution contains Fluorescein Sodium (equivalent to Fluorescein 10% or 25%), Sodium Hydroxide and/or Hydrochloric Acid (to adjust pH), and Water for Injection.
Clinical Pharmacology: The yellowish-green fluorescence of the drug demarcates the vascular area under observation distinguishing it from adjacent areas.
Indications and Usage: Indicated in diagnostic fluorescein angiography or angioscopy of the fundus and of the iris vasculature.
Contraindications: Contraindicated in those persons who have shown hypersensitivity to any component of this preparation.
Warning: Care must be taken to avoid extravasation during injection as the high pH of fluorescein solution can result in severe local tissue damage. The following complications resulting from extravasation of fluorescein have been noted to occur: sloughing of the skin; superficial phlebitis; subcutaneous granuloma; and toxic neuritis along the median curve in the antecubital area. Complications resulting from extravasation can cause severe pain in the arm for up to several hours. When significant extravasation occurs, the injection should be discontinued and conservative measures to treat damaged tissue and to relieve pain should be implemented.
Precautions: Caution is to be exercised in patients with a history of allergy or bronchial asthma. An emergency tray including such items as 0.1% epinephrine for intravenous or intramuscular use; an antihistamine, soluble steroid, and aminophyllene for IV use; and

Continued on next page

Alcon—Cont.

oxygen should always be available in the event of possible reaction to fluorescein injection.[1]

Use in Pregnancy: Avoid angiography on patients who are pregnant, especially those in first trimester. There have been no reports of fetal complications for fluorescein injection during pregnancy.

Patient Warning: Skin will attain a temporary yellowish discoloration. Urine attains a bright yellow color. Discoloration of the skin fades in 6 to 12 hours; urine fluorescein in 24 to 36 hours.

Adverse Reactions: Nausea and headache, gastrointestinal distress, syncope, vomiting, hypotension, and other symptoms and signs of hypersensitivity have occurred. Cardiac arrest, basilar artery ischemia, severe shock, convulsions, and thrombophlebitis at the injection site and rare cases of death have been reported. Extravasation of the solution at the injection site causes intense pain at the site and a dull aching pain in the injected arm. (SEE WARNING.) Generalized hives and itching, bronchospasm and anaphylaxis have been reported. A strong taste may develop after injection.

Dosage and Administration: Inject the contents of the ampule or pre-filled syringe rapidly into the antecubital vein, *after taking precautions to avoid extravasation.* A syringe, filled with fluorescein, is attached to transparent tubing and a 25 gauge scalp vein needle for injection. Insert the needle and draw the patient's blood to the hub of the syringe so that a *small* air bubble separates the patient's blood in the tubing from the fluorescein. With the room lights on, slowly inject the blood back into the vein while watching the skin over the needle tip. If the needle has extravasated, the patient's blood will be seen to bulge the skin and the injection should be stopped before any fluorescein is injected. When assured that extravasation has not occurred, the room light may be turned off and the fluorescein injection completed. Luminescence appears in the retina and choroidal vessels in 9 to 14 seconds and can be observed by standard viewing equipment. If potential allergy is suspected, an intradermal skin test may be performed prior to intravenous administration, i.e., 0.05 mL injected intradermally to be evaluated 30 to 60 minutes following injection. For children, the dose is calculated on the basis of 35 mg for each ten pounds of body weight.

In patients with inaccessible veins where early phases of an angiogram are not necessary, such as cystoid macular edema, one gram of FLUORESCITE (fluorescein) has been administered orally. Ten to fifteen minutes is usually required before evidence of dye appears in the fundus.

How Supplied: 5 mL of 10% in pre-filled syringe, 10% in 5 mL ampule and 25% in 2 mL ampule.

10% NDC 0065-0092-05
10% NDC 0065-0093-05 syringe
25% NDC 0065-0094-02

Storage: Store at 46°–80°F.

Reference:

1. Schatz, Burton, Yannuzzi, Rabb. Interpretation of Fundus Fluorescein Angiography, Page 38, C. V. Mosby Co., Saint Louis, 1978.

GLAUCON® ℞
(epinephrine)
Sterile Ophthalmic Solution

Description: GLAUCON® (epinephrine) is a sterile topical ophthalmic solution. The active ingredient is represented by the chemical structure:

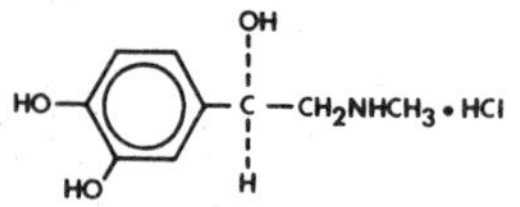

Established name:
Epinephrine Hydrochloride

Chemical name:
1,2-Benzenediol, 4-[1-hydroxy-2-(methylamino)ethyl]-, (*R*)-, monohydrochloride.

Each mL contains: Active: Epinephrine Hydrochloride equivalent to 1.0% or 2.0% Epinephrine base. **Preservative:** Benzalkonium Chloride 0.01%. **Inactive:** Sodium Metabisulfite, Edetate Disodium, Sodium Chloride in 1% solution only, Hydrochloric Acid, Sodium Hydroxide (to adjust pH), Purified Water.

Clinical Pharmacology: Lowers intraocular pressure by reducing the production of aqueous and increasing the facility of outflow.

Indications and Usage: For the control of simple (open angle) glaucoma. It may be used in combination with miotics, beta blockers, hyperosmotic agents, or carbonic anhydrase inhibitors when indicated.

Contraindications: Do not use in narrow or shallow angle (angle closure) glaucoma. Contraindicated in those persons who have shown hypersensitivity to any component of this preparation.

Warnings: For topical eye use only—not for injection. To avoid inducing angle closure glaucoma, an estimation of the depth of the angle of the anterior chamber should be made. Use with caution in individuals with history of hyperthyroidism, hypertension, organic cardiac disease and long-standing bronchial asthma. Maculopathy with associated decrease in visual acuity may occur in the aphakic eye; in this event, administration should be discontinued promptly. Do not use if solution is brown or contains a precipitate. Contains sodium metabisulfite, a sulfite that may cause allergic-type reactions including anaphylactic symptoms and life-threatening or less severe asthmatic episodes in certain susceptible people. The overall prevalence of sulfite sensitivity in the general population is unknown and probably low. Sulfite sensitivity is seen more frequently in asthmatic than in nonasthmatic people.

Precautions: General. Do not use this preparation while wearing soft contact lenses.

Information For Patients: Do not touch dropper tip to any surface, as this may contaminate the solution.

Carcinogenesis, Mutagenesis, Impairment of Fertility: There have been no long-term studies done using GLAUCON® (epinephrine) in animals to evaluate carcinogenic potential.

Pregnancy: Pregnancy Category C. Animal reproduction studies have not been conducted with epinephrine. It is also not known whether epinephrine can cause fetal harm when administered to a pregnant woman or can affect reproduction capacity. GLAUCON Ophthalmic Solution should be given to a pregnant women only if clearly needed.

Nursing Mothers: It is not known whether these drugs are excreted in human milk. Because many drugs are excreted in human milk, caution should be exercised when epinephrine is administered to a nursing woman.

Adverse Reactions: Transient symptoms of stinging and burning may occur. Prolonged use may be associated with conjunctival or corneal pigmentation. Following prolonged administration, ocular irritation (hypersensitivity) may develop. Systemic side effects such as headache, palpitation, faintness, tachycardia, and extrasystoles may occur. Severe side effects such as hypertension and cardiac arrhythmia have been reported.

Dosage and Administration: Usual dosage is one drop topically in the eye(s) one or two times daily for the control of glaucoma.

How Supplied: 10 mL in 15 mL plastic DROP-TAINER® dispenser.

1% NDC 0998-0249-10
2% NDC 0998-0250-10

Storage: Store at 36° to 75°F. (2° - 24° C).

Caution: Federal (USA) law prohibits dispensing without prescription.

GONIOSCOPIC PRISM SOLUTION ℞
Sterile prism solution

Description: A sterile buffered isotonic solution containing hydroxyethylcellulose, preserved with thimerosal 0.004% and edetate disodium 0.1%.

Storage: Store at room temperature.

Indications and Usage: For professional use only. To be used in accordance with directions for bonding gonioscopic prisms to the eye. Refractive index approximately 1.35.

Warning: This product contains thimerosal. Do not use with patients allergic to thimerosal or any other ingredient containing mercury.

How Supplied: In 15mL (½ fl. oz.) plastic dispensers, NDC 0065-0259-15.

ISOPTO® ATROPINE ℞
(atropine sulfate)
Ophthalmic Solution

Description: ISOPTO® ATROPINE (atropine sulfate) is an anticholinergic prepared as a sterile topical ophthalmic solution supplied in three strengths. The active ingredient is represented by the chemical structure:

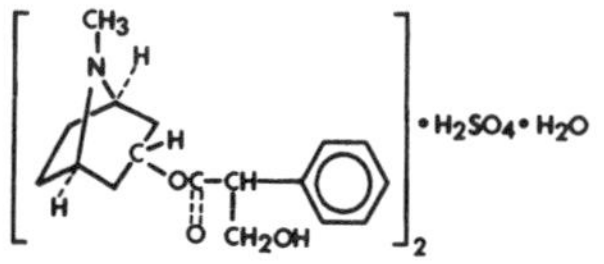

Established name:
Atropine Sulfate

Chemical name:
Benzeneacetic acid, α-(hydroxymethyl)-, 8-methyl-8-aza-bicyclo-[3.2.1]oct-3-yl ester, *endo*-(±)-, sulfate (2:1) (salt), monohydrate.

Each mL contains: **Active:** Atropine Sulfate 0.5%, 1.0% or 3.0%. **Preservative:** Benzalkonium Chloride 0.01%. **Vehicle:** 0.5% Hydroxypropyl Methylcellulose 2910. **Inactive:** Boric Acid, Sodium Hydroxide and/or Hydrochloric Acid (to adjust pH), Purified Water.

Clinical Pharmacology: This anticholinergic preparation blocks the responses of the sphincter muscle of the iris and the accommodative muscle of the ciliary body to cholinergic stimulation, producing pupillary dilation (mydriasis) and paralysis of accommodation (cycloplegia).

Indications and Usage: For mydriasis and/or cycloplegia. For cycloplegic refraction, for pupillary dilation desired in inflammatory conditions of the iris and uveal tract.

Contraindications: Contraindicated in persons with primary glaucoma or a tendency toward glaucoma, e.g., narrow anterior chamber angle, and in those persons showing hypersensitivity to any component of this preparation.

Warnings: For topical use only—not for injection. In infants and small children, use with extreme caution. Excessive use in children or in certain individuals with a previous history of susceptibility to belladonna alkaloids may produce systemic symptoms of atropine poisoning.

Precautions: General: To avoid excessive systemic absorption, the lacrimal sac should be compressed by digital pressure for two to three minutes after instillation. To avoid inducing angle closure glaucoma, an estimation of the depth of the angle of the anterior chamber should be made. Administration of atropine in infants requires great caution.
Information for Patients: Do not touch dropper tip to any surface, as this may contaminate the solution.
Carcinogenesis, mutagenesis, impairment of fertility: No studies have been conducted in animals or in humans to evaluate the potential of these effects.
Pregnancy Category C: Animal reproduction studies have not been performed with atropine. It is also not known whether atropine can cause fetal harm when administered to a pregnant woman or can affect reproduction capacity. Atropine should be given to pregnant women only if clearly needed.
Nursing Mothers: It is not known whether this drug is excreted in human milk. Because many drugs are excreted in human milk, caution should be exercised when atropine is administered to a nursing woman.
Patient Warning: Patient should be advised not to drive or engage in other hazardous activities while pupils are dilated. Patient may experience sensitivity to light and should protect eyes in bright illumination during dilation. Parents should be warned not to get this preparation in their child's mouth and to wash their own hands and the child's hands following administration.
Adverse Reactions: Prolonged use may produce local irritation characterized by follicular conjunctivitis, vascular congestion, edema, exudate, and an eczematoid dermatitis. Severe reactions are manifested by hypotension with progressive respiratory depression. Coma and death have been reported in the very young.
Overdosage: Systemic atropine toxicity is manifested by flushing and dryness of the skin (a rash may be present in children), blurred vision, a rapid and irregular pulse, fever, abdominal distention in infants, mental aberration (hallucinosis) and loss of neuromuscular coordination.
Atropine poisoning, although distressing, is rarely fatal, even with large doses of atropine, and is self-limited if the cause is recognized and the atropine medication is discontinued. In severe intoxication, physostigmine salicylate may be administered parenterally to provide more prompt relief of the intoxication.
Give physostigmine salicylate as 1–5 mL IV of dilution containing 1 mg in 5 mL of saline. The smaller dose is for children, and injection should take not less than two minutes. EKG control is advisable. Dosage can be repeated every five minutes up to a total dose of 2 mg in children and 6 mg in adults every 30 minutes. Physostigmine is contraindicated in hypotensive reactions. Atropine (1 mg) should be available for immediate injection if physostigmine causes bradycardia, convulsions or bronchconstriction.[1] In infants and small children, the body surface must be kept moist.
Dosage and Administration: Adults: For uveitis, administer one or two drops topically to the eye(s) up to four times daily.
Children: For refraction, administer one or two drops of 0.5% solution to each eye twice daily for one to three days prior to examination. For uveitis, administer one or two drops of 0.5% solution to each eye up to three times daily. The lacrimal sac should be compressed by digital pressure for two to three minutes after instillation. Heavily pigmented irides may require larger doses.
How Supplied: In 5mL (1% also available in 15mL) plastic DROP-TAINER® dispenser.
0.5%: 5mL: NDC 0998-0302-05
1%: 5mL: NDC 0998-0303-05
15mL: NDC 0998-0303-15
3%: 5mL: NDC 0998-0305-05
Storage: Store at 46°–80°F.
Caution: Federal (USA) law prohibits dispensing without prescription.
Reference:

1. This treatment regimen for severe atropine toxicoses is from "Handbook of Poisoning," Ninth Edition by Robert Dreisbach, Lange Medical Publications, Los Altos, California, 1977.

ISOPTO® CARBACHOL ℞
(carbachol)
Sterile Ophthalmic Solution

Description: ISOPTO® CARBACHOL is a cholinergic prepared as a sterile topical ophthalmic solution. The active ingredient is represented by the chemical structure: $[NH_2COOCH_2CH_2N(CH_3)_3]^+Cl^-$
Established name: Carbachol
Chemical name: 2-[(Aminocarbonyl) oxy]-*N,N,N*-trimethylethanaminium chloride.
Each mL contains: Active: Carbachol 0.75%, 1.5%, 2.25%, or 3.0%. **Preservative:** Benzalkonium Chloride 0.005%. **Vehicle:** Hydroxypropyl Methylcellulose 1.0%. **Inactive:** Boric Acid, Sodium Chloride, Sodium Borate, Purified Water.
Clinical Pharmacology: A cholinergic (parasympathomimetic) agent. Carbachol has a double action; it not only stimulates the motor endplate of the muscle cell, as do all cholinesters, but it also partially inhibits cholinesterase.
Indications and Usage: For lowering intraocular pressure in the treatment of glaucoma.
Contraindications: Miotics are contraindicated where constriction is undesirable such as acute iritis. Contraindicated in those persons showing hypersensitivity to any component of this preparation.
Warnings: For topical use only. Not for injection. Carbachol should be used with caution in the presence of corneal abrasion to avoid excessive penetration which can produce systemic toxicity and in patients with acute cardiac failure, bronchial asthma, active peptic ulcer, hyperthyroidism, gastrointestinal spasm, urinary tract obstruction, and Parkinson's disease. As with all miotics, retinal detachment has been reported when used in certain susceptible individuals.
Precautions: Information for Patients. Avoid overdosage. The miosis usually causes difficulty in dark adaptation. Patient should be advised to exercise caution in night driving and other hazardous occupations in poor light. Do not touch dropper tip to any surface, as this may contaminate the solution.
Carcinogenesis, Mutagenesis, Impairment of Fertility. There have been no long-term studies done using carbachol in animals to evaluate carcinogenic potential.
Pregnancy. Pregnancy Category C. Animal reproduction studies have not been conducted with carbachol. It is also not known whether carbachol can cause fetal harm when administered to a pregnant woman or can affect reproduction capacity. Carbachol should be given to a pregnant woman only if clearly needed.
Nursing Mothers. It is not known whether this drug is excreted in human milk. Because many drugs are excreted in human milk, caution should be exercised when carbachol is administered to a nursing woman.
Adverse Reactions: Transient symptoms of stinging and burning may occur. This preparation is capable of producing systemic symptoms of a cholinesterase inhibitor even when the epithelium is intact. Transient ciliary and conjunctival injection, headache, and ciliary spasm with resultant temporary decrease of visual acuity may occur. Salivation, syncope, cardiac arrhythmia, gastrointestinal cramping, vomiting, asthma, diarrhea, frequent urge to urinate, increased sweating, and irritation of eyes may occur.
Overdosage: Atropine should be administered parenterally (for dosage refer to Goodman & Gilman or other pharmacology reference).
Dosage and Administration: Instill two drops topically in the eye(s) up to three times daily or as indicated by physician.
How Supplied: 15mL and 30mL in plastic DROP-TAINER® dispensers.
0.075% **ISOPTO CARBACHOL**
15 mL NDC 0998-0221-15
30 mL NDC 0998-0221-30
1.5% **ISOPTO CARBACHOL**
15 mL NDC 0998-0223-15
30 mL NDC 0998-0223-30
2.25% **ISOPTO CARBACHOL**
15 mL NDC 0998-0224-15
3% **ISOPTO CARBACHOL**
15 mL NDC 0998-0225-15
30 mL NDC 0998-0225-30
Storage: Store at 46°–80°F. (8°–27°C).
Caution: Federal (USA) law prohibits dispensing without prescription.

ISOPTO® CARPINE ℞
(pilocarpine hydrochloride)
Sterile Ophthalmic Solution

Description: ISOPTO® CARPINE (Pilocarpine Hydrochloride) is a cholinergic prepared as a sterile topical ophthalmic solution. The active ingredient is represented by the chemical structure:

Established name:
Pilocarpine Hydrochloride

Chemical name:
2(3*H*)-Furanone, 3-ethyldihydro-4-[(1-methyl-1*H*-imidazol-5-yl)-methyl]-, monohydrochloride, (3*S*-*cis*)-.

Each mL contains: Active: Pilocarpine Hydrochloride 0.25%, 0.5%, 1%, 2%, 3%, 4%, 5%, 6%, 8% or 10%. **Preservative:** Benzalkonium Chloride 0.01%. **Vehicle:** 0.5% Hydroxypropyl Methycellulose 2910. **Inactive:** Boric Acid, Sodium Citrate, Sodium Chloride (present in 0.25%, 0.5%, and 1% only); Hydrochloric Acid and/or Sodium Hydroxide (to adjust pH in 1%, 2%, 3%, 4%, 5%, 6%, 8% and 10%); Citric Acid, Hydrochloric Acid and/or Sodium Hydroxide (to adjust pH in 0.25% and 0.5%); Purified Water.
Clinical Pharmacology: Pilocarpine is a direct acting cholinergic parasympathomimetic agent which acts through direct stimulation of muscarinic neuro receptors and smooth muscle such as the iris and secretory glands. Pilocarpine produces miosis through contraction of the iris sphincter, causing increased tension on the scleral spur and opening of the trabecular meshwork spaces to facilitate outflow of aqueous humor. Outflow resistance is thereby reduced, lowering intraocular pressure.
Indications and Usage: Pilocarpine Hydrochloride is a miotic (parasympathomimetic) used to control intraocular pressure. It may be used in combination with other miotics, beta blockers, carbonic anhydrase inhibitors, sympathomimetics, or hyperosmotic agents.
Contraindications: Miotics are contraindicated where constriction is undesirable such as

Continued on next page

Alcon—Cont.

in acute iritis in those persons showing hypersensitivity to any of their components, and in pupillary block glaucoma.

Warnings: For topical use only. NOT FOR INJECTION.

Precautions: **General.** The miosis usually causes difficulty in dark adaptation. Patient should be advised to exercise caution in night driving and other hazardous occupations in poor illumination.

Carcinogenesis, Mutagenesis, Impairment of Fertility: There have been no long-term studies done using pilocarpine in animals to evaluate carcinogenic potential.

Pregnancy: Pregnancy Category C. Animal reproduction studies have not been conducted with pilocarpine. It is also not known whether pilocarpine can cause fetal harm when administered to a pregnant woman or can affect reproduction capacity. Pilocarpine should be given to a pregnant woman only if clearly needed.

Nursing Mothers: It is not known whether this drug is excreted in human milk. Because many drugs are excreted in human milk, caution should be exercised when pilocarpine is administered to a nursing woman.

Information for Patients: Do not touch dropper tip to any surface, as this may contaminate the solution.

Adverse Reactions: Transient symptoms of stinging and burning may occur. Ciliary spasm, conjunctival vascular congestion, temporal or supraorbital headache, and induced myopia may occur. This is especially true in younger individuals who have recently started administration. Reduced visual acuity in poor illumination is frequently experienced by older individuals and individuals with lens opacity. As with all miotics, rare cases of retinal detachment have been reported when used in certain susceptible individuals. Lens opacity may occur with prolonged use of pilocarpine.

Overdosage: Systemic reactions following topical administration are extremely rare.

Dosage and Administration: Two drops topically in the eye(s) up to three or four times daily or as directed by a physician. Under selected conditions, more frequent instillations may be indicated. Individuals with heavily pigmented irides may require higher strengths.

How Supplied: In 15mL and 30mL plastic DROP-TAINER® dispensers.

0.25%—15mL: NDC 0998-0201-15
0.5%—15mL: NDC 0998-0202-15
30mL: NDC 0998-0202-30
1%—15mL: NDC 0998-0203-15
30mL: NDC 0998-0203-30
2%—15mL: NDC 0998-0204-15
30mL: NDC 0998-0204-30
3%—15mL: NDC 0998-0205-15
30mL: NDC 0998-0205-30
4%—15mL: NDC 0998-0206-15
30mL: NDC 0998-0206-30
5%—15mL: NDC 0998-0207-15
6%—15mL: NDC 0998-0208-15
30mL: NDC 0998-0208-30
8%—15mL: NDC 0998-0209-15
10%—15mL: NDC 0998-0211-15

Storage: Store at 46° to 80°F.

Caution: Federal (USA) law prohibits dispensing without prescription.

ISOPTO CETAMIDE® ℞
(sulfacetamide sodium 15%)
Sterile Ophthalmic Solution
and

CETAMIDE™ ℞
(sulfacetamide sodium 10%)
Sterile Ophthalmic Ointment

Description: ISOPTO CETAMIDE® (15% Sulfacetamide Sodium) is a sterile topical ophthalmic antibacterial solution formulated in a viscous vehicle to delay medication washout. CETAMIDE™ (10% Sulfacetamide Sodium) is a sterile topical ophthalmic antibacterial ointment formulated to melt at body temperature. The active ingredient is represented by the chemical structure:

NH_2–C₆H₄–$SO_2N(Na)COCH_3 \cdot H_2O$

Established name:
Sulfacetamide Sodium

Chemical name:
Acetamide, *N*-[(4-aminophenyl) sulfonyl]-, monosodium salt, monohydrate.

Each mL of solution contains: Active: Sulfacetamide Sodium 15%. Preservatives: Methylparaben 0.05%, Propylparaben 0.01%. Vehicle: 0.5% Hydroxypropyl Methylcellulose 2910 (viscosity type, 4000cps). Inactive: Sodium Thiosulfate 0.3%, Dibasic Sodium Phosphate and /or Monobasic Sodium Phosphate (to adjust pH), Purified Water.

Each gram of ointment contains: Active: Sulfacetamide Sodium 10%. Preservatives: Methylparaben 0.05%, Propylparaben 0.01%. Inactive: White Petrolatum, Anhydrous Liquid Lanolin, Mineral Oil.

Clinical Pharmacology: Sulfonamides exert a bacteriostatic effect against a wide range of gram-positive and gram-negative microorganisms by restricting, through competition with para-aminobenzoic acid, the synthesis of folic acid which bacteria require for growth.

Indications and Usage: For the treatment of conjunctivitis, corneal ulcer, and other superficial ocular infections due to susceptible microorganisms, and as an adjunctive in systemic sulfonamide therapy of trachoma.

Contraindications: Hypersensitivity to sulfonamides or to any ingredient of the preparation.

Warnings: For topical eye use only—not for injection. As with all sulfonamide preparations, severe sensitivity reactions, e.g., Stevens-Johnson syndrome, fever, skin rash, G.I. disturbance and bone marrow depression, have been identified in individuals with no prior history of sulfonamide hypersensitivity.

A significant percentage of staphylococcal isolater are completely resistant to sulfa drugs.

Precautions: **General.** The solutions are incompatible with silver preparations. Ophthalmic ointments may retard corneal wound healing. Non-susceptible organisms, including fungi, may proliferate with the use of this preparation. Sulfonamides are inactivated by the para-aminobenzoic acid present in the purulent exudates. Use with caution in patients with severe dry eye. Sensitization may recur when a sulfonamide is readministered irrespective of the route of administration, and cross-sensitivity between different sulfonamides may occur. If signs of sensitivity or other untoward reactions occur, discontinue use of the preparation.

Information for Patients: Do not touch tube or dropper tip to any surface as this may contaminate the contents.

Adverse Reactions: Sulfacetamide sodium may cause local irritation.

Although sensitivity reactions to sulfacetamide sodium are rare, an isolated incident of Stevens-Johnson syndrome was reported in a patient who had experienced a previous bullous drug reaction to an orally administered sulfonamide, and a single instance of local hypersensitivity was reported which progressed to a fatal syndrome resembling systemic lupus erythematous.

The development of secondary infection has occurred after the use of antimicrobials.

Dosage and Administration: SOLUTION: Instill one or two drops into the conjunctival sac(s) every one to two hours initially, increasing time interval as condition responds. OINTMENT: Apply a small amount into the conjunctival sac(s) at night in conjunction with the use of drops during the day, or before an eye is patched. A ribbon one-half to one inch long should be used to insure adequate dosage.

How to apply CETAMIDE™ Ointment:

1. Tilt your head back.
2. Place a finger on your cheek just under your eye and gently pull down until a "V" pocket is formed between your eyeball and your lower lid.
3. Place a small amount (about ½ inch) of CETAMIDE™ ointment in the "V" pocket. Do not let the tip of the tube touch your eye.
4. Look downward before closing your eye.

How Supplied: Solution in 5mL and 15mL plastic DROP-TAINER® dispensers. Ointment in 3.5 g ophthalmic tube.

5mL solution— NDC 0998-0522-05
15mL solution—NDC 0998-0522-15
3.5g ointment— NDC 0065-0526-35

Storage:
Solution—Store at 46°–75°F. Protect from light. Do not use if solution is discolored (dark brown).
Ointment—Store at 46°–80°F.

ISOPTO® CETAPRED® ℞
(sulfacetamide sodium
and prednisolone acetate)
Ophthalmic Suspension

CETAPRED® ℞
(sulfacetamide sodium and
prednisolone acetate)
Ophthalmic Ointment

Description: ISOPTO® CETAPRED® is a sterile topical ophthalmic suspension combining an antibacterial and an adrenocortical steroid. This combination is also supplied in ointment form as CETAPRED® Ointment. The active ingredients are represented by the chemical structures:

NH_2–C₆H₄–$SO_2N(Na)COCH_3 \cdot H_2O$

Established name:
Sulfacetamide Sodium

Chemical name:
Acetamide, *N*-[(4-aminophenyl) sulfonyl]-, monosodium salt, monohydrate.

Chemical formula:
$C_8H_9N_2NaO_3S \cdot H_2O$

[Structure: prednisolone acetate — HO, CH_3, CH_3, OH, C=O, HC–O–C(=O)–CH_3, O]

Established name:
Prednisolone Acetate

Chemical name:
Pregna-1,4-diene-3,20-dione, 21-(acetyloxy)-11,17-dihydroxy-,(11β)-.
Chemical formula:
$C_{23}H_{30}O_6$

Each mL of suspension contains: Active: Sulfacetamide Sodium 10%, Prednisolone Acetate 0.25%. **Preservatives:** Benzalkonium Chloride 0.025%, Methylparaben 0.05%, Propylparaben 0.01%. **Vehicle:** 0.5% Hydroxypropyl Methylcellulose 2910 (viscosity type 4000cps). **Inactive:** Dibasic Sodium Phosphate, Monobasic Sodium Phosphate, Sodium Thiosulfate, Polysorbate 80, Edetate Disodium, Hydrochloric Acid and/or Sodium Hydroxide (to adjust pH), Purified Water.

Each gram of ointment contains: Active: Sulfacetamide Sodium 10%, Prednisolone Acetate 0.25%. **Preservatives:** Methylparaben 0.05%, Propylparaben 0.01%. **Inactive:** White Petrolatum, Anhydrous Liquid Lanolin, Mineral Oil.

Clinical Pharmacology: Corticoids suppress the inflammatory response to a variety of agents, and they probably delay or slow healing. Since corticoids may inhibit the body's defense mechanism against infection, a concomitant antibacterial drug may be used when this inhibition is considered to be clinically significant in a particular case.

The antibacterial component in the combination is included to provide action against specific organisms susceptible to it.

When a decision to administer both a corticoid and an antibacterial is made, the administration of such drugs in combination has the advantage of greater patient compliance and convenience, with the added assurance that the appropriate dosage of both drugs is administered, plus assured compatibility of ingredients when both types of drugs are in the same formulation and, particularly, that the correct volume of drug is delivered and retained.

The relative potency of corticosteroids depends on the molecular structure, concentration, and release from the vehicle.

Indications and Usage: For steroid-responsive inflammatory ocular conditions for which a corticosteroid is indicated and where bacterial infection or a risk of bacterial ocular infection exists.

Ocular steroids are indicated in inflammatory conditions of the palpebral and bulbar conjunctiva, cornea, and anterior segment of the globe where the inherent risk of steroid use in certain infective conjunctivitises is accepted to obtain a diminution in edema and inflammation. They are also indicated in chronic anterior uveitis and corneal injury from chemical, radiation or thermal burns, or penetration of foreign bodies.

The use of a combination drug with an antibacterial component is indicated where the risk of infection is high or where there is an expectation that potentially dangerous numbers of bacteria will be present in the eye.

The particular antibacterial drug in this product is active against the following common bacterial eye pathogens: *Escherichia coli, Staphylococcus aureus, Streptococcus pneumoniae, Streptococcus (viridans* group), *Pseudomonas* species, *Haemophilus influenzae, Klebsiella* species, and *Enterobacter* species.

The product does not provide adequate coverage against: *Neisseria* species and *Serratia marcescens.*

Contraindications: Epithelial herpes simplex keratitis (dendritic keratitis), vaccinia, varicella, and many other viral diseases of the cornea and conjunctiva. Mycobacterial infection of the eye. Fungal diseases of ocular structures. Hypersensitivity to a component of the medication. (Hypersensitivity to the antibacterial component occurs at a higher rate than for the corticosteroid component.)

The use of these combinations is always contraindicated after uncomplicated removal of a corneal foreign body.

Warnings: Prolonged use may result in glaucoma, with damage to the optic nerve, defects in visual acuity and fields of vision, and in posterior subcapsular cataract formation. Prolonged use may suppress the host response and thus increase the hazard of secondary ocular infections. In those diseases causing thinning of the cornea or sclera, perforation has been known to occur with the use of topical steroids. In acute purulent conditions of the eye, steroids may mask infection or enhance existing infection. If these products are used for 10 days or longer, intraocular pressure should be routinely monitored even though it may be difficult in children and uncooperative patients.

Employment of steroid medication in the treatment of herpes simplex requires great caution.

A significant percentage of staphylococcal isolates are completely resistant to sulfa drugs.

As with all sulfonamide preparations, severe sensitivity reactions, e.g., Stevens-Johnson syndrome, fever, skin rash, gastrointestinal disturbance and bone marrow depression have been identified in individuals with no prior history of sulfonamide hypersensitivity.

Precautions: General: The initial prescription and renewal of the medication order beyond 20 mL or 8 g should be made by a physician only after examination of the patient with the aid of magnification, such as slit-lamp biomicroscopy, and, where appropriate, fluorescein staining.

The possibility of fungal infections of the cornea should be considered after prolonged steroid dosing. Use with caution in patients with severe dry eye.

Information for Patients: Do not touch dropper or tube tip to any surface, as this may contaminate the contents.

Adverse Reactions: Adverse reactions have occurred with steroid/antibacterial combination drugs which can be attributed to the steroid component, the antibacterial component, or the combination. Exact incidence figures are not available since no denominator of treated patients is available.

Reactions occurring most often from the presence of the antibacterial ingredient are allergic sensitizations. The reactions due to the steroid component are: elevation of intraocular pressure (IOP) with possible development of glaucoma, and infrequent optic nerve damage; posterior subcapsular cataract formation; and delayed wound healing.

Secondary infection. The development of secondary infection has occurred after use of combinations containing steroids and antibacterials. Fungal infections of the cornea are particularly prone to develop coincidentally with long-term applications of steroid. The possibility of fungal invasion must be considered in any persistent corneal ulceration where steroid treatment has been used. Secondary bacterial ocular infection following suppression of host responses also occurs.

Dosage and Administration:
ISOPTO® CETAPRED® Ophthalmic Suspension: SHAKE WELL BEFORE USING. Two or three drops should be instilled into the conjunctival sac every one to two hours during the day and at bedtime until a favorable response is obtained.

CETAPRED® Ophthalmic Ointment: A thin film should be applied three or four times daily and once at bedtime until a favorable response is obtained. The initial prescription should **not** be more than 20 mL of the Suspension or 8 g of the Ointment and the prescription should not be refilled without further evaluation as outlined in PRECAUTIONS.

Dosage should be adjusted according to the specific needs of the patient.

ISOPTO® CETAPRED® Ophthalmic Suspension or CETAPRED Ointment dosage may be reduced, but care should be taken not to discontinue therapy prematurely. In chronic conditions, withdrawal of treatment should be carried out by gradually decreasing the frequency of application.

How Supplied: Suspension in 5mL and 15mL plastic DROP-TAINER® dispensers. Ointment in 3.5 g ophthalmic tube.
5 mL suspension—NDC 0998-0613-05
15mL suspension—NDC 0998-0613-15
3.5g ointment— NDC 0065-0607-35

Storage: Store CETAPRED® Ointment at 46°–80°F and ISOPTO® CETAPRED® Suspension at 46°–75°F in an upright position.

Caution: Federal (USA) law prohibits dispensing without prescription.

ISOPTO® HOMATROPINE ℞
(homatropine hydrobromide)
Sterile Ophthalmic Solution

Description: ISOPTO® HOMATROPINE (homatropine hydrobromide) is an anticholinergic prepared as a sterile topical ophthalmic solution supplied in two strengths. The active ingredient is represented by the chemical structure:

Established name:
Homatropine Hydrobromide

Chemical name:
Benzeneacetic acid, α-hydroxy-, 8-methyl-8-azabicyclo[3.2.1]-oct-3-yl ester, hydrobromide, *endo*-(±)-.

Each mL contains: Active: Homatropine Hydrobromide 2.0% or 5.0%. Preservatives: Benzalkonium Chloride 0.01% in 2% strength, Benzethonium Chloride 0.005% in 5% strength. Vehicle: Hydroxypropyl Methylcellulose 0.5%. Inactive: Sodium Chloride, Polysorbate 80 (in 2% strength), Sodium Hydroxide and/or Hydrochloric Acid (to adjust pH), Purified Water.

Clinical Pharmacology: This anticholinergic preparation blocks the responses of the sphincter muscle of the iris and the accommodative muscle of the ciliary body to cholinergic stimulation, producing pupillary dilation (mydriasis) and paralysis of accommodation (cycloplegia).

Indications and Usage: A moderately long-acting mydriatic and cycloplegic for cycloplegic refraction and in the treatment of inflammatory conditions of the uveal tract. For pre- and postoperative states when mydriasis is required. Use as an optical aid in some cases of axial lens opacities.

Contraindications: Contraindicated in persons with primary glaucoma or a tendency toward glaucoma, e.g., narrow anterior chamber angle, and in those persons showing hypersensitivity to any component of this preparation.

Warnings: For topical use only—not for injection. In infants and small children, use with extreme caution.

Precautions: General: To avoid excessive systemic absorption, the lacrimal sac should be compressed by digital pressure for two to three minutes after instillation. To avoid inducing angle closure glaucoma, an estimation of the depth of the angle of the anterior chamber should be made. Excessive topical use of this drug can potentially lead to a confusional state

Continued on next page

Alcon—Cont.

characterized by delirium, agitation, and rarely coma. This state is more apt to occur in the pediatric and geriatric age groups. The specific anti-dote for this systemic anticholinergic syndrome is injectable physostigmine salicylate.

Information for Patients. Patient should be advised not to drive or engage in other hazardous activities while pupils are dilated. Patient may experience sensitivity to light and should protect eyes in bright illumination during dilation. Parents should be warned not to get this preparation in their child's mouth and to wash their own hands and the child's hands following administration. Do not touch dropper tip to any surface, as this may contaminate the solution.

Carcinogenesis, Mutagenesis, Impairment of Fertility. There have been no long-term studies done using homatropine hydrobromide in animals to evaluate carcinogenic potential.

Pregnancy. Pregnancy Category C. Animal reproduction studies have not been conducted with homatropine hydrobromide. It is also not known whether homatropine hydrobromide can cause fetal harm when administered to a pregnant woman or can affect reproduction capacity. Homatropine hydrobromide should be given to a pregnant woman only if clearly needed.

Nursing Mothers. It is not known whether this drug is excreted in human milk. Because many drugs are excreted in human milk, caution should be exercised when homatropine hydrobromide is administered to a nursing woman.

Adverse Reactions: Transient symptoms of stinging and burning may occur. Prolonged use may produce local irritation characterized by follicular conjunctivitis, vascular congestion, edema, exudate, and an eczematoid dermatitis.

Dosage and Administration: For refraction, instill one or two drops topically in the eye(s). May be repeated in five to ten minutes if necessary. For uveitis, instill one or two drops topically up to every three to four hours. Individuals with heavily pigmented irides may require larger doses. Only the 2% strength should be used in pediatric patients.

How Supplied: In 5mL and 15mL plastic DROP-TAINER® dispensers.
2% ISOPTO HOMATROPINE
5mL NDC 0998-0311-05
15mL NDC 0998-0311-15
5% ISOPTO HOMATROPINE
5mL NDC 0998-0315-05
15mL NDC 0998-0315-15

Storage: Store at 46° to 75°F.

Caution: Federal (USA) law prohibits dispensing without prescription.

ISOPTO® HYOSCINE ℞
(scopolamine hydrobromide)
Sterile Ophthalmic Solution

Description: ISOPTO® HYOSCINE (scopolamine hydrobromide) is an anticholinergic prepared as a sterile topical ophthalmic solution. The active ingredient is represented by the chemical structure:

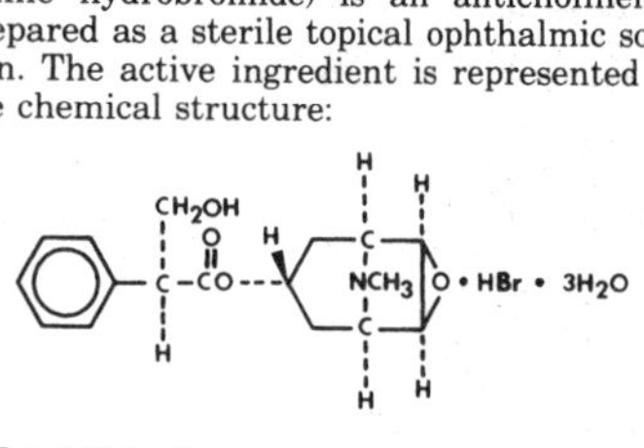

Established name:
Scopolamine Hydrobromide

Chemical name:
Benzeneacetic acid, α-(hydroxymethyl)-, 9-methyl-3-oxa-9-azatricyclo[3.3.1.$0^{2,4}$]non-7-yl ester, hydrobromide, trihydrate, [7(S)-(1α,2β,4β,5α,7β)]-.

Each mL contains: Active: Scopolamine Hydrobromide 0.25%. Preservative: Benzalkonium Chloride 0.01%. Vehicle: Hydroxypropyl Methylcellulose 0.5%. Inactive: Sodium Chloride, Glacial Acetic Acid, Sodium Acetate (to adjust pH), Purified Water.

Clinical Pharmacology: This anticholinergic preparation blocks the responses of the sphincter muscle of the iris and the accommodative muscle of the ciliary body to cholinergic stimulation, producing pupillary dilation (mydriasis) and paralysis of accommodation (cycloplegia).

Indications and Usage: For mydriasis and cycloplegia in diagnostic procedures. For some pre- and postoperative states when a mydriatic and cycloplegic is needed in the treatment of iridocyclitis.

Contraindications: Contraindicated in persons with primary glaucoma or a tendency toward glaucoma, e.g., narrow anterior chamber angle; and in those showing hypersensitivity to any component of this preparation.

Warnings: Do not touch dropper tip to any surface, as this may contaminate the solution. For topical use only—not for injection. In infants and small children, use with extreme caution.

Precautions: To avoid excessive absorption, the lacrimal sac should be compressed by digital pressure for two to three minutes after instillation. To avoid inducing angle closure glaucoma, an estimation of the depth of the angle of the anterior chamber should be made.

Patient Warning: Patient should be advised not to drive or engage in other hazardous activities when drowsy or while pupils are dilated. Patient may experience sensitivity to light and should protect eyes in bright illumination during dilation. Parents should be warned not to get this preparation in their child's mouth and to wash their own hands and the child's hands following administration.

Adverse Reactions: Prolonged use may produce local irritation, characterized by follicular conjunctivitis, vascular congestion, edema, exudate, and an eczematoid dermatitis. Somnolence, dryness of the mouth, or visual hallucinations may occur.

Dosage and Administration: For refraction, administer one or two drops topically in the eye(s) one hour before refracting. For uveitis, administer one or two drops topically in the eye(s) up to four times daily.

How Supplied: In 5 mL and 15mL plastic DROP-TAINER® dispensers.
5mL NDC 0998-0331-05
15mL NDC 0998-0331-15

Storage: Store at 46° to 80°F. Protect from light.

MAXIDEX® ℞
(dexamethasone sodium phosphate)
Sterile Ophthalmic Ointment

Description: MAXIDEX® (dexamethasone sodium phosphate) is an adrenocortical steroid prepared as a sterile ophthalmic ointment. The active ingredient is represented by the chemical structure:

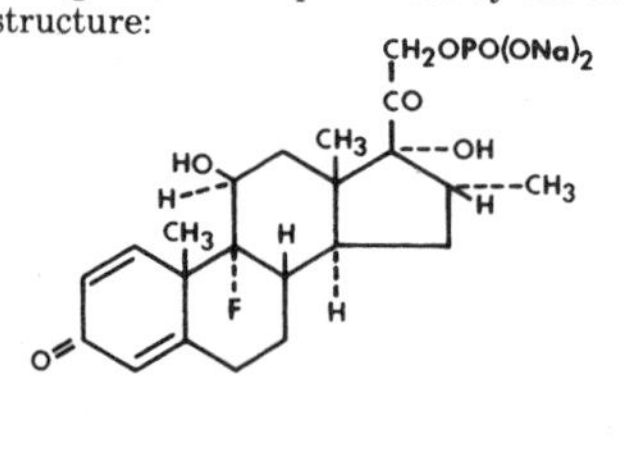

Established name:
Dexamethasone Sodium Phosphate

Chemical name:
Pregn-4-ene-3,20-dione, 9-fluoro-11,17-dihydroxy-16-methyl-21-(phosphonooxy)-, disodium salt, (11β,16α)-.

Each gram contains: **Active:** Dexamethasone Sodium Phosphate equivalent to Dexamethasone Phosphate 0.5mg (0.05%). **Inactive:** Mineral Oil, White Petrolatum.

Clinical Pharmacology: Dexamethasone sodium phosphate suppresses the inflammatory response to a variety of agents and it probably delays or slows healing. No generally accepted explanation of these steroid properties has been advanced.

Indications and Usage: Steroid responsive inflammatory conditions of the palpebral and bulbar conjunctiva, cornea, and anterior segment of the globe. These include allergic conjunctivitis, acne rosacea, superficial punctate keratitis, herpes zoster keratitis, iritis, cyclitis, selected infective conjunctivitises when the inherent hazard of steroid use is accepted to obtain an advisable diminution in edema and inflammation; corneal injury from chemical or thermal burns, or penetration of foreign bodies.

Contraindications: Contraindicated in epithelial herpes simplex keratitis (dendritic keratitis); fungal diseases of ocular structures; acute infectious stages of vaccinia, varicella and many other viral diseases of the cornea and conjunctiva; mycobacterial infection of the eye and in those persons who have shown hypersensitivity to any component of this preparation.

Warnings: Prolonged use may result in ocular hypertension and/or glaucoma, with damage to the optic nerve, defects in visual acuity and fields of vision, and posterior subcapsular cataract formation. Prolonged use may suppress the host response and thus increase the hazard of secondary ocular infections. In those diseases causing thinning of the cornea or sclera, perforations have been known to occur with the use of topical corticosteroids. In acute purulent conditions of the eye, corticosteroids may mask infection or enhance existing infection. If these products are used for 10 days or longer, intraocular pressure should be routinely monitored even though it may be difficult in children and uncooperative patients. Employment of corticosteroid medication in the treatment of herpes simplex other than epithelial herpes simplex keratitis, in which it is contraindicated, requires great caution; periodic slit-lamp microscopy is essential.

Precautions:

General:
The possibility of persistent fungal infections of the cornea should be considered after prolonged corticosteroid dosing.

Information for Patients: Do not touch tube tip to any surface, as this may contaminate the contents.

Carcinogenesis, Mutagenesis, Impairment of Fertility: Long-term animal studies have not been performed to evaluate the carcinogenic potential or the effect on fertility of MAXIDEX® Ointment.

Pregnancy: Pregnancy Category C. Dexamethasone has been shown to be teratogenic in mice and rabbits following topical ophthalmic application in multiples of the therapeutic dose. In the mouse, corticosteroids produce fetal resorptions and a specific abnormality, cleft palate. In the rabbit, corticosteroids have produced fetal resorptions and multiple abnormalities involving the head, ears, limbs, palate, etc. There are no adequate or well-controlled studies in pregnant women. MAXIDEX Ointment should be used during pregnancy only if the potential benefit to the mother justifies the potential risk to the embryo or fetus. Infants born of mothers who have received substantial doses of corticosteroids during pregnancy should be observed carefully for signs of hypoadrenalism.

Nursing Mothers: Topically applied steroids are absorbed systemically. Therefore, because of the potential for serious adverse reactions in nursing infants from dexamethasone sodium phosphate, a decision should be made whether to discontinue nursing or discontinue the drug, taking into account the importance of the drug to the mother.

Pediatric Use: Safety and effectiveness in children have not been establshed.

Adverse Reactions: The following adverse reactions have been reported: glaucoma with optic nerve damage, visual acuity and field defects, posterior subcapsular cataract formation, secondary ocular infections from pathogens including herpes simplex, and perforation of the globe. Rarely, filtering blebs have been reported when topical steroids have been used following cataract surgery. Rarely, stinging or burning may occur.

Dosage and Administration: The duration of treatment will vary with the type of lesion and may extend from a few days to several weeks, according to therapeutic response. Relapses, more common in chronic active lesions than in self-limited conditions, usually respond to treatment.

Apply a one-half to one inch ribbon of ointment into the conjunctival sac(s) up to four times daily. When a favorable response is observed, dosage may be reduced gradually to once a day application for several days. MAXIDEX® Ointment may be used in conjunction with MAXIDEX® Suspension.

How To Apply MAXIDEX® OINTMENT:

1. Tilt your head back.
2. Place a finger on your cheek just under your eye and gently pull down until a "V" pocket is formed between your eyeball and your lower lid.
3. Place a small amount (about ½ inch) of MAXIDEX® in the "V" pocket. Do not let the tip of the tube touch your eye.
4. Look downward before closing your eye.

How Supplied: In 3.5 g ophthalmic tubes. NDC 0065-0616-35

Storage: Store at 8°–27°C (46° to 80°F).

Caution: Federal (USA) law prohibits dispensing without prescription.

MAXIDEX® ℞

(dexamethasone 0.1%)
Sterile Ophthalmic Suspension

Description: MAXIDEX® (dexamethasone 0.1%) is an adrenocortical steroid prepared as a sterile topical ophthalmic suspension. The active ingredient is represented by the chemical structure:

Established name:
Dexamethasone

Chemical name:
Pregna-1,4-diene-3,20-dione,
9-fluoro-11,17,21-trihydroxy-16-
methyl-, (11β,16α)-.

Each mL contains: **Active:** Dexamethasone 0.1%. **Preservative:** Benzalkonium Chloride 0.01%. **Vehicle:** Hydroxypropyl Methylcellulose 0.5%. **Inactive:** Sodium Chloride, Dibasic Sodium Phosphate, Polysorbate 80, Edetate Disodium, Citric Acid and/or Sodium Hydroxide (to adjust pH), Purified Water.

Clinical Pharmacology: Dexamethasone suppresses the inflammatory response to a variety of agents and it probably delays or slows healing. No generally accepted explanation of these steroid properties has been advanced.

Indications and Usage: Steroid responsive inflammatory conditions of the palpebral and bulbar conjunctiva, cornea, and anterior segment of the globe, such as allergic conjunctivitis, acne rosacea, superficial punctate keratitis, herpes zoster keratitis, iritis, cyclitis, selected infective conjunctivitides when the inherent hazard of steroid use is accepted to obtain an advisable dimunition in edema and inflammation; corneal injury from chemical, radiation or thermal burns, or penetration of foreign bodies.

Contraindications: Contraindicated in epithelial herpes simplex (dendritic keratitis), vaccinia, varicella, and most other viral diseases of the cornea and conjunctiva; tuberculosis of the eye; fungal disease of ocular structures; and in those persons who have shown hypersensitivity to any component of this preparation. Steroids should not be used after uncomplicated removal of a corneal foreign body.

Warnings: Prolonged use may result in ocular hypertension and/or glaucoma, with damage to the optic nerve, defects in visual acuity and fields of vision, and posterior subcapsular cataract formation. Prolonged use may suppress the host response and thus increase the hazard of secondary ocular infections. In those diseases causing thinning of the cornea or sclera, perforations have been known to occur with the use of topical corticosteroids. In acute purulent conditions of the eye, corticosteroids may mask infection or enhance existing infection. If these products are used for 10 days or longer, intraocular pressure should be routinely monitored even though it may be difficult in children and uncooperative patients. Employment of corticosteroid medication in the treatment of herpes simplex other than epithelial herpes simplex keratitis, in which it is contraindicated, requires great caution; periodic slit-lamp microscopy is essential.

Precautions: General. The possibility of persistent fungal infections of the cornea should be considered after prolonged corticosteroid dosing.

Information for Patients. Do not touch dropper tip to any surface, as this may contaminate the contents.

Carcinogenesis, Mutagenesis, Impairment of Fertility. Long-term animal studies have not been performed to evaluate the carcinogenic potential or the effect on fertility of MAXIDEX® Suspension.

Pregnancy. Pregnancy Category C. Dexamethasone has been shown to be teratogenic in mice and rabbits following topical ophthalmic application in multiples of the therapeutic dose.

In the mouse, corticosteroids produce fetal resorptions and a specific abnormality, cleft palate. In the rabbit, corticosteroids have produced fetal resorptions and multiple abnormalities involving the head, ears, limbs, palate, etc.

There are no adequate or well-controlled studies in pregnant women. MAXIDEX Suspension should be used during pregnancy only if the potential benefit to the mother justifies the potential risk to the embryo or fetus. Infants born to mothers who have received substantial doses of coerticosteroids during pregnancy should be observed carefully for signs of hypoadrenalism.

Nursing Mothers. Topically applied steroids are absorbed systemically. Therefore, because of the potential for serious adverse reactions in nursing infants from dexamethasone, a decision should be made whether to discontinue nursing or discontinue the drug, taking into account the importance of the drug to the mother.

Pediatric Use. Safety and effectiveness in children have not been established.

Adverse Reactions: Glaucoma with optic nerve damage, visual acuity and field defects; cataract formation; secondary ocular infection following suppression of host response; and perforation of the globe may occur.

Dosage and Administration: SHAKE WELL BEFORE USING. One or two drops topically in the conjunctival sac(s). In severe disease, drops may be used hourly, being tapered to discontinuation as the inflammation subsides. In mild disease, drops may be used up to four to six times daily.

How Supplied: In 5 mL NDC 0998-0615-05 and 15 mL NDC 0998-0615-15 plastic DROP-TAINER® dispensers.

Storage: Store upright at 46° to 80°F.

Caution: Federal (USA) law prohibits dispensing without prescription.

MAXITROL® ℞

(neomycin and polymyxin b sulfates and dexamethasone)
Sterile Ophthalmic
Suspension and Ointment

Description: MAXITROL® (Neomycin and Polymyxin B Sulfates and Dexamethasone) is a multiple dose anti-infective steroid combination in sterile suspension and sterile ointment forms for topical application. The chemical structure for the active ingredient, Dexamethasone, is:

Established name:
Dexamethasone

Chemical name:
Pregna-1,4-diene-3,20-dione,
9-fluoro-11,17,21-trihydroxy-16-
methyl-, (11β,16α)-.

The other active ingredients are Neomycin Sulfate and Polymyxin B Sulfate.

Each mL of suspension contains: Active: Neomycin Sulfate equivalent to Neomycin 3.5 mg, Polymyxin B Sulfate 10,000 units, Dexamethasone 0.1%. Preservative: Benzalkonium Chloride 0.004%. Vehicle: Hydroxypropyl Methylcellulose 2910 0.5%. Inactive: Sodium Chloride, Polysorbate 20, Hydrochloric Acid and/or Sodium Hydroxide (to adjust pH), Purified Water.

Each gram of ointment contains: Active: Neomycin Sulfate equivalent to Neomycin 3.5 mg, Polymyxin B Sulfate 10,000 units, Dexamethasone 0.1%. Preservatives: Methylparaben 0.05%, Propylparaben 0.01%. Inactive: White Petrolatum, Anhydrous Liquid Lanolin.

Clinical Pharmacology: Corticoids suppress the inflammatory response to a variety of agents and they probably delay or slow healing. Since corticoids may inhibit the body's defense mechanism against infection, a concomitant antimicrobial drug may be used when this inhibition is considered to be clinically significant in a particular case.

When a decision to administer both a corticoid and an antimicrobial is made, the administration of such drugs in combination has the advantage of greater patient compliance and con-

Continued on next page

Alcon—Cont.

venience, with the added assurance that the appropriate dosage of both drugs is administered, plus assured compatibility of ingredients when both types of drugs are in the same formulation and, particularly, that the correct volume of drug is delivered and retained.

The relative potency of corticosteroids depends on the molecular structure, concentration and release from the vehicle.

Indications and Usage: For steroid-responsive inflammatory ocular conditions for which a corticosteroid is indicated and where bacterial infection or a risk of bacterial ocular infection exists.

Ocular steroids are indicated in inflammatory conditions of the palpebral and bulbar conjunctiva, cornea, and anterior segment of the globe where the inherent risk of steroid use in certain infective conjunctivitises is accepted to obtain a diminution in edema and inflammation. They are also indicated in chronic anterior uveitis and corneal injury from chemical, radiation or thermal burns; or penetration of foreign bodies.

The use of a combination drug with an anti-infective component is indicated where the risk of infection is high or where there is an expectation that potentially dangerous numbers of bacteria will be present in the eye.

The particular anti-infective drug in this product is active against the following common bacterial eye pathogens: *Staphylococcus aureus, Escherichia coli, Haemophilus influenzae, Klebsiella/Enterobacter* species, *Neisseria* species, and *Pseudomonas aeruginosa.*

This product does not provide adequate coverage against: *Serratia marcescens* and Streptococci, including *Streptococcus pneumoniae.*

Contraindications: Epithelial herpes simplex keratitis (dendritic keratitis), vaccinia, varicella, and many other viral diseases of the cornea and conjunctiva. Mycobacterial infection of the eye. Fungal diseases of ocular structures. Hypersensitivity to a component of the medication. (Hypersensitivity to the antibiotic component occurs at a higher rate than for other components.)

The use of these combinations is always contraindicated after uncomplicated removal of a corneal foreign body.

Warnings: NOT FOR INJECTION. Do not touch dropper or tube tip to any surface, as this may contaminate the contents. Prolonged use may result in glaucoma, with damage to the optic nerve, defects in visual acuity and fields of vision, and posterior subcapsular cataract formation. Prolonged use may suppress the host response and thus increase the hazard of secondary ocular infections. In those diseases causing thinning of the cornea or sclera, perforations have been known to occur with the use of topical steroids. In acute purulent conditions of the eye, steroids may mask infection or enhance existing infection. If these products are used for 10 days or longer, intraocular pressure should be routinely monitored even though it may be difficult in children and uncooperative patients.

Products containing neomycin sulfate may cause cutaneous sensitization.

Employment of steroid medication in the treatment of herpes simplex requires great caution.

Precautions: The initial prescription and renewal of the medication order beyond 20 mL or 8 g should be made by a physician only after examination of the patient with the aid of magnification, such as slit lamp biomicroscopy and, where appropriate, fluorescein staining.

The possibility of persistent fungal infections of the cornea should be considered after prolonged steroid dosing.

Usage in Pregnancy: The safety of intensive or protracted use of topical steroids in pregnancy has not been studied.

Adverse Reactions: Adverse reactions have occurred with steroid/anti-infective combination drugs which can be attributed to the steroid component, the anti-infective component, or the combination. Exact incidence figures are not available since no denominator of treated patients is available.

Reactions occurring most often from the presence of the anti-infective ingredient are allergic sensitizations. The reactions due to the steroid component are: elevation of intraocular pressure (IOP) with possible development of glaucoma, and infrequent optic nerve damage; posterior subcapsular cataract formation; and delayed wound healing.

Secondary Infection: The development of secondary infection has occurred after use of combinations containing steroids and antimicrobials. Fungal infections of the cornea are particularly prone to develop coincidentally with long-term applications of steroid. The possibility of fungal invasion must be considered in any persistent corneal ulceration where steroid treatment has been used.

Secondary bacterial ocular infection following suppression of host responses also occurs.

Dosage and Administration:

MAXITROL ® Suspension: One to two drops topically in the conjunctival sac(s). In severe disease, drops may be used hourly, being tapered to discontinuation as the inflammation subsides. In mild disease, drops may be used up to four to six times daily. *MAXITROL ® Ointment:* Apply a small amount into the conjunctival sac(s) up to three or four times daily, or may be used adjunctively with drops at bedtime.

How to apply MAXITROL Ointment:

1. Tilt your head back.
2. Place a finger on your cheek just under your eye and gently pull down until a "V" pocket is formed between your eyeball and your lower lid.
3. Place a small amount (about ½ inch) of MAXITROL Ointment in the "V" pocket. Do not let the tip of the tube touch your eye.
4. Look downward before closing your eye.

Not more than 20 mL or 8 g should be prescribed initially and the prescription should not be refilled without further evaluation as outlined in PRECAUTIONS above.

How Supplied:

Suspension (**NDC** 0998-0630-06) in 5 mL plastic DROP-TAINER® dispenser.

Ointment (**NDC** 0065-0631-36) in 3.5 g ophthalmic tube.

Storage: Store at 46°–80°F.

MYDFRIN® 2.5% ℞

(phenylephrine hydrochloride Ophthalmic Solution)
Vasoconstrictor and Mydriatic
For Use in Ophthalmology

WARNING: PHYSICIANS SHOULD COMPLETELY FAMILIARIZE THEMSELVES WITH THE COMPLETE CONTENTS OF THIS LEAFLET BEFORE PRESCRIBING PHENYLEPHRINE HYDROCHLORIDE.

Description: MYDFRIN® 2.5% is a sterile topical ophthalmic solution. The active ingredient is represented by the chemical structure:

Established name:
Phenylephrine Hydrochloride

Chemical name:
Benzenemethanol, 3-hydroxy-α-[(methylamino)methyl]-, hydrochloride (*R*)-.

Each mL contains: Active: Penylephrine HCl 2.5%. **Preservative:** Benzalkonium Chloride 0.01%. **Inactive:** Boric Acid, Sodium Bisulfite, Edetate Disodium, Sodium Hydroxide and/or Hydrochloric Acid (to adjust pH), Purified Water.

Clinical Pharmacology: MYDFRIN 2.5% Ophthalmic Solution is an alpha receptor sympathetic agonist used in local ocular disorders because of its vasoconstrictor and mydriatic action. It exhibits rapid and moderately prolonged action, and it produces little rebound vasodilation. Systemic side effects are uncommon.

Indications and Usage: MYDFRIN 2.5% Ophthalmic Solution is recommended as a vasoconstrictor, decongestant, and mydriatic in a variety of ophthalmic conditions and procedures. Some of its uses are for pupillary dilation in uveitis (to prevent or aid in the disruption of posterior synechiae formation), for many ophthalmic surgical procedures and for refraction without cycloplegia. MYDFRIN 2.5% Ophthalmic Solution may also be used for funduscopy and other diagnostic procedures.

Contraindications: Ophthalmic solutions of phenylephrine HCl are contraindicated in patients with anatomically narrow angles or narrow angle glaucoma. Phenylephrine HCl may be contraindicated in low birth weight infants and in some elderly adults with severe arteriosclerotic cardiovascular or cerebrovascular disease. Phenylephrine HCl may be contraindicated during intraocular operative procedures when the corneal epithelial barrier has been disturbed. This preparation is also contraindicated in persons with a known sensitivity to phenylephrine HCl or any of its components.

Warnings: Not for intraocular use. As with other adrenergic drugs, when MYDFRIN 2.5% Ophthalmic Solution is administered simultaneously with, or up to 21 days after, administration of monoamine oxidase (MAO) inhibitors, careful supervision and adjustment of dosages are required since exaggerated adrenergic effects may result. The pressor response of adrenergic agents may also be potentiated by tricyclic antidepressants.

Systemic side effects are more common in patients taking beta adrenergic blocking agents such as propanolol. Concomitant use of phenylephrine and atropine may enhance the pressor effects and induce tachycardia in some patients, especially infants.[1] Contains sodium bisulfite, a sulfite that may cause allergic-type reactions including anaphylactic symptoms and life-threatening or less severe asthmatic episodes in certain susceptible people. The overall prevalence of sulfite sensitivity in the general population is unknown and probably low. Sulfite sensitivity is seen more frequently in asthmatic than in nonasthmatic people.

Precautions: Ordinarily, any mydriatic, including phenylephrine HCl, is contraindicated in patients with glaucoma, since it may occasionally raise intraocular pressure. However, when temporary dilation of the pupil may free adhesions, this advantage may temporarily outweigh the danger from coincident dilation of the pupil. Rebound miosis has been reported in older persons one day after receiving phenylephrine HCl ophthalmic solutions, and reinstillation of the drug may produce less mydriasis than previously. This may be of clinical importance in dilating the pupils of older subjects prior to retinal detachment or cataract surgery.

The lacrimal sac should be compressed by digital pressure for two to three minutes after instillation to avoid excessive systemic absorption.

Due to a strong action of the drug on the dilator muscle, older individuals may also develop transient pigment floaters in the aqueous humor 40 to 45 minutes following the administration of phenylephrine HCl ophthalmic solution. The appearance may be similar to anterior uveitis or to a microscopic hyphema.

To prevent pain, a drop of suitable topical anesthetic may be applied before using MYDFRIN 2.5% Ophthalmic Solution. Prolonged exposure to air or strong light may cause oxidation and discoloration. Do not use if solution is brown or contains a precipitate.

Monitor blood pressure in geriatric patients with known cardiac disease. Use caution in infants with known cardiac anomalies. Exceeding recommended dosages or applying MYDFRIN® 2.5% Ophthalmic Solution to the instrumented, traumatized, diseased or postsurgical eye or adnexa, or to patients with suppressed lacrimation, as during anesthesia, may result in the absorption of sufficient quantities of phenylephrine to produce a systemic vasopressor response.

Information for Patients: Do not touch dropper tip to any surface, as this may contaminate the solution.

Carcinogenesis, Mutagenesis, Impairment of Fertility: There have been no long-term studies done using phenylephrine HCl in animals to evaluate carcinogenic potential.

Pregnancy: Pregnancy Category C. Animal reproduction studies have not been conducted with phenylephrine HCl. It is also not known whether phenylephrine HCl can cause fetal harm when administered to a pregnant woman or can affect reproduction capacity. MYDFRIN Ophthalmic Solution should be given to a pregnant woman only if clearly needed.

Nursing Mothers: It is not known whether these drugs are excreted in human milk. Because many drugs are excreted in human milk, caution should be exercised when MYDFRIN Ophthalmic Solution is administered to a nursing woman.

Adverse Reactions: A marked increase in blood pressure has been reported in low-weight premature neonates, infants and adult patients with idiopathic orthostatic hypotension. Cardiovascular reactions which have occurred primarily in elderly patients include marked increase in blood pressure, syncope, myocardial infarction, tachycardia, arrythmia, and fatal subarachnoid hemorrhage.[2]

Dosage and Administration:

Vasoconstriction and Pupil Dilation:
MYDFRIN 2.5% Ophthalmic Solution is especially useful when rapid and powerful dilation of the pupil without cycloplegia and reduction of congestion in the capillary bed are desired. A drop of a suitable topical anesthetic may be applied, followed in a few minutes by 1 drop of MYDFRIN 2.5% Ophthalmic Solution on the upper limbus. The anesthetic prevents stinging and consequent dilution of the solution by lacrimation. It may occasionally be necessary to repeat the instillation after one hour, again preceded by the use of the topical anesthetic.

Uveitis: Posterior Synechiae: MYDFRIN 2.5% Ophthalmic Solution may be used in patients with uveitis when synechiae are present or may develop. The formation of synechiae may be prevented by the use of this solution and atropine or other cycloplegics to produce wide dilation of the pupil. For recently formed posterior synechiae one drop of MYDFRIN 2.5% Ophthalmic Solution may be applied to the upper surface of the cornea and be repeated as necessary, not to exceed three times. Treatment may be continued the following day, if necessary. Atropine sulfate and the application of hot compresses should also be used if indicated.

Glaucoma: MYDFRIN 2.5% Ophthalmic Solution may be used with miotics in patients with open angle glaucoma. It reduces the difficulties experienced by the patient because of the small field produced by miosis, and still it permits and often supports the effect of the miotic in lowering the intraocular pressure in open angle glaucoma. Hence, there may be marked improvement in visual acuity after using MYDFRIN 2.5% Ophthalmic Solution in conjunction with miotic drugs.

Surgery: When a short-acting mydriatic is needed for wide dilation of the pupil before intraocular surgery, MYDFRIN 2.5% Ophthalmic Solution may be applied topically from 30 to 60 minutes before the operation.

Refraction: MYDFRIN 2.5% Ophthalmic Solution may be used effectively to increase mydriasis with homatropine hydrobromide, cyclopentolate hydrochloride, tropicamide hydrochloride and atropine sulfate.

FOR ADULTS:

One drop of the preferred cycloplegic is placed in each eye, followed in 5 minutes by one drop of MYDFRIN 2.5% Ophthalmic Solution.

Since adequate cycloplegia is achieved at different time intervals after the instillation of the necessary number of drops, different cycloplegics will require different waiting periods to achieve adequate cycloplegia.

FOR CHILDREN:

For a "one application method,"MYDFRIN 2.5% Ophthalmic Solution may be combined with one of the preferred rapid acting cycloplegics to produce adequate cycloplegia.

Ophthalmoscopic Examination: One drop of MYDFRIN 2.5% Ophthalmic Solution is placed in each eye. Sufficient mydriasis to permit examination is produced in 15 to 30 minutes. Dilation lasts from one to three hours.

Diagnostic Procedures: Provocative Test for Angle Closure Glaucoma: MYDFRIN 2.5% Ophthalmic Solution may be used cautiously as a provocative test when interval narrow angle closure glaucoma is suspected. Intraocular tension and gonioscopy are performed prior to and after dilation of the pupil with phenylephrine HCl. A "significant" intraocular pressure (IOP) rise combined with gonioscopic evidence of angle closure indicates an anterior segment anatomy capable of angle closure. A negative test does not rule this out. This pharmacologically induced angle closure glaucoma may not simulate real life conditions and other causes for transient elevations of IOP should be excluded.

Retinoscopy (Shadow Test): When dilation of the pupil without cycloplegic action is desired for retinoscopy, MYDFRIN 2.5% Ophthalmic Solution may be used.

NOTE: Heavily pigmented irides may require larger doses in all of the above procedures.

Blanching Test: One or two drops of MYDFRIN 2.5% Ophthalmic Solution should be applied to the injected eye. After five minutes, examine for perilimbal blanching. If blanching occurs, the congestion is superficial and probably does not indicate iridocyclitis.

How Supplied: MYDFRIN 2.5% Ophthalmic Solution in plastic DROP-TAINER® dispensers:

3 mL: NDC 0065-0342-03
5 mL: NDC 0998-0342-05

Storage: Store at 36° to 80°F. Protect from light and excessive heat.

References:

1. Fraunfelder, F. T., and Meyer, S. M.: Possible Cardiovascular Effects Secondary to Topical Ophthalmic 2.5% Phenylephrine, *Am. J. Oph.* 99:3:362, 1985.
2. Ibid.

Caution: Federal (USA) law prohibits dispensing without prescription.

MYDRIACYL® ℞

(tropicamide)
Sterile Ophthalmic Solution

Description: MYDRIACYL® (Tropicamide) is an anticholinergic prepared as a sterile topical ophthalmic solution in two strengths. The active ingredient is represented by the chemical structure:

Established name:
Tropicamide

Chemical name:
Benzeneacetamide, *N*-ethyl-α-(hydroxymethyl)-*N*-(4-pyridinylmethyl)-.

Each mL contains: **Active:** Tropicamide 0.5% or 1.0%. **Preservative:** Benzalkonium Chloride 0.01%. **Inactive:** Sodium Chloride, Edetate Disodium, Hydrochloric Acid and/or Sodium Hydroxide (to adjust pH), Purified Water.

Clinical Pharmacology: This anticholinergic preparation blocks the responses of the sphincter muscle of the iris and the ciliary muscle to cholinergic stimulation, dilating the pupil (mydriasis). The stronger preparation (1.0%) also paralyzes accommodation. This preparation acts rapidly and the duration of activity is relatively short. The weaker strength may be useful in producing mydriasis with only slight cycloplegia.

Indications and Usage: For mydriasis and cycloplegia for diagnostic procedures.

Contraindications: Contraindicated in persons with primary glaucoma or a tendency toward glaucoma (e.g. narrow anterior chamber angle) and in persons showing hypersensitivity to any component of this preparation.

Warnings: For topical use only—not for injection. Reproductive studies have not been performed in animals. There is not adequate information on whether this drug may affect fertility in human males or females or have a teratogenic potential or other adverse effect on the fetus. This preparation may cause CNS disturbances which may be dangerous in infants and children. Possibility of occurrence of psychotic reaction and behavioral disturbance due to hypersensitivity to anticholinergic drugs should be borne in mind.

Precautions: In the elderly and others where increased intraocular pressure may be encountered, mydriatics and cycloplegics should be used cautiously. To avoid inducing angle closure glaucoma, an estimation of the depth of the angle of the anterior chamber should be made. The lacrimal sac should be compressed by digital pressure for two to three minutes after instillation to avoid excessive systemic absorption.

Patient Warning: Do not touch dropper tip to any surface, as this may contaminate the solution. Patient should be advised not to drive or engage in other hazardous activities while pupils are dilated. Patient may experience sensitivity to light and should protect eyes in bright illumination during dilation. Parents should be warned not to get this preparation in their child's mouth and to wash their own hands and the child's hands following administration.

Adverse Reactions: Increased intraocular pressure. Psychotic reactions, behavioral disturbances, and cardiorespiratory collapse in children and some adults with this class of drugs have been reported. Transient stinging, dryness of the mouth, blurred vision, photophobia with or without corneal staining, tachycardia, headache, parasympathetic stimulation, or allergic reaction may occur.

Continued on next page

Alcon—Cont.

Dosage and Administration: For refraction, one or two drops of 1.0% solution in the eye(s), repeated in five minutes. If patient is not seen within 20 to 30 minutes, an additional drop may be instilled to prolong mydriatic effect. For examination of fundus, one or two drops of 0.5% solution 15 or 20 minutes prior to examination. Individuals with heavily pigmented irides may require larger doses.
How Supplied: 0.5% and 1.0% in 15 mL plastic DROP-TAINER® dispensers.
0.5% NDC 0998-0354-15
1.0% NDC 0998-0355-15
1.0% in 3 mL plastic DROP-TAINER® dispensers.
1.0% NDC 0065-0355-03
Storage: Store at 46° to 80° F. Do not refrigerate or store at high temperatures. Keep container tightly closed.
Caution: Federal (USA) law prohibits dispensing without prescription.

NAPHCON® OTC
(Naphazoline Hydrochloride Ophthalmic Solution)
Redness Reliever Eye Drops
Sterile

Ingredients: Each mL contains: **Active:** Naphazoline Hydrochloride 0.012%. **Preservative:** Benzalkonium Chloride 0.01%. **Inactives:** Boric Acid, Sodium Chloride, Potassium Chloride, Edetate Disodium, Sodium Carbonate and/or Hydrochloric Acid (to adjust pH), Purified Water.
Indications:

> FDA APPROVED USE
> Relieves redness of the eye due to minor eye irritations.

For topical eye use only.
Warnings: If you experience eye pain, changes in vision, continued redness or irritation of the eye, or if the condition worsens or persists for more than 72 hours, discontinue use and consult a doctor. If you have glaucoma, do not use this product except under the advice and supervision of a doctor. Overuse of this product may produce increased redness of the eye. If solution changes color or becomes cloudy, do not use.
To avoid contamination, do not touch tip of container to any surface. Replace cap after using. Keep this and all drugs out of the reach of children. In case of accidental ingestion, seek professional assistance or contact a Poison Control Center immediately.
Directions: Instill 1 to 2 drops in the affected eye(s) up to four times daily.
How Supplied: In 15 mL DROP-TAINER® dispenser. NDC 0998-0078-15
Storage: Store at room temperature.

NAPHCON® FORTE ℞
brand of Naphazoline Hydrochloride Ophthalmic Solution, USP

Description: NAPHCON® FORTE brand of Naphazoline Hydrochloride Ophthalmic Solution, USP is a sterile preparation. Naphazoline HCl, an ocular vasoconstrictor, is an imidazoline derivative sympathomimetic amine. It occurs as a white, odorless crystalline powder having a bitter taste and is freely soluble in water and in alcohol. The active ingredient is represented by the structural formula:
[See chemical formula at top of next column.]

Chemical name:
2-(1-naphthylmethyl)-2-imidazoline monohydrochloride

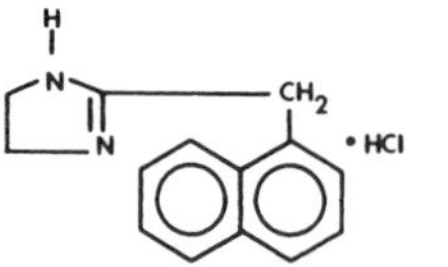

$C_{14}H_{14}N_2HCl$

Each mL contains: Active: Naphazoline Hydrochloride 0.1%. Preservative: Benzalkonium Chloride 0.01%. Inactive: Boric Acid, Sodium Chloride, Potassium Chloride, Edetate Disodium, Sodium Carbonate and/or Hydrochloric Acid (to adjust pH), Purified Water. It has a pH of 5.5 to 7.0.
Clinical Pharmacology: Naphazoline constricts the vascular system of the conjunctiva. It is presumed that this effect is due to direct stimulation action of the drug upon the alpha adrenergic receptors in the arterioles of the conjunctiva resulting in decreased conjunctival congestion. Naphazoline belongs to the imidazoline class of sympathomimetics.
Indications and Usage: NAPHCON® FORTE brand of Naphazoline Hydrochloride Ophthalmic Solution is indicated for use as a topical ocular vasoconstrictor.
Contraindications: Contraindicated in the presence of an anatomically narrow angle or in narrow angle glaucoma or in persons who have shown hypersensitivity to any component of this preparation.
Warnings: Patients under therapy with MAO inhibitors may experience a severe hypertensive crisis if given a sympathomimetic drug. Use in children, especially infants may result in CNS depression leading to coma and marked reduction in body temperature.
Precautions:
General: For topical ophthalmic use only. Use with caution in the presence of hypertension, cardiovascular abnormalities, hyperglycemia (diabetes), hyperthyroidism, infection or injury.
Patient Information: Patients should be advised to discontinue the drug and consult a physician if relief is not obtained within 48 hours of therapy; if irritation, blurring or redness persists, or increases; or if symptoms of systemic absorption occur, i.e., dizziness, headache, nausea, decrease in body temperature, or drowsiness.
To prevent contaminating the dropper tip and solution, do not touch the eyelids or the surrounding area with the dropper tip of the bottle. If solution changes color or becomes cloudy, do not use.
Drug Interactions: Concurrent use of maprotiline or tricyclic antidepressants and naphazoline may potentiate the pressor effect of naphazoline. Patients under therapy with MAO inhibitors may experience a severe hypertensive crisis if given a sympathomimetic drug. (See WARNINGS).
Pregnancy Category C: Animal reproduction studies have not been conducted with naphazoline. It is also not known whether naphazoline can cause fetal harm when administered to a pregnant woman or can affect reproduction capacity. Naphazoline should be given to a pregnant woman only if clearly needed.
Nursing Mothers: It is not known whether naphazoline is excreted in human milk. Because many drugs are excreted in human milk, caution should be exercised when naphazoline is administered to a nursing woman.
Pediatric Use: Safety and effectiveness in children have not been established. See "WARNINGS" and "CONTRAINDICATIONS."
Adverse Reactions:
Ocular: Mydriasis, increased redness, irritation, discomfort, blurring, punctate keratitis, lacrimation, increased intraocular pressure.
Systemic: Dizziness, headache, nausea sweating, nervousness, drowsiness, weakness hypertension, cardiac irregularities, and hyperglycemia.
Dosage and Administration: Instill one or two drops in the conjunctival sac(s) every three to four hours as needed.
How Supplied: In 15 mL DROP-TAINER® dispenser.
NDC 0998-0079-15.
Storage: Store at 46°–80°F.

NAPHCON–A® ℞
(naphazoline hydrochloride and pheniramine maleate)
Sterile Ophthalmic Solution

Description: NAPHCON–A® (naphazoline hydrochloride, pheniramine maleate) is a combination of an antihistamine and a decongestant prepared as a sterile topical ophthalmic solution. The active ingredients are represented by the chemical structures:

Established name:
Naphazoline Hydrochloride

Chemical Name:
1*H*-Imidazole, 4,5-dihydro-2-(1-naphthalenylmethyl)-, monohydrochloride.

Established name:
Pheniramine Maleate

Chemical name:
N,N-Dimethyl-γ-phenyl-2-pyridine-propanamine, (*Z*)-Butenedioic acid.

Each mL contains: Active: Naphazoline Hydrochloride 0.025%, Pheniramine Maleate 0.3%. Preservative: Benzalkonium Chloride 0.01%. Inactive: Boric Acid, Sodium Borate, Edetate Disodium, Sodium Chloride, Sodium Hydroxide and/or Hydrochloric Acid (to adjust pH), and Purified Water.
Clinical Pharmacology: NAPHCON–A® combines the effects of the antihistamine, pheniramine maleate, and the decongestant, naphazoline.

> **Indications and Usage:** Based on a review of a related combination of drugs by the National Academy of Sciences—National Research Council and/or other information, FDA has classified the indications as follows: "Possibly" effective: For relief of ocular irritation and/or congestion or for the treatment of allergic or inflammatory ocular conditions. Final classification of the less-than-effective indication requires further investigation.

Contraindications: Hypersensitivity to one or more of the components of this preparation. Do not use in the presence of narrow angle glaucoma or in patients predisposed to narrow angle glaucoma.
Warnings: Patients under MAO inhibitors may experience a severe hypertensive crisis if given a sympathomimetic drug such as Naphazoline HCl. Use in infants and children may result in CNS depression leading to coma and marked reduction in body temperature.

Precautions: General: For topical eye use only—not for injection. This preparation should be used with caution in patients with severe cardiovascular disease including cardiac arrhythmias, patients with poorly controlled hypertension, patients with diabetes, especially those with a tendency toward diabetic ketoacidosis.

Information for Patients: To prevent contaminating the dropper tip and solution, care should be taken not to touch the eyelids or surrounding area with the dropper tip of the bottle.

Carcinogenesis, Mutagenesis, Impairment of Fertility: There have been no long-term studies done using naphazoline hydrochloride and/or pheniramine maleate in animals to evaluate carcinogenic potential.

Pregnancy: Pregnancy Category C. Animal reproduction studies have not been conducted with naphazoline hydrochloride and/or pheniramine maleate. It is also not known whether naphazoline hydrochloride and/or pheniramine maleate can cause fetal harm when administered to a pregnant woman or can affect reproduction capacity. NAPHCON-A® Ophthalmic Solution should be given to a pregnant woman only if clearly needed.

Nursing Mothers: It is not known whether these drugs are excreted in human milk. Because many drugs are excreted in human milk, caution should be exercised when NAPHCON-A Ophthalmic Solution is administered to a nursing woman.

Adverse Reactions: The following adverse reactions may occur: Pupillary dilation, increase in intraocular pressure, systemic effects due to absorption (i.e., hypertension, cardiac irregularities, hyperglycemia). Drowsiness may be experienced by some patients.

Dosage and Administration: One or two drops instilled in each eye every 3 to 4 hours or less frequently, as required to relieve symptoms.

How Supplied: In 15 mL plastic DROP-TAINER® Dispenser.
NDC 0998-0080-15.

Storage: Store at 36° to 80°F. Keep bottle tightly closed when not in use. Protect from light and excessive heat.

Caution: Federal (USA) law prohibits dispensing without prescription.

NATACYN® ℞
(natamycin 5%)
Ophthalmic Suspension

Description: Natamycin 5% Ophthalmic Suspension is a sterile, anti-fungal drug for topical ophthalmic administration. The active ingredient is represented by the chemical structure:

Established name:
Natamycin

Chemical name:
Stereoisomer of 22-[(3-amino-3,6-dideoxy-β-D-mannopyranosyl)oxy]-1,3,26-trihydroxy-12-methyl-10-oxo-6,11,28-trioxatricyclo[22.3.1.$0^{5,7}$]octacosa-8,14,16,18,20-pentaene-25-carboxylic acid.
Other: pimaricin

Each mL of the suspension contains: Active: Natamycin 5% (50 mg). Preservative: Benzalkonium Chloride 0.02%. Inactive: Sodium Hydroxide and/or Hydrochloric Acid (neutralized to adjust the pH); Purified Water.

Clinical Pharmacology: Natamycin is a tetraene polyene antibiotic derived from *Streptomyces natalensis*. It possesses *in vitro* activity against a variety of yeast and filamentous fungi, including *Candida, Aspergillus, Cephalosporium, Fusarium,* and *Penicillium.* The mechanism of action appears to be through binding of the molecule to the sterol moiety of the fungal cell membrane. The polyenesterol complex alters the permeability of the membrane to produce depletion of essential cellular constituents. Although the activity against fungi is dose-related, natamycin is predominantly fungicidal.‡ Natamycin is not effective *in vitro* against gram-positive or gram-negative bacteria. Topical administration appears to produce effective concentrations of natamycin within the corneal stroma, but not in intraocular fluid. Systemic absorption should not be expected following topical administration of Natamycin 5% Ophthalmic Suspension. As with other polyene antibiotics, absorption from the gastrointestinal tract is very poor. Studies in rabbits receiving topical natamycin revealed no measurable compound in the aqueous humor or sera but the sensitivity of the measurement was no greater than 2 mg/mL.

Indications and Usage: Natamycin 5% Ophthalmic Suspension is indicated for treatment of fungal blepharitis, conjunctivitis, and keratitis caused by susceptible organisms. Natamycin has proven to be the initial drug of choice in *Fusarium solani* keratitis. As in other forms of suppurative keratitis, initial and sustained therapy of fungal keratitis should be determined by the clinical diagnosis, laboratory diagnosis by smear and culture of corneal scrapings, and drug response. Whenever possible, the *in vitro* activity of natamycin against the responsible fungus should be determined. The effectiveness of natamycin as a single agent in fungal endophthalmitis has not been established.

Contraindication: Natamycin 5% Ophthalmic Suspension is contraindicated in individuals with a history of hypersensitivity to any of its components.

Precautions: General. For topical eye use only—NOT FOR INJECTION. Failure of improvement of keratitis following 7–10 days of administration of the drug suggests that the infection may be caused by a microorganism not susceptible to natamycin. Continuation of therapy should be based on clinical re-evaluation and additional laboratory studies.
Adherence of the suspension to areas of epithelial ulceration or retention of the suspension in the fornices occurs regularly. There has only been a limited number of cases in which natamycin has been used; therefore, it is possible that adverse reactions of which we have no knowledge at present may occur. For this reason, patients on this drug should be monitored at least twice weekly. Should suspicion of drug toxicity occur, the drug should be discontinued.

Information for Patients: Do not touch dropper tip to any surface, as this may contaminate the suspension.

Usage in Pregnancy: The safety of Natamycin 5% Ophthalmic Suspension in pregnancy has not been evaluated; therefore, caution should be used during administration in such situations.

Adverse Reactions: One case of conjunctival chemosis and hyperemia, thought to be allergic in nature, has been reported.

Dosage and Administration: SHAKE WELL BEFORE USING. The preferred initial dosage in fungal keratitis is one drop of Natamycin 5% Ophthalmic Suspension instilled in the conjunctival sac at hourly or two-hourly intervals. The frequency of application can usually be reduced to one drop 6 to 8 times daily after the first 3 to 4 days. Therapy should generally be continued for 14 to 21 days or until there is resolution of active fungal keratitis. In many cases, it may be helpful to reduce the dosage gradually at 4 to 7 day intervals to assure that the replicating organism has been eliminated. Less frequent initial dosage (4 to 6 daily applications) may be sufficient in fungal blepharitis and conjunctivitis.

How Supplied: 15 mL in glass bottles with sterile dropper assembly. **NDC 0065-0645-15.**

Storage: May be stored in refrigerator (36–46° F) or at room temperature (46–75° F). *Do not freeze.* Avoid exposure to light and excessive heat.

‡ Laupen, J. O.; McLellan, W. L.; El Nakeeb, M.A.; "Antibiotics and Fungal Physiology," Antimicrobial Agents and Chemotherapy, 1965:1006, 1965.

References:

1. Barckhausen, B.: Die Behandlung der Probleminfektionen das vorderen Augenabschnittes in der Praxis. Landarzt 46:842, 1970.
2. Cuendet, J. F.; Nouri, A.: Traitement local en ophthalmologie par un nouvel antibiotique fungicide, la "pimaricine". Ophthalmologica 145:297, 1963.
3. Forster, R. K.; Rebell, G.: "The Diagnosis and Management of Keratomycoses". Arch. Ophth. 93:1134, 1975.
4. Francois, J.; de Vos, E.: Traitement des mycoses oculaires par la pimaricine. Bull. Soc. beige Ophthal. 131:382, 1962.
5. Jones, D. B.; Sexton, R.; Rebell, G.: "Mycotic keratitis in South Florida: A Review of Thirty-nine Cases". Transactions ophthal. Soc. U. K. 89:781, 1969.
6. Jones, D. B.; Forster, R. K.; Rebell, G.: "*Fusarium solani* keratitis treated with Natamycin (pimaricin), 18 consecutive cases". Arch. Ophth. 88:147, 1972.
7. L'Editeur: Traitement des mycoses oculaires. Presse med. 77:147, 1969.
8. Vozza, R.; Bagolini, B.: Su di un caso di grave ulcerazione bilaterale delle palpebra de Candida albicans. Bol. Oculist. 43:433, 1964.

Caution: Federal (USA) Law prohibits dispensing without prescription.
Manufactured under License from Gist-Brocades, N.V., Delft, Holland

---

PILOPINE HS® Gel ℞
(pilocarpine hydrochloride) 4%
Sterile Ophthalmic Gel

Description: PILOPINE HS® (Pilocarpine Hydrochloride) 4% Gel is a sterile topical ophthalmic aqueous gel which contains more than 90% water and employs CARBOPOL 940, a synthetic high molecular weight crosslinked polymer of acrylic acid to impart a high viscosity. The active ingredient, Pilocarpine Hydrochloride, is a cholinergic and is represented by the chemical structure:

Established name:
Pilocarpine Hydrochloride
Chemical name:
2(3*H*)-Furanone, 3-ethyldihydro-4-[(1-methyl-1*H*-imidazol-5-yl)-methyl]-, monohydrochloride, (3S-*cis*)-.

Continued on next page

Alcon—Cont.

PILOPINE HS Gel—Each Gram Contains: **Active:** Pilocarpine Hydrochloride 4% (40 mg). **Preservative:** Benzalkonium Chloride 0.008%. **Inactive:** Carbopol 940, Edetate Disodium, Hydrochloric Acid and/or Sodium Hydroxide (to adjust pH) and Purified Water.

Clinical Pharmacology: Pilocarpine is a direct acting cholinergic parasympathomimetic agent which acts through direct stimulation of muscarinic neuro receptors and smooth muscle such as the iris and secretory glands. Pilocarpine produces miosis through contraction of the iris sphincter causing increased tension on the scleral spur and opening of the trabecular meshwork spaces to facilitate outflow of aqueous humor. Outflow resistance is thereby reduced, lowering intraocular pressure.

Indications and Usage: Pilocarpine Hydrochloride is a miotic (parasympathomimetic) used to control intraocular pressure. It may be used in combination with other miotics, beta blockers, carbonic anhydrase inhibitors, sympathomimetics or hyperosmotic agents.

Contraindications: Miotics are contraindicated where constriction is undesirable, such as in acute iritis, and in those persons showing hypersensitivity to any of their components.

Warnings: For topical use only.

Precautions: General. The miosis usually causes difficulty in dark adaptation. Patient should be advised to exercise caution in night driving and other hazardous occupations in poor illumination.

Information For Patients. Do not touch tube tip to any surface, as this may contaminate the gel.

Carcinogenesis, Mutagenesis, Impairment of Fertility. There have been no long-term studies done using Pilocarpine Hydrochloride in animals to evaluate carcinogenic potential.

Pregnancy. Pregnancy Category C. Animal reproduction studies have not been conducted with Pilocarpine Hydrochloride. It is also not known whether Pilocarpine Hydrochloride can cause fetal harm when administered to a pregnant woman or can affect reproduction capacity. PILOPINE HS Gel should be given to a pregnant woman only if clearly needed.

Nursing Mothers. It is not known whether this drug is excreted in human milk. Because many drugs are excreted in human milk, caution should be exercised when Pilocarpine Hydrochloride is administered to a nursing woman.

Adverse Reactions: PILOPINE HS® Gel is usually well tolerated. In a controlled clinical study in 78 glaucomatous patients treated for 30 days, there were no significant differences in the type or severity of adverse effects associated with the instillation of PILOPINE HS Gel at bedtime or the four daily instillations of pilocarpine 4% drops. The following adverse experiences associated with pilocarpine therapy have been reported: lacrimation, burning or discomfort, temporal or periorbital headache, ciliary spasm, conjunctival vascular congestion, superficial keratitis and induced myopia. Ocular reactions usually occur during initiation of therapy and often will not persist with continued therapy. Reduced visual acuity in poor illumination is frequently experienced by older individuals and in those with lens opacity. A subtle corneal granularity was observed in about 10% of patients treated with PILOPINE HS Gel. In a control patient group treated with other therapies including pilocarpine drops, timolol, or epinephrine, the incidence was the same as reported among the individuals treated with PILOPINE HS Gel. In both groups, the corneal granularity was asymptomatic and visual acuity was not affected. Rare cases of retinal detachment have been reported during treatment with miotic agents; thus care should be exercised with all miotic therapy, especially in young myopic patients. Lens opacity may occur with prolonged use of pilocarpine.

Overdosage: Systemic reactions following topical administration are extremely rare.

Dosage and Administration: Apply a one-half inch ribbon in the lower conjunctival sac of the affected eye(s) once a day at bedtime. Under selected conditions, more frequent instillations may be indicated.

How Supplied: PILOPINE HS Gel is supplied as a 4% sterile aqueous gel in 5 gram tubes with ophthalmic tip.

5g: NDC 0065-0215-05

Storage: Store in a refrigerator (36°F–46°F) until dispensed to patient. Do not freeze. Patient may store at room temperature and should discard any unused portion after eight weeks.

Caution: Federal (USA) law prohibits dispensing without prescription.

Patented. U.S. Patent No. 4,271,143

TEARS NATURALE® II — OTC
Lubricant Eye Drops
TEARS NATURALE® FREE
Lubricant Eye Drops

Description: TEARS NATURALE II is the only lubricant eye drop preserved with safe, nonsensitizing POLYQUAD 0.001%. *In vitro* studies have shown that POLYQUAD substantially avoids the damaging effects of epithelial cell toxicity possible with other tear substitute preservatives and allows epithelial cell growth. POLYQUAD has been shown to be 99% reaction-free in normal subjects and 97% reaction-free in subjects known to be preservative sensitive. TEARS NATURALE FREE is a preservative-free version of TEARS NATURALE II.

With their unique mucin like polymeric formulation, and with their natural pH, low viscosity, and isotonicity, TEARS NATURALE II and TEARS NATURALE FREE provide dry eye patients with comfort and prompt relief of dry eye symptoms.

Sterile-For Topical Eye Use Only

Ingredients: TEARS NATURALE II: each mL contains:

Active: DUASORB®, a water soluble polymeric system containing Dextran 70 0.1% and Hydroxypropyl Methylcellulose 2910 0.3%. **Preservative:** POLYQUAD®* (Polyquaternium-1) 0.001%. **Inactive:** Sodium Borate, Potassium Chloride, Sodium Chloride, Purified Water. May contain Hydrochloric Acid and/or Sodium Hydroxide to adjust pH.

TEARS NATURALE FREE:

Active: DUASORB, a water soluble polymeric system containing Dextran 70 0.1% and Hydroxypropyl Methylcellulose 2910 0.3%. **Inactive:** Sodium Borate, Potassium Chloride, Sodium Chloride, Purified Water. May contain Hydrochloric Acid and/or Sodium Hydroxide to adjust pH.

Indications: For the temporary relief of burning and irritation due to dryness of the eye and for use as a protectant against further irritation. For temporary relief of discomfort due to minor irritations of the eye or to exposure to wind or sun.

Directions: TEARS NATURALE II: Instill 1 or 2 drops in the affected eye(s) as needed. TEARS NATURALE FREE: Completely twist off tab: do not pull. Instill 1 or 2 drops in the affected eye(s) as needed.

Warnings: If you experience eye pain, changes in vision, continued redness or irritation of the eye, or if the condition worsens or persists for more than 72 hours, discontinue use and consult a doctor. If solution changes color or becomes cloudy, do not use.

To avoid contamination, do not touch tip of container to any surface. TEARS NATURALE II: Replace cap after using. TEARS NATURALE FREE: Do not reuse. Once opened, discard. Keep this and all drugs out of the reach of children. In case of accidental ingestion, seek professional assistance or contact a Poison Control Center immediately.

How Supplied: TEARS NATURALE II Lubricant Eye Drops are supplied in 15 mL and 30 mL plastic DROP-TAINER® bottles.

15 mL NDC 0065-0418-15
30 mL NDC 0065-0418-30

TEARS NATURALE FREE Lubricant Eye Drops are supplied in boxes of 24 0.02 fl. oz. single-use containers.

NDC 0998-0416-24

Storage: Store at room temperature.

*U.S. Patent No. 3,931,319 and others.

TOBRADEX® — ℞
(Tobramycin and Dexamethasone)
Sterile Ophthalmic Suspension and Ointment

Description: TOBRADEX® (Tobramycin and Dexamethasone) Ophthalmic Suspension and Ointment are sterile, multiple dose antibiotic and steroid combinations for topical ophthalmic use.

The chemical structures for tobramycin and dexamethasone are presented below:

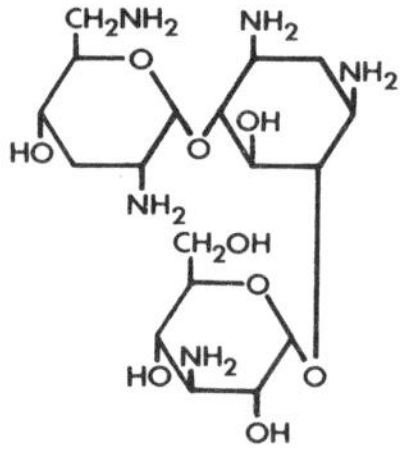

Tobramycin
Empirical Formula: $C_{18}H_{37}N_5O_9$
Chemical name:
O-3-Amino-3-deoxy-α-D-glucopyranosyl-(1→4)-*O*-[2,6-diamino-2,3,6-trideoxy-α-D-*ribo*-hexopyranosyl-(1→6)]-2-deoxy-L-streptamine

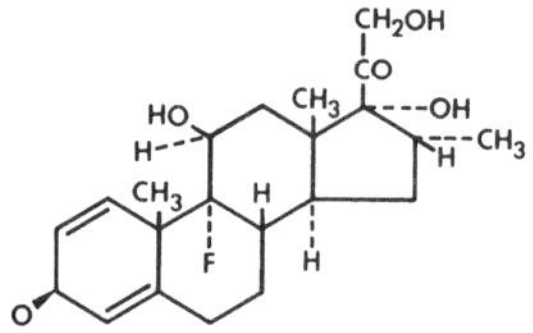

Dexamethasone
Empirical Formula: $C_{22}H_{29}FO_5$
Chemical Name:
9-Fluoro-11β,17,21-trihydroxy-16α-methylpregna-1,4-diene-3,20-dione

Each mL of TOBRADEX® Suspension contains: Active: Tobramycin 0.3% (3 mg) and Dexamethasone 0.1% (1 mg). Preservative: Benzalkonium Chloride 0.01%. Inactive: Tyloxapol, Edetate Disodium, Sodium Chloride, Hydroxyethyl Cellulose, Sodium Sulfate, Sulfuric Acid and/or Sodium Hydroxide (to adjust pH) and Purified Water.

Each gram of TOBRADEX® Ointment contains: Active: Tobramycin 0.3% (3 mg) and Dexamethasone 0.1% (1 mg). Preservative: Chlorobutanol 0.5%. Inactive: Mineral Oil and White Petrolatum.

Clinical Pharmacology: Corticoids suppress the inflammatory response to a variety of agents and they probably delay or slow healing. Since corticoids may inhibit the body's defense mechanism against infection, a concomitant antimicrobial drug may be used when this inhibition is considered to be clinially significant. Dexamethasone is a potent corticoid.

The antibiotic component in the combination (tobramycin) is included to provide action against susceptible organisms. *In vitro* studies have demonstrated that tobramycin is active against susceptible strains of the following microorganisms:

Staphylococci, including *S. aureus* and *S. epidermidis* (coagulase-positive and coagulase-negative), including penicillin-resistant strains.

Streptococci, including some of the Group A beta-hemolytic species, some nonhemolytic species, and some *Streptococcus pneumoniae*.

Pseudomonas aeruginosa, Escherichia coli, Klebsiella pneumoniae, Enterobacter aerogenes, Proteus mirabilis, Morganella morganii, most *Proteus vulgaris* strains, *Haemophilus influenzae* and *H. aegyptius, Moraxella lacunata,* and *Acinetobacter calcoaceticus* and some *Neisseria* species.

Bacterial susceptibility studies demonstrate that in some cases microorganisms resistant to gentamicin remain susceptible to tobramycin. A significant bacterial population resistant to tobramycin has not yet emerged; however, bacterial resistance may develop upon prolonged use.

No data are available on the extent of systemic absorption from TOBRADEX® Ophthalmic Suspension or Ointment; however, it is known that some systemic absorption can occur with ocularly applied drugs. If the maximum dose of TOBRADEX Ophthalmic Suspension is given for the first 48 hours (two drops in each eye every 2 hours) and complete systemic absorption occurs, which is highly unlikely, the daily dose of dexamethasone would be 2.4 mg. The usual physiological replacement dose is 0.75 mg daily. If TOBRADEX Ophthalmic Suspension is given after the first 48 hours as two drops in each eye every 4 hours, the administered dose of dexamethasone would be 1.2 mg daily. The administered dose for TOBRADEX Ophthalmic Ointment in both eyes four times daily would be 0.4 mg of dexamethasone daily.

Indications and Usage: TOBRADEX® Ophthalmic Suspension and Ointment are indicated for steroid-responsive inflammatory ocular conditions for which a corticosteroid is indicated and where superficial bacterial ocular infection or a risk of bacterial ocular infection exists.

Ocular steroids are indicated in inflammatory conditions of the palpebral and bulbar conjunctiva, cornea and anterior segment of the globe where the inherent risk of steroid use in certain infective conjunctivitides is accepted to obtain a diminution in edema and inflammation. They are also indicated in chronic anterior uveitis and corneal injury from chemical, radiation or thermal burns, or penetration of foreign bodies.

The use of a combination drug with an anti-infective component is indicated where the risk of superficial ocular infection is high or where there is an expectation that potentially dangerous numbers of bacteria will be present in the eye.

The particular anti-infective drug in this product is active against the following common bacterial eye pathogens:

Staphylococci, including *S. aureus* and *S. epidermidis* (coagulase-positive and coagulase-negative), including penicillin-resistant strains.

Streptococci, including some of the Group A beta-hemolytic species, some nonhemolytic species, and some *Streptococcus pneumoniae*.

Pseudomonas aeruginosa, Escherichia coli, Klebsiella pneumoniae, Enterobacter aerogenes, Proteus mirabilis, Morganella morganii, most *Proteus vulgaris* strains, *Haemophilus influenzae* and *H. aegyptius, Moraxella lacunata,* and *Acinetobacter calcoaceticus* and some *Neisseria* species.

Contraindications: Epithelial herpes simplex keratitis (dendritic keratitis), vaccinia, varicella, and many other viral diseases of the cornea and conjunctiva. Mycobacterial infection of the eye. Fungal diseases of ocular structures. Hypersensitivity to a component of the medication.

The use of this combination is always contraindicated after uncomplicated removal of a corneal foreign body.

Warnings: NOT FOR INJECTION INTO THE EYE. Sensitivity to topically applied aminoglycosides may occur in some patients. If a sensitivity reaction does occur, discontinue use.

Prolonged use of steroids may result in glaucoma, with damage to the optic nerve, defects in visual acuity and fields of vision, and posterior subcapsular cataract formation. Intraocular pressure should be routinely monitored even though it may be difficult in children and uncooperative patients. Prolonged use may suppress the host response and thus increase the hazard of secondary ocular infections. In those diseases causing thinning of the cornea or sclera, perforations have been known to occur with the use of topical steroids. In acute purulent conditions of the eye, steroids may mask infection or enhance existing infection.

Precautions:

General. The possibility of fungal infections of the cornea should be considered after long-term steroid dosing. As with other antibiotic preparations, prolonged use may result in overgrowth of nonsusceptible organisms, including fungi. If superinfection occurs, appropriate therapy should be initiated. When multiple prescriptions are required, or whenever clinical judgement dictates, the patient should be examined with the aid of magnification, such as slit lamp biomicroscopy and, where appropriate, fluorescein staining.

Information for Patients: Do not touch dropper or tube tip to any surface as this may contaminate the contents.

Carcinogenesis, Mutagenesis, Impairment of Fertility. No studies have been conducted to evaluate the carcinogenic or mutagenic potential. No impairment of fertility was noted in studies of subcutaneous tobramycin in rats at doses of 50 and 100 mg/kg/day.

Pregnancy Category C. Corticosteroids have been found to be teratogenic in animal studies. Ocular administration of 0.1% dexamethasone resulted in 15.6% and 32.3% incidence of fetal anomalies in two groups of pregnant rabbits. Fetal growth retardation and increased mortality rates have been observed in rats with chronic dexamethasone therapy. Reproduction studies have been performed in rats and rabbits with tobramycin at doses up to 100 mg/kg/day parenterally and have revealed no evidence of impaired fertility or harm to the fetus. There are no adequate and well-controlled studies in pregnant women. TOBRADEX® Ophthalmic Suspension and Ointment should be used during pregnancy only if the potential benefit justifies the potential risk to the fetus.

Nursing Mothers. It is not known whether this drug is excreted in human milk. Because many drugs are excreted in human milk, a decision should be considered to discontinue nursing temporarily while using TOBRADEX Ophthalmic Suspension or Ointment.

Pediatric Use. Safety and effectiveness in children have not been established.

Adverse Reactions: Adverse reactions have occurred with steroid/anti-infective combination drugs which can be attributed to the steroid component, the anti-infective component, or the combination. Exact incidence figures are not available. The most frequent adverse reactions to topical ocular tobramycin (TOBREX®) are localized ocular toxicity and hypersensitivity, including lid itching and swelling, and conjunctival erythema. These reactions occur in less than 4% of patients. Similar reactions may occur with the topical use of other aminoglycoside antibiotics. Other adverse reactions have not been reported; however, if topical ocular tobramycin is administered concomitantly with systemic aminoglycoside antibiotics, care should be taken to monitor the total serum concentration. The reactions due to the steroid component are: elevation of intraocular pressure (IOP) with possible development of glaucoma, and infrequent optic nerve damage; posterior subcapsular cataract formation; and delayed wound healing.

Secondary Infection. The development of secondary infection has occurred after use of combinations containing steroids and antimicrobials. Fungal infections of the cornea are particularly prone to develop coincidentally with long-term applications of steroids. The possibility of fungal invasion must be considered in any persistent corneal ulceration where steroid treatment has been used. Secondary bacterial ocular infection following suppression of host responses also occurs.

Dosage and Administration: Suspension: One or two drops instilled into the conjunctival sac(s) every four to six hours. During the initial 24 to 48 hours, the dosage may be increased to one or two drops every two (2) hours. Frequency should be decreased gradually as warranted by improvement in clinical signs. Care should be taken not to discontinue therapy prematurely. **Ointment:** Apply a small amount (approximately ½ inch ribbon) into the conjunctival sac(s) up to three or four times daily. TOBRADEX Ophthalmic Ointment may be used at bedtime in conjunction with TOBRADEX Ophthalmic Suspension used during the day. Not more than 20 mL or 8 g should be prescribed initially and the prescription should not be refilled without further evaluation as outlined in PRECAUTIONS above.

How Supplied: Sterile ophthalmic suspension in 2.5 mL (NDC 0065-0647-25) and 5 mL (NDC 0065-0647-05) DROP-TAINER® dispensers. Sterile ophthalmic ointment in 3.5 g ophthalmic tube (NDC 0065-0648-35).

Storage: Store 46° to 80°F (8° to 27°C).

Store suspension upright and shake well before using.

Caution: Federal (USA) law prohibits dispensing without prescription.

Patent Pending.

TOBREX® ℞

(tobramycin 0.3%)

Ophthalmic Solution and Ointment

Description: TOBREX® (tobramycin 0.3%) is a sterile topical ophthalmic antibiotic formulation prepared specifically for topical therapy of external infections. This product is supplied in solution and ointment forms.

Each mL of TOBREX Ophthalmic solution contains: Active: Tobramycin 0.3% (3 mg). Preservative: Benzalkonium Chloride 0.01%. Inactive: Boric Acid, Sodium Sulfate, Sodium Chloride, Tyloxapol, Sodium Hydroxide and/or Sulfuric Acid (to adjust pH), and Purified Water.

Each gram of TOBREX Ophthalmic ointment contains: Active: Tobramycin 0.3% (3 mg). Preservative: Chlorobutanol 0.5%. Inactive: Mineral Oil and White Petrolatum.

Continued on next page

Alcon—Cont.

The chemical structure of tobramycin is presented below.

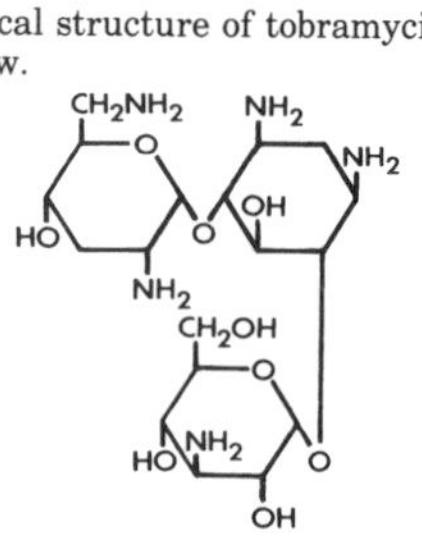

Chemical name: O-{3-amino-3-deoxy-α-D-gluco-pyranosyl-(1→4)}-O-{2,6-diamino- 2,3,6-trideoxy-αD-ribohexo-pyranosyll-(1→6)}- 2-de-oxy-streptamine.

Tobramycin is a water-soluble aminoglycoside antibiotic active against a wide variety of gram-negative and gram-positive ophthalmic pathogens.

Clinical Pharmacology: *In Vitro Data: In vitro* studies have demonstrated tobramycin is active against susceptible strains of the following microorganisms:

Staphylococci, including *S. aureus* and *S. epidermidis* (coagulase-positive and coagulase-negative), including penicillin-resistant strains.

Streptococci, including some of the Group A beta-hemolytic species, some nonhemolytic species, and some *Streptococcus pneumoniae.*

Pseudomonas aeruginosa, Escherichia coli, Klebsiella pneumoniae, Enterobacter aerogenes, Proteus mirabilis, Morganella morganii, most *Proteus vulgaris* strains, *Haemophilus influenzae* and *H. aegyptius, Moraxella lacunata, Acinetobacter calcoaceticus* and some *Neisseria* species. Bacterial susceptibility studies demonstrate that in some cases, microorganisms resistant to gentamicin retain susceptibility to tobramycin. A significant bacterial population resistant to tobramycin has not yet emerged; however, bacterial resistance may develop upon prolonged use.

Indications and Usage: TOBREX® is a topical antibiotic indicated in the treatment of external infections of the eye and its adnexa caused by susceptible bacteria. Appropriate monitoring of bacterial response to topical antibiotic therapy should accompany the use of TOBREX.

Clinical studies have shown tobramycin to be safe and effective for use in children.

Contraindications: TOBREX Ophthalmic Solution and Ointment are contraindicated in patients with known hypersensitivity to any of their components.

Warnings: NOT FOR INJECTION INTO THE EYE. Do not touch tube or dropper tip to any surface, as this may contaminate the contents. Sensitivity to topically applied aminoglycosides may occur in some patients. If a sensitivity reaction to TOBREX occurs, discontinue use.

Precautions: As with other antibiotic preparations, prolonged use may result in overgrowth of nonsusceptible organisms, including fungi. If superinfection occurs, appropriate therapy should be initiated. Ophthalmic ointments may retard corneal wound healing.

Pregnancy Category B. Reproduction studies in three types of animals at doses up to thirty-three times the normal human systemic dose have revealed no evidence of impaired fertility or harm to the fetus due to tobramycin. There are, however, no adequate and well-controlled studies in pregnant women. Because animal studies are not always predictive of human response, this drug should be used during pregnancy only if clearly needed.

Nursing Mothers: Because of the potential for adverse reactions in nursing infants from TOBREX, a decision should be made whether to discontinue nursing the infant or discontinue the drug, taking into account the importance of the drug to the mother.

Adverse Reactions: The most frequent adverse reactions to TOBREX Ophthalmic Solution and Ointment are localized ocular toxicity and hypersensitivity, including lid itching and swelling, and conjunctival erythema. These reactions occur in less than three of 100 patients treated with TOBREX. Similar reactions may occur with the topical use of other aminoglycoside antibiotics.

Other adverse reactions have not been reported from TOBREX therapy; however, if topical ocular tobramycin is administered concomitantly with systemic aminoglycoside antibiotics, care should be taken to monitor the total serum concentration. In clinical trials, TOBREX Ophthalmic Ointment produced significantly fewer adverse reactions (3.7%) than did GARAMYCIN® Ophthalmic Ointment (10.6%).

Overdosage: Clinically apparent signs and symptoms of an overdose of TOBREX Ophthalmic Solution or Ointment (punctate keratitis, erythema, increased lacrimation, edema and lid itching) may be similar to adverse reaction effects seen in some patients.

Dosage and Administration: Solution: In mild to moderate disease, instill one or two drops into the affected eye(s) every four hours. In severe infections, instill two drops into the eye(s) hourly until improvement, following which treatment should be reduced prior to discontinuation.

Ointment: In mild to moderate disease, apply a half-inch ribbon into the affected eye(s) two or three times per day. In severe infections, instill a half-inch ribbon into the affected eye(s) every three to four hours until improvement, following which treatment should be reduced prior to discontinuation.

How to Apply TOBREX® Ointment

1. Tilt your head back.
2. Place a finger on your cheek just under your eye and gently pull down until a "V" pocket is formed between your eyeball and your lower lid.
3. Place a small amount (about ½ inch) of TOBREX in the "V" pocket. Do not let the tip of the tube touch your eye.
4. Look downward before closing your eye.

Tobrex Ointment may be used in conjunction with Tobrex Solution.

How Supplied: 5 mL STERILE solution in DROP-TAINER® dispenser (NDC 0998-0643-05), containing tobramycin 0.3% (3 mg/mL) and 3.5 g STERILE ointment in ophthalmic tube (NDC 0065-0644-35), containing tobramycin 0.3% (3 mg/g).

Storage: Store at 8°–27°C (46°–80°F.)

Caution: Federal (USA) law prohibits dispensing without prescription.

ZINCFRIN® OTC

Redness Reliever/Astringent Eye Drops

Indications: For the temporary relief of redness and discomfort due to minor eye irritations.

Sterile—For topical eye use only.

Ingredients: Each mL contains: Active: Zinc Sulfate 0.25%, Phenylephrine Hydrochloride 0.12%. **Preservative:** Benzalkonium Chloride 0.01%. **Inactives:** Sodium Citrate, Polysorbate 80, Citric Acid and/or Sodium Hydroxide (to adjust pH), Purified Water.

Warnings: If you experience eye pain, changes in vision, continued redness or irritation of the eye, or if the condition worsens or persists for more than 72 hours, discontinue use and consult a doctor. If you have glaucoma, do not use this product except under the advice and supervision of a doctor. Overuse of this product may produce increased redness of the eye. If solution changes color or becomes cloudy, do not use. To avoid contamination, do not touch tip of container to any surface. Replace cap after using. Keep this and all drugs out of the reach of children. In case of accidental ingestion, seek professional assistance or contact a Poison Control Center immediately.

Directions: Instill 1 to 2 drops in the affected eye(s) up to four times daily.

How Supplied: In ½ fl. oz DROP-TAINER® dispenser.
NDC 0998-0512-15

Storage: Store at 46° to 80° F.

Alcon Surgical, Inc.

6201 SOUTH FREEWAY
FT. WORTH, TX 76134

BSS® ℞

(balanced salt solution)
Sterile Irrigating Solution

Description: BSS® Sterile Irrigating Solution is a sterile physiological balanced salt solution, each mL containing Sodium Chloride (NaCl) 0.64%, Potassium Chloride (KCl) 0.075%, Calcium Chloride Dihydrate ($CaCl_2 \cdot 2H_2O$) 0.048%, Magnesium Chloride Hexahydrate ($MgCl_2 \cdot 6H_2O$) 0.03%, Sodium Acetate Trihydrate ($C_2H_3NaO_2 \cdot 3H_2O$) 0.39%, Sodium Citrate Dihydrate ($C_6H_5Na_3O_7 \cdot 2H_2O$) 0.17%, Sodium Hydroxide and/or Hydrochloric Acid (to adjust pH), and Water for Injection. BSS Sterile Irrigating Solution is isotonic to the tissues of the eyes. It is a lint-free solution containing essential ions for normal cell metabolism.

Clinical Pharmacology: A physiologic irrigating solution.

Indications and Usage: For irrigation during various surgical procedures of the eyes, ears, nose, and/or throat.

Warnings: If blister or paper backing is damaged or broken, sterility of the enclosed bottle cannot be assured. Open under aseptic conditions only.

NOT FOR INJECTION OR INTRAVENOUS INFUSION.

Precautions: This solution contains no preservative and should not be used for more than one patient. Prior to use, check the following: tip should be firmly in place, irrigating needle should be properly seated; squeeze out several drops before inserting into anterior chamber. The needle should be removed from the anterior chamber prior to releasing pressure to prevent suction.

The addition of any medication to BSS solution may result in damage to intraocular tissue. Studies suggest that intraocular irrigating solutions which are iso-osmotic with normal aqueous fluids should be used with caution in diabetic patients undergoing vitrectomy since intraoperative lens changes have been observed.[1,2]

There have been reports of corneal clouding or edema following ocular surgery in which BSS solution was used as an irrigating solution. As in all surgical procedures appropriate measures should be taken to minimize trauma to the cornea and other ocular tissues.

Adverse Reactions: When the corneal endothelium is abnormal, irrigation or any other trauma may result in bullous keratopathy. Postoperative inflammatory reactions as well as incidents of corneal edema and corneal decompensation have been reported. Their relationship to the use of BSS solution has not been established.

Dosage and Administration: The adapter plug is designed to accept an irrigating needle. Tissues may be irrigated by attaching the needle to the DROP-TAINER® bottle as explained below. External irrigation may be done without the irrigating needle.

Method of using Adapter Plug for LUER-LOK® Hub Ophthalmic Irrigating Needle:

1. Aseptically remove DROP-TAINER bottle from blister by peeling paper backing.
2. Snap on surgeon's sterile irrigation needle. Push until firmly in place and twist slightly.
3. Test assembly for proper function before use.

NOTE: LUER-LOK is a registered trademark of Becton, Dickinson and Company.

How Supplied: In 15 mL and 30 mL sterile DROP-TAINER bottles.

15 mL NDC 0065-0795-15
30 mL NDC 0065-0795-30

Storage: Store at 46° to 80° F (8° to 27° C).

References:

1. Faulborn, J., Conway, B.P., Machemer, R., Surgical Complications of Pars Plana Vitreous Surgery. Ophthalmology 85: 116–125, 1978.
2. Haimann, M.H. and Abrams, G. W., Prevention of Lens Opacification During Diabetic Vitrectomy. Ophthalmology 91: 116–121, 1984.

BSS® ℞

(Balanced Salt Solution)
Sterile Irrigating Solution
(250 mL and 500 mL)

Description: BSS® Sterile Irrigating Solution is a sterile physiological balanced salt solution, each mL containing Sodium Chloride (NaCl) 0.64%, Potassium Chloride (KCl) 0.075%, Calcium Chloride Dihydrate ($CaCl_2 \cdot 2H_2O$) 0.048%, Magnesium Chloride Hexahydrate ($MgCl_2 \cdot 6H_2O$) 0.03%, Sodium Acetate Trihydrate ($C_2H_3NaO_2 \cdot 3H_2O$) 0.39%, Sodium Citrate Dihydrate ($C_6H_5Na_3O_7 \cdot 2H_2O$) 0.17%, Sodium Hydroxide and/or Hydrochloric Acid (to adjust pH), and Water for Injection.

BSS Sterile Irrigating Solution is isotonic to the tissues of the eyes. It is a lint-free solution containing essential ions for normal cell metabolism.

Clinical Pharmacology: A physiologic irrigation solution.

Indications and Usage: For irrigation during various surgical procedures of the eyes, ears, nose and/or throat.

Warning: Not for injection or intravenous infusion.

Precautions: This solution contains no preservative and should not be used for more than one patient. Use only if vacuum is present and if container and seal are undamaged and solution is clear.

The addition of any medication to BSS sterile irrigating solution may result in damage to intraocular tissue. Studies suggest that intraocular irrigating solutions which are iso-osmotic with normal aqueous fluids should be used with caution in diabetic patients undergoing vitrectomy since intraoperative lens changes have been observed.[1,2] There have been reports of corneal clouding or edema following ocular surgery in which BSS sterile irrigating solution was used as an irrigating solution. As in all surgical procedures appropriate measures should be taken to minimize trauma to the cornea and other ocular tissues.

Adverse Reactions: When the corneal endothelium is abnormal, irrigation or any other trauma may result in bullous keratopathy. Postoperative inflammatory reactions as well as incidents of corneal edema and corneal decompensation have been reported. Their relationship to the use of BSS sterile irrigating solution has not been established.

Dosage and Administration: This irrigating solution should be used according to standard format for each surgical procedure.

Note:

Use an administration set with an air inlet in the plastic spike since the bottle does not contain a separate airway tube. Follow directions of the particular administration set to be used. Pull the tab to remove the outer aluminum ring and dust cover. Insert the spike aseptically into the bottle through the target area of the rubber stopper. Allow the fluid to flow and remove air from the tubing before irrigation begins.

How Supplied: In 250 mL bottle **NDC** 0065-0795-25 and in 500 mL bottle **NDC** 0065-0795-50.

Storage: Store at 46° to 80° F (8° to 27° C).

References:

1. Faulborn, J., Conway, B.P., Machemer, R., Surgical Complications of Pars Plana Vitreous Surgery. Ophthalmology 85: 116–125, 1978.
2. Haimann, M.H. and Abrams, G. W., Prevention of Lens Opacification During Diabetic Vitrectomy. Ophthalmology 91: 116–121, 1984.

BSS PLUS® ℞

(Balanced Salt Solution Enriched with Bicarbonate, Dextrose and Glutathione)
Sterile Intraocular Irrigating Solution
U.S. Patent Nos. 4,443,432 and 4,550,022

Description: BSS PLUS® is a sterile intraocular irrigating solution for use during all intraocular surgical procedures, even those requiring a relatively long intraocular perfusion time (e.g., pars plana vitrectomy, phacoemulsification, extracapsular cataract extraction/lens aspiration, anterior segment reconstruction, etc.). The solution does not contain a preservative and should be prepared just prior to use in surgery.

PART I: Part I is a sterile 480 mL solution in a 500 mL single-dose bottle to which the Part II concentrate is added. Each mL of Part I contains: Sodium Chloride 7.44 mg, Potassium Chloride 0.395 mg, Dibasic Sodium Phosphate 0.433 mg, Sodium Bicarbonate 2.19 mg, Hydrochloric Acid and/or Sodium Hydroxide (to adjust pH), in Water for Injection.

Part II: Part II is a sterile concentrate in a 20 mL single-dose vial for addition to Part I. Each mL of Part II contains: Calcium Chloride Dihydrate 3.85 mg, Magnesium Chloride Hexahydrate 5 mg, Dextrose 23 mg, Glutathione Disulfide (Oxidized Glutathione) 4.6 mg, in Water for Injection.

After addition of BSS PLUS® Part II to the Part I bottle, each mL of the reconstituted product contains: Sodium Chloride 7.14 mg, Potassium Chloride 0.38 mg, Calcium Chloride Dihydrate 0.154 mg, Magnesium Chloride Hexahydrate 0.2 mg, Dibasic Sodium Phosphate 0.42 mg, Sodium Bicarbonate 2.1 mg, Dextrose 0.92 mg, Glutathione Disulfide (Oxidized Glutathione) 0.184 mg, Hydrochloric Acid and/or Sodium Hydroxide (to adjust pH), in Water for Injection.

The reconstituted product has a pH of approximately 7.4. Osmolality is approximately 305 mOsm.

Clinical Pharmacology: None of the components of BSS PLUS are foreign to the eye, and BSS PLUS has no pharmacological action. Human perfused cornea studies[1-3] have shown BSS PLUS to be an effective irrigation solution for providing corneal detumescence and maintaining corneal endothelial integrity during intraocular perfusion. An *in vivo* study[4] in rabbits has shown that BSS PLUS is more suitable than normal saline or Balanced Salt Solution for intravitreal irrigation because BSS PLUS contains the appropriate bicarbonate, pH, and ionic composition necessary for the maintenance of normal retinal electrical activity. Human *in vivo* studies have demonstrated BSS PLUS to be safe and effective when used during surgical procedures such as pars plana vitrectomy, phacoemulsification, cataract extraction/lens aspiration and anterior segment reconstruction.

Indications and Usage: BSS PLUS® is indicated for use as an intraocular irrigating solution during intraocular surgical procedures involving perfusion of the eye.

Contraindications: There are no specific contraindications to the use of BSS PLUS; however, contraindications for the surgical procedure during which BSS PLUS is to be used should be strictly adhered to.

Warnings: For IRRIGATION during ophthalmic surgery only. BSS PLUS is **NOT** for injection or intravenous infusion.

Precautions: DO NOT USE BSS PLUS UNTIL RECONSTITUTED. Do not use Part I if it does not contain a vacuum. **Do not use additives other than Part II.** Do not use if the reconstituted solution is discolored or contains a precipitate. SINCE BSS PLUS® IS INTENDED FOR INTRAOCULAR IRRIGATION, IT DOES NOT CONTAIN A PRESERVATIVE AND, THEREFORE, SHOULD NOT BE USED FOR MORE THAN ONE PATIENT. DISCARD ANY UNUSED PORTION SIX HOURS AFTER PREPARATION. Studies suggest that intraocular irrigating solutions which are iso-osmotic with normal aqueous fluids should be used with caution in diabetic patients undergoing vitrectomy since intraoperative lens changes have been observed.[5,6] There have been reports of corneal clouding or edema following ocular surgery in which BSS PLUS was used as an irrigating solution. As in all surgical procedures appropriate measures should be taken to minimize trauma to the cornea and other ocular tissues.

Preparation: Reconstitute BSS PLUS just prior to use in surgery. Follow the same strict aseptic procedures in the reconstitution of BSS PLUS as is used for intravenous additives. Pull the tab to remove the outer aluminum ring and dust cover from the BSS PLUS Part I (480 mL) bottle. Remove the blue flip-off seal from the BSS PLUS Part II (20 mL) vial. Clean and disinfect the rubber stoppers on both containers by using sterile alcohol wipes. Transfer the contents of the Part II vial to the Part I bottle using a BSS PLUS Vacuum Transfer Device (provided). An alternative method of solution transfer may be accomplished by using a 20 mL syringe to remove the Part II solution from the vial and transferring exactly 20 mL to the Part I container through the target area of the rubber stopper. An excess volume of Part II is provided in each vial. Gently agitate the contents to mix the solution. Place a sterile cap on the bottle. Remove the tear-off portion of the label. Record the time and date of reconstitution and the patient's name on the bottle label.

Adverse Reactions: Postoperative inflammatory reactions as well as incidents of corneal edema and corneal decompensation have been reported. Their relationship to the use of BSS PLUS has not been established.

Overdosage: The solution has no pharmacological action and thus has no potential for overdosage. However, as with any intraocular surgical procedure, the duration of intraocular manipulation should be kept to a minimum.

Dosage and Administration: The solution should be used according to the technique standardly employed by the operating surgeon. Use an administration set with an air inlet in the plastic spike since the bottle does not contain a separate airway tube. Follow the directions for the particular administration set to be used. Insert the spike aseptically into the bottle through the target area of the rubber stopper. Allow the fluid to flow to remove air from the tubing before intraocular irrigation begins. If a second bottle is necessary to complete the surgical procedure, insure that the vacuum is

Continued on next page

Alcon Surgical—Cont.

vented from the second bottle BEFORE attachment to the administration set.

How Supplied: BSS PLUS is supplied in two packages for reconstitution prior to use: a 500 mL bottle containing 480 mL (Part I) and a 20 mL vial (Part II). See the **Precautions** and **Preparation** sections for information concerning reconstitution of the solution.

NDC 0065-0800-50.

Storage: Store Part I and Part II at 46°–80°F. Discard prepared solution after six hours.

References:

1. Edelhauser, H. F., Van Horn, D. L., Hyndiuk, R. A., Schultz, R. O., Intraocular Irrigating Solutions: Their Effect on the Corneal Endothelium. **Arch. Ophthalmol., 93,** 648, 1975.
2. Edelhauser, H. F., Van Horn, D. L., Schultz, R. O., Hyndiuk, R. A., Comparative Toxicity of Intraocular Irrigating Solutions on the Corneal Endothelium, **Am. J. Ophthalmol., 81,** 473, 1976.
3. Edelhauser, H. F., Gonnering, R., Van Horn, D. L., Intraocular Irrigating Solutions: A Comparative Study of BSS PLUS and Lactated Ringer's Solution, **Arch. Ophthalmol., 96,** 516, 1978.
4. Moorhead, L. C., Redburn, D. A., Merritt, J., Garcia, C. A., The Effects of Intravitreal Irrigation During Vitrectomy on the Electroretinogram, **Am. J. Ophthalmol., 88,** 239, 1979.
5. Faulborn, J., Conway, B.P., Machemer, R., Surgical Complications of Pars Plana Vitreous Surgery. Ophthalmology 85: 116–125, 1978.
6. Haimann, M.H. and Abrams, G. W., Prevention of Lens Opacification During Diabetic Vitrectomy. Ophthalmology 91: 116–121, 1984.

ENUCLENE® OTC

Cleaning/Lubricating Solution for Artificial Eyes

Ingredients: Each mL contains: Active: Tyloxapol 0.25%, Benzalkonium Chloride 0.02%.

Description: ENUCLENE® is a sterile, buffered, isotonic solution formulated especially for artificial eye wearers. ENUCLENE Solution lubricates, cleans, and wets the artificial eye, thereby increasing the wearing comfort to the patient. In addition, ENUCLENE Solution contains sufficient concentration of the antibacterial agent, Benzalkonium Chloride, to kill most germs which are commonly found in the eye socket of artificial eye wearers.

ENUCLENE Solution contains a special ingredient, Tyloxapol, which is a detergent. It liquefies the solid matter so that it is less irritating. Laboratory tests show that ENUCLENE Solution causes no harmful effects to artificial eyes. Benzalkonium Chloride, in addition to its germ killing action, aids Tyloxapol in wetting the artificial eye so that it is completely covered. This combination of wetting, cleansing, and lubricating, and also the softening of thickened matter, makes ENUCLENE Solution an ideal drug for artificial eye wearers.

ENUCLENE Solution is recommended for wearers of artificial eyes. In clinical studies, the use of this preparation was found to improve the wearing effects of the artificial eye by its soothing action, thus reducing the undesirable effects of secretions of the glands in the mucous membrane of the eye socket.

Contraindications: Contraindicated in those persons who have shown hypersensitivity to any component of this preparation.

Caution: If irritation persists or increases, discontinue use and consult physician. Keep container tightly closed. Keep out of reach of children.

Warning: Do not touch dropper tip to any surface since this may contaminate solution.

Directions: The drops should be used just as ordinary eye drops are used. With the artificial eye in place, drop 1 to 2 drops onto it, 3 to 4 times daily. The artificial eye may be removed periodically if advised by the physician and 2 to 3 drops applied to remove oily or mucous materials. The artificial eye is then rubbed between the fingers and rinsed with tap water. Then 1 to 2 drops may then be applied to the artificial eye, either prior to or after reinsertion.

How Supplied: ½ fl. oz. (15 mL) in sterile DROP-TAINER® Dispenser.

Storage: Store at 46°–80°F (8°–27°C.)

IOPIDINE® ℞

(apraclonidine hydrochloride)
1% As Base
Sterile Ophthalmic Solution

Description: IOPIDINE® Ophthalmic Solution contains apraclonidine hydrochloride, an alpha adrenergic agonist, in a sterile isotonic solution for topical application to the eye. Apraclonidine hydrochloride is a white to off-white powder and is highly soluble in water. Its chemical name is 2-[(4-amino-2,6 dichlorophenyl) imino]imidazolidine monohydrochloride with an empirical formula of $C_9H_{11}Cl_3N_4$ and a molecular weight of 281.6. The chemical structure of apraclonidine hydrochloride is:

[Chemical structure: NH_2–phenyl(Cl, Cl)–N=imidazolidine (H, N, N, H) • HCl]

Each mL of IOPIDINE Ophthalmic Solution contains: Active: Apraclonidine hydrochloride 11.5 mg equivalent to apraclonidine base 10 mg; Preservative: Benzalkonium chloride 0.01%. Inactive: Sodium chloride, sodium acetate, sodium hydroxide and/or hydrochloric acid (pH 4.4–7.8) and purified water.

Clinical Pharmacology: Apraclonidine is a relatively selective, alpha adrenergic agonist and does not have significant membrane stabilizing (local anesthetic) activity. When instilled into the eye, IOPIDINE (apraclonidine hydrochloride) Ophthalmic Solution has the action of reducing intraocular pressure. Ophthalmic apraclonidine has minimal effect on cardiovascular parameters.

Optic nerve head damage and visual field loss may result from an acute elevation in intraocular pressure that can occur after argon or Nd:YAG Laser surgical procedures. Elevated intraocular pressure, whether acute or chronic in duration, is a major risk factor in the pathogenesis of visual field loss. The higher the peak or spike of intraocular pressure, the greater the likelihood of visual field loss and optic nerve damage especially in patients with previously compromised optic nerves. The onset of action with IOPIDINE Ophthalmic Solution can usually be noted within one hour and the maximum intraocular pressure reduction usually occurs three to five hours after application of a single dose. The precise mechanism of the ocular hypotensive action of IOPIDINE Ophthalmic Solution is not completely established at this time. Aqueous fluorophotometry studies in man suggest that its predominant action may be related to a reduction of aqueous formation. Controlled clinical studies of patients requiring argon laser trabeculoplasty or argon laser iridotomy or Nd:YAG posterior capsulotomy showed that IOPIDINE Ophthalmic Solution controlled or prevented the postsurgical intraocular pressure rise typically observed in patients after undergoing those procedures. After surgery, the mean intraocular pressure was 1.2 to 4.0 mmHg below the corresponding presurgical baseline pressure before IOPIDINE Ophthalmic Solution treatment. With placebo treatment, postsurgical pressures were 2.5 to 8.4 mmHg higher than their corresponding presurgical baselines. Overall, only 2% of patients treated with IOPIDINE Ophthalmic Solution had severe intraocular pressure elevations (spike ≥ 10 mmHg) during the first three hours after laser surgery, whereas 22% of placebo-treated patients responded with severe pressure spikes (Table 1). Of the patients that experienced a pressure spike after surgery, the peak intraocular pressure was above 30 mmHg in most patients (Table 2) and was above 50 mmHg in seven placebo-treated patients and one IOPIDINE Ophthalmic Solution-treated patient.

[See table below.]

Indications and Usage: IOPIDINE (apraclonidine hydrochloride) Ophthalmic Solution is indicated to control or prevent postsurgical elevations in intraocular pressure that occur in patients after argon laser trabeculoplasty, argon laser iridotomy or Nd:YAG posterior capsulotomy.

Table 1
Incidence of Intraocular Pressure Spikes ≥ 10 mmHg

Study	Laser Procedure	P-Value	Treatment: Apraclonidine [a]N	(%)	Placebo [a]N	(%)
1	Trabeculoplasty	<0.05	0/40	(0%)	6/35	(17%)
2	Trabeculoplasty	=0.06	2/41	(5%)	8/42	(19%)
1	Iridotomy	<0.05	0/11	(0%)	4/10	(40%)
2	Iridotomy	=0.05	0/17	(0%)	4/19	(21%)
1	Nd:YAG Capsulotomy	<0.05	3/80	(4%)	19/83	(23%)
2	Nd:YAG Capsulotomy	<0.05	0/83	(0%)	22/81	(27%)

[a]N = Number Spikes/Number Eyes.

Table 2
Magnitude of Postsurgical Intraocular Pressure in Trabeculoplasty, Iridotomy and Nd:YAG Capsulotomy Patients With Severe Pressure Spikes ≥ 10 mmHg

Treatment	Total Spikes	Maximum Postsurgical Intraocular Pressure (mmHg): 20–29 mmHg	30–39 mmHg	40–49 mmHg	>50 mmHg
IOPIDINE	8	1	4	2	1
Placebo	78	16	47	8	7

Contraindication: IOPIDINE Ophthalmic Solution is contraindicated for patients receiving monoamine oxidase inhibitor therapy and for patients with hypersensitivity to any component of this medication or to clonidine.

Precautions:

General: Since IOPIDINE Ophthalmic Solution is a potent depressor of intraocular pressure, patients who develop exaggerated reductions in intraocular pressure should be closely monitored.

Although the acute administration of two drops of IOPIDINE® Ophthalmic Solution has minimal effect on heart rate or blood pressure in clinical studies evaluating patients undergoing anterior segment laser surgery, the preclinical pharmacologic profile of this drug suggests that caution should be observed in treating patients with severe cardiovascular disease including hypertension.

The possibility of a vasovagal attack occurring during laser surgery should be considered and caution used in patients with history of such episodes.

Topical ocular administration of two drops of 0.5%, 1.0% and 1.5% IOPIDINE Ophthalmic Solution to New Zealand Albino rabbits three times daily for one month resulted in sporadic and transient instances of minimal corneal cloudiness in the 1.5% group only. No histopathological changes were noted in those eyes. No adverse ocular effects were observed in cynomolgus monkeys treated with two drops of 1.5% IOPIDINE Ophthalmic Solution applied three times daily for three months. No corneal changes were observed in 320 humans given at least one dose of 1.0% IOPIDINE Ophthalmic Solution.

Drug Interactions: Interactions with other agents have not been investigated.

Carcinogenesis, Mutagenesis, Impairment of Fertility: In a variety of *in vitro* cell assays, apraclonidine was nonmutagenic. Studies addressing carcinogenesis and the impairment of fertility have not been conducted.

Pregnancy: Pregnancy Category C: There are no adequate and well controlled studies of IOPIDINE Ophthalmic Solution in pregnant women. Animal reproduction studies have not been conducted with apraclonidine hydrochloride. This medication should be used in pregnancy only if the potential benefit to the mother justifies the potential risk to the fetus.

Nursing Mothers: It is not known if topically applied IOPIDINE Ophthalmic Solution is excreted in human milk. A decision should be considered to discontinue nursing temporarily for the one day on which IOPIDINE Ophthalmic Solution is used.

Pediatric Use: Safety and effectiveness in children have not been established.

Adverse Reactions: The following adverse events were reported in association with the use of IOPIDINE Ophthalmic Solution in laser surgery: ocular injection (1.8%),upper lid elevation (1.3%), irregular heart rate (0.7%), ocular inflammation (0.45%), nasal decongestion (0.45%),conjunctival blanching (0.4%) and mydriasis (0.4%).

The following adverse events were observed in investigational studies dosing IOPIDINE Ophthalmic Solution once or twice daily for up to 28 days in nonlaser studies:

Ocular: Conjunctival blanching, upper lid elevation, mydriasis, burning, discomfort, foreign body sensation, dryness, itching, hypotony, blurred or dimmed vision, allergic response, conjunctival microhemorrhage;
Gastrointestinal: Abdominal pain, diarrhea, stomach discomfort, emesis;
Cardiovascular: Bradycardia, vasovagal attack, palpitations, orthostatic episode;
Central Nervous System: Insomnia, dream disturbances, irritability, decreased libido;
Other: Taste abnormalities, dry mouth, nasal burning or dryness, headache, head cold sensation, chest heaviness or burning, clammy or sweaty palms, body heat sensation, shortness of breath, increased pharyngeal secretion, extremity pain or numbness, fatigue, paresthesia, pruritus not associated with rash.

Overdosage: No information is available on overdosage in humans. The oral LD_{50} of the drug ranged from 3–8 mg/kg in mice and 38–107 mg/kg in rats. The intravenous LD_{50} of the drug ranged from 6–9 mg/kg in mice and 9–21 mg/kg in rats. LD_{50} values in these ranges are indicative of a drug with a high degree of toxicity.

Dosage and Administration: One drop of IOPIDINE Ophthalmic Solution should be instilled in the scheduled operative eye one hour before initiating anterior segment laser surgery and a second drop should be instilled to the same eye immediately upon completion of the laser surgical procedure. Use a separate container for each single-drop dose and discard each container after use.

How Supplied: IOPIDINE (apraclonidine hydrochloride) Ophthalmic Solution 1% as base is a sterile, isotonic, aqueous solution containing apraclonidine hydrochloride.

Supplied as follows: 0.1 mL in plastic ophthalmic dispensers, packaged two per pouch. These dispensers are enclosed in a foil overwrap as an added barrier to evaporation.

0.1 mL: **NDC** 0065-0660-10

Storage: Store at room temperature. Protect from light.

U.S. Patent No. 4,517,199

ISMOTIC® ℞

(Isosorbide Solution)
45% w/v Solution

Description: ISMOTIC® is a 45% w/v solution of isosorbide in a vanilla-mint flavored vehicle. ISMOTIC is a caramel colored aqueous solution that is chemically stable at room temperature.

Each mL contains: Isosorbide 45% w/v (Isosorbide Concentrate 60.6%), Alcohol 0.3% w/v, Caramel, Creme de Menthe, Malic Acid, Potassium Citrate, Potassium Sorbate, Saccharin Calcium, Sodium Citrate, Sorbitol Solution, Vanilla Concentrate Imitation #20, Potassium Hydroxide (to adjust pH) and Purified Water.

Typical analysis of electrolyte content:
4.6 meq. of Sodium/220 mL ISMOTIC Solution
0.9 meq. of Potassium/220 mL ISMOTIC Solution

Isosorbide, the osmotic agent in ISMOTIC, is a dihydric alcohol with the formula $C_6H_{10}O_4$ represented by the chemical structure:

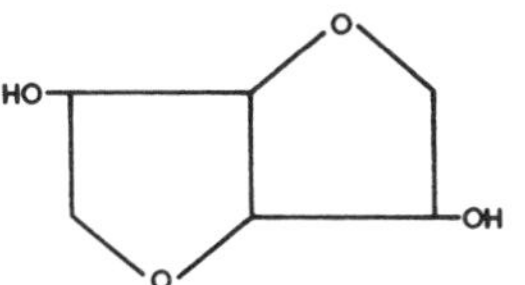

Established name:
Isosorbide

Chemical name:
1,4:3,6-dianhydro-D-glucitol

Clinical Pharmacology: Isosorbide is rapidly absorbed after oral administration. It is essentially non-metabolized, and in the circulation, it contributes to the tonicity of the blood until it is eliminated by the kidney unchanged. While in the blood, isosorbide acts as an osmotic agent to promote redistribution of water toward the circulation with ultimate elimination in the urine. The physical action of ISMOTIC is similar to that of other osmotic agents.

Indications and Usage: For the short-term reduction of intraocular pressure. May be used prior to and after intraocular surgery. May be used to interrupt an acute attack of glaucoma. Use where less risk of nausea and vomiting than that posed by other oral hyperosmotic agents is needed.

Contraindications:
1. Well-established anuria.
2. Severe dehydration.
3. Frank or impending acute pulmonary edema.
4. Severe cardiac decompensation.
5. Hypersensitivity to any component of this preparation.

Warnings:
1. With repeated doses, consideration should be given to maintenance of adequate fluid and electrolyte balance.
2. If urinary output continues to decrease, the patient's clinical status should be closely reviewed. Accumulation of ISMOTIC may result in over-expansion of the extracellular fluid.

Precautions: For oral use only—not for injection. Repetitive doses should be used with caution particularly in patients with diseases associated with salt retention. Ensure that patient's bladder has been emptied prior to surgery.

Usage in Pregnancy: Pregnancy Category B: Reproduction studies have been performed in rats and rabbits and there was no evidence of impaired fertility or harm to the animal fetus due to isosorbide. There are no adequate or well controlled studies on whether this drug may affect fertility in human males or females or have a teratogenic potential or other adverse effect on the fetus. Because animal reproduction studies are not always predictive of human responses, this drug should be used during pregnancy only if clearly needed.

Adverse Reactions: Nausea, vomiting, headache, confusion and disorientation may occur. Occurrences of syncope, gastric discomfort, lethargy, vertigo, thirst, dizziness, hiccups, hypernatremia, hyperosmolarity, irritability, rash, and light-headedness have been reported.

Dosage and Administration: The recommended initial dose 1.5 gm/kg body weight of isosorbide (equivalent to 1.5 mL of ISMOTIC/lb of body weight). The onset of action is usually within 30 minutes while the maximum effect is expected at 1 to $1\frac{1}{2}$ hours. The useful dose range is 1 to 3 gm/kg body weight and the drug effect will persist up to 5 to 6 hours. Use two to four times a day as indicated. Palatability may be improved if the medication is poured over cracked ice and sipped.

Recommended Dosages Are:

Pounds	Milliliters	Pounds	Milliliters
100	150	155	235
105	155	160	240
110	165	165	250
115	170	170	255
120	180	175	265
125	190	180	270
130	195	185	280
135	205	190	285
140	210	195	295
145	220	200	300
150	225		

Storage: Store at room temperature.

How Supplied: Disposable plastic bottles of 220 mL (100 gm of isosorbide/220 mL) for oral use only. NDC 0065-0034-08

MIOSTAT® ℞

(carbachol 0.01%)
Intraocular Solution

Description: MIOSTAT® (Carbachol 0.01%) is a sterile balanced salt solution of Carbachol for intraocular injection. The active ingredient

Continued on next page

Alcon Surgical—Cont.

is represented by the chemical structure: $[NH_2COOCH_2CH_2N^+(CH_3)_3]Cl^-$
Established name: Carbachol
Chemical name: Ethanaminium, 2-[(aminocarbonyl)oxy]-*N,N,N*-trimethyl-, chloride.
Each mL contains: Active: Carbachol 0.01%. Inactive: Sodium Chloride 0.64%, Potassium Chloride 0.075%, Calcium Chloride Dihydrate 0.048%, Magnesium Chloride Hexahydrate 0.03%, Sodium Acetate Trihydrate 0.39%, Sodium Citrate Dihydrate 0.17%, Sodium Hydroxide and/or Hydrochloric Acid (to adjust pH) and Water for Injection.
Clinical Pharmacology: Carbachol is a potent cholinergic (parasympathomimetic) agent.
Indications and Usage: Intraocular use for miosis during surgery.
Contraindications: Should not be used in those persons showing hypersensitivity to any of the components of this preparation.
Warnings: For single-dose intraocular use only. Discard unused portion. Intraocular carbachol 0.01% should be used with caution in patients with acute cardiac failure, bronchial asthma, peptic ulcer, hyperthyroidism, G. I. spasm, urinary tract obstruction and Parkinson's disease.
Adverse Reactions: Side effects such as flushing, sweating, epigastric distress, abdominal cramps, tightness in urinary bladder, and headache have been reported after systemic or topical use of carbachol. These symptoms were not reported following intraocular use of carbachol 0.01% in pre-marketing studies.
Corneal clouding, persistent bullous keratopathy and post-operative iritis following cataract extraction with utilization of intraocular carbachol have been reported in an occasional patient. As with all miotics, retinal detachment has been reported when miotics are used in certain susceptible individuals.
Overdosage: Atropine should be administered parenterally (for dosage refer to Goodman & Gilman or other pharmacology reference).
Dosage and Administration: Aseptically remove the sterile vial from the blister package by peeling the backing paper and dropping the vial onto a sterile tray. Withdraw the contents into a dry sterile syringe, and replace the needle with an atraumatic cannula prior to intraocular irrigation. **No more than one-half milliliter** should be gently instilled into the anterior chamber for the production of satisfactory miosis. It may be instilled before or after securing sutures. Miosis is usually maximal within two to five minutes after application.
How Supplied: In 1.5 mL sterile glass vials packaged twelve to a carton.
NDC 0065-0023-15
Storage: Store at controlled room temperature 15°–30°C (59°–86°F).
Caution: Federal (USA) law prohibits dispensing without prescription.

OSMOGLYN® ℞
[50% Glycerin (volume/volume)]
Oral Osmotic Agent

OSMOGLYN® Oral Osmotic Agent is a 50% v/v (0.628 g/mL) solution of Glycerin in a pleasantly lime flavored aqueous vehicle. It is administered orally, thereby avoiding the hazards of hypertonic agents that must be given intravenously.
Description: Active: glycerin 50% v/v (0.628 g/mL). Preservative: potassium sorbate 0.05%. Inactive: lime flavor, purified water.
Linear structure of Glycerin is: $CH_2OH \cdot CHOH \cdot CH_2OH$.
Chemical name: 1,2,3-Propanetriol.
CAUTION: FEDERAL (USA) LAW PROHIBITS DISPENSING WITHOUT PRESCRIPTION.
Clinical Pharmacology: An oral osmotic agent for reducing intraocular pressure. It adds to the tonicity of the blood until metabolized and eliminated by the kidneys.
Indications and Usage: For the short term reduction of intraocular pressure. May be used prior to and after intraocular surgery. May be used to interrupt an acute attack of glaucoma.
Contraindications: Contraindicated in patients with well-established anuria; severe dehydration; frank or impending acute pulmonary edema; severe cardiac decompensation; and in those with hypersensitivity to any component of this preparation.
Warnings: For oral use only. Not for injection. Caution should be exercised in hypervolemia, confused mental states, and congestive heart disease; and in the dehydrated patient, e.g., certain diabetics.
Precautions: When administered prior to surgery, ensure that the patient's bladder is emptied. Prolonged use may cause excess weight gain. Glycerin should be administered with caution to patients with cardiac, renal or hepatic diseases. Altered hydration may lead to pulmonary edema and/or congestive heart failure.
PREGNACY CATEGORY C. Animal reproduction studies have not been conducted with OSMOGLYN®. It is also not known whether OSMOGLYN can cause fetal harm when administered to a pregnant woman or can affect reproduction capacity. This drug should be given to a pregnant woman only if clearly needed.
Adverse Reactions: Nausea, vomiting, headache, confusion, and disorientation may occur. Severe dehydration, cardiac arrhythmia, or hyperosmolar nonketotic coma which can result in death have been reported.
Dosage and Administration: Usual dosage is 2 to 3 mL of OSMOGLYN per kg of body weight (approximately 4 to 6 oz. per individual), given 1 to 1½ hours prior to surgery.
Storage: Store at room temperature.
How Supplied: 220 mL NDC 0065-0035-08.
Serving over cracked ice with a soda straw improves palatability.

PROFENAL® 1% ℞
(Suprofen)
Sterile Ophthalmic Solution

Description: PROFENAL® (suprofen) 1% ophthalmic solution is a topical nonsteroidal anti-inflammatory product for ophthalmic use. Suprofen chemically is α-methyl-4-(2-thienylcarbonyl) benzeneacetic acid, with an empirical formula of $C_{14}H_{12}O_3S$, and a molecular weight of 260.3. The chemical structure of suprofen is:

PROFENAL Sterile Ophthalmic Solution contains suprofen 1.0% (10 mg/mL), thimerosal 0.005% (0.05 mg/mL), caffeine 2% (20 mg/mL), edetate disodium, dibasic sodium phosphate, monobasic sodium phosphate, sodium chloride, sodium hydroxide and/or hydrochloric acid (to adjust pH to 7.4) and purified water. DM-00
Clincal Pharmacology: Suprofen is one of a series of phenylalkanoic acids that have shown analgesic, antipyretic, and anti-inflammatory activity in animal inflammatory diseases. Its mechanism of action is believed to be through inhibition of the cyclo-oxygenase enzyme that is essential in the biosynthesis of prostaglandins.
Prostaglandins have been shown in many animal models to be mediators of certain kinds of intraocular inflammation. In studies performed on animal eyes, prostaglandins have been shown to produce disruption of the blood aqueous humor barrier, vasodilatation, increased vascular permeability, leukocytosis, and increased intraocular pressure. Prostaglandins appear to play a role in the miotic response produced during ocular surgery by constricting the iris sphincter independently of cholinergic mechanisms. In clinical studies PROFENAL has been shown to inhibit the miosis induced during the course of cataract surgery. PROFENAL could possibly interfere with the miotic effect of intraoperatively administered acetylcholine chloride.
Results from clinical studies indicate that PROFENAL Ophthalmic Solution has no significant effect on intraocular pressure.
There are no data available on the systemic absorption of ocularly applied suprofen. The oral dose of suprofen is 200 mg every four to six hours. If PROFENAL 1% Ophthalmic Solution is applied as two drops (1 mg suprofen) to one eye five times on the day prior to surgery and three times on the day of surgery, the total applied dose over the two days would be about 25 times less than a single 200 mg oral dose.
Indications and Usage: PROFENAL Ophthalmic Solution is indicated for inhibition of intraoperative miosis.
Contraindications: PROFENAL is contraindicated in epithelial herpes simplex keratitis (dendritic keratitis) and in individuals hypersensitive to any component of the medication.
Warnings: The potential exists for cross sensitivity to acetylsalicylic acid and other nonsteroidal anti-inflammatory drugs. Therefore, caution should be used when treating individuals who have previously exhibited sensitivities to these drugs.
With nonsteroidal anti-inflammatory drugs, the potential exists for increased bleeding time due to interference with thrombocyte aggregation. There have been reports that ocularly applied nonsteroidal anti-inflammatory drugs may cause increased bleeding tendency of ocular tissues in conjunction with ocular surgery.
Precautions:
General. Use of oral suprofen has been associated with a syndrome of acute flank pain and generally reversible renal insufficiency, which may present as acute uric acid nephropathy. This syndrome occurs in approximately 1 in 3500 patients and has been reported with as few as one to two doses of a 200 mg capsule. If PROFENAL 1% Ophthalmic Solution is applied as two drops (1 mg suprofen) to one eye five times on the day prior to surgery and three times on the day of surgery, the total applied dose over the two days would be about 25 times less than a single 200 mg oral dose.
Ocular. Patients with histories of herpes simplex keratitis should be monitored closely. PROFENAL is contraindicated in patients with active herpes simplex keratitis.
The possibility of increased ocular bleeding during surgery associated with nonsteroidal anti-inflammatory drugs should be considered.
Carcinogenesis, Mutagenesis, Impairment of Fertility. In an 18-month study in mice, an increased incidence of benign hepatomas occurred in females at a dose of 40 mg/kg/day. Male mice, treated at doses of 2, 5, 10 and 40 mg/kg/day, also had an increased incidence of hepatomas when compared to control animals. No evidence of carcinogenicity was found in long term studies in doses as high as 40 mg/kg/day in the rat and mouse. Based on a battery of mutagenicity tests (Ames, micronucleus, and dominant lethal) suprofen does not appear to have mutagenic potential. Reproductive studies in rats at a dose of up to 40 mg/kg/day revealed no impairment of fertility and only slight reductions of fertility at doses of 80

ng/kg/day. However, testicular atrophy/hypoplasia was observed in a six-month dog study at 80 mg/kg/day) and a 12-month rat study (at 40 mg/kg/day).

Pregnancy Category C. Reproductive studies have been performed in rabbits at doses up to 200 mg/kg/day and in rats at doses up to 80 mg/kg/day. In rats, doses of 40 mg/kg/day and above, and in rabbits, doses of 80 mg/kg/day and above, resulted in an increased incidence of fetal resorption associated with maternal toxicity. There was an increase in stillbirths and a decrease in postnatal survival in pregnant rats treated with suprofen at 2.5 mg/kg/day and above. An increased incidence of delayed parturition occurred in rats. As there are no adequate and well-controlled studies in pregnant women, this drug should be used during pregnancy only if the potential benefit justifies the potential risk to the fetus. Because of the known effect of nonsteroidal anti-inflammatory drugs on the fetal cardiovascular system (closure of ductus arteriosus), use during late pregnancy should be avoided.

Nursing Mothers. Suprofen is excreted in human milk after a single oral dose. Based on measurements of plasma and milk levels in women taking oral suprofen, the milk concentration is about 1% of the plasma level. Because systemic absorption may occur from topical ocular administration, a decision should be considered to discontinue nursing while receiving PROFENAL since the safety of suprofen in human neonates has not been established.

Pediatric Use. Safety and effectiveness in children have not been established.

Drug Interations. Clinical studies with acetylcholine chloride revealed no interference, and there is no known, pharmacological basis for such an interaction. However, with other topical nonsteroidal anti-inflammatory products, there have been reports that acetylcholine chloride and carbachol have been ineffective when used in patients treated with these agents.

Interaction of PROFENAL with other topical ophthalmic medications has not been fully investigated.

Adverse Reactions: **Ocular** —The most frequent adverse reactions reported are burning and stinging of short duration. Instances of discomfort, itching and redness have been reported. Other reactions occurring in less than 0.5% of patients include allergy, iritis, pain, chemosis, photophobia, irritation, and punctate epithelial staining.

Systemic —Systemic reactions related to therapy were not reported in the clinical studies. It is known that some systemic absorption does occur with ocularly applied drugs, and that nonsteroidal anti-inflammatory drugs have been shown to increase bleeding time by interference with thrombocyte aggregation. It is recommended that PROFENAL be used with caution in patients with bleeding tendencies and those taking anticoagulants.

Overdosage: Overdosage will not ordinarily cause acute problems. If accidently ingested, drink fluids to dilute.

Dosage and Administration: On the day of surgery, instill two drops into the conjunctival sac at three, two and one hour prior to surgery. Two drops may be instilled into the conjunctival sac every four hours, while awake, the day preceding surgery.

How Supplied: Sterile ophthalmic solution, 2.5 mL in plastic DROP-TAINER® dispensers.

2.5mL NDC 0065-0348-25

Storage: Store at room temperature.

U.S. Patent Nos. 4,035,376; 4,559,343

STERI-UNITS® Solutions ℞

Description:

STERILE OPHTHALMIC SOLUTIONS FOR SINGLE USE ONLY.

Packaged in Pre-Sterilized Ready to Use Units.

Sterile Unless Opened or Damaged

Except for 2% Fluorescein Sodium, no preservatives are added to the solutions.

Ophthalmic solutions available in STERI-UNITS containers are:

1% or 2% Atropine Sulfate
1%, 2%, 4%, or 8% Pilocarpine Hydrochloride
0.5% Tetracaine Hydrochloride
15% Sulfacetamide Sodium
0.5% Eserine (Physostigmine Salicylate)
5% Homatropine Hydrobromide
2% Fluorescein Sodium

How Supplied: In 2 mL sterile blister packs, packaged 12 to a carton.

VISCOAT® ℞

(Sodium Chondroitin Sulfate-Sodium Hyaluronate)

Sterile Ophthalmic Viscoelastic

Description: VISCOAT® is a sterile, nonpyrogenic, viscoelastic solution of a highly purified, non-inflammatory medium molecular weight fraction of sodium chondroitin sulfate and sodium hyaluronate. VISCOAT® is formulated to a viscosity of 40,000 ± 20,000 cps (at shear rate of 2 sec^{-1}, 25° C). Each 1 mL of VISCOAT® solution contains not more than 40 mg sodium chondroitin sulfate, 30 mg sodium hyaluronate, 0.45 mg sodium dihydrogen phosphate hydrate, 2.00 mg disodium hydrogen phosphate, 4.3 mg sodium chloride (with Water For Injection, USP grade, q.s.). The osmolarity of VISCOAT® is 325mOsM ± 40mOsM; the pH is 7.2 ± 0.2.

Sodium chondroitin sulfate and sodium hyaluronate are quite similar in regard to chemical and physical composition, as each occurs as a large, unbranched chain structure of medium to high molecular weight. Sodium chondroitin sulfate has a mean molecular weight of approximately 22,500 daltons, while sodium hyaluronate exhibits a molecular weight of over 500,000 daltons.

The sugar moieties of these two compounds occur as repeating disaccharide subunits consisting of glucoronic acid in $\beta 1 \rightarrow 3$ linkage with N-acetylgalactosamine for sodium chondroitin sulfate and N-acetylglucosamine for sodium hyaluronate. The subunits are then combined by $\beta 1 \rightarrow 4$ linkage of the amino sugar residue to the glucuronic residue of the next subunit to form large polymers. The two compounds differ in that sodium chondroitin sulfate possesses a sulfate group and a double, rather than a single, negative charge (as in the case of sodium hyaluronate) per repeating disaccharide subunit.

Sodium chondroitin sulfate and sodium hyaluronate are biological polymers centered in the extracellular matrix of animals and humans. The cornea is the ocular tissue having the greatest concentration of sodium chondroitin sulfate, while the vitreous and aqueous humor contain the greatest concentration of sodium hyaluronate.

VISCOAT® is a specific fraction of sodium chondroitin sulfate-sodium hyaluronate that has been developed for use as an ophthalmosurgical aid in anterior segment surgery.

VISCOAT® is completely transparent and exhibits excellent flow properties.

Indications: VISCOAT® is indicated for use as a surgical aid in anterior segment procedures including cataract extraction and intraocular lens implantation. VISCOAT® maintains a deep chamber during anterior segment surgeries, enhances visualization during the surgical procedure, and protects the corneal endothelium and other ocular tissues. The viscoelasticity of the solution maintains the normal position of the vitreous face, thus preventing formation of a postoperative flat chamber.

Contraindications: At the present time, there are no known contraindications to the use of VISCOAT® when used as recommended.

Precautions: Precautions are limited to those normally associated with the surgical procedure being performed. Although sodium hyaluronate and sodium chondroitin sulfate are highly purified biological polymers, the physician should be aware of the potential allergic risks inherent in the use of any biological material.

Adverse Reactions: VISCOAT® has been extremely well tolerated in human and animal studies. A transient rise in intraocular pressure may be expected due to the presence of sodium hyaluronate, which has been shown to effect such a rise (9.8% > 25mmHg during 1–3 days after surgery in human clinical trials).

Clinical Applications: For cataract surgery and intraocular lens implantation, VISCOAT® should be carefully introduced (using a 27 gauge cannula) into the anterior chamber. VISCOAT® may be injected into the chamber prior to or following delivery of the crystalline lens. Instillation of VISCOAT® prior to lens delivery will provide additional protection to the corneal endothelium. Instillation of the solution at this point is significant in that a coating of VISCOAT® may protect the corneal endothelium from possible damage arising from surgical instrumentation during the cataract extraction surgery. VISCOAT® may also be used to coat an intraocular lens as well as the tips of surgical instruments prior to implantation surgery. Additional solution may be injected during anterior segment surgery to fully maintain the chamber or replace any solution lost during the surgical procedure. At the end of the surgical procedure, VISCOAT® may be removed from the eye by thoroughly irrigating and aspirating with a balanced salt solution. Alternatively, VISCOAT® may be left in the eye, when used as directed.

How Supplied: VISCOAT® is a sterile, nonpyrogenic, 0.5 mL, viscoelastic preparation supplied in a disposable syringe with a threaded luer tip. A sterile 27-gauge, disposable, bent, blunt-tip cannula is provided separately. The cannula sheath should be used to firmly attach the cannula to the syringe.

Directions For Use—Syringe Activation

NOTICE: THIS VISCOAT® DELIVERY SYSTEM IS NOT DESIGNED OR INTENDED TO BE ATTACHED TO REUSABLE (METAL-HUBBED) INSTRUMENTS OR TO DISPOSABLE INSTRUMENTS OTHER THAN THE ONE PROVIDED WITH THE PRODUCT.

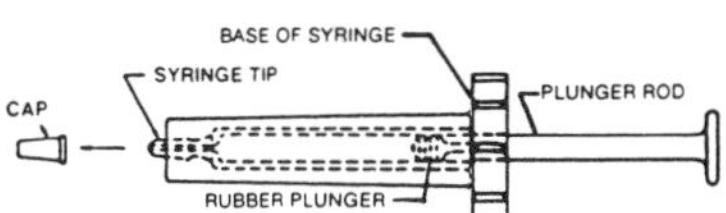

1. PEEL LID FROM BLISTER PACK UNDER ASEPTIC CONDITIONS.
2. REMOVE CAP FROM SYRINGE TIP. (CAP IS ON TIGHTLY.)

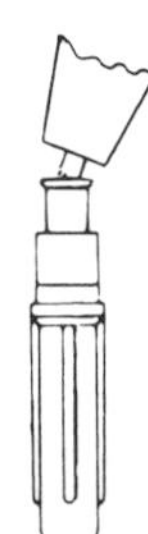

Continued on next page

Alcon Surgical—Cont.

3. INJECT VISCOAT® INTO THE CANNULA HUB UNTIL IT IS ¾ FULL.

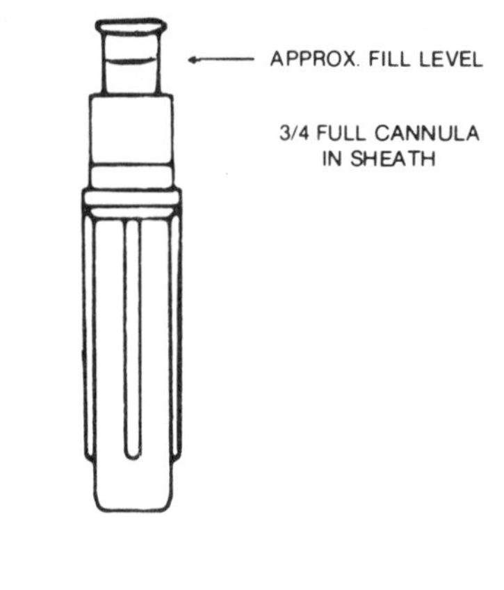

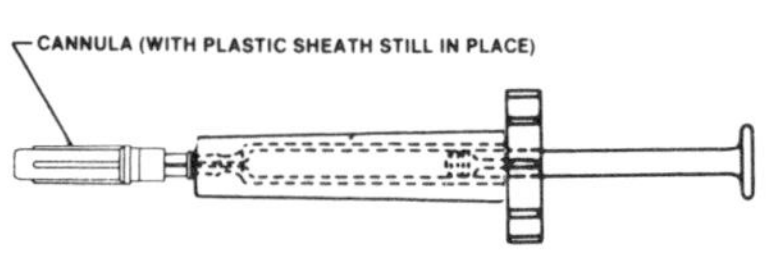

4. INSTALL THE STERILE 27 GAUGE CANNULA. TWIST INTO PLACE AS TIGHTLY AS POSSIBLE.
5. REMOVE PLASTIC SHEATH FROM CANNULA.

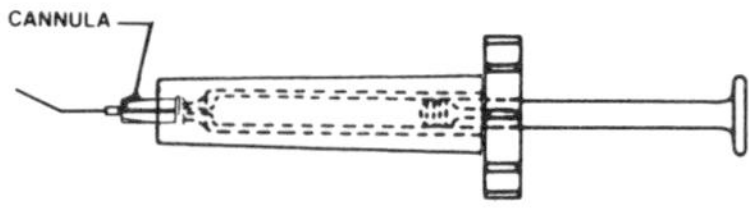

6. GENTLY PUSH PLUNGER ROD TO EXPEL AIR BUBBLES FROM SYRINGE TIP AND CANNULA.

Directions For Use:
FOR INTRAOCULAR USE.
BOTH VISCOAT® AND CANNULA ARE FOR SINGLE USE ONLY.

The syringe assembly is designed only for the injection of the VISCOAT® viscoelastic solution it contains. Use of the syringe assembly for aspiration is not advised.

STORE BETWEEN 2° to 8°C (36° to 46°F). DO NOT FREEZE.

Caution: Federal (USA) law restricts this device to sale by, or on the order of, a licensed physician.

References:

1. CILCO, Inc. Study "Preclinical evaluation of CDS-PLUS: Measurement of intraocular pressure variation after instillation into artifical eyes" (1983).
2. CILCO, Inc. Study "Preclinical evaluation of the protective efficacy of CDS-PLUS on rabbit corneal buttons" (1983).
3. CILCO, Inc. Study "Evaluation of CDS for induction of anaphylaxis in guinea pigs" (1981).
4. Richter, W., Ryde, M. and Zetterstrom, O. Nonimmunogenicity of purified sodium hyaluronate preparation in man. Int Arch Allergy Appl Immunol 59:45–48, 1979.
5. Richter, W. Nonimmunogenicity of purified hyaluronic acid preparations tested by passive cutaneous anaphylaxis. Int Arch Allergy Appl Immunol 47:211–217, 1974.
6. CILCO, Inc. Study "Evaluation of CDS for induction of antibodies in rabbits" (1982).
7. Balazs, E. A. Ultrapure hyaluronic acid and the use thereof. U.S. patent 4,141,973 (1979).
8. CILCO, Inc. Summary of Safety and Efficacy for VISCOAT (1984).

ZOLYSE® ℞
(chymotrypsin)
for Ophthalmic Solution

Description: ZOLYSE® is a lyophilized form of crystalline chymotrypsin, a proteolytic enzyme obtained from the pancreas of the ox. The diluent is a sterile balanced salt solution to be used for reconstituting crystals. Package includes one vial chymotrypsin, 750 U.S.P. Units; and one 9 mL vial of diluent containing: Sodium Chloride 0.49%, Sodium Acetate Trihydrate 0.39%, Sodium Citrate Dihydrate 0.17%, Potassium Chloride 0.075%, Calcium Chloride Dihydrate 0.048%, Magnesium Chloride Hexahydrate 0.03%, Hydrochloric Acid and/or Sodium Hydroxide (to adjust pH), Water for Injection.

Clinical Pharmacology: When instilled into the posterior chamber of the eye, its enzymatic action causes dissolution of zonular fibers attached to the lens.

Indications and Usage: For enzymatic zonulysis in intracapsular lens extraction.

Contraindications: Contraindicated in significant anterior displacement of the lens iris diaphragm with impending vitreous loss or other conditions in which loss of vitreous is a significant problem (e.g., intracapsular extraction of congenital cataracts); and in those persons who have shown hypersensitivity to any component of this preparation.

Warnings: Do not use the reconstituted solution if cloudy or if it contains a precipitate. Do not autoclave the powder or the reconstituted solution—excessive heat, alcohol, and other chemicals used for sterilization inactivate the enzyme. After the operation, discard any unused portion including the diluent. The solution contains no preservative and should not be used for more than one patient.

Precautions: ZOLYSE may produce an acute rise in intraocular pressure following surgery. This is especially true in patients with poor facility of outflow. Use of ZOLYSE is not advised in patients under 20 years of age. Ensure that the synechiae are separated, since this enzyme will not lyse them.

Adverse Reactions: Increases in intraocular pressure, moderate uveitis, corneal edema, and striation have been reported.

Dosage and Administration: Reconstitute immediately prior to the start of surgery. Utilize aseptic technique when inserting a syringe into the rubber stopper of the diluent bottle. It is recommended that the ZOLYSE be reconstituted with 5mL of the diluent to provide the dilution of 150 units of chymotrypsin per mL which is comparable to a 1:5,000 dilution. Following cataract section, irrigate the posterior chamber with the reconstituted ZOLYSE using 0.25 to 0.5 mL (evenly distribute around circumference of the lens). Wait two to four minutes from time of irrigation with ZOLYSE then irrigate the anterior chamber and the corneal wound edges with at least 2mL of the diluent or balanced salt solution.

Note: If zonules are still intact, irrigate with additional ZOLYSE and wait an additional two minutes before flushing with diluent.

How Supplied: Single dose unit carton containing one vial of 750 U.S.P. Units of lyophilized ZOLYSE (chymotrypsin) and one 9mL vial of balanced salt solution diluent. NDC 0065-3020-09.

Storage: Store at 46° to 75°F (8° to 24°C).

Caution: Federal (USA) law prohibits dispensing without prescription.

Allergan Medical Optics
9701 JERONIMO ROAD
IRVINE, CA 92718

AMO® VITRAX® SOLUTION ℞
(SODIUM HYALURONATE)
FOR USE IN ANTERIOR SEGMENT SURGERY ONLY

Description: VITRAX® is a sterile, nonpyrogenic, viscoelastic preparation of a highly purified, noninflammatory, fraction of sodium hyaluronate. VITRAX® contains 30 mg/mL of sodium hyaluronate, dissolved in a physiologically balanced salt solution (pH 7.0 to 7.5). This polymer is made up of repeating disaccharide units of N-acetylglucosamine and sodium glucuronate linked by glycosidic bonds.
Sodium hyaluronate is a physiological substance that is widely distributed in the extracellular matrix of connective tissues in both animals and man. For example, it is present in the vitreous and aqueous humor of the eye, the synovial fluid, the skin and the umbilical cord. Sodium hyaluronates prepared from various human and animal tissues are not chemically different from each other.
VITRAX® SODIUM HYALURONATE HAS BEEN DEVELOPED AS AN OPHTHALMIC SURGICAL AID FOR USE IN ANTERIOR SEGMENT SURGERY.

Indications: VITRAX® sodium hyaluronate is indicated for use as a surgical aid in the following ophthalmic surgical procedures:

- Cataract surgery with an intraocular lens
- Cataract surgery without an intraocular lens
- Secondary intraocular lens implantation
- Corneal transplant surgery
- Glaucoma filtration surgery

VITRAX® aids in filling space left by the loss of ocular fluid or tissues during or after these surgical procedures and reduces endothelial cell damage during these procedures by acting as a protective layer, reducing endothelial trauma from instruments or intraocular lens touch.

Contraindications: There are no known contraindications for the use of VITRAX® Sodium Hyaluronate, other than contraindications for the specific surgical procedure.

Applications:

1. **Cataract Surgery and IOL Implantation**
The required amount of VITRAX® is slowly infused through a needle or cannula into the anterior chamber. The protective effect of VITRAX® as an aid is optimized when the injection is performed prior to cataract extraction and insertion of the IOL and may be performed prior to both intra- and extra capsular cataract procedures. VITRAX® may also be used to coat surgical instruments and the IOL prior to insertion. Additional VITRAX® may be injected during surgery to replace any that is lost during manipulation (see **Precautions**).
2. **Corneal Transplant Surgery**
The corneal button is removed and the anterior chamber filled with VITRAX® until it is level with the surface of the cornea. The donor graft is then placed on top of the VITRAX® and sutured into place. Additional VITRAX® can be used as required to aid in the surgical procedure (see **Precautions**).

3. **Glaucoma Filtration Surgery**
VITRAX® is injected through a corneal paracentesis to restore and maintain the anterior chamber volume during the performance of the trabeculectomy. Additional VITRAX® can be used as required to aid in the surgical procedure (see **Precautions**).

Precautions: Those precautions normally considered during ophthalmic surgery procedure are recommended. There have been reports of significantly increased intraocular pressure following the use of sodium hyaluronate as an ophthalmic surgical aid. For this reason, the following precautions should be considered:

- The intraocular pressure of postoperative patients should be carefully monitored.
- An excess quantity of VITRAX® should not be used.
- VITRAX® should be removed from the anterior chamber at the end of surgery by irrigation or aspiration.
- If the postoperative intraocular pressure increases above expected values, correcting therapy should be administered.

Denaturation and particulate formation in viscoelastics with the repeated use of a reusable cannula has been reported in some studies. A single use cannula such as the one provided in this package should be used when instilling VITRAX® into the eye.

Because VITRAX® is a highly purified fraction extracted from avian tissues and may contain minute amounts of protein, the physician should be aware of potential risks of the type that can occur with the injection of biological material.

Adverse Reactions: The following adverse reactions have been reported following the use of sodium hyaluronate: increased intraocular pressure, secondary glaucoma, postoperative inflammatory reactions.

How Supplied: VITRAX® is a sterile, nonpyrogenic viscoelastic preparation of sodium hyaluronate. It is supplied in a disposable glass syringe delivering 0.65 mL sodium hyaluronate dissolved in a balanced salt solution. Each 1 mL of VITRAX® contains 30 mg sodium hyaluronate, 3.2 mg sodium chloride, 0.75 mg potassium chloride, 0.48 mg calcium chloride, 0.30 mg magnesium chloride, 3.9 mg sodium acetate, 1.7 mg sodium citrate and sterile water for injection USP. The viscosity of VITRAX® is approximately 40,000 cp and the osmolality is nominally 310 mOsm/kg. VITRAX® syringes are aseptically filled and terminally sterilized using ethylene oxide. A single use, 23 gauge blunt tip cannula is also included in the package.

FOR INTRAOCULAR USE

Store at room temperature: 15–30°C (59–86°F).
Protect from freezing.
Protect from light.

References:

1. Bourne, W., Liesegang, T., Walter, R., Illstrup, D: "The effect of sodium hyaluronate on endothelial cell damage during estracapsular cataract extraction and posterior chamber lens implantation." **Am. J. Ophthalmol,** 98:759–762, 1984.
2. Genstler, D., Keates, R. "Am-Visc in extracapsular cataract extraction, "**J. Am. Intraocul. Implant Soc.,** 9:317–320, 1983.
3. Miller, D., Stegmann, R.: "Use of Na-hyaluronate in anterior segment eye surgery," **Am. Intra-Ocular Implant Soc. J.,** 6:13–15, 1980.
4. Richter, W.: "Non-immunogenicity of purified hyaluronic acid preparations tested by passive cutaneous anaphylaxis," **Int. Arch. All,** 47:211–217, 1974.
5. Richter, W., Ryde, M., Zetterston, O.: "Non-immunogenicity of a purified sodium hyaluronate preparation in man," **Int. Arch Appl Immun,** 59:45–48, 1979.
6. Swann, D. A.: "Studies on Hyaluronic Acid. 1. The preparation and properties of rooster comb hyaluronic acid." **Biochim, Biophys. Acta,** 156:17–30, 1968.

Caution: Federal (USA) law restricts this device to sale, distribution, or use by or on the order of a physician.

Distributed By:
ALLERGAN MEDICAL OPTICS
Subsidiary of Allergan, Inc.
Irvine, CA 92718, U.S.A.
Telephone: 1 (800) 366-6554
In Canada Distributed By:
ALLERGAN MEDICAL OPTICS
Div. of ALLERGAN Inc.
625 Cochrane Drive, Suite 1000,
Markham, Ontario, Canada, L3R 9R9
Telephone: 1-800-668-6472

OCUFEN® ℞
(flurbiprofen sodium) 0.03%
LIQUIFILM®
sterile ophthalmic solution

Description: OCUFEN® (flurbiprofen sodium) 0.03% LIQUIFILM® sterile ophthalmic solution is a topical nonsteroidal anti-inflammatory product for ophthalmic use.

Chemical Name: Sodium (±)-2-fluoro-α-methyl-4-biphenyl-acetate dihydrate.

Contains: flurbiprofen sodium ....0.03% with: LIQUIFILM® (polyvinyl alcohol) 1.4%; thimerosal 0.005%; edetate disodium; potassium chloride; sodium chloride; sodium citrate; citric acid; hydrochloric acid and/or sodium hydroxide to adjust the pH; and purified water.

Clinical Pharmacology: Flurbiprofen sodium is one of a series of phenylalkanoic acids that have shown analgesic, antipyretic, and anti-inflammatory activity in animal inflammatory diseases. Its mechanism of action is believed to be through inhibition of the cyclo-oxygenase enzyme that is essential in the biosynthesis of prostaglandins.

Prostaglandins have been shown in many animal models to be mediators of certain kinds of intraocular inflammation. In studies performed on animal eyes, prostaglandins have been shown to produce disruption of the blood-aqueous humor barrier, vasodilatation, increased vascular permeability, leukocytosis, and increased intraocular pressure.

Prostaglandins also appear to play a role in the miotic response produced during ocular surgery by constricting the iris sphincter independently of cholinergic mechanisms. In clinical studies, OCUFEN has been shown to inhibit the miosis induced during the course of cataract surgery.

Results from clinical studies indicate that flurbiprofen sodium has no significant effect upon intraocular pressure.

Indications and Usage: OCUFEN is indicated for the inhibition of intraoperative miosis.

Contraindications: OCUFEN is contraindicated in epithelial herpes simplex keratitis (dendritic keratitis) and in individuals who are hypersensitive to any components of the medication.

Warnings: With nonsteroidal anti-inflammatory drugs, there exists the potential for increased bleeding due to interference with thrombocyte aggregation. There have been reports that OCUFEN may cause increased bleeding of ocular tissues (including hyphemas) in conjunction with ocular surgery. There exists the potential for cross-sensitivity to acetylsalicylic acid and other nonsteroidal anti-inflammatory drugs. Therefore, caution should be used when treating individuals who have previously exhibited sensitivities to these drugs.

Precautions: General: Patients with histories of herpes simplex keratitis should be monitored closely. OCUFEN® is contraindicated in patients with active herpes simplex keratitis. Wound healing may be delayed with the use of OCUFEN . It is recommended that OCUFEN® (flurbiprofen sodium) 0.03% LIQUIFILM® sterile ophthalmic solution be used with caution in surgical patients with known bleeding tendencies or who are receiving other medications which may prolong bleeding time.

Drug Interactions: Interaction of OCUFEN with other topical ophthalmic medications has not been fully investigated.

Although clinical studies with acetylcholine chloride and animal studies with acetylcholine chloride or carbachol revealed no interference, and there is no known pharmacological basis for an interaction, there have been reports that acetylcholine chloride and carbachol have been ineffective when used in patients treated with OCUFEN .

Carcinogenesis, mutagenesis, impairment of fertility: Long-term studies in mice and/or rats have shown no evidence of carcinogenicity or impairment of fertility with flurbiprofen. Long-term mutagenicity studies in animals have not been performed.

Pregnancy:

Pregnancy category C. Flurbiprofen has been shown to be embryocidal, delay parturition, prolong gestation, reduce weight, and/or slightly retard growth of fetuses when given to rats in daily oral doses of 0.4 mg/kg (approximately 185 times the human daily topical dose) and above. There are no adequate and well-controlled studies in pregnant women. OCUFEN should be used during pregnancy only if the potential benefit justifies the potential risk to the fetus.

Nursing Mothers: It is not known whether this drug is excreted in human milk. Because many drugs are excreted in human milk and because of the potential for serious adverse reactions in nursing infants from flurbiprofen sodium, a decision should be made whether to discontinue nursing or to discontinue the drug, taking into account the importance of the drug to the mother.

Pediatric use: Safety and effectiveness in children have not been established.

Adverse Reactions: The most frequent adverse reactions reported with the use of OCUFEN are transient burning and stinging upon instillation and other minor symptoms of ocular irritation.

Increased bleeding tendency of ocular tissues in conjunction with ocular surgery has also been reported.

Overdosage: Overdosage will not ordinarily cause acute problems. If accidentally ingested, drink fluids to dilute.

Dosage and Administration: A total of four (4) drops of OCUFEN should be administered by instilling 1 drop approximately every ½ hour beginning 2 hours before surgery.

How Supplied: OCUFEN® (flurbiprofen sodium) 0.03% solution is supplied in plastic dropper bottles in the following size:

2.5 mL—NDC 11980-801-03

Note: Store at room temperature.

Caution: Federal (U.S.A.) law prohibits dispensing without prescription.

Refer to contents page
for information on
Pharmaceutical Products.

Allergan Pharmaceuticals
A Division of Allergan, Inc.
2525 DUPONT DRIVE
P.O. BOX 19534
IRVINE, CA 92713-9534

ALBALON® ℞
(naphazoline hydrochloride ophthalmic solution) 0.1% with Liquifilm® (polyvinyl alcohol) 1.4% sterile

Description: Naphazoline hydrochloride, an ocular vasoconstrictor, is an imidazoline derivative sympathomimetic amine. It occurs as a white, odorless crystalline powder having a bitter taste and is freely soluble in water and in alcohol.

Chemical Name:
2-(1-Naphthylmethyl)-2-imidazoline monohydrochloride

Contains:
naphazoline HCl..0.1%
with: Liquifilm (polyvinyl alcohol) 1.4%; benzalkonium chloride 0.004%; edetate disodium; citric acid, monohydrate; sodium citrate, dihydrate; sodium chloride; sodium hydroxide to adjust the pH; and purified water. It has a pH of 5.5 to 7.0.

Clinical Pharmacology: Naphazoline constricts the vascular system of the conjunctiva. It is presumed that this effect is due to direct stimulation action of the drug upon the alpha-adrenergic receptors in the arterioles of the conjunctiva, resulting in decreased conjunctival congestion. Naphazoline belongs to the imidazoline class of sympathomimetics.

Indications and Usage: Albalon (naphazoline hydrochloride ophthalmic solution) 0.1% is indicated for use as a topical ocular vasoconstrictor.

Contraindications: Albalon ophthalmic solution is contraindicated in the presence of an anatomically narrow angle or in narrow-angle glaucoma or in persons who have shown hypersensitivity to any component of this preparation.

Warnings: Patients under therapy with MAO inhibitors may experience a severe hypertensive crisis if given a sympathomimetic drug. Use in children, especially infants, may result in CNS depression leading to coma and marked reduction in body temperature.

Precautions:
General: Use with caution in the presence of hypertension, cardiovascular abnormalities, hyperglycemia (diabetes), hyperthyroidism, infection or injury.
Patient Information: Patients should be advised to discontinue the drug and consult a physician if relief is not obtained within 48 hours of therapy. If irritation, blurring or redness persists or increases, or if symptoms of systemic absorption occur, i.e., dizziness, headache, nausea, decrease in body temperature, or drowsiness.
To prevent contaminating the dropper tip and solution, do not touch the eyelids or the surrounding area with the dropper tip of the bottle. If solution changes color or becomes cloudy, do not use.
Drug Interactions: Concurrent use of maprotiline or tricyclic antidepressants and naphazoline may potentiate the pressor effect of naphazoline. Patients under therapy with MAO inhibitors may experience a severe hypertensive crisis if given a sympathomimetic drug. (See WARNINGS).
Pregnancy: Pregnancy Category C: Animal reproduction studies have not been conducted with naphazoline. It is also not known whether naphazoline can cause fetal harm when administered to a pregnant woman or can affect reproduction capacity. Naphazoline should be given to a pregnant woman only if clearly needed.
Nursing Mothers: It is not known whether naphazoline is excreted in human milk. Because many drugs are excreted in human milk, caution should be exercised when naphazoline is administered to a nursing woman.
Pediatric Use: Safety and effectiveness in children have not been established. See "WARNINGS" AND "CONTRAINDICATIONS."

Adverse Reactions:
Ocular: Mydriasis, increased redness, irritation, discomfort, blurring, punctate keratitis, lacrimation, increased intraocular pressure.
Systemic: Dizziness, headache, nausea, sweating, nervousness, drowsiness, weakness, hypertension, cardiac irregularities, and hyperglycemia.

Dosage and Administration: Instill one or two drops in the conjunctival sac(s) every three to four hours as needed.

How Supplied: Albalon® (naphazoline hydrochloride ophthalmic solution) 0.1% with Liquifilm® (polyvinyl alcohol) 1.4% is supplied sterile in plastic dropper bottles in the following size:
15 mL—NDC 11980-154-15

Note: Store at room temperature.
Caution: Federal (U.S.A.) law prohibits dispensing without prescription.

ALBALON-A™ ℞
(naphazoline HCl 0.05%, antazoline phosphate 0.5%) LIQUIFILM® sterile ophthalmic solution

Description: ALBALON-A (naphazoline HCl 0.05%, antazoline phosphate 0.5%) LIQUIFILM® sterile ophthalmic solution is a decongestant/antihistamine for topical ophthalmic use.

Chemical Names:
Naphazoline HCl:
1H-Imidazole,4,5-dihydro-2-(1-naphthalenyl-methyl)-, monohydrochloride.
Antazoline Phosphate:
1H-Imidazole -2- methanamine, 4, 5-dihydro- -N-phenyl-N-(phenylmethyl)-, phosphate (1:1).

Contains:
naphazoline HCl 0.05%
antazoline phosphate 0.5%
with: LIQUIFILM® (polyvinyl alcohol) 1.4%; benzalkonium chloride 0.004%; edetate disodium; povidone; sodium chloride; sodium acetate, acetic acid and/or sodium hydroxide to adjust the pH; and purified water.

Clinical Pharmacology: ALBALON-A combines the effects of the antihistamine, antazoline, and the decongestant, naphazoline. Naphazoline acts as a vasoconstrictor on the conjunctival blood vessels, presumably due to direct action of the drug upon the alpha-adrenergic receptors of the vascular smooth muscle. It is characterized by a relatively long duration of action and belongs to the imidazoline class of sympathomimetics. Antazoline is an H_1-receptor blocking agent which inhibits most smooth muscle responses to histamine.

> **Indications and Usage**
> Based on a review of a related combination of drugs by the National Academy of Sciences—National Research Council and/or other information, the FDA has classified the indications as follows:
> "Possibly" effective: For relief of ocular irritation and/or congestion or for the treatment of allergic, inflammatory, or infectious ocular conditions. Final classification of the less-than-effective indications requires further investigation.

Contraindications: ALBALON-A™ LIQUIFILM® sterile ophthalmic solution is contraindicated in the presence of an anatomically narrow angle or in narrow-angle glaucoma, or in persons hypersensitive to any component in the medication.

Warnings: A severe hypertensive crisis may ensue in patients under MAO inhibitor medication from use of a sympathomimetic drug. CNS depression leading to coma and marked reduction in body temperature may occur in children, especially infants.

Precautions:
General: Use only with caution in the presence of hypertension, cardiac irregularities, hyperglycemia (diabetes), hyperthyroidism, and when other medications are being used.
Information for patients: Do not touch dropper tip to any surface since this may contaminate the solution. Keep bottle tightly closed when not in use. Protect from light.
Carcinogenesis, mutagenesis, impairment of fertility: No studies have been conducted in animals or in humans using naphazoline and/or antazoline to evaluate the potential of these effects.
Pregnancy Category C: Animal reproduction studies have not been conducted with naphazoline and/or antazoline. It is also not known whether naphazoline and/or antazoline can cause fetal harm when administered to a pregnant woman or can affect reproduction capacity. Naphazoline and/or antazoline should be given to a pregnant woman only if clearly needed.
Nursing mothers: It is not known whether these drugs are excreted in human milk. Because many drugs are excreted in human milk, caution should be exercised when naphazoline and/or antazoline is administered to a nursing woman.
Pediatric use: See "Warnings."

Adverse Reactions: Pupillary dilation may occur with an increase in intraocular pressure. Rarely, systemic effects due to absorption may include hypertension, cardiac irregularities, and hyperglycemia. Drowsiness may be experienced in some patients.

Dosage and Administration: One or two drops instilled in each eye every 3 or 4 hours or less frequently, as required to relieve symptoms.

How Supplied: ALBALON-A™ LIQUIFILM® sterile ophthalmic solution is supplied in plastic dropper bottles in the following size:
15 mL—NDC 11980-137-15

Note: Protect from light.
Caution: Federal (U.S.A.) law prohibits dispensing without prescription.

ALLERGAN® EYEWASH OTC

Contains: Benzalkonium chloride 0.004%, edetate disodium 0.01%, mono- and dibasic sodium phosphates, potassium chloride, purified water, sodium chloride.

FDA APPROVED USES

Indications: FOR IRRIGATING THE EYE TO REMOVE LOOSE FOREIGN MATERIAL.

Directions: Flush the affected eye(s) as needed, controlling the flow rate of solution by pressure on the bottle.

Warnings: To avoid contamination, do not touch tip of container to any surface. Replace cap after using. If you experience eye pain, changes in vision, continued redness or irritation of the eye, or if the condition worsens or persists, consult a doctor. Obtain immediate medical treatment for all open wounds in or near the eyes. If the solution changes color or becomes cloudy, do not use. Keep this and all drugs out of the reach of children. In case of accidental ingestion, seek professional assistance or contact a poison control center immediately.

Description: A sterile, buffered, isotonic solution for flushing or irrigating the eye postoperatively or following diagnostic procedures to remove loose foreign material.

How Supplied: 2 fl oz in the Allergan Custom Care Kits.

ATROPINE SULFATE ℞
sterile ophthalmic solution
and
ATROPINE SULFATE S.O.P.®
sterile ophthalmic ointment

Description: ATROPINE SULFATE sterile ophthalmic solution and sterile ophthalmic ointment are topical anticholinergics for ophthalmic use.
Chemical Name: Benzeneacetic acid, α-(hydroxymethyl)-,8-methyl-8-azabicyclo-[3.2.1]oct-3-yl ester, endo-(±)-, sulfate (2:1) (salt), monohydrate.
ATROPINE SULFATE sterile ophthalmic solution contains:
atropine sulfate 1%
with: chlorobutanol (chloral deriv.) 0.5%, boric acid, sodium citrate, hydrochloric acid and/or sodium hydroxide to adjust the pH, and purified water.
ATROPINE SULFATE S.O.P. sterile ophthalmic ointment contains:
atropine sulfate 0.5%, 1%
with: chlorobutanol (chloral deriv.) 0.5%, white petrolatum, mineral oil, petrolatum (and) lanolin alcohol, and purified water.
Clinical Pharmacology: Anticholinergics act directly on the smooth muscles and secretory glands innervated by postganglionic cholinergic nerves. They act by blocking the parasympathomimetic (muscarinic) effects of acetylcholine and parasympathomimetic drugs at these sites.
Indications and Usage: ATROPINE SULFATE is used to produce mydriasis and cycloplegia for refraction, or for iris dilation and relaxation of the ciliary muscle desirable in acute inflammatory conditions of the anterior uveal tract.
Contraindications: Should not be used in patients with glaucoma or a predisposition to narrow-angle glaucoma. Should not be used in children who have previously had a severe systemic reaction to atropine.
Warnings: Excessive use in children and certain susceptible individuals may produce general toxic symptoms. If this occurs, discontinue medication and use appropriate therapy as outlined in "Overdosage" section.
Precautions: Information for patients: Keep out of the reach of children.
Carcinogenesis, mutagenesis, impairment of fertility: No studies have been conducted in animals or in humans to evaluate the potential of these effects.
Pregnancy Category C: Animal reproduction studies have not been performed with atropine. It is also not known whether atropine can cause fetal harm when administered to a pregnant woman or can affect reproduction capacity. Atropine should be given to pregnant women only if clearly needed.
Pediatric use: See "Contraindications" and "Warnings" sections.
Adverse Reactions: Prolonged use may cause general systemic reactions, allergic lid reactions, local irritation, hyperemia, edema, follicular conjunctivitis or dermatitis.
Overdosage: General signs and symptoms of atropine toxicity include dryness of mouth and skin, fever, irritability or delirium, tachycardia, and flushing of the face. Should overdosage in the eye(s) occur, flush the eye(s) with water or normal saline. Use of a topical miotic may be required.
If accidentally ingested induce emesis or gastric lavage with 4% tannic acid. Five mg of pilocarpine should be administered orally at repeated intervals until the mouth is moist. General supportive measures should be used if needed as listed below:
respiratory depression—oxygen and artificial respiration
urinary retention—catheterization
fever—alcohol sponge baths.
Use extreme caution when employing short-acting barbiturates to control excitement.
Dosage and Administration: Solution: 1 or 2 drops in the eyes three times a day or as directed by physician.
Ointment: A small amount in the conjunctival sac once or twice a day or as directed by physician.
How Supplied: ATROPINE SULFATE sterile ophthalmic solution is supplied in plastic dropper bottles in the following concentration and size:
1%–15 mL—NDC 11980-002-15
ATROPINE SULFATE S.O.P.® sterile ophthalmic ointment is supplied in ophthalmic ointment tubes in the following concentrations and sizes:
½%–3.5 g—NDC 0023-0306-04
1%–3.5 g—NDC 0023-0305-04
Note: Store ointment away from heat.
Caution: Federal (U.S.A.) law prohibits dispensing without prescription.

BALANCED SALT SOLUTION ℞

Description: Allergan Balanced Salt Solution is a sterile, physiologically balanced salt solution containing essential ions (Na^+, K^+, Ca^{++}, Mg^{++}, Cl^-, acetate and citrate) to irrigate and help maintain the integrity of the ocular tissues during ophthalmic surgical procedures.
Allergan® Balanced Salt Solution contains:
Sodium Chloride (NaCl) 0.64%
Potassium Chloride (KCl) 0.075%
Calcium Chloride, Dihydrate 0.048%
($CaCl_2 \cdot 2H_2O$)
Magnesium Chloride, Hexahydrate 0.03%
($MgCl_2 \cdot 6H_2O$)
Sodium Acetate, Trihydrate 0.39%
($C_2H_3NaO_2 \cdot 3H_2O$)
Sodium Citrate, Dihydrate 0.17%
($C_6H_5Na_3O_7 \cdot 2H_2O$)
and Water for Injection, with Sodium Hydroxide and/or Hydrochloric Acid to adjust the solution to physiologic pH. The solution is isotonic and has the following electrolyte content (mEq/liter): Na^+156, K^+10, Ca^{++} 6.5, Mg^{++}3, Cl^-129, acetate 29, and citrate 17.
Allergan® Balanced Salt Solution contains no bacteriostat or antimicrobial agent and is intended for use only as a single-dose or short procedure irrigant.
Clinical Pharmacology: Allergan Balanced Salt Solution is a physiological irrigating solution. It does not contain organic agents with pharmacological activity.
Indications and Usage: For irrigation during ophthalmic surgery, and surgical procedures of ears, nose or throat requiring a physiological irrigant.
Warnings: Not for parenteral injection or infusion.
Precautions: Allergan Balanced Salt Solution does not contain a preservative and should not be reused after opening. Do not use if seal assembly or bottle is damaged. Do not use 18 mL bottle if blister package is opened or damaged. Open only under aseptic conditions. Do not use the product unless product is clear.
Adverse Reactions: When used for intraocular surgery in cases where the corneal endothelium is abnormal, excessive intraocular irrigation (as well as other intraocular manipulations) may contribute to endothelial damage and result in bullous keratopathy.
Dosage and Administration: Allergan® Balanced Salt Solution should be used according to standard format for each surgical procedure. Irrigating solutions should be visually inspected for particulate matter and discoloration prior to administration, whenever solution container permits. Tissue damage could result if other drugs are added to product.

- **For 500 mL plastic bottles**

An administration set equipped with an air inlet device in the plastic spike end should be used since the container does not have an airway tube.
1. Flip off plastic cap from the aluminum seal assembly.
2. Using aseptic technique, it is recommended to insert the spike through the larger circular, indented area of the rubber plug.
3. Prior to irrigating, invert the bottle and allow solution to flow entire length of tubing so air is purged from the tubing.

- **For 18 mL plastic bottles**

The Luer-Lok® adapter is designed to accept a needle or other device with reciprocal fitting. For external irrigation, attachment of any device may not be necessary. To use the container in an aseptic field:
1. Remove the backing material to expose the container of Allergan® Balanced Salt Solution.
2. Aseptically transfer the container out of the plastic tray and remove the protective cap with a brisk twist to reveal the adapter.
3. Attach needle or appropriate attachment by pushing it firmly onto the adapter and twisting into place.
4. Prior to use, test the assembly to ensure proper function.

How Supplied: Allergan® Balanced Salt Solution is supplied in sterile plastic bottles:
18 mL NDC 0023-0997-18
500 mL NDC 0023-0997-05
Caution: Federal (U.S.A.) law prohibits dispensing without prescription.
Recommended storage: Room temperature ranges from 46°F to 80°F (8°C–27°C). Avoid excessive heat. Protect from freezing.
Luer-Lok is a registered trademark of Becton-Dickinson.

BETAGAN® ℞
(levobunolol HCl)
Liquifilm®
sterile ophthalmic solution
with C Cap™ Compliance Cap Q.D. and B.I.D.

Description: BETAGAN® (levobunolol HCl) Liquifilm® sterile ophthalmic solution is a noncardioselective beta-adrenoceptor blocking agent for ophthalmic use.
Chemical Name: (-)-5-[3-(*tert*-Butylamino)-2- hydroxypropoxy]-3,4-dihydro- 1(2*H*)-naphthalenone hydrochloride.
Contains:
levobunolol HCl 0.25%, 0.5%
with: Liquifilm® (polyvinyl alcohol) 1.4%; benzalkonium chloride 0.004%; edetate disodium; sodium metabisulfite; sodium phosphate, dibasic; potassium phosphate, monobasic; sodium chloride; hydrochloric acid or sodium hydroxide to adjust the pH; and purified water.
Clinical Pharmacology: Levobunolol HCl is a noncardioselective beta-adrenoceptor blocking agent, equipotent at both $beta_1$ and $beta_2$ receptors. Levobunolol HCl is greater than 60 times more potent than its dextro isomer in its beta-blocking activity, yet equipotent in its potential for direct myocardial depression. Accordingly, the levo isomer, levobunolol HCl, is used. Levobunolol HCl does not have significant local anesthetic (membrane-stabilizing) or intrinsic sympathomimetic activity.
Beta-adrenergic receptor blockade reduces cardiac output in both healthy subjects and patients with heart disease. In patients with severe impairment of myocardial function, beta-adrenergic receptor blockade may inhibit the stimulatory effect of the sympathetic ner-

Continued on next page

Allergan Pharm—Cont.

vous system necessary to maintain adequate cardiac function.
Beta-adrenergic receptor blockade in the bronchi and bronchioles results in increased airway resistance from unopposed para-sympathetic activity. Such an effect in patients with asthma or other bronchospastic conditions is potentially dangerous.
BETAGAN® (levobunolol HCl) has been shown to be an active agent in lowering elevated as well as normal intraocular pressure (IOP) whether or not accompanied by glaucoma. Elevated IOP presents a major risk factor in glaucomatous field loss. The higher the level of IOP, the greater the likelihood of optic nerve damage and visual field loss.
In controlled clinical studies of approximately two years duration, intraocular pressure was well-controlled in approximately 80% of subjects treated with BETAGAN® 0.5% b.i.d. The mean IOP decrease from baseline was between 6.87 mm Hg and 7.81 mm Hg. No significant effects on pupil size, tear production or corneal sensitivity were observed. BETAGAN® at the concentrations tested, when applied topically, decreased heart rate and blood pressure in some patients. The IOP-lowering effect of BETAGAN® was well maintained over the course of these studies.
In a three month clinical study, a single daily application of BETAGAN® 0.5% controlled the IOP of 72% of subjects achieving an overall mean decrease in IOP of 7.0 mm Hg.
In two, separate, controlled studies (one three month and one up to 12 months duration) BETAGAN® 0.25% b.i.d. controlled the IOP of approximately 64% and 70% of the subjects. The overall mean decrease from baseline was 5.4 mm Hg and 5.1 mm Hg respectively. In an open-label study BETAGAN 0.25% q.d. controlled the IOP of 72% of the subjects while achieving an overall mean decrease of 5.9 mm Hg.
The onset of action with one drop of BETAGAN can be detected within one hour after treatment, with maximum effect seen between 2 and 6 hours.
A significant decrease in IOP can be maintained for up to 24 hours following a single dose.
The primary mechanism of the ocular hypotensive action of levobunolol HCl in reducing IOP is most likely a decrease in aqueous humor production. BETAGAN® reduces IOP with little or no effect on pupil size or accommodation, in contrast to the miosis which cholinergic agents are known to produce. The blurred vision and night blindness often associated with miotics would not be expected and have not been reported with the use of BETAGAN®. This is particularly important in cataract patients with central lens opacities who would experience decreased visual acuity with pupillary constriction.
Indications and Usage: BETAGAN® 0.25% and 0.5% have been shown to be effective in lowering intraocular pressure and may be used in patients with chronic open-angle glaucoma or ocular hypertension.
Contraindications: BETAGAN® is contraindicated in those individuals with bronchial asthma or with a history of bronchial asthma, or severe chronic obstructive pulmonary disease (see WARNINGS); sinus bradycardia, second and third degree atrioventricular block, overt cardiac failure (see WARNINGS), cardiogenic shock; or hypersensitivity to any component of this product.
Warnings: As with other topically applied ophthalmic drugs, BETAGAN® may be absorbed systemically. The same adverse reactions found with systemic administration of beta-adrenergic blocking agents may occur with topical administration. For example, severe respiratory reactions and cardiac reactions, including death due to bronchospasm in patients with asthma, and rarely death in association with cardiac failure, have been reported with topical application of beta-adrenergic blocking agents (see CONTRAINDICATIONS).
Cardiac Failure: Sympathetic stimulation may be essential for support of the circulation in individuals with diminished myocardial contractility, and its inhibition by beta-adrenergic receptor blockade may precipitate more severe failure.
In Patients Without a History of Cardiac Failure: Continued depression of the myocardium with beta-blocking agents over a period of time can, in some cases, lead to cardiac failure. At the first sign or symptom of cardiac failure, BETAGAN® should be discontinued.
Non-allergic Bronchospasm: In patients with non-allergic bronchospasm or with a history of non-allergic bronchospasm (e.g., chronic bronchitis, emphysema), BETAGAN® should be administered with caution since it may block bronchodilation produced by endogenous and exogenous catecholamine stimulation of $beta_2$ receptors.
Major Surgery: The necessity or desirability of withdrawal of beta-adrenergic blocking agents prior to major surgery is controversial. Beta-adrenergic receptor blockade impairs the ability of the heart to respond to beta-adrenergically mediated reflex stimuli. This may augment the risk of general anesthesia in surgical procedures. Some patients receiving beta-adrenergic receptor blocking agents have been subject to protracted severe hypotension during anesthesia. For these reasons, in patients undergoing elective surgery, gradual withdrawal of beta-adrenergic receptor blocking agents may be appropriate.
If necessary during surgery, the effects of beta-adrenergic blocking agents may be reversed by sufficient doses of such agonists as isoproterenol, dopamine, dobutamine or levarterenol (See OVERDOSAGE).
Diabetes Mellitus: Beta-adrenergic blocking agents should be administered with caution in patients subject to spontaneous hypoglycemia or to diabetic patients (especially those with labile diabetes) who are receiving insulin or oral hypoglycemic agents. Beta-adrenergic receptor blocking agents may mask the signs and symptoms of acute hypoglycemia.
Thyrotoxicosis: Beta-adrenergic blocking agents may mask certain clinical signs (e.g., tachycardia) of hyperthyroidism. Patients suspected of developing thyrotoxicosis should be managed carefully to avoid abrupt withdrawal of beta-adrenergic blocking agents, which might precipitate a thyroid storm.
Contains sodium metabisulfite, a sulfite that may cause allergic-type reactions including anaphylactic symptoms and life-threatening or less severe asthmatic episodes in certain susceptible people. The overall prevalence of sulfite sensitivity in the general population is unknown and probably low. Sulfite sensitivity is seen more frequently in asthmatic than in nonasthmatic people.
Precautions:
General: BETAGAN® (levobunolol HCl) Liquifilm® sterile ophthalmic solution should be used with caution in patients with known hypersensitivity to other beta-adrenoceptor blocking agents.
Use with caution in patients with known diminished pulmonary function.
In patients with angle-closure glaucoma, the immediate objective of treatment is to reopen the angle. This requires, in most cases, constricting the pupil with a miotic. BETAGAN® has little or no effect on the pupil. When BETAGAN® is used to reduce elevated intraocular pressure in angle-closure glaucoma, it should be used with a miotic and not alone.
Muscle Weakness: Beta-adrenergic blockade has been reported to potentiate muscle weakness consistent with certain myasthenic symptoms (e.g., diplopia, ptosis and generalized weakness).
Drug Interactions: BETAGAN® should be used with caution in patients who are receiving a beta-adrenergic blocking agent orally, because of the potential for additive effects on systemic beta-blockade.
Although BETAGAN® used alone has little or no effect on pupil size, mydriasis resulting from concomitant therapy with BETAGAN® and epinephrine may occur.
Close observation of the patient is recommended when a beta-blocker is administered to patients receiving catecholamine-depleting drugs such as reserpine, because of possible additive effects and the production of hypotension and/or marked bradycardia, which may produce vertigo, syncope, or postural hypotension.
Animal Studies: No adverse ocular effects were observed in rabbits administered BETAGAN® topically in studies lasting one year in concentrations up to 10 times the human dose concentration.
Carcinogenesis, mutagenesis, impairment of fertility: In a lifetime oral study in mice, there were statistically significant ($p \leq 0.05$) increases in the incidence of benign leiomyomas in female mice at 200 mg/kg/day (14,000 times the recommended human dose for glaucoma), but not at 12 or 50 mg/kg/day (850 and 3,500 times the human dose). In a two-year oral study of levobunolol HCl in rats, there was a statistically significant ($p \leq 0.05$) increase in the incidence of benign hepatomas in male rats administered 12,800 times the recommended human dose for glaucoma. Similar differences were not observed in rats administered oral doses equivalent to 350 times to 2,000 times the recommended human dose for glaucoma.
Levobunolol did not show evidence of mutagenic activity in a battery of microbiological and mammalian *in vitro* and *in vivo* assays.
Reproduction and fertility studies in rats showed no adverse effect on male or female fertility at doses up to 1,800 times the recommended human dose for glaucoma.
Pregnancy Category C: Fetotoxicity (as evidenced by a greater number of resorption sites) has been observed in rabbits when doses of levobunolol HCl equivalent to 200 and 700 times the recommended dose for the treatment of glaucoma were given. No fetotoxic effects have been observed in similar studies with rats at up to 1,800 times the human dose for glaucoma. Teratogenic studies with levobunolol in rats at doses up to 25 mg/kg/day (1,800 times the recommended human dose for glaucoma) showed no evidence of fetal malformations. There were no adverse effects on postnatal development of offspring. It appears when results from studies using rats and studies with other beta-adrenergic blockers are examined, that the rabbit may be a particularly sensitive species. There are no adequate and well-controlled studies in pregnant women. BETAGAN® should be used during pregnancy only if the potential benefit justifies the potential risk to the fetus.
Nursing Mothers: It is not known whether this drug is excreted in human milk. Systemic beta-blockers and topical timolol maleate are known to be excreted in human milk. Caution should be exercised when BETAGAN® is administered to a nursing woman.
Pediatric Use: Safety and effectiveness in children have not been established.
Adverse Reactions: In clinical trials, the use of BETAGAN® has been associated with transient ocular burning and stinging in about

1 in 3 patients, and with blepharoconjunctivitis in about 1 in 20 patients. Decreases in heart rate and blood pressure have been reported (see CONTRAINDICATIONS and WARNINGS).

The following adverse effects have been reported rarely with the use of BETAGAN®: iridocyclitis, headache, transient ataxia, dizziness, lethargy, urticaria and pruritus.

Decreased corneal sensitivity has been noted in a small number of patients. Although levobunolol has minimal membrane-stabilizing activity, there remains a possibility of decreased corneal sensitivity after prolonged use.

The following additional adverse reactions have been reported with ophthalmic use of $beta_1$ and $beta_2$ (non-selective) adrenergic receptor blocking agents: BODY AS A WHOLE: Headache. CARDIOVASCULAR: Arrhythmia, syncope, heart block, cerebral vascular accident, cerebral ischemia, congestive heart failure, palpitation. DIGESTIVE: Nausea. PSYCHIATRIC: Depression. SKIN: Hypersensitivity, including localized and generalized rash. RESPIRATORY: Bronchospasm (predominantly in patients with pre-existing bronchospastic disease), respiratory failure. ENDOCRINE: Masked symptoms of hypoglycemia in insulin-dependent diabetics (see WARNINGS). SPECIAL SENSES: Signs and symptoms of keratitis, blepharoptosis, visual disturbances including refractive changes (due to withdrawal of miotic therapy in some cases), diplopia, ptosis.

Other reactions associated with the oral use of non-selective adrenergic receptor blocking agents should be considered potential effects with ophthalmic use of these agents.

Overdosage: No data are available regarding overdosage in humans. Should accidental ocular overdosage occur, flush eye(s) with water or normal saline. If accidentally ingested, efforts to decrease further absorption may be appropriate (gastric lavage).

The most common signs and symptoms to be expected with overdosage with administration of a systemic beta-adrenergic blocking agent are symptomatic bradycardia, hypotension, bronchospasm, and acute cardiac failure. Should these symptoms occur, discontinue BETAGAN® therapy and initiate appropriate supportive therapy. The following supportive measures should be considered:

1. Symptomatic bradycardia: Use atropine sulfate intravenously in a dosage of 0.25 mg to 2 mg to induce vagal blockade. If bradycardia persists, intravenous isoproterenol hydrochloride should be administered cautiously. In refractory cases, the use of a transvenous cardiac pacemaker should be considered.
2. Hypotension: Use sympathomimetic pressor drug therapy, such as dopamine, dobutamine or levarterenol. In refractory cases, the use of glucagon hydrochloride may be useful.
3. Bronchospasm: Use isoproterenol hydrochloride. Additional therapy with aminophylline may be considered.
4. Acute cardiac failure: Conventional therapy with digitalis, diuretics and oxygen should be instituted immediately. In refractory cases, the use of intravenous aminophylline is suggested. This may be followed, if necessary, by glucagon hydrochloride, which may be useful.
5. Heart block (second or third degree): Use isoproterenol hydrochloride or a transvenous cardiac pacemaker.

Dosage and Administration: The recommended starting dose is one to two drops of BETAGAN® 0.5% in the affected eye(s) once a day. Typical dosing with BETAGAN 0.25% is one to two drops twice daily. In patients with more severe or uncontrolled glaucoma, BETAGAN 0.5% can be administered b.i.d. As with any new medication, careful monitoring of patients is advised.

Dosages above one drop of Betagan 0.5% b.i.d. are not generally more effective. If the patient's IOP is not at a satisfactory level on this regimen, concomitant therapy with dipivefrin and/or epinephrine, and/or pilocarpine and other miotics, and/or systemically administered carbonic anhydrase inhibitors, such as acetazolamide, can be instituted.

How Supplied: BETAGAN® (levobunolol HCl) Liquifilm® sterile ophthalmic solution is supplied in white opaque plastic dropper bottles as follows:

Betagan 0.25%:
C Cap™ Compliance Cap
B.I.D. (twice daily)
5 mL—11980-469-25
10 mL—11980-469-20

Betagan 0.5%:
Standard Cap
2 mL—NDC 11980-252-02
C CAP™ Compliance Cap
Q.D. (once daily)
5 mL—NDC 11980-252-65
10 mL—NDC 11980-252-60
15 mL—NDC 11980-252-61
C Cap™ Compliance Cap
B.I.D. (twice daily)
5 mL—NDC 11980-252-25
10 mL—NDC 11980-252-20
15 mL—NDC 11980-252-21

NOTE: Protect from light. Store at controlled room temperature 15°–30°C (59°–86°F).

Caution: Federal (U.S.A.) law prohibits dispensing without prescription.

C Cap™ Compliance Cap Patient Instructions

Instructions for use:

1. On the first usage, make sure the number "1" or the correct day of the week appears in the window. If not, click the cap to the right station.
2. Remove the cap and apply medication.
3. Replace the cap. Hold the C Cap between your thumb and forefinger. Now rotate the bottle until the cap clicks to the next station.
4. When it's time to take your next dose, repeat steps 2 and 3.

Important Notes: Don't try to catch up on missed doses by applying more than one dose at a time. Each time you replace the cap, turn it until you hear the click. The number in the window specifies your next dosage.

BLEPH®-10 ℞

(sulfacetamide sodium)
Liquifilm **®**
sterile ophthalmic solution

Description: Bleph-10 (sulfacetamide sodium) Liquifilm sterile ophthalmic solution is a topical anti-infective agent for ophthalmic use.

Structural Formula:

$$NH_2-C_6H_4-SO_2N(Na)COCH_3 \cdot H_2O$$

Chemical Name:
N-Sulfanilylacetamide monosodium salt monohydrate.

Contains:
Sulfacetamide sodium 10.0%
with: Liquifilm® (polyvinyl alcohol) 1.4%; thimerosal (0.005%); polysorbate 80; sodium thiosulfate; potassium phosphate monobasic; edetate disodium; sodium phosphate dibasic, anhydrous; hydrochloric acid to adjust the pH; and purified water.

Clinical Pharmacology: Sulfonamides exert a bacteriostatic effect against a wide range of gram-positive and gram-negative organisms including pyogenic cocci, gonococcus, *Escherichia coli* and Koch-Weeks bacillus. Sulfonamides act by restricting, through competition with para-amino-benzoic acid, the synthesis of folic acid which bacteria require for growth.

Indications and Usage: Bleph-10 is indicated for the treatment of conjunctivitis, corneal ulcer and other superficial ocular infections from susceptible microorganisms, and as adjunctive treatment in systemic sulfonamide therapy of trachoma.

Contraindications: Bleph-10 is contraindicated in individuals who have a hypersensitivity to sulfonamide preparations or to any of the ingredients of the preparation.

Warnings: A significant percentage of staphylococcal isolates are completely resistant to sulfa drugs.

Precautions: Sulfacetamide preparations are incompatible with silver preparations. Nonsusceptible organisms, including fungi, may proliferate with the use of this preparation. Sulfonamides are inactivated by the amino-benzoic acid present in purulent exudates. Sensitization may occur when a sulfonamide is readministered irrespective of the route of administration, and cross sensitivity between different sulfonamides may occur. If signs of sensitivity or other untoward reactions occur, discontinue use of the preparation.

Adverse Reactions: Exact incidence figures are not available since no denominator of treated patients is available. Reactions occurring most often from anti-infective agents are allergic sensitizations. Instances of Stevens-Johnson syndrome and systemic lupus erythematosus (in one case producing a fatal outcome) have been reported following the use of ophthalmic sulfonamide-containing preparations.

The development of secondary infection has occurred after the use of antimicrobials.

Dosage and Administration: One or two drops into lower conjunctival sac every 2 to 3 hours during the day, less often at night.

How Supplied: Bleph®-10 (sulfacetamide sodium) Liquifilm® sterile ophthalmic solution is supplied in plastic dropper bottles in the following sizes:

2.5 mL—**NDC 0023-0011-03**
5 mL—**NDC 0023-0011-05**
15 mL—**NDC 0023-0011-15**

Note: Store between 8°–25°C (46°–77°F). Protect from light. Do not use if solution is discolored (dark brown).

Caution: Federal law prohibits dispensing without description.

BLEPH®-10 ℞

(sulfacetamide sodium ophthalmic ointment) 10%

Description: BLEPH®-10 (sulfacetamide sodium ophthalmic ointment) 10% is a topical anti-infective agent for ophthalmic use.

Chemical Name: N-Sulfanilylacetamide monosodium salt monohydrate.

Contains:
Sulfacetamide sodium 10%
with: phenylmercuric acetate (0.0008%), white petrolatum, mineral oil, and petrolatum (and) lanolin alcohol.

Clinical Pharmacology: Sulfonamides exert a bacteriostatic effect against a wide range of gram-positive and gram-negative organisms by restricting, through competition with para-aminobenzoic acid, the synthesis of folic acid which bacteria require for growth.

Indications and Usage: BLEPH-10 is indicated for the treatment of conjunctivitis, corneal ulcer and other superficial ocular infections caused by susceptible microorganisms, and as adjunctive treatment in systemic sulfonamide therapy of trachoma.

Contraindications: BLEPH-10 is contraindicated in individuals who have a hypersensi-

Continued on next page

Allergan Pharm—Cont.

tivity to sulfonamide preparations or to any of the ingredients of the preparation.

Precautions: Sulfacetamide preparations are incompatible with silver preparations. Nonsusceptible organisms, including fungi, may proliferate with the use of this preparation. Sulfonamides are inactivated by the aminobenzoic acid present in purulent exudates. Sensitization may occur when a sulfonamide is readministered irrespective of the route of administration, and cross-sensitivity between different sulfonamides may occur. If signs of sensitivity or other untoward reactions occur, discontinue use of the preparation.

Ophthalmic ointments may retard corneal healing.

Adverse Reactions: Sulfacetamide sodium may cause local irritation, stinging and burning. While the irritation may be transient, occasionally, use of the medication has to be discontinued.

Although sensitivity reactions to sulfacetamide sodium are rare, an isolated incident of Stevens-Johnson syndrome was reported in a patient who had experienced a previous bullous drug reaction to an orally administered sulfonamide, and a single instance of local hypersensitivity was reported which progressed to a fatal syndrome resembling systemic lupus erythematosus.

Dosage and Administration: Apply a small amount of ointment in the conjunctival sac 4 times daily and at bedtime.

How Supplied: BLEPH®-10 (sulfacetamide sodium ophthalmic ointment) 10% is supplied sterile in ophthalmic ointment tubes in the following size:

3.5 g—NDC 0023-0311-04

Note: Store away from heat.

Caution: Federal (U.S.A.) law prohibits dispensing without description.

BLEPHAMIDE® ℞
(sulfacetamide sodium - prednisolone acetate)
LIQUIFILM®
sterile ophthalmic suspension
and
BLEPHAMIDE®
(sulfacetamide sodium—prednisolone acetate)
S.O.P.®
sterile ophthalmic ointment

Description: BLEPHAMIDE® is a topical anti-inflammatory/anti-infective combination product for ophthalmic use.

Chemical Names:

Sulfacetamide sodium: N-Sulfanilylacetamide monosodium salt monohydrate

Prednisolone acetate: 11β, 17, 21-Trihydroxypregna-1, 4-diene-3, 20-dione 21-acetate

BLEPHAMIDE LIQUIFILM sterile ophthalmic suspension contains:

sulfacetamide sodium 10.0%
prednisolone acetate
(microfine suspension) 0.2%

with: LIQUIFILM® (polyvinyl alcohol) 1.4%; benzalkonium chloride; polysorbate 80; edetate disodium; sodium phosphate; potassium phosphate, monobasic; sodium thiosulfate; hydrochloric acid and/or sodium hydroxide to adjust the pH; and purified water.

BLEPHAMIDE SOP sterile ophthalmic ointment contains:

sulfacetamide sodium 10.0%
prednisolone acetate 0.2%
(microfine suspension)

with: phenylmercuric acetate (0.0008%), mineral oil, white petrolatum and petrolatum (and) lanolin alcohol.

Clinical Pharmacology: Corticosteroids suppress the inflammatory response to a variety of agents and they probably delay or slow healing. Since corticosteroids may inhibit the body's defense mechanism against infection, a concomitant antimicrobial drug may be used when this inhibition is considered to be clinically significant in a particular case.

The anti-infective component in BLEPHAMIDE is included to provide action against specific organisms susceptible to it. Sulfacetamide sodium is considered active against the following microorganisms: **Escherichia coli, Staphylococcus aureus, Streptococcus pneumoniae, Streptococcus (viridans group), Pseudomonas** species, **Haemophilus influenzae, Klebsiella** species, and **Enterobacter** species.

When a decision to administer both a corticosteroid and an antimicrobial is made, the administration of such drugs in combination has the advantage of greater patient compliance and convenience, with the added assurance that the appropriate dosage of both drugs is administered. When both types of drugs are in the same formulation, compatibility of ingredients is assured and the correct volume of drug is delivered and retained. The relative potency of corticosteroids depends on the molecular structure, concentration, and release from the vehicle.

Indications and Usage: A steroid/anti-infective combination is indicated for steroid-responsive inflammatory ocular conditions for which a corticosteroid is indicated and where bacterial infection or a risk of bacterial ocular infection exists.

Ocular steroids are indicated in inflammatory conditions of the palpebral and bulbar conjunctiva, cornea, and anterior segment of the globe where the inherent risk of steroid use in certain infective conjunctivitides is accepted to obtain a diminution in edema and inflammation. They are also indicated in chronic anterior uveitis and corneal injury from chemical, radiation, or thermal burns or penetration of foreign bodies.

The use of a combination drug with an anti-infective component is indicated where the risk of infection is high or where there is an expectation that potentially dangerous numbers of bacteria will be present in the eye.

The particular anti-infective drug in this product is active against the following common bacterial eye pathogens: **Escherichia coli, Staphylococcus aureus, Streptococcus pneumoniae, Streptococcus (viridans group), Pseudomonas** species, **Haemophilus influenzae, Klebsiella** species, and **Enterobacter** species. This product does not provide adequate coverage against **Neisseria** species and **Serratia marcescens.**

Contraindications: Epithelial herpes simplex keratitis (dendritic keratitis), vaccinia, varicella, and many other viral diseases of the cornea and conjunctiva. Mycobacterial infection of the eye. Fungal diseases of the ocular structures. Hypersensitivity to a component of the medication. (Hypersensitivity to the antimicrobial component occurs at a higher rate than for other components.)

The use of these combinations is always contra-indicated after uncomplicated removal of a corneal foreign body.

Warnings: Prolonged use may result in glaucoma, with damage to the optic nerve, defects in visual acuity and fields of vision, and in posterior subcapsular cataract formation. Prolonged use may suppress the host response and thus increase the hazard of secondary ocular infections. In those diseases causing thinning of the cornea or sclera, perforations have been known to occur with the use of topical steroids. In acute purulent conditions of the eye, steroids may mask infection or enhance existing infection. If these products are used for 10 days or longer, intraocular pressure should be routinely monitored even though it may be difficult in children and uncooperative patients. Employment of a steroid medication in the treatment of herpes simplex requires great caution.

A significant percentage of staphylococcal isolates are completely resistant to sulfa drugs.

Precautions: The initial prescription and renewal of the medication order beyond 20 milliliters (BLEPHAMIDE suspension) or 8 grams (BLEPHAMIDE ointment) should be made by a physician only after examination of the patient with the aid of magnification, such as slit lamp biomicroscopy and, where appropriate, fluorescein staining.

The possibility of fungal infections of the cornea should be considered after prolonged steroid dosing.

Ophthalmic ointments may retard corneal healing.

Adverse Reactions: Adverse reactions have occurred with steroid/anti-infective combination drugs which can be attributed to the steroid component, the anti-infective component, or the combination. Exact incidence figures are not available since no denominator of treated patients is available.

Reactions occurring most often from the presence of the anti-infective ingredient are allergic sensitizations. The reactions due to the steroid component in decreasing order of frequency are: elevation of intraocular pressure (IOP) with possible development of glaucoma, and infrequent optic nerve damage; posterior subcapsular cataract formation; and delayed wound healing.

Secondary infection: The development of secondary infection has occurred after use of combinations containing steroids and antimicrobials. Fungal infections of the cornea are particularly prone to develop coincidentally with long-term applications of steroid. The possibility of fungal invasion must be considered in any persistent corneal ulceration where steroid treatment has been used.

Secondary bacterial ocular infection following suppression of host responses also occurs.

Dosage and Administration: BLEPHAMIDE suspension: Optimal dosage is 1 drop two to four times daily, depending upon the severity of the condition.

In general, during early or acute stages of blepharitis, BLEPHAMIDE® LIQUIFILM® sterile ophthalmic suspension produces results most rapidly—and most efficiently—with instillation directly into the eye, with the excess spread on the lid (Method I). When the condition is confined to the lid, however, BLEPHAMIDE may be applied directly to the site of the lesions (Method II).

METHOD I: In the Eye and On the Lid

1. Wash hands carefully. Tilt head back and drop **1 drop** into the eye.
2. Close the eye and spread the excess medication present after closing the eye on the full length of the upper and lower lids.
3. Do not wipe any of the medication off the lids. It will dry completely in 4 or 5 minutes to a clear film that remains on the lids for several hours—it cannot be seen by others, nor will it interfere with vision.
4. The medication should be washed off the lids once or twice a day. **However, it should be reapplied after each washing.**

METHOD II: On the Lid

1. Wash hands carefully. With head tilted back and **eye closed,** drop 1 drop onto the lid—preferably at the corner of the eye close to the nose.
2. Spread the medication over the full length of the upper and lower lids.
3. Do not wipe away any medication—it will dry in 4 to 5 minutes to a clear, invisible film which will remain on the lids for several hours.
4. The medication should be washed off the lids once or twice a day. **However, it should be reapplied after each washing.**

Not more than 20 milliliters should be prescribed initially and the prescription should not be refilled without further evaluation as outlined in **Precautions** above.

Dosage and Administration: BLEPHAMIDE ointment: A small amount should be applied in the conjunctival sac three or four times daily and once or twice at night. Not more than 8 grams should be prescribed initially and the prescription should not be refilled without further evaluation as outlined in **Precautions** above.

How Supplied: BLEPHAMIDE® LIQUIFILM® is supplied in plastic dropper bottles in the following sizes:

2.5 mL—NDC 11980-022-03
5 mL—NDC 11980-022-05
10 mL—NDC 11980-022-10

Note: Protect from freezing. Shake well before using.

How Supplied: BLEPHAMIDE® S.O.P.® sterile ophthalmic ointment is supplied in ophthalmic ointment tubes in the following size:

3.5 g—NDC 0023-0313-04

Note: Store away from heat.

Caution: Federal (U.S.A.) law prohibits dispensing without prescription.

CELLUFRESH™ OTC

(carboxymethylcellulose sodium) 0.5%
Lubricant Ophthalmic Solution

Contains: Active: Carboxymethylcellulose sodium 0.5%. Inactive: calcium chloride, magnesium chloride, potassium chloride, purified water, sodium chloride, and sodium lactate. May also contain hydrochloric acid or sodium hydroxide to adjust pH.

FDA APPROVED USES

INDICATIONS: FOR USE AS A LUBRICANT TO PREVENT FURTHER IRRITATION OR TO RELIEVE DRYNESS OF THE EYE.

Warnings: To avoid contamination, do not touch tip of container to any surface. Do not reuse. Once opened, discard. If you experience eye pain, changes in vision, continued redness or irritation of the eye, or if the condition worsens or persists for more than 72 hours, discontinue use and consult a doctor. If solution changes color or becomes cloudy, do not use. Keep this and all medications out of the reach of children. In case of accidental ingestion, seek professional assistance or contact a Poison Control Center immediately.

Directions: Instill 1 or 2 drops in the affected eye(s) as needed.

Note: Do not touch unit-dose tip to eye.

How Supplied: In sterile, preservative-free, disposable, single-use containers of 0.01 fluid ounce each in the following size:

30 single-use containers—NDC 0023-5487-30

CELLUVISC® OTC

(carboxymethylcellulose sodium) 1%
Lubricant Ophthalmic Solution

Celluvisc is a preservative free ophthalmic lubricant formulated specifically for the patient who needs frequent relief from dryness of the eye:

- Special lubricating formula helps maintain the natural electrolyte balance of your tears.
- Preservative free for no preservative-induced irritation.
- Single, unit-dose containers for greater convenience.

Contains: Active: Carboxymethylcellulose sodium 1%. Inactives: calcium chloride, potassium chloride, purified water, sodium chloride, and sodium lactate.

FDA APPROVED USES

Indications: FOR USE AS A LUBRICANT TO PREVENT FURTHER IRRITATION OR TO RELIEVE DRYNESS OF THE EYE.

Warnings: To avoid contamination, do not touch tip of container to any surface. Do not reuse. Once opened, discard. If you experience eye pain, changes in vision, continued redness or irritation of the eye, or if the condition worsens or persists for more than 72 hours, discontinue use and consult a doctor. If solution changes color or becomes cloudy, do not use. Keep this and all drugs out of the reach of children. In case of accidental ingestion, seek professional assistance or contact a poison control center immediately.

Directions: Instill 1 or 2 drops in the affected eye(s) as needed.

Note: Do not touch unit-dose tip to eye. Celluvisc may cause temporary blurring due to its viscosity.

How Supplied: Celluvisc (carboxymethylcellulose sodium) 1% Lubricant Ophthalmic Solution is supplied in sterile, preservative-free, disposable, single-use containers of 0.01 fluid ounces each, in the following size:

30 SINGLE-USE CONTAINERS—NDC 0023-4554-30.

CHLOROPTIC®* ℞

(chloramphenicol 0.5%)
sterile ophthalmic solution

Contains:
chloramphenicol .... 0.5% (5 mg/mL)
with: chlorobutanol (chloral deriv. as a preservative) 0.5%; polyethylene glycol 300; polyoxyl 40 stearate; sodium hydroxide or hydrochloric acid to adjust the pH and purified water.

Actions: CHLOROPTIC® (chloramphenicol) has a wide spectrum of antimicrobial activity and is effective against many gram-negative and gram-positive organisms such as **Escherichia coli, Haemophilus influenzae, Staphylococcus aureus, Streptococcus hemolyticus,** and **Moraxella lacunata** (Morax-Axenfeld bacillus).

Indications: For the treatment of superficial ocular infections involving the conjunctiva and/or cornea caused by chloramphenicol-susceptible organisms.

Contraindications: Contraindicated in patients who are hypersensitive to chloramphenicol.

Warnings: As with other antibiotics, prolonged use may result in overgrowth of non-susceptible organisms. If superinfection occurs, or if clinical improvement is not noted within a reasonable period, discontinue use and institute appropriate therapy. Sensitivity reactions such as stinging, itching, angioneurotic edema, urticaria, vesicular and maculopapular dermatitis may also occur in some patients. Occasionally one sees hematopoietic toxicity with the use of systemic chloramphenicol, and rarely with topical administration. This type of blood dyscrasia is generally a dose related toxic effect on bone marrow and is usually reversible on cessation of the drug. Rare cases of aplastic anemia have been reported with prolonged (months to years) or frequent intermittent (over months and years) use of topical chloramphenicol.

Adverse Reactions: The most serious reaction reported following prolonged or frequent intermittent use of topical chloramphenicol is bone marrow aplasia.

Dosage and Administration: One or two drops 4 to 6 times a day for the first 72 hours, depending upon the severity of the condition. Intervals between applications may be increased after the first two days. Since the action of the drug is primarily bacteriostatic, therapy should be continued for 48 hours after an apparent cure has been attained.

How Supplied: CHLOROPTIC® (chloramphenicol) sterile ophthalmic solution is supplied in plastic dropper bottles in the following sizes:

2.5 mL—NDC 11980-109-03
7.5 mL—NDC 11980-109-08

Refrigerate until dispensed.

Caution: Federal (U.S.A.) law prohibits dispensing without prescription.

*U.S. Patent 3,702,364

CHLOROPTIC® ℞

(chloramphenicol) 1.0%
S.O.P.®
sterile ophthalmic ointment

Description: CHLOROPTIC® (chloramphenicol) 1.0% S.O.P.® sterile ophthalmic ointment is a topical anti-infective product for ophthalmic use.

Chemical Name: D-*threo* -(-)-2,2-Dichloro-N-[β-hydroxy-α-(hydroxymethyl)-p-nitrophenethyl] acetamide

Contains:
chloramphenicol .... 1.0% (10 mg/g)
with: chlorobutanol (chloral deriv.) 0.5%; white petrolatum; mineral oil; polyoxyl 40 stearate; polyethylene glycol 300; and petrolatum (and) lanolin alcohol.

Clinical Pharmacology: Chloramphenicol inhibits protein synthesis by interfering with the transfer of activated amino acids from soluble RNA to ribosomes. Chloramphenicol is a broad-spectrum antibiotic originally isolated from **Streptomyces venezuelae.** It is primarily bacteriostatic and useful in the treatment of bacterial infections caused by organisms such as **Haemophilus influenzae, Staphylococcus aureus, Streptococcus hemolyticus** and **Moraxella lacunata** (Morax-Axenfeld bacillus). Chloramphenicol also has an effect on the rickettsiae and the mycoplasma (PPLO) groups of organisms.

Indications and Usage: Chloramphenicol should be used only in those serious infections for which less potent drugs are ineffective or contraindicated.

CHLOROPTIC is indicated for the treatment of ocular infections involving the conjunctiva and/or cornea caused by chloramphenicol-susceptible organisms.

The particular anti-infective drug in the product is active against the following common eye pathogens: **Staphylococcus aureus;** Streptococci, including **Streptococcus pneumoniae; Escherichia coli; Haemophilus influenzae; Klebsiella/Enterobacter** species; **Neisseria** species; **Moraxella lacunata** (Morax-Axenfeld bacillus).

The product does not provide adequate coverage against: **Pseudomonas aeruginosa** and **Serratia marcescens.**

Contraindications: This product is contraindicated in persons sensitive to any of the components.

Warnings: Occasionally one sees hematopoietic toxicity with the use of systemic chloramphenicol and rarely with topical administration. This type of blood dyscrasia is generally a dose related toxic effect on bone marrow and is usually reversible on cessation of the drug. Rare cases of aplastic anemia have been reported with prolonged (months to years) or frequent intermittent (over months and years) use of topical chloramphenicol.

As with other antibiotics, prolonged use may result in overgrowth of non-susceptible organisms. If superinfection occurs, or if clinical improvement is not noted within a reasonable period, discontinue use and institute appropriate therapy.

Precautions: Ophthalmic ointments may retard corneal healing.

Adverse Reactions: Exact incidence figures are not available since no denominator of treated patients is available.

Continued on next page

Allergan Pharm—Cont.

The most serious reaction occurring from the presence of chloramphenicol is bone marrow aplasia. Three cases, including one fatality, have been reported following prolonged or frequent intermittent use of topical chloramphenicol.
Reactions occurring most often from the use of topical anti-infectives are allergic sensitizations. These reactions include stinging, itching, angioneurotic edema, urticaria, vesicular and maculopapular dermatitis.
Dosage and Administration: Place a small amount of ointment in the conjunctival sac every 3 hours, or more often if required, day and night for the first 48 hours. Intervals between applications may be increased after the first two days. Since the action of chloramphenicol is primarily bacteriostatic, therapy should be continued for 48 hours after an apparent cure has been obtained.
How Supplied: CHLOROPTIC® (chloramphenicol) 1.0% S.O.P.® sterile ophthalmic ointment is supplied in ophthalmic ointment tubes in the following size:

3.5 g—**NDC** 0023-0301-04

Note: Store away from heat.
Caution: Federal (U.S.A.) law prohibits dispensing without prescription.

EPIFRIN® ℞
(epinephrine, USP)
sterile ophthalmic solution

Description: EPIFRIN® (epinephrine, USP) sterile ophthalmic solution is a topical sympathomimetic agent for ophthalmic use.
Chemical Name: 1, 2- Benzenediol, 4- [1- hydroxy-2-(methylamino)ethyl]-, (R) -.
Contains: epinephrine, USP 0.25%,* 0.5%, 1%, 2% with: benzalkonium chloride; sodium metabisulfite; edetate disodium; hydrochloric acid; and purified water.
Clinical Pharmacology: Epinephrine is an adrenergic agonist that stimulates α- and β-adrenergic receptors. The capacity of EPIFRIN (epinephrine, USP) to decrease the aqueous inflow in open-angle glaucoma has been well documented. Studies have also shown that prolonged topical epinephrine therapy offers significant improvement in the coefficient of aqueous outflow.
EPIFRIN is effective alone in reducing intraocular pressure and is particularly useful in combination with miotics or beta-adrenergic blocking agents for the difficult-to-control patients. The addition of EPIFRIN to the patient's regimen often provides better control of intraocular pressure than the original agent alone.
Indications and Usage: EPIFRIN is indicated for the treatment of chronic simple glaucoma.
Contraindications: EPIFRIN should not be used in patients who have had an attack of narrow-angle glaucoma, since dilation of the pupil may trigger an acute attack. Do not use if hypersensitive to any ingredient.
Warnings:

1. EPIFRIN should be used with caution in patients with a narrow angle, since dilation of the pupil may trigger an acute attack of narrow-angle glaucoma.
2. Use with caution in patients with hypertensive cardiovascular disease or coronary artery disease.
3. Epinephrine has been reported to produce reversible macular edema in some aphakic patients and should be used with caution in these patients.

Contains sodium metabisulfite, a sulfite that may cause allergic-type reactions, including anaphylactic symptoms and life-threatening or less severe asthmatic episodes in certain susceptible people. The overall prevalence of sulfite sensitivity in the general population is unknown and probably low. Sulfite sensitivity is seen more frequently in asthmatic than in non-asthmatic people.
Precautions:
General: Epinephrine in any form is relatively uncomfortable upon instillation. However, discomfort lessens as the concentration of epinephrine decreases. EPIFRIN is not for injection.
Carcinogenesis, mutagenesis and impairment of fertility: No studies have been conducted in animals or in humans to evaluate the potential of these effects.
Pregnancy Category C: Animal reproduction studies have not been conducted with epinephrine. It is also not known whether epinephrine can cause fetal harm when administered to a pregnant woman or if it can affect reproduction capacity. Epinephrine should be given to a pregnant woman only if clearly needed.
Pediatric Use: Safety and effectiveness in children have not been established.
Adverse Reactions: Undesirable reactions to topical epinephrine include eye pain or ache, browache, headache, conjunctival hyperemia and allergic lid reactions.
Adrenochrome deposits in the conjunctiva and cornea after prolonged epinephrine therapy have been reported. Topical epinephrine has been reported to produce reversible macular edema in some aphakic patients.
Overdosage: Accidental ingestion will not cause problems because pharmacologically active concentrations of epinephrine cannot be achieved orally in man. Should accidental overdosage in the eye(s) occur, flush eye(s) with water or normal saline.
Dosage and Administration: The usual dosage is 1 drop in the affected eye(s) once or twice daily. However, the dosage should be adjusted to meet the needs of the individual patients. This is made easier with EPIFRIN® (epinephrine, USP) sterile ophthalmic solution available in four strengths.
How Supplied: EPIFRIN® is available on prescription only in plastic dropper bottles in the following concentrations and sizes:

0.25%	15 mL—NDC 11980-220-15
0.50%	15 mL—NDC 11980-119-15
1%	15 mL—NDC 11980-122-15
2%	15 mL—NDC 11980-058-15

Note: Protect from light and excessive heat. If the solution discolors or a precipitate forms, it should be discarded.

*The 0.25% formulation also contains sodium chloride.

FML® ℞
(fluorometholone) 0.1%
LIQUIFILM®
sterile ophthalmic suspension

Description: FML (fluorometholone) 0.1% LIQUIFILM sterile ophthalmic suspension is a topical anti-inflammatory agent for ophthalmic use.
Chemical Name: 9-fluoro-11β,17-dihydroxy-6α-methylpregna-1,4-diene-3,20-dione.
Contains:
fluorometholone 0.1%
with: LIQUIFILM (polyvinyl alcohol) 1.4%; benzalkonium chloride 0.004%; edetate disodium; sodium chloride; sodium phosphate monobasic; sodium phosphate dibasic; polysorbate 80; sodium hydroxide to adjust the pH, and purified water.
Clinical Pharmacology: Corticosteroids inhibit the inflammatory response to a variety of inciting agents. They inhibit the edema, fibrin deposition, capillary dilation, leukocyte migration, phagocytic activity, capillary proliferation, fibroblast proliferation, deposition of collagen, and scar formation associated with inflammation.
No generally accepted explanation of steroid action is available. However, corticosteroids are thought to act by the induction of phospholipase A_2 inhibitory proteins, collectively called lipocortins. It is postulated that these proteins control the biosynthesis of potent mediators of inflammation such as prostaglandins and leukotrienes by inhibiting the release of their common precursor, arachidonic acid. Arachidonic acid is released from membrane phospholipids by phospholipase A_2.
Corticosteroids are capable of producing a rise in intraocular pressure. In clinical studies on patients' eyes treated with both dexamethasone and fluorometholone suspensions, fluorometholone demonstrated a lower propensity to increase intraocular pressure than did dexamethasone.
Indications and Usage: FML is indicated for the treatment of corticosteroid-responsive inflammation of the palpebral and bulbar conjunctiva, cornea and anterior segment of the globe.
Contraindications: FML is contraindicated in the following conditions:
Epithelial herpes simplex keratitis (dendritic keratitis), vaccinia, varicella and other viral diseases of the cornea and conjunctiva.
Tuberculosis of the eye.
Fungal diseases of the ocular structures.
Hypersensitivity to any ingredient of the medication.
Warnings: Corticosteroid medication in the treatment of patients with a history of herpes simplex keratitis (involving the stroma) requires great caution; frequent slit lamp microscopy is mandatory.
Prolonged use may result in elevation of IOP, with damage to the optic nerve, defects in visual acuity and fields of vision, and/or in posterior subcapsular cataract formation. It may also aid in the establishment of secondary ocular infections from fungi or viruses liberated from ocular tissues.
Various ocular diseases and long-term use of topical corticosteroids have been known to cause corneal and scleral thinning. Use of topical corticosteroids in the presence of thin corneal or scleral tissue may lead to perforation.
Acute purulent untreated infection of the eye may be masked or activity enhanced by presence of corticosteroid medication.
Precautions: General: As fungal infections of the cornea are particularly prone to develop coincidentally with long-term local corticosteroid applications, fungal invasion must be suspected in any persistent corneal ulceration where a corticosteroid has been used or is in use.
Intraocular pressure should be checked frequently.
Carcinogenesis, mutagenesis, impairment of fertility: No studies have been conducted in animals or in humans to evaluate the possibility of these effects with fluorometholone.
Pregnancy Category C: Fluorometholone has been shown to be teratogenic and embryocidal in rabbits when given in doses approximating the human dose and above. There are no adequate, well-controlled studies in pregnant women. Fluorometholone should be used during pregnancy only if the potential benefit outweighs the potential risk to the fetus.
Fluorometholone was ocularly applied to both eyes of pregnant rabbits at various dosage levels on days 6 to 18 of gestation. A significant dose-related increase in fetal abnormalities and in fetal loss was observed.
Nursing Mothers: It is not known whether topical ophthalmic administration of corticosteroids could result in sufficient systemic absorption to produce detectable quantities in breast milk, nevertheless, the physician should consider the patient discontinuing nursing while the drug is being administered.

Pediatric Use: Safety and effectiveness in children have not been established.

Adverse Reactions: Adverse reactions include, in decreasing order of frequency, elevation of intraocular pressure (IOP) with possible development of optic nerve damage; loss of visual acuity or defects in fields of vision; posterior subcapsular cataract formation; and delayed wound healing.

The following have also been reported after the use of topical corticosteroids: Secondary ocular infection from pathogens liberated from ocular tissues and, rarely, perforation of the globe when used in conditions where there is thinning of the cornea or sclera.

Dosage and Administration: Instill one drop into the conjunctival sac two to four times daily. During the initial 24 to 48 hours, the frequency of dosing may be safely increased if necessary. Care should be taken not to discontinue therapy prematurely.

How Supplied: FML® (fluorometholone) 0.1% LIQUIFILM® sterile ophthalmic suspension is supplied in plastic dropper bottles in the following sizes:

1 mL—NDC 11980-211-01
5 mL—NDC 11980-211-05
10 mL—NDC 11980-211-10
15 mL—NDC 11980-211-15

Note: Protect from freezing. **Shake well before using.**

Caution: Federal (U.S.A.) law prohibits dispensing without prescription.

FML® ℞
(fluorometholone) 0.1%
S.O.P.®
sterile ophthalmic ointment

Description: FML® (fluorometholone) 0.1% S.O.P.® sterile ophthalmic ointment is a topical anti-inflammatory agent for ophthalmic use.

Chemical Name:
9-Fluoro-11β,17-dihydroxy-6α-methylpregna-1,4-diene-3,20-dione.

Contains:
fluorometholone 0.1%
with: phenylmercuric acetate (0.0008%), white petrolatum, mineral oil, and petrolatum (and) lanolin alcohol.

Clinical Pharmacology: Corticosteroids inhibit the inflammatory reponse to inciting agents of mechanical, chemical or immunological nature of edema, fibrin deposition, capillary dilation and leukocyte migration, capillary proliferation, deposition of collagen and scar formation. Corticosteroids and their derivatives are capable of producing a rise in intraocular pressure. In clinical studies on patients' eyes treated with both dexamethasone and fluorometholone suspensions, fluorometholone demonstrated a lower propensity to increase intraocular pressure than did dexamethasone.

Indications and Usage: FML S.O.P. is indicated for the treatment of corticosteroid-responsive inflammation of the palpebral and bulbar conjunctiva, cornea and anterior segment of the globe.

Contraindications: FML S.O.P. is contraindicated in the following conditions:

Acute superficial herpes simplex keratitis
Fungal diseases of ocular structures
Vaccinia, varicella and most other viral diseases of the cornea and conjunctiva
Tuberculosis of the eye
Hypersensitivity to the constituents of this medication

Warnings: Corticosteroid medication in the treatment of herpes simplex keratitis (involving the stroma) requires great caution; frequent slit-lamp microscopy is mandatory.

Prolonged use may result in glaucoma, with damage to the optic nerve, defects in visual acuity and fields of vision, posterior subcapsular cataract formation, or may aid in the establishment of secondary ocular infections from fungi or viruses liberated from ocular tissues.

In those diseases causing thinning of the cornea or sclera, perforations have been known to occur with the use of topical corticosteroids.

Acute purulent untreated infection of the eye may be masked or activity enhanced by presence of corticosteroid medication.

Precautions:

General: As fungal infections of the cornea are particularly prone to develop coincidentally with long-term local corticosteroid applications, fungal invasion must be suspected in any persistent corneal ulceration where a corticosteroid has been used or is in use.

Intraocular pressure should be checked frequently.

Ophthalmic ointments may retard corneal healing.

Carcinogenesis, mutagenesis, impairment of fertility: No studies have been conducted in animals or in humans to evaluate the potential of these effects.

Pregnancy Category C: Fluorometholone has been shown to be teratogenic and embryocidal in rabbits when given in doses approximating the human dose and above. There are no adequate, well-controlled studies in pregnant women. Fluorometholone should be used during pregnancy only if the potential benefit justifies the potential risk to the fetus.

Fluorometholone was ocularly applied to both eyes of pregnant rabbits at various dosage levels on days 6 to 18 of gestation. A significant dose-related increase in fetal abnormalities and in fetal loss was observed.

Pediatric Use: Safety and effectiveness in children below the age of 2 years have not been established.

Adverse Reactions: Adverse reactions include glaucoma, with optic nerve damage, visual acuity or field defects, and posterior subcapsular cataract formation may occur rarely with the use of topical corticosteroids. Secondary ocular infection from pathogens liberated from ocular tissues and perforation of the globe have also been reported following use of topical corticosteroids.

Overdosage: Overdosage will not ordinarily cause acute problems. If accidentally ingested, drink fluids to dilute.

Dosage and Administration: A small amount (approximately ½ inch ribbon) of ointment should be applied in the conjunctival sac one to three times daily. During the initial 24 to 48 hours, the dosage may be increased to one application every four hours. Care should be taken not to discontinue therapy prematurely.

How Supplied: FML® (fluorometholone) 0.1% S.O.P.® sterile ophthalmic ointment is supplied in ophthalmic ointment tubes in the following size:

3.5 g—NDC 0023-0316-04

Note: Store away from heat.

Caution: Federal (U.S.A.) law prohibits dispensing without prescription.

FML Forte® ℞
(fluorometholone) 0.25%
Liquifilm®
sterile ophthalmic suspension

Description: FML Forte® Liquifilm® sterile ophthalmic suspension is a topical anti-inflammatory product for ophthalmic use.

Chemical Name:
Fluorometholone: 9-Fluoro-11β, 17-dihydroxy-6α-methylpregna-1,4-diene-3,20-dione.

Contains:
fluorometholone 0.25%
with: Liquifilm (polyvinyl alcohol) 1.4%; benzalkonium chloride 0.005%; edetate disodium; sodium chloride; sodium biphosphate; sodium phosphate; polysorbate 80; sodium hydroxide to adjust the pH; and purified water.

Clinical Pharmacology: Corticosteroids inhibit the inflammatory response to a variety of inciting agents. They inhibit the edema, fibrin deposition, capillary dilation, leukocyte migration, phagocytic activity, capillary proliferation, fibroblast proliferation, deposition of collagen, and scar formation associated with inflammation.

No generally accepted explanation of steroid action is available. However, corticosteroids are thought to act by the induction of phospholipase A_2 inhibitory proteins, collectively called lipocortins. It is postulated these proteins control the biosynthesis of potent mediators of inflammation such as prostaglandins and leukotrienes by inhibiting the release of their common precursor, arachidonic acid. Arachidonic acid is released from membrane phospholipids by phospholipase A_2.

Corticosteroids are capable of producing a rise in intraocular pressure. In clinical studies of documented steroid-responders, fluorometholone demonstrated a significantly longer average time to produce a rise in intraocular pressure than dexamethasone phosphate; however, in a small percentage of individuals a significant rise in intraocular pressure occurred within one week. The ultimate magnitude of the rise was equivalent for both drugs.

Indications and Usage: FML Forte® is indicated for the treatment of corticosteroid-responsive inflammation of the palpebral and bulbar conjunctiva, cornea and anterior segment of the globe.

Contraindications:

- Epithelial herpes simplex keratitis (dendritic keratitis), vaccinia, varicella, and other viral diseases of the cornea and conjunctiva.
- Tuberculosis of the eye
- Fungal diseases of the ocular structures
- Hypersensitivity to any component of the medication

Warnings: Corticosteroid medication in the treatment of patients with a history of herpes simplex keratitis (involving the stroma) requires great caution; frequent slit-lamp microscopy is mandatory.

Prolonged use may result in glaucoma, with damage to the optic nerve, defects in visual acuity and fields of vision, and/or in posterior subcapsular cataract formation. It may also aid in the establishment of secondary ocular infections from fungi or viruses liberated from ocular tissues.

In diseases causing thinning of the cornea or sclera, perforations have been known to occur with the use of topical corticosteroids.

Acute purulent untreated infection of the eye may be masked or activity enhanced by presence of corticosteroid medication.

Precautions: General: As fungal infections of the cornea are particularly prone to develop coincidentally with long-term local corticosteroid applications, fungal invasion must be suspected in any persistent corneal ulceration where a corticosteroid has been used or is in use.

As with other corticosteroids, frequent intraocular pressure checks are warranted since a significant increase in IOP may occur in a small percentage of patients treated with FML Forte.

Carcinogenesis, mutagenesis, impairment of fertility: No studies have been conducted in animals or in humans to evaluate the possibility of these effects with fluorometholone.

Pregnancy Category C: Fluorometholone has been shown to be teratogenic and embryocidal in rabbits when given in doses approximating the human dose and above. There are no adequate and well-controlled studies in pregnant women. Fluorometholone should be used dur-

Continued on next page

Allergan Pharm—Cont.

ing pregnancy only if the potential benefit outweighs the potential risk to the fetus.
Fluorometholone was ocularly applied to both eyes of pregnant rabbits at various dosage levels on days 6 to 18 of gestation. A significant dose-related increase in fetal abnormalities and in fetal loss was observed.
Nursing Mothers: It is not known whether topical ophthalmic administration of corticosteroids could result in sufficient systemic absorption to produce detectable quantities in breast milk, nevertheless, the physician should consider having the patient discontinue nursing while the drug is being administered.
Pediatric Use: Safety and effectiveness in children have not been established.
Adverse Reactions: Adverse reactions include, in decreasing order of frequency, elevation of intraocular pressure (IOP) with possible development of glaucoma and infrequent optic nerve damage; loss of visual acuity or defects in fields of vision; posterior subcapsular cataract formation; delayed wound healing; and conjunctival erythema.
The following have also been reported after the use of topical corticosteroids: Secondary ocular infection from pathogens liberated from ocular tissues and, rarely, perforation of the globe when used in conditions where there is thinning of the cornea or sclera.
Dosage and Administration: Instill one drop into the conjunctival sac two to four times daily. Care should be taken not to discontinue therapy prematurely. Patients should be instructed to consult their physician for re-evaluation if the condition persists after two weeks of treatment.
How Supplied: FML Forte® (fluorometholone) 0.25% Liquifilm® sterile ophthalmic suspension is supplied in plastic dropper bottles in the following sizes:

2 mL—NDC 11980-228-02
5 mL—NDC 11980-228-05
10 mL—NDC 11980-228-10
15 mL—NDC 11980-228-15

Note: Protect from freezing. **(Shake well before using.)**
Caution: Federal (U.S.A.) law prohibits dispensing without prescription.

FML-S® ℞
(fluorometholone, sulfacetamide sodium)
LIQUIFILM®
sterile ophthalmic suspension

Description: FML-S LIQUIFILM sterile ophthalmic suspension is a topical anti-inflammatory/anti-infective combination product for ophthalmic use.
Chemical Names: Fluorometholone: 9-Fluoro-11β, 17-dihydroxy-6α-methylpregna-1,4-diene-3, 20-dione.
Sulfacetamide sodium: N-Sulfanilylacetamide monosodium salt monohydrate.
Contains:
fluorometholone 0.1%
sulfacetamide sodium 10%
with: LIQUIFILM® (polyvinyl alcohol) 1.4%; benzalkonium chloride 0.006%; edetate disodium; polysorbate 80; povidone; sodium chloride; sodium phosphate, dibasic; sodium phosphate, monobasic; sodium thiosulfate; hydrochloric acid and/or sodium hydroxide to adjust the pH; and purified water.
Clinical Pharmacology: Corticosteroids suppress the inflammatory response to a variety of agents and they probably delay or slow healing. Corticosteroids and their derivatives are capable of producing a rise in intraocular pressure. Since corticosteroids may inhibit the body's defense mechanism against infection, a concomitant antimicrobial drug may be used when this inhibition is considered to be clinically significant in a particular case.
In clinical studies of documented steroid-responders, fluorometholone demonstrated a significantly longer average time to produce a rise in intraocular pressure than dexamethasone phosphate; however, in a small percentage of individuals, a significant rise in intraocular pressure occurred within one week. The ultimate magnitude of the rise was equivalent for both drugs.
The anti-infective component in FML-S is included to provide action against specific organisms susceptible to it. Sulfacetamide sodium is active *in-vitro* against susceptible strains of the following microorganisms: *Escherichia coli, Staphylococcus aureus, Streptococcus pneumoniae, Streptococcus* (viridans group), *Haemophilus influenzae, Klebsiella* species, and *Enterobacter* species. Some strains of these bacteria may be resistant to sulfacetamide or resistant strains may emerge *in-vivo*.
When a decision to administer both a corticosteroid and an antimicrobial is made, the administration of such drugs in combination has the advantage of greater patient compliance and convenience, with the added assurance that the appropriate dosage of both drugs is administered. When both types of drugs are in the same formulation, compatibility of ingredients is assured and the correct volume of drug is delivered and retained.
The relative potency of corticosteroid formulations depends on the molecular structure, concentration, and release from the vehicle.
Indications and Usage: FML-S is indicated for steroid-responsive inflammatory ocular conditions for which a corticosteroid is indicated and where superficial bacterial ocular infection or a risk of bacterial ocular infection exists.
Ocular steroids are indicated in inflammatory conditions of the palpebral and bulbar conjunctiva, cornea, and anterior segment of the globe where the inherent risk of steroid use in certain infective conjunctivitides is accepted to obtain a diminution in edema and inflammation. They are also indicated in chronic anterior uveitis and corneal injury from chemical, radiation or thermal burns or penetration of foreign bodies.
The use of a combination drug with an anti-infective component is indicated where the risk of superficial ocular infection is high or where there is an expectation that potentially dangerous numbers of bacteria will be present in the eye.
The anti-infective drug in this product, sulfacetamide, is active against the following common bacterial eye pathogens: *Escherichia coli, Staphylococcus aureus, Streptococcus pneumoniae, Streptococcus* (viridans group), *Haemophilus influenzae, Klebsiella* species, and *Enterobacter* species.
The product does not provide adequate coverage against: *Neisseria* species and *Serratia marcescens*. A significant percentage of Staphylococcal isolates are completely resistant to sulfa drugs.
Contraindications: Epithelial herpes simplex keratitis (dendritic keratitis), and vaccinia. Fungal diseases of the ocular structures. Hypersensitivity to any component of the medication.
Warnings: NOT FOR INJECTION INTO THE EYE.
Prolonged use of steroids may result in glaucoma, with damage to the optic nerve, defects in visual acuity and fields of vision, and in posterior subcapsular cataract formation. If used for longer than 10 days, intraocular pressure should be routinely monitored even though it may be difficult in children and uncooperative patients.
Prolonged use of steroids may suppress the host immune response in ocular tissues and thus increase the hazard of secondary ocular infections. Various ocular diseases and long term use of topical corticosteroids have been known to cause corneal and scleral thinning. Use of topical corticosteroids in the presence of thin corneal or scleral tissue may lead to perforation. In acute purulent conditions of the eye, corticosteroids may mask infection or enhance existing infection.
Use of ocular steroids may prolong the course and may exacerbate the severity of many viral infections of the eye.
Employment of a corticosteroid medication in the treatment of patients with a history of herpes simplex requires great caution.
Fatalities have occurred, although rarely, due to severe reactions to sulfonamides including Stevens-Johnson syndrome, toxic epidermal necrolysis, fulminant hepatic necrosis, agranulocytosis, aplastic anemia, and other blood dyscrasias. Sensitizations may recur when a sulfonamide is readministered, irrespective of the route of administration. If signs of hypersensitivity or other serious reactions occur, discontinue use of this preparation. (see **Adverse Reactions**). Cross-sensitivity among corticosteroids has been demonstrated.
A significant percentage of staphylococcal isolates are completely resistant to sulfa drugs.
Precautions: General: The initial prescription and renewal of the medication order beyond 20 milliliters should be made only by a physician after evaluation of the patient's intraocular pressure, examination of the patient with the aid of magnification, such as slit lamp biomicroscopy and, where appropriate, fluorescein staining.
Keep this and all drugs out of the reach of children.
Drug Interactions: Sulfacetamide preparations are incompatible with silver preparations.
Carcinogenesis, mutagenesis, impairment of fertility: No studies have been conducted in animals or in humans to evaluate the possibility of these effects with fluorometholone or sulfacetamide.
Pregnancy: Pregnancy Category C: Animal studies have not been conducted with FML-S Liquifilm Ophthalmic Suspension. Fluorometholone has been shown to be embryocidal and teratogenic in rabbits when administered at low multiples of the human dose. Fluorometholone was applied ocularly to rabbits daily on days 6-18 of gestation, and dose-related fetal loss and fetal abnormalities including cleft palate, deformed rib cage, anomalous limbs and neural abnormalities such as encephalocele, craniorachischisis, and spina bifida were observed. Kernicterus may be precipitated in infants by sulfonamides being given systemically during the third trimester of pregnancy. There are no adequate and well-controlled studies of FML-S Liquifilm Ophthalmic Suspension in pregnant women, and it is not known whether FML-S can cause fetal harm when administered to a pregnant woman. FML-S Liquifilm Ophthalmic Suspension should be used during pregnancy only if the potential benefit justifies the potential risk to the fetus.
Nursing Mothers: It is not known whether topical administration of corticosteroids could result in sufficient systemic absorption to produce detectable quantities in breast milk. Systemically administered corticosteroids appear in breast milk and could suppress growth, interfere with endogenous corticosteroid production, or cause other untoward effects. Systemically administered sulfonamides are capable of producing kernicterus in infants of lactating women. Because of the potential for serious adverse reactions in nursing infants from FML-S, a decision should be made whether to discontinue nursing or to discontinue the medication.

Pediatric Use: Safety and effectiveness in children have not been established.

Adverse Reactions: Adverse reactions have occurred with corticosteroid/anti-infective combination drugs which can be attributed to the corticosteroid component, the anti-infective component, or the combination. Exact incidence figures are not available since no denominator of treated patients is available.

Reactions occurring most often from the presence of the anti-infective ingredient are allergic sensitizations. Fatalities have occurred, although rarely, due to severe reactions to sulfonamides including Stevens-Johnson syndrome, toxic epidermal necrolysis, fulminant hepatic necrosis, agranulocytosis, aplastic anemia, and other blood dyscrasias (see **Warnings**). Sulfacetamide sodium may cause local irritation.

The reactions due to the corticosteroid component in decreasing order of frequency are: elevation of intraocular pressure (IOP) with possible development of glaucoma, and infrequent optic nerve damage; posterior subcapsular cataract formation; and delayed wound healing.

Secondary Infection: The development of secondary infection has occurred after use of combinations containing corticosteroids and antimicrobials. Fungal infections of the cornea are particularly prone to develop coincidentally with long-term application of corticosteroids. When signs of chronic ocular inflammation persist following prolonged corticosteroid dosing, the possibility of fungal infections of the cornea should be considered.

Secondary bacterial ocular infection following suppression of host responses also occurs.

Dosage and Administration: One drop of FML-S® should be instilled into the conjunctival sac four times daily. Care should be taken not to discontinue therapy prematurely.

Not more than 20 milliliters should be prescribed initially and the prescription should not be refilled without further evaluation as outlined in **Precautions** above.

How Supplied: FML-S® (fluorometholone, sulfacetamide sodium) Liquifilm® Sterile Ophthalmic Suspension is supplied in plastic dropper bottles in the following sizes:

5 mL—NDC 11980-422-05
10 mL—NDC 11980-422-10

Note: Store at controlled room temperature 15°-30°C (59°-86°F). Protect from freezing and light. **SHAKE WELL BEFORE USING.** Do not use suspension if it is dark brown.

Caution: Federal (U.S.A.) law prohibits dispensing without prescription.

GENOPTIC® ℞

(gentamicin sulfate, USP)
LIQUIFILM®
sterile ophthalmic solution

Description: GENOPTIC® LIQUIFILM® sterile ophthalmic solution is a topical anti-infective agent for ophthalmic use.

Contains: gentamicin sulfate, USP equivalent to 0.3% gentamicin base with: LIQUIFILM (polyvinyl alcohol) 1.4%; benzalkonium chloride; edetate disodium; sodium phosphate, dibasic; sodium chloride; hydrochloric acid and/or sodium hydroxide to adjust the pH; and purified water.

Clinical Pharmacology: Gentamicin sulfate is a water-soluble antibiotic of the aminoglycoside group active against a wide variety of pathogenic gram-negative and gram-positive bacteria. The gram-positive bacteria against which gentamicin sulfate is active include coagulase-positive and coagulase-negative staphylococci, including certain strains that are resistant to penicillin; Group A beta-hemolytic and nonhemolytic streptococci; and **Diplococcus pneumoniae.** The gram-negative bacteria against which gentamicin sulfate is active include certain strains of **Pseudomonas aeruginosa,** indole-positive and indole-negative **Proteus** species, **Escherichia coli, Klebsiella pneumoniae** (Friedlander's bacillus), **Haemophilus influenzae** and **Haemophilus aegyptius** (Koch-Weeks bacillus), **Aerobacter aerogenes, Moraxella lacunata** (diplobacillus of Morax-Axenfeld), and **Neisseria** species, including **Neisseria gonorrhoeae.** Although significant resistant organisms have not been isolated from patients treated with gentamicin at the present time, this may occur in the future as resistance has been produced with difficulty **in vitro** by repeated exposures.

Indications and Usage: GENOPTIC LIQUIFILM sterile ophthalmic solution is indicated in the topical treatment of infections of the external eye and its adnexa caused by susceptible bacteria. Such infections include conjunctivitis, keratitis and keratoconjunctivitis, corneal ulcers, blepharitis and blepharoconjunctivitis, acute meibomianitis, and dacryocystitis.

Contraindications: This product is contraindicated in patients with known hypersensitivities to any of its components.

Warnings: GENOPTIC® LIQUIFILM® is not for injection. It should never be injected subconjunctivally, nor should it be introduced directly into the anterior chamber of the eye.

Precautions:

General: Prolonged use of topical antibiotics may give rise to overgrowth of nonsusceptible microorganisms, such as fungi. Should this occur, or if irritation or hypersensitivity to any component of the drug develops, discontinue use of the preparation and institute appropriate therapy.

Carcinogenesis, mutagenesis, impairment of fertility: There are no published carcinogenicity or impairment of fertility studies on gentamicin. Negative results have been reported on the mutagenicity of aminoglycoside antibiotics.

Pregnancy Category C: Gentamicin has been shown to depress newborn body weights, kidney weights and median glomerular counts in rats when administered systemically in daily doses of approximately 500 times the maximum recommended ophthalmic dose in humans.

There are no adequate and well-controlled studies in pregnant women. Gentamicin should be used during pregnancy only if the potential benefit justifies the potential risk to the fetus.

Adverse Reactions: Transient irritation has been reported with the use of topical ophthalmic gentamicin sulfate.

Dosage and Administration: Instill one or two drops into the affected eye(s) every four hours. In severe infections, dosage may be increased to as much as two drops once every hour.

How Supplied: GENOPTIC® (gentamicin sulfate, USP) LIQUIFILM® sterile ophthalmic solution is supplied in plastic dropper bottles in the following sizes:

1 mL—NDC 11980-117-01
5 mL—NDC 11980-117-05

Note: Store at room temperature.

Caution: Federal (U.S.A.) law prohibits dispensing without prescription.

GENOPTIC® ℞

(gentamicin sulfate)
S.O.P.®
sterile ophthalmic ointment, USP
Each gram contains gentamicin sulfate, USP equivalent to 3.0 mg gentamicin

Description: Gentamicin sulfate is a water-soluble antibiotic of the aminoglycoside group active against a wide variety of pathogenic gram-negative and gram-positive bacteria.

GENOPTIC® S.O.P.® sterile ophthalmic ointment contains gentamicin sulfate, USP (equivalent to 0.3% gentamicin) in a bland base of white petrolatum, with methylparaben and propylparaben as preservatives.

Actions: The gram-positive bacteria against which gentamicin sulfate is active include coagulase-positive and coagulase-negative staphylococci, including certain strains that are resistant to penicillin; Group A beta-hemolytic and non-hemolytic streptococci; and **Diplococcus pneumoniae.** The gram-negative bacteria against which gentamicin sulfate is active include certain strains of **Pseudomonas aeruginosa,** indole-positive and indole-negative **Proteus** species, **Escherichia coli, Klebsiella pneumoniae** (Friedländer's bacillus), **Haemophilus influenzae** and **Haemophilus aegyptius** (Koch-Weeks bacillus), **Aerobacter aerogenes, Moraxella lacunata** (diplobacillus of Morax-Axenfeld), and **Neisseria** species, including **Neisseria gonorrhoeae.** Although significant resistant organisms have not been isolated from patients treated with gentamicin at the present time, this may occur in the future as resistance has been produced with difficulty **in vitro** by repeated exposures.

Indications: GENOPTIC S.O.P. sterile ophthalmic ointment is indicated in the topical treatment of infections of the external eye and its adnexa caused by susceptible bacteria. Such infections embrace conjunctivitis, keratitis and keratoconjunctivitis, corneal ulcers, blepharitis and blepharoconjunctivitis, acute meibomianitis, and dacryocystitis.

Contraindications: GENOPTIC S.O.P. sterile ophthalmic ointment is contraindicated in patients with known hypersensitivity to any of the components.

Precautions: Prolonged use of topical antibiotics may give rise to overgrowth of nonsusceptible organisms, such as fungi. Should this occur, or if irritation or hypersensitivity to any component of the drug develops, discontinue use of the preparation and institute appropriate therapy.

Ophthalmic ointments may retard corneal healing.

Adverse Reactions: Occasional burning or stinging may occur with the use of GENOPTIC S.O.P. sterile ophthalmic ointment.

Dosage and Administration: Apply a small amount to the affected eye two to three times a day.

How Supplied: GENOPTIC® S.O.P.® sterile ophthalmic ointment is available in 3.5 g tubes, **NDC** 0023-0320-04.

Store between 2° and 30°C (36° and 86°F).

Caution: Federal (U.S.A.) law prohibits dispensing without prescription.

HMS® ℞

(medrysone) 1.0%
LIQUIFILM®
sterile ophthalmic suspension

Description: HMS® (medrysone) 1.0% LIQUIFILM® sterile ophthalmic suspension is a topical anti-inflammatory agent for ophthalmic use.

Chemical Name: 11β-Hydroxy-6α-methylpregn-4-ene-3, 20-dione.

Contains:

medrysone..1.0%

with: LIQUIFILM (polyvinyl alcohol) 1.4%; benzalkonium chloride 0.004%; edetate disodium; sodium chloride; potassium chloride; sodium phosphate monobasic; sodium phosphate dibasic; hydroxypropyl methylcellulose; sodium hydroxide to adjust the pH; and purified water.

Clinical Pharmacology: HMS (medrysone) is a synthetic corticosteroid with topical anti-inflammatory and anti-allergic activity. Corticosteroids inhibit the inflammatory response to inciting agents of mechanical, chemical, or immunological nature of edema, fibrin deposi-

Continued on next page

Allergan Pharm—Cont.

tion, capillary dilation and leukocyte migration, capillary proliferation, deposition of collagen and scar formation. HMS (medrysone) has less anti-inflammatory potency than 0.1% dexamethasone. Data from 2 uncontrolled studies[1-2] indicate that in patients with increased intraocular pressure and in those susceptible to a rise in intraocular pressure, there is less effect on pressure with HMS than with dexamethasone or betamethasone.

Indications and Usage: HMS is indicated for the treatment of allergic conjunctivitis, vernal conjunctivitis, episcleritis, and epinephrine sensitivity.

Contraindications: HMS is contraindicated in the following conditions:
Acute superficial herpes simplex
Viral diseases of the conjunctiva and cornea
Ocular tuberculosis
Fungal diseases of the eye
Hypersensitivity to any of the components of the drug

Warnings:
Acute purulent untreated infections of the eye may be masked, enhanced or activated by the presence of corticosteroid medication.
Corneal or scleral perforation occasionally has been reported with prolonged use of topical corticosteroids. In high dosages, they have been associated with corneal thinning.
Prolonged use of topical corticosteroids may increase intraocular pressure, with resultant glaucoma, damage to the optic nerve, and defects in visual acuity and fields of vision. However, data from 2 uncontrolled studies[1-2] indicate that in patients with increased intraocular pressure and in those susceptible to a rise in intraocular pressure upon application of topical corticosteroids, there is less effect on pressure with HMS® than with dexamethasone or betamethasone.
Prolonged use of topical corticosteroids may rarely be associated with development of posterior subcapsular cataracts.
Systemic absorption and systemic side effects may result with the use of topical corticosteroids.
HMS is not recommended for use in iritis and uveitis as its therapeutic effectiveness has not been demonstrated in these conditions.
Corticosteroid medication in the presence of stromal herpes simplex requires great caution; frequent slit-lamp microscopy is suggested.
Prolonged use may aid in the establishment of secondary ocular infections from fungi and viruses liberated from ocular tissue.

Precautions:
General: With prolonged use of HMS, the intraocular pressure and the lens should be examined periodically.
In persistent corneal ulceration where a corticosteroid has been used, or is in use, fungal infection should be suspected.
Carcinogenesis, mutagenesis, impairment of fertility: No studies have been conducted in animals or in humans to evaluate the potential of these effects.
Pregnancy Category C: Medrysone has been shown to be embryocidal in rabbits when given in doses 10 and 30 times the human dose. Medrysone was ocularly applied to both eyes of pregnant rabbits 2 drops 4 times per day on day 6 through 18 of gestation. A significant increase in early resorptions was observed in the treated rabbits. There are no adequate or well-controlled studies in pregnant women. Medrysone should be used during pregnancy only if the potential benefit justifies the potential risk to the fetus.
Pediatric Use: Safety and effectiveness in children have not been established.

Adverse Reactions: Adverse reactions include occasional transient stinging and burning on instillation. Increased intraocular pressure, which may be associated with optic nerve damage and defects in the visual fields, and posterior subcapsular cataract formation have been reported rarely with the use of HMS.

Overdosage: Overdosage will not ordinarily cause acute problems. If accidentally ingested, drink fluids to dilute.

Dosage and Administration: **Shake well before using.** Instill one drop in the conjunctival sac up to every four hours.

How Supplied: HMS® (medrysone) is supplied in plastic dropper bottles in the following sizes:

5 mL—NDC 11980-074-05
10 mL—NDC 11980-074-10

Note: Protect from freezing.

Caution: Federal (U.S.A.) law prohibits dispensing without a prescription.

References:

1. Becker B, Kolker AE. Intraocular pressure response to topical corticosteroids. In: Leopold IH, ed. Ocular therapy, complications and management. St. Louis: CV Mosby, 1967.
2. Spaeth G. Hydroxymethylprogesterone. Arch Ophthalmol 1966;75:783–787.

HERPLEX® ℞
(idoxuridine) 0.1%
LIQUIFILM®
sterile ophthalmic solution

For Ophthalmic Use Only

Description: A topical ophthalmic antiviral chemotherapeutic preparation.

Chemical Name: 2′-Deoxy-5-iodouridine.

Contains:
idoxuridine 0.1%
with: LIQUIFILM® (polyvinyl alcohol) 1.4%, benzalkonium chloride, sodium chloride, edetate disodium, and purified water.

Clinical Pharmacology: In chemical structure, idoxuridine closely approximates the configuration of thymidine, one of the four building blocks of DNA—the genetic material of the herpes virus. As a result, idoxuridine is able to replace thymidine in the enzymatic step of viral replication or "growth". The consequent production of faulty DNA results in a pseudo-structure which cannot infect or destroy tissue. In short, by preempting a vital building block in the genetic material of the herpes simplex virus, idoxuridine destroys the infective and destructive capacity of the viral material.

Indications and Usage: HERPLEX LIQUIFILM is indicated for the treatment of keratitis caused by the herpes simplex virus.

Contraindications: HERPLEX LIQUIFILM is contraindicated for those who have a hypersensitivity to the active ingredient or other components of this medication.

Warnings: Recurrence may occur if medication is not continued 5 to 7 days after lesion is apparently healed (does not stain).

Precautions: **General:** Some strains of herpes simplex virus appear resistant to the action of idoxuridine. If there is no lessening of fluorescein staining in 14 days, another form of therapy should be undertaken.
Drug Interactions: Boric acid should not be administered during the course of therapy. The potential exists for interaction between boric acid and ingredients in HERPLEX LIQUIFILM which may result in precipitate formation.
Carcinogenesis, mutagenesis, impairment of fertility: The studies performed to date on idoxuridine are inadequate for assessment of carcinogenicity. This cytotoxic drug should be regarded as being potentially carcinogenic. It can inhibit DNA synthesis or function and is incorporated into the DNA of mammalian cells as well as into the genome of DNA viruses. Idoxuridine has been reported to induce RNA tumor virus (type C particles) production from virus-negative mouse cells. The degree of oncogenic activity of idoxuridine-induced oncornaviruses has not been documented. However, several idoxuridine-activated oncornaviruses have caused *in vitro* cell transformation and induction of specific neoplasms (lymphatic leukemias and carcinomas) upon inoculation into syngeneic mice.
Idoxuridine has been reported to cause chromosome aberrations in mice and to be mutagenic in mammalian cells in culture (e.g., diploid human lymphoblasts and mouse lymphoma cells), Drosophila melanogaster and in host-mediated assay system utilizing mammalian cells.
Pregnancy Category C: Idoxuridine has been reported to cross the placental barrier and to produce fetal malformations in rabbits when administered topically to the eyes of pregnant females in doses similar to those used clinically. Idoxuridine has also been reported to produce fetal malformations in the rat after intraperitoneal and oral administration and in the mouse after subcutaneous administration. There are no adequate and well-controlled studies in pregnant women. Idoxuridine should be used during pregnancy only if the potential benefit justifies the potential risk to the fetus.
Nursing Mothers: It is not known whether this drug is excreted in human milk. Because of the potential for tumorigenicity shown for idoxuridine in animal studies, a decision should be made whether to discontinue nursing or to discontinue the drug, taking into account the importance of the drug to the mother.
Pediatric Use: Safety and effectiveness in children have not been established.

Adverse Reactions: Exact incidence figures are not available since no denominator of treated patients is available.
Adverse reactions associated with topical idoxuridine administration include occasional irritation, pain, pruritus, inflammation, edema of the eyes or lids, allergic reactions, photophobia, occasional corneal clouding, stippling, and punctate defects of the epithelium.

Overdosage: Overdosage will not ordinarily cause acute problems. Should accidental overdosage in the eye(s) occur, flush the eye(s) with water or normal saline. If accidentally ingested, drink fluids to dilute.

Dosage and Administration: For optimal results, the infected tissues should be kept "saturated" with HERPLEX LIQUIFILM. Under practical, clinical conditions, one of the following "high frequency" dosage schedules is recommended.
1. Instill one drop in the infected eye(s) every hour during the day. At night, the dosage may be reduced to one drop every other hour.
2. Instill one drop every minute for 5 minutes. This schedule should be repeated every four hours—night and day.

How Supplied: HERPLEX® (idoxuridine) 0.1% LIQUIFILM® sterile ophthalmic solution is supplied in plastic dropper bottles in the following size: 15 mL—NDC 0023-0033-15.

Note: Store at controlled room temperature (59°– 86°F). Protect from light.

Caution: Federal (U.S.A.) law prohibits dispensing without prescription.

LACRIL® OTC
(hydroxypropyl methylcellulose 0.5%, gelatin A 0.01%)
Lubricant Ophthalmic Solution

Contains: Actives: Hydroxypropyl methylcellulose 0.5% and gelatin A 0.01%. Inactives: calcium chloride, chlorobutanol (chloral deriv.) 0.5%, dextrose, magnesium chloride, polysorbate 80, potassium chloride, purified water, sodium acetate, sodium borate, sodium chloride, and sodium citrate. May also contain acetic acid to adjust pH.

FDA APPROVED USES

Indications: FOR USE AS A LUBRICANT TO PREVENT FURTHER IRRITATION OR TO RELIEVE DRYNESS OF THE EYE.

Warnings: To avoid contamination, do not touch tip of container to any surface. Replace cap after using. If you experience eye pain, changes in vision, continued redness or irritation of the eye, or if the condition worsens or persists for more than 72 hours, discontinue use and consult a doctor. If solution changes color or becomes cloudy, do not use. Keep this and all drugs out of the reach of children. In case of accidental ingestion, seek professional assistance or contact a poison control center immediately.

Directions: Instill 1 or 2 drops in the affected eye(s) as needed.

NOTE: Not for use while wearing soft contact lenses.

How Supplied: LACRIL® (hydroxypropyl methylcellulose 0.5%, gelatin A 0.01%) Lubricant Ophthalmic Solution is supplied in sterile plastic dropper bottles in the following size:

½ fl oz—NDC 11980-045-15

LACRI-LUBE® NP — OTC

(white petrolatum 57.3%, mineral oil 42.5%)
Lubricant Ophthalmic Ointment

Contains: Actives: white petrolatum 57.3%, mineral oil 42.5%; Inactive: lanolin alcohols.

FDA APPROVED USES

Indications: FOR USE AS A LUBRICANT TO PREVENT FURTHER IRRITATION OR TO RELIEVE DRYNESS OF THE EYE.

Warnings: To avoid contamination, do not touch tip of container to any surface. Do not reuse. Once opened, discard. If you experience eye pain, changes in vision, continued redness or irritation of the eye, or if the condition worsens or persists for more than 72 hours, discontinue use and consult a doctor. Keep this and all drugs out of the reach of children. In case of accidental ingestion, seek professional assistance or contact a poison control center immediately.

Directions: Pull down the lower lid of the affected eye and apply a small amount (one-fourth inch) of ointment to the inside of the eyelid.

How Supplied: As a sterile ophthalmic ointment in 0.7 g unit-dose containers (24 units).
0.7 g—NDC 0023-0240-01

Note: Store away from heat.

LACRI-LUBE® S.O.P.® — OTC

(white petrolatum 56.8%, mineral oil 42.5%)
Lubricant Ophthalmic Ointment

Contains: Actives: white petrolatum 56.8%, mineral oil 42.5%; Inactives: chlorobutanol (chloral deriv.) 0.5% and lanolin alcohols.

FDA APPROVED USES

Indications: FOR USE AS A LUBRICANT TO PREVENT FURTHER IRRITATION OR TO RELIEVE DRYNESS OF THE EYE.

Warnings: To avoid contamination, do not touch tip of container to any surface. Replace cap after using. If you experience eye pain, changes in vision, continued redness or irritation of the eye, or if the condition worsens or persists for more than 72 hours, discontinue use and consult a doctor. Keep this and all drugs out of the reach of children. In case of accidental ingestion, seek professional assistance or contact a poison control center immediately.

Directions: Pull down the lower lid of the affected eye and apply a small amount (one-fourth inch) of ointment to the inside of the eyelid.

How Supplied: As a sterile ophthalmic ointment in 3.5 g and 7 g ophthalmic ointment tubes and 0.7 g unit-dose containers (24 units).
0.7 g—NDC 0023-0312-01
3.5 g—NDC 0023-0312-04
7.0 g—NDC 0023-0312-07

Note: Store away from heat.

LIQUIFILM FORTE® — OTC

(polyvinyl alcohol) 3.0%
Lubricant Ophthalmic Solution

Contains: Active: Polyvinyl alcohol 3.0%. Inactives: edetate disodium, mono- and dibasic sodium phosphates, purified water, sodium chloride, and thimerosal 0.002%. May also contain hydrochloric acid or sodium hydroxide to adjust pH.

FDA APPROVED USES

Indications: FOR USE AS A LUBRICANT TO PREVENT FURTHER IRRITATION OR TO RELIEVE DRYNESS OF THE EYE.

Warnings: To avoid contamination, do not touch tip of container to any surface. Replace cap after using. If you experience eye pain, changes in vision, continued redness or irritation of the eye, or if the condition worsens or persists for more than 72 hours, discontinue use and consult a doctor. If solution changes color or becomes cloudy, do not use. This product contains thimerosal 0.002% as a preservative. Do not use this product if you are sensitive to mercury. Keep this and all drugs out of the reach of children. In case of accidental ingestion, seek professional assistance or contact a poison control center immediately.

Directions: Instill 1 or 2 drops in the affected eye(s) as needed.

Note: Not for use while wearing soft contact lenses.

How Supplied: LIQUIFILM FORTE® (polyvinyl alcohol) 3.0% Lubricant Ophthalmic Solution is supplied in sterile plastic dropper bottles in the following sizes:

½ fl oz—NDC 11980-187-15
1 fl oz—NDC 11980-187-30

LIQUIFILM TEARS® — OTC

(polyvinyl alcohol) 1.4%
Lubricant Ophthalmic Solution

Contains: Active: Polyvinyl alcohol 1.4%. Inactives: chlorobutanol (chloral deriv.) 0.5%, purified water, and sodium chloride. May also contain hydrochloric acid or sodium hydroxide to adjust pH.

FDA APPROVED USES

Indications: FOR USE AS A LUBRICANT TO PREVENT FURTHER IRRITATION OR TO RELIEVE DRYNESS OF THE EYE. LIQUIFILM TEARS® Lubricant Ophthalmic Solution hypotonic formula is recommended by eye care professionals to soothe and lubricate scratchy, irritated, dry eyes. LIQUIFILM TEARS acts as a supplement to your normal tears.

Warnings: To avoid contamination, do not touch tip of container to any surface. Replace cap after using. If you experience eye pain, changes in vision, continued redness or irritation of the eye, or if the condition worsens or persists for more than 72 hours, discontinue use and consult a doctor. If solution changes color or becomes cloudy, do not use. Keep this and all drugs out of the reach of children. In case of accidental ingestion, seek professional assistance or contact a poison control center immediately.

Directions: Instill 1 or 2 drops in the affected eye(s) as needed.

Note: Not for use while wearing soft contact lenses.

How Supplied: LIQUIFILM TEARS® (polyvinyl alcohol) 1.4% Lubricant Ophthalmic Solution is supplied in sterile plastic dropper bottles in the following sizes:

½ fl oz—NDC 11980-025-15
1 fl oz—NDC 11980-025-30

OPHTHETIC® — ℞

(proparacaine HCl) 0.5%
sterile ophthalmic solution

Description: OPHTHETIC® (proparacaine HCl) 0.5% sterile ophthalmic solution is a topical local anesthetic for ophthalmic use.

Chemical Name:
Benzoic acid, 3-amino-4-propoxy-,2-(diethylamino)ethyl ester, monohydrochloride.

Contains:
proparacaine HCl 0.5%
with: benzalkonium chloride (0.01%), glycerin, sodium chloride and purified water.

Clinical Pharmacology: OPHTHETIC sterile ophthalmic solution is a rapidly-acting topical anesthetic, with induced anesthesia lasting 15 minutes or longer.

Indications and Usage: OPHTHETIC sterile ophthalmic solution is indicated for procedures in which a topical ophthalmic anesthetic is indicated: corneal anesthesia of short duration, e.g., tonometry, gonioscopy, removal of corneal foreign bodies, and for short corneal and conjunctival procedures.

Contraindications: OPHTHETIC sterile ophthalmic solution should be considered contraindicated in patients with known hypersensitivity to any of the ingredients of this preparation.

Warnings: Prolonged use of a topical ocular anesthetic is not recommended. It may produce permanent corneal opacification with accompanying visual loss.

Precautions:

Carcinogenesis, Mutagenesis, Impairment of Fertility: Long-term studies in animals have not been performed to evaluate carcinogenic potential, mutagenicity, or possible impairment of fertility in males or females.

Pregnancy: Pregnancy Category C: Animal reproduction studies have not been conducted with OPHTHETIC ophthalmic solution (proparacaine hydrochloride). It is also not known whether proparacaine hydrochloride can cause fetal harm when administered to a pregnant woman or can affect reproduction capacity. Proparacaine hydrochloride should be administered to a pregnant woman only if clearly needed.

Nursing Mothers: It is not known whether this drug is excreted in human milk. Because many drugs are excreted in human milk, caution should be exercised when proparacaine hydrochloride is administered to a nursing woman.

Pediatric Use: Safety and effectiveness in children have not been established.

Adverse Reactions: Occasional temporary stinging, burning, and conjunctival redness may occur with the use of proparacaine. A rare, severe, immediate-type, apparently hyperallergic corneal reaction, characterized by acute, intense and diffuse epithelial keratitis, a gray, ground glass appearance, sloughing of large areas of necrotic epithelium, corneal filaments and sometimes, iritis with descemetitis has been reported.

Allergic contact dermatitis from proparacaine with drying and fissuring of the fingertips has also been reported.

Dosage and Administration:

Usual Dosage: Removal of foreign bodies and sutures, and for tonometry: 1 to 2 drops (in single instillations) in each eye before operating.

Deep Ophthalmic Anesthesia: 1 drop in each eye every 5 to 10 minutes for 5–7 doses.

Note: Do not use if solution is discolored (amber).

Continued on next page

Allergan Pharm—Cont.

How Supplied:
OPHTHETIC® sterile ophthalmic solution is supplied in plastic dropper bottles in the following sizes:

15 mL—NDC 11980-048-15

Bottle must be stored in unit carton to protect contents from light. Store unopened bottle at controlled room temperature 15°-30°C (59°-86°F). Opened bottle should be refrigerated.
Caution: Federal (U.S.A.) law prohibits dispensing without prescription.

PILAGAN™ ℞
(pilocarpine nitrate)
Liquifilm®
sterile ophthalmic solution
with C Cap™ Compliance Cap Q.I.D.

Description: **PILAGAN™** (pilocarpine nitrate) Liquifilm® sterile ophthalmic solution is a topical parasympathomimetic agent for ophthalmic use.
Chemical Name: 2(3*H*)-Furanone, 3-ethyldihydro-4-[(1-methyl-1*H*-imidazol-5-yl)methyl]-,(3S-*cis*)-,mononitrate.
Contains: pilocarpine nitrate ...1%, 2%, 4% with Liquifilm® (polyvinyl alcohol) 1.4%; chlorobutanol (chloral derivative) 0.5% as a preservative; sodium acetate; sodium chloride; citric acid; menthol; camphor; phenol; eucalyptol; and purified water.
Clinical Pharmacology: Pilocarpine is a direct-acting parasympathomimetic drug which duplicates the muscarinic effects of acetylcholine, but has no nicotinic effects. Pilocarpine stimulates secretory glands and smooth muscles and has no effect on striated muscle. Pilocarpine is effective in the treatment of glaucoma by improving the facility of outflow and by decreasing aqueous secretion.
Indications and Usage: PILAGAN Liquifilm is indicated for:
1. The control of intraocular pressure in glaucoma.
2. Emergency relief of mydriasis in an acutely glaucomatous situation.
3. To reverse mydriasis caused by cycloplegic agents.

Contraindications: PILAGAN Liquifilm is contraindicated in persons showing hypersensitivity to any of its ingredients.
Warnings: Pilocarpine is readily absorbed systemically through the conjunctiva. Excessive application (instillation) may elicit systemic toxicity symptoms in some individuals.
Precautions: **General:** Pilocarpine has been reported to elicit retinal detachment in individuals with pre-existing retinal disease or predisposed to retinal tears. Fundus examination is advised for all patients prior to initiation of pilocarpine therapy.
Carcinogenesis, mutagenesis and impairment of fertility: No studies have been conducted in animals or in humans to evaluate the potential of these effects.
Pregnancy Category C: Animal reproduction studies have not been conducted with pilocarpine. It is also not known whether pilocarpine can cause fetal harm when administered to a pregnant woman or can affect reproduction capacity. Pilocarpine should be given to a pregnant woman only if clearly needed.
Pediatric Use: Safety and effectiveness in children have not been established.
Adverse Reactions: Adverse reactions associated with topical pilocarpine therapy include: visual blurring due to miosis and accommodative spasm, poor dark adaptation caused by the failure of the pupil to dilate in reduced illumination, and conjunctival hyperemia. Miotics have been reported to cause lens opacities in susceptible individuals after prolonged use.
Systemic reactions following topical use of pilocarpine are rare.
Overdosage: Should accidental overdosage in the eye(s) occur, flush eye(s) with water or normal saline. If accidentally ingested, induce emesis or perform gastric lavage. Observe patients for signs of pilocarpine toxicity, i.e., salivation, lacrimation, sweating, nausea, vomiting and diarrhea. If these occur, therapy with anticholinergics (atropine) may be necessary. Bronchial constriction may be a problem in asthmatic patients.
Dosage and Administration:
1. For glaucoma, the recommended dosage is 1 to 2 drops two or four times a day of the selected concentration; patient response may be variable.
2. To aid in emergency miosis, 1 to 2 drops of one of the higher concentrations should be used.
3. The dosage and strength required to reverse mydriasis depends on the cycloplegic used.

How Supplied: PILAGAN™ (pilocarpine nitrate) Liquifilm® sterile ophthalmic solution is available in 15 mL plastic dropper bottles with the C Cap™ Compliance Cap.

1%—NDC 11980-879-45
2%—NDC 11980-878-45
4%—NDC 11980-877-45

Note: Shake well before use. Protect from freezing. Keep out of the reach of children.
Caution: Federal (U.S.A.) law prohibits dispensing without prescription.

POLY-PRED® ℞
(prednisolone acetate—neomycin sulfate—polymyxin B sulfate)
Liquifilm®
sterile ophthalmic suspension

Description: POLY-PRED Liquifilm sterile ophthalmic suspension is a topical anti-inflammatory/anti-infective combination product for ophthalmic use.
Chemical Name: Prednisolone acetate: 11β, 17, 21-Trihydroxypregna-1, 4-diene-3, 20-dione 21-acetate.
Neomycin sulfate is the sulfate salt of neomycin B and neomycin C which are produced by the growth of **Streptomyces fradiae** (Fam. **Streptomycetaceae**). It has a potency equivalent to not less than 600 micrograms per milligram of neomycin base, calculated on an anhydrous basis.
Polymyxin B sulfate is the sulfate salt of polymyxin B_1 and polymyxin B_2 which are produced by the growth of **Bacillus polymyxa** (Prazmowski) Migula (Fam. **Bacillaceae**). It has a potency of not less than 6,000 polymyxin B units per milligram, calculated on an anhydrous basis.
Contains: prednisolone acetate (microfine suspension) 0.5%
neomycin sulfate equivalent to 0.35% neomycin base
polymyxin B sulfate ....10,000 units/mL
with: Liquifilm (polyvinyl alcohol) 1.4%; thimerosal 0.001%; polysorbate 80; propylene glycol; sodium acetate; and purified water.
Clinical Pharmacology: Corticosteroids suppress the inflammatory response to a variety of agents and they probably delay or slow healing. Since corticosteroids may inhibit the body's defense mechanism against infection, a concomitant antimicrobial drug may be used when this inhibition is considered to be clinically significant in a particular case.
The anti-infective components in POLY-PRED are included to provide action against specific organisms susceptible to them. Neomycin sulfate and polymyxin B sulfate are considered active against the following microorganisms: **Staphylococcus aureus; Escherichia coli; Hemophilus influenzae; Klebsiella/Enterobacter** species; **Neisseria** species; and **Pseudomonas aeruginosa.**
When a decision to administer both a corticosteroid and an antimicrobial is made, the administration of such drugs in combination has the advantage of greater patient compliance and convenience, with the added assurance that the appropriate dosage of both drugs is administered. When both types of drugs are in the same formulation, compatibility of ingredients is assured and the correct volume of drug is delivered and retained.
The relative potency of corticosteroids depends on the molecular structure, concentration, and release from the vehicle.
Indications and Usage: A steroid/anti-infective combination is indicated for steroid-responsive inflammatory ocular conditions for which a corticosteroid is indicated and where bacterial infection or a risk of bacterial ocular infection exists.
Ocular steroids are indicated in inflammatory conditions of the palpebral and bulbar conjunctiva, cornea, and anterior segment of the globe where the inherent risk of steroid use in certain infective conjunctivitides is accepted to obtain a diminution in edema and inflammation. They are also indicated in chronic anterior uveitis and corneal injury from chemical, radiation or thermal burns, or penetration of foreign bodies.
The use of a combination drug with an anti-infective component is indicated where the risk of infection is high or where there is an expectation that potentially dangerous numbers of bacteria will be present in the eye.
The particular anti-infective drugs in this product are active against the following common bacterial eye pathogens: **Staphylococcus aureus; Escherichia coli; Hemophilus influenzae; Klebsiella/Enterobacter** species; **Neisseria** species; and **Pseudomonas aeruginosa.**
The product does not provide adequate coverage against: **Serratia marcescens;** Streptococci, including **Streptococcus pneumoniae.**
Contraindications: Epithelial herpes simplex keratitis (dendritic keratitis), vaccinia, varicella, and many other viral diseases of the cornea and conjunctiva. Mycobacterial infection of the eye. Fungal diseases of the ocular structures. Hypersensitivity to a component of the medication. (Hypersensitivity to the antibiotic component occurs at a higher rate than for other components.)
The use of these combinations is always contraindicated after uncomplicated removal of a corneal foreign body.
Warnings: Prolonged use may result in glaucoma, with damage to the optic nerve, defects in visual acuity and fields of vision, and in posterior subcapsular cataract formation. Prolonged use may suppress the host response and thus increase the hazard of secondary ocular infections. In those diseases causing thinning of the cornea or sclera, perforations have been known to occur with the use of topical steroids. In acute purulent conditions of the eye, steroids may mask infection or enhance existing infection. If these products are used for 10 days or longer, intraocular pressure should be routinely monitored even though it may be difficult in children and uncooperative patients.
Employment of a steroid medication in the treatment of herpes simplex requires great caution.
There exists a potential for neomycin sulfate to cause cutaneous sensitization. The exact incidence of this reaction is unknown.
Precautions: The initial prescription and renewal of the medication order beyond 20 milliliters should be made by a physician only after examination of the patient with the aid of magnification, such as slit lamp biomicroscopy and, where appropriate, fluorescein staining.

The possibility of persistent fungal infections of the cornea should be considered after prolonged steroid dosing.

Adverse Reactions: Adverse reactions have occurred with steroid/anti-infective combination drugs which can be attributed to the steroid component, the anti-infective component, or the combination. Exact incidence figures are not available since no denominator of treated patients is available.

Reactions occurring most often from the presence of the anti-infective ingredients are allergic sensitizations. The reactions due to the steroid component in decreasing order of frequency are: elevation of intraocular pressure (IOP) with possible development of glaucoma, and infrequent optic nerve damage; posterior subcapsular cataract formation; and delayed wound healing.

Secondary Infection: The development of secondary infection has occurred after use of combinations containing steroids and antimicrobials. Fungal infections of the cornea are particularly prone to develop coincidentally with long-term applications of steroid. The possibility of fungal invasion must be considered in any persistent corneal ulceration where steroid treatment has been used.

Secondary bacterial ocular infection following suppression of host responses also occurs.

Dosage and Administration: TO TREAT THE EYE: 1 or 2 drops every 3 or 4 hours, or more frequently as required. Acute infections may require administration every 30 minutes, with frequency of administration reduced as the infection is brought under control. TO TREAT THE LIDS: Instill 1 or 2 drops in the eye every 3 to 4 hours, close the eye and rub the excess on the lids and lid margins.

Not more than 20 milliliters should be prescribed initially and the prescription should not be refilled without further evaluation as outlined in the **Precautions** section above.

How Supplied: POLY-PRED® Liquifilm® sterile ophthalmic suspension is supplied in plastic dropper bottles in the following sizes:

5 mL—NDC 0023-0028-05
10 mL—NDC 0023-0028-15

Note: Protect from freezing. **Shake well before using.**

Caution: Federal (U.S.A.) law prohibits dispensing without prescription.

POLYTRIM® OPHTHALMIC SOLUTION ℞
Sterile
(TRIMETHOPRIM SULFATE AND POLYMYXIN B SULFATE)

Description: Polytrim® Ophthalmic Solution (trimethoprim sulfate and polymyxin B sulfate) is a sterile antimicrobial solution for topical ophthalmic use. Each mL contains trimethoprim sulfate equivalent to 1 mg trimethoprim and polymyxin B sulfate 10,000 units. The vehicle contains benzalkonium chloride 0.004% (added as preservative) and the inactive ingredients sodium chloride, sodium hydroxide or sulfuric acid (added to adjust pH), and Water for Injection.

Trimethoprim sulfate, 2,4-diamino-5-(3,4,5-trimethoxybenzyl)pyrimidine sulfate (2:1), is a white, odorless, crystalline powder with a molecular weight of 678.72.

Polymyxin B sulfate is the sulfate salt of polymyxin B_1 and B_2 which are produced by the growth of *Bacillus polymyxa* (Prazmowski) Migula (Fam. Bacillaceae). It has a potency of not less than 6,000 polymyxin B units per mg, calculated on an anhydrous basis.

Clinical Pharmacology: Trimethoprim is a synthetic antibacterial drug active against a wide variety of aerobic gram-positive and gram-negative ophthalmic pathogens. Trimethoprim blocks the production of tetrahydrofolic acid from dihydrofolic acid by binding to and reversibly inhibiting the enzyme dihydrofolate reductase. This binding is very much stronger for the bacterial enzyme than for the corresponding mammalian enzyme. For that reason, trimethoprim selectively interferes with bacterial biosynthesis of nucleic acids and proteins.

Polymyxin B, a cyclic lipopeptide antibiotic, is rapidly bactericidal for a variety of gram-negative organisms, especially *Pseudomonas aeruginosa*. It increases the permeability of the bacterial cell membrane by interacting with the phospholipid components of the membrane.

When used topically, trimethoprim and polymyxin B absorption through intact skin and mucous membranes is insignificant.

Blood samples were obtained from 11 human volunteers at 20 minutes, 1 hour and 3 hours following instillation in the eye of 2 drops of ophthalmic solution containing 1 mg trimethoprim and 10,000 units polymyxin B per mL. Peak serum concentrations were approximately 0.03 μg/mL trimethoprim and 1 unit/mL polymyxin B.

Microbiology: *In vitro* studies have demonstrated that the anti-infective components of Polytrim are active against the following bacterial pathogens that are capable of causing external infections of the eye:

Trimethoprim: *Staphylococcus aureus* and *Staphylococcus epidermidis, Streptococcus pyogenes, Streptococcus faecalis, Streptococcus pneumoniae, Haemophilus influenzae, Haemophilus aegyptius, Escherichia coli, Klebsiella pneumoniae, Proteus mirabilis* (indole-negative), *Proteus vulgaris* (indole-positive), *Enterobacter aerogenes,* and *Serratia marcescens.*

Polymyxin B: *Pseudomonas aeruginosa, Escherichia coli, Klebsiella pneumoniae, Enterobacter aerogenes* and *Haemophilus influenzae.*

Indications and Usage: Polytrim Ophthalmic Solution is indicated in the treatment of surface ocular bacterial infections, including acute bacterial conjunctivitis, and blepharoconjunctivitis, caused by susceptible strains of the following microorganisms: *Staphylococcus aureus, Staphylococcus epidermidis, Streptococcus pneumoniae, Streptococcus viridans, Haemophilus influenzae* and *Pseudomonas aeruginosa.**

Contraindications: Polytrim Ophthalmic Solution is contraindicated in patients with known hypersensitivity to any of its components.

Warnings: NOT FOR INJECTION INTO THE EYE. If a sensitivity reaction to Polytrim occurs, discontinue use. Polytrim Ophthalmic Solution is not indicated for the prophylaxis or treatment of ophthalmia neonatorum.

Precautions:

General: As with other antimicrobial preparations, prolonged use may result in overgrowth of nonsusceptible organisms, including fungi. If superinfection occurs, appropriate therapy should be initiated.

Information for Patients: Avoid contaminating the applicator tip with material from the eye, fingers, or other source. This precaution is necessary if the sterility of the drops is to be maintained.

If redness, irritation, swelling or pain persists or increases, discontinue use immediately and contact your physician.

Carcinogenesis, Mutagenesis, Impairment of Fertility:

Carcinogenesis: Long-term studies in animals to evaluate carcinogenic potential have not been conducted with polymyxin B sulfate or trimethoprim.

Mutagenesis: Trimethoprim was demonstrated to be non-mutagenic in the Ames assay. In studies at two laboratories no chromosomal damage was detected in cultured Chinese hamster ovary cells at concentrations approximately 500 times human plasma levels after oral administration; at concentrations approximately 1000 times human plasma levels after oral administration in these same cells a low level of chromosomal damage was induced at one of the laboratories. Studies to evaluate mutagenic potential have not been conducted with polymyxin B sulfate.

Impairment of Fertility: Polymyxin B sulfate has been reported to impair the motility of equine sperm, but its effects on male or female fertility are unknown.

No adverse effects on fertility or general reproductive performance were observed in rats given trimethoprim in oral dosages as high as 70 mg/kg/day for males and 14 mg/kg/day for females.

Pregnancy: ***Teratogenic Effects:*** Pregnancy Category C. Animal reproduction studies have not been conducted with polymyxin B sulfate. It is not known whether polymyxin B sulfate can cause fetal harm when administered to a pregnant woman or can affect reproduction capacity.

Trimethoprim has been shown to be teratogenic in the rat when given in oral doses 40 times the human dose. In some rabbit studies, the overall increase in fetal loss (dead and resorbed and malformed conceptuses) was associated with oral doses 6 times the human therapeutic dose.

While there are no large well-controlled studies on the use of trimethoprim in pregnant women, Brumfitt and Pursell, in a retrospective study, reported the outcome of 186 pregnancies during which the mother received either placebo or oral trimethoprim in combination with sulfamethoxazole. The incidence of congenital abnormalities was 4.5% (3 of 66) in those who received placebo and 3.3% (4 of 120) in those receiving trimethoprim and sulfamethoxazole. There were no abnormalities in the 10 children whose mothers received the drug during the first trimester. In a separate survey, Brumfitt and Pursell also found no congenital abnormalities in 35 children whose mothers had received oral trimethoprim and sulfamethoxazole at the time of conception or shortly thereafter.

Because trimethoprim may interfere with folic acid metabolism, trimethoprim should be used during pregnancy only if the potential benefit justifies the potential risk to the fetus.

Nonteratogenic Effects: The oral administration of trimethoprim to rats at a dose of 70 mg/kg/day commencing with the last third of gestation and continuing through parturition and lactation caused no deleterious effects on gestation or pup growth and survival.

Pediatric Use: Safety and effectiveness in children below the age of 2 months have not been established (see WARNINGS).

Adverse Reactions: The most frequent adverse reaction to Polytrim Ophthalmic Solution is local irritation consisting of transient burning or stinging, itching or increased redness on instillation. These reactions occur in less than 4 of 100 patients treated. Polytrim has a low incidence of hypersensitivity reactions (less than 2 of 100 patients treated) consisting of lid edema, itching, increased redness, tearing and/or circumocular rash.

Although sensitivity reactions to trimethoprim are rare, an isolated incident of photosensitivity was reported in a patient who received the drug orally.

Dosage and Administration:

Adults: In mild to moderate infections, instill one drop in the affected eye(s) every three hours (maximum of 6 doses per day) for a period of 7 to 10 days.

Pediatric Use: Clinical studies have shown Polytrim to be safe and effective for use in children over two months of age. The dosage regimen is the same as for adults.

Continued on next page

*Efficacy for this organism in this organ system was studied in fewer than 10 infections.

Allergan Pharm—Cont.

How Supplied: A sterile ophthalmic solution, each mL contains trimethoprim sulfate** equivalent to 1 mg trimethoprim and polymyxin B sulfate 10,000 units in a plastic dropper bottle of 10 mL (NDC 0023-7824-10).
Store at 15°–25°C (59°–77°F) and protect from light.
**Mfd. under U.S. Patent No. 3,956,327.

PRED FORTE® ℞
(prednisolone acetate) 1%
sterile ophthalmic suspension

Description: PRED FORTE® (prednisolone acetate) 1% sterile ophthalmic suspension is a topical anti-inflammatory agent for ophthalmic use.
Chemical Name: 11β, 17, 21-Trihydroxypregna-1,4-diene-3,20-dione 21-acetate
Contains:
prednisolone acetate (microfine suspension) 1.0%
with: benzalkonium chloride, polysorbate 80, boric acid, sodium citrate, sodium bisulfite, sodium chloride, edetate disodium, hydroxypropyl methylcellulose and purified water.
Clinical Pharmacology: Prednisolone acetate is a glucocorticoid that, on the basis of weight, has 3 to 5 times the anti-inflammatory potency of hydrocortisone. Glucocorticoids inhibit the edema, fibrin deposition, capillary dilation and phagocytic migration of the acute inflammatory response as well as capillary proliferation, deposition of collagen and scar formation.
Indications and Usage: PRED FORTE is indicated for the treatment of steroid responsive inflammation of the palpebral and bulbar conjunctiva, cornea and anterior segment of the globe.
Contraindications: PRED FORTE is contraindicated in acute untreated purulent ocular infections, acute superficial herpes simplex (dendritic keratitis), vaccinia, varicella and most other viral diseases of the cornea and conjunctiva, ocular tuberculosis, and fungal diseases of the eye. It is also contraindicated for individuals sensitive to any components of the formulation.
Warnings: In those diseases causing thinning of the cornea, perforation has been reported with the use of topical steroids.
Since PRED FORTE contains no antimicrobial, if infection is present, appropriate measures must be taken to counteract the organisms involved.
Acute purulent infections of the eye may be masked or enhanced by the use of topical steroids.
Use of steroid medication in the presence of stromal herpes simplex requires caution and should be followed by frequent mandatory slit-lamp microscopy.
As fungal infections of the cornea have been reported coincidentally with long-term local steroid applications, fungal invasion may be suspected in any persistent corneal ulceration where a steroid has been used, or is in use.
Use of topical corticosteroids may cause increased intraocular pressure in certain individuals. This may result in damage to the optic nerve, with defects in the visual fields. It is advisable that the intraocular pressure be checked frequently.
Posterior subcapsular cataract formation has been reported after heavy or protracted use of topical ophthalmic corticosteroids.
Contains sodium bisulfite, a sulfite that may cause allergic-type reactions, including anaphylactic symptoms and life-threatening or less severe asthmatic episodes in certain susceptible people. The overall prevalence of sulfite sensitivity in the general population is unknown and probably low. Sulfite sensitivity is seen more frequently in asthmatic than in nonasthmatic people.
Precautions: General: Patients with histories of herpes simplex keratitis should be treated with caution.
Carcinogenesis, mutagenesis, Impairment of fertility: No studies have been conducted in animals or in humans to evaluate the potential of these effects.
Pregnancy Category C: Prednisolone has been shown to be teratogenic in mice when given in doses 1–10 times the human dose. There are no adequate well-controlled studies in pregnant women. Prednisolone should be used during pregnancy only if the potential benefit justifies the potential risk to the fetus. Dexamethasone, hydrocortisone and prednisolone were ocularly applied to both eyes of pregnant mice five times per day on days 10 through 13 of gestation. A significant increase in the incidence of cleft palate was observed in the fetuses of the treated mice.
Nursing Mothers: It is not known whether topical administration of corticosteroids could result in sufficient systemic absorption to produce detectable quantities in breast milk. Systemically administered corticosteroids are secreted into breast milk in quantities not likely to have a deleterious effect on the infant. Nevertheless, caution should be exercised when topical corticosteroids are administered to a nursing woman.
Pediatric Use: Safety and effectiveness in children have not been established.
Adverse Reactions: Adverse reactions include increased intraocular pressure, which may be associated with optic nerve damage and defects in the visual fields, posterior subcapsular cataract formation, secondary ocular infections from fungi or viruses liberated from ocular tissues and perforation of the globe when used in conditions where there is thinning of the cornea or sclera. Systemic side effects may occur rarely with extensive use of topical steroids.
Overdosage: Overdosage will not ordinarily cause acute problems. If accidentally ingested, drink fluids to dilute.
Dosage and Administration: Shake well before using. Instill one to two drops into the conjunctival sac two to four times daily. During the initial 24 to 48 hours, the dosing frequency may be increased if necessary. Care should be taken not to discontinue therapy prematurely.
NOTE: Keep this and all medications out of the reach of children.
How Supplied: PRED FORTE® (prednisolone acetate) 1% sterile ophthalmic suspension is supplied in plastic dropper bottles in the following sizes:

1 mL—**NDC** 11980-180-01
5 mL—**NDC** 11980-180-05
10 mL—**NDC** 11980-180-10
15 mL—**NDC** 11980-180-15

Note: Protect from freezing.
Caution: Federal (U.S.A.) law prohibits dispensing without prescription.

PRED–G® ℞
(prednisolone acetate, gentamicin sulfate) Liquifilm®
sterile ophthalmic suspension

Description: PRED-G® Liquifilm® sterile ophthalmic suspension is a topical anti-inflammatory/anti-infective combination product for ophthalmic use.
Chemical Names: Prednisolone acetate: 11β, 17,21-Trihydroxypregna-1,4-diene-3,20-dione 21-acetate.
Gentamicin sulfate is the sulfate salt of gentamicin C_1, gentamicin C_2, and gentamicin C_{1A} which are produced by the growth of **Micromonospora purpurea.**
Contains: prednisolone acetate ....1.0% (microfine suspension)
gentamicin sulfate ....equivalent to 0.3% gentamicin base
with: Liquifilm® (polyvinyl alcohol) 1.4%; benzalkonium chloride 0.005%; edetate disodium; hydroxypropyl methylcellulose; polysorbate 80; sodium citrate, dihydrate; sodium chloride; sodium hydroxide and/or hydrochloric acid to adjust the pH; and purified water.
Clinical Pharmacology: Corticosteroids suppress the inflammatory response to a variety of agents and they probably delay or slow healing. Since corticosteroids may inhibit the body's defense mechanism against infection, a concomitant antimicrobial drug may be used when this inhibition is considered to be clinically significant in a particular case.
The anti-infective component in PRED-G is included to provide action against specific organisms susceptible to it. Gentamicin sulfate is active *in vitro* against susceptible strains of the following microorganisms: coagulase-positive and coagulase-negative staphylococci, including **S. aureus,** and certain strains that are resistant to penicillin; Group A beta-hemolytic and non-hemolytic streptococci, and **Streptococcus pneumoniae; Escherichia coli; Hemophilus influenzae; Klebsiella/Enterobacter** species; **Neisseria** species, including **Neisseria gonorrhoeae; Pseudomonas aeruginosa;** indole-positive and indole-negative **Proteus** species; and **Serratia marcescens.**
When a decision to administer both a corticosteroid and an antimicrobial is made, the administration of such drugs in combination has the advantage of greater patient compliance and convenience, with the added assurance that the appropriate dosage of both drugs is administered. When both types of drugs are in the same formulation, compatibility of ingredients is assured and the correct volume of drug is delivered and retained.
The relative potency of corticosteroids depends on the molecular structure, concentration, and release from the vehicle.
Indications and Usage: PRED-G suspension is indicated for steroid-responsive inflammatory ocular conditions for which a corticosteroid is indicated and where superficial bacterial ocular infection or a risk of bacterial ocular infection exists.
Ocular steroids are indicated in inflammatory conditions of the palpebral and bulbar conjunctiva, cornea, and anterior segment of the globe where the inherent risk of steroid use in certain infective conjunctivitides is accepted to obtain a diminution in edema and inflammation. They are also indicated in chronic anterior uveitis and corneal injury from chemical, radiation, or thermal burns or penetration of foreign bodies.
The use of a combination drug with an anti-infective component is indicated where the risk of superficial ocular infection is high or where there is an expectation that potentially dangerous numbers of bacteria will be present in the eye.
The particular anti-infective drug in this product is active against the following common bacterial eye pathogens: coagulase-positive and coagulase-negative staphyloccocci, including **Staphylococcus aureus,** and certain strains that are resistant to penicillin; Group A beta-hemolytic and nonhemolytic streptococci, and **Streptococcus pneumoniae; Escherichia coli; Hemophilus influenzae; Klebsiella/Enterobacter** species; **Neisseria** species, including **Neisseria gonorrhoeae; Pseudomonas aeruginosa;** indole-positive and indole-negative **Proteus** species; and **Serratia marcescens.**
Contraindications: Epithelial herpes simplex keratitis (dendritic keratitis), vaccinia, varicella, and many other viral diseases of the cornea and conjunctiva. Mycobacterial infection of the eye. Fungal diseases of the ocular

structures. Hypersensitivity to a component of the medication. (Hypersensitivity to the antibiotic component occurs at a higher rate than for other components.)

PRED-G suspension is always contraindicated after uncomplicated removal of a corneal foreign body.

Warnings: Prolonged use may result in glaucoma, with damage to the optic nerve, defects in visual acuity and fields of vision, and in posterior subcapsular cataract formation. Prolonged use may suppress the host response and thus increase the hazard of secondary ocular infections. In those diseases causing thinning of the cornea or sclera, perforations have been known to occur with the use of topical steroids. In acute purulent conditions of the eye, steroids may mask infection or enhance existing infection. If these products are used for 10 days or longer, intraocular pressure should be routinely monitored even though it may be difficult in children and uncooperative patients.

Employment of a steroid medication in the treatment of patients with a history of herpes simplex requires great caution. PRED-G is contraindicated in patients with active herpes simplex keratitis.

PRED-G Liquifilm sterile ophthalmic suspension is not for injection. It should never be injected subconjunctivally, nor should it be directly introduced into the anterior chamber of the eye.

Precautions: The initial prescription and renewal of the medication order beyond 20 milliliters should be made by a physician only after examination of the patient with the aid of magnification, such as slit lamp biomicroscopy and, where appropriate, fluorescein staining. The possibility of fungal infections of the cornea should be considered after prolonged steroid dosing.

Adverse Reactions: Adverse reactions have occurred with steroid/anti-infective combination drugs which can be attributed to the steroid component, the anti-infective component, or the combination. Exact incidence figures are not available since no denominator of treated patients is available.

Reactions occurring most often from the presence of the anti-infective ingredient are allergic sensitizations. The reactions due to the steroid component in decreasing order of frequency are: elevation of intraocular pressure (IOP) with possible development of glaucoma, and infrequent optic nerve damage; posterior subcapsular cataract formation; and delayed wound healing.

Burning, stinging and other symptoms of irritation have been reported with PRED-G. Superficial punctate keratitis has been reported occasionally with onset occurring typically after several days of use.

Secondary Infection: The development of secondary infection has occurred after use of combinations containing steroids and antimicrobials. Fungal infections of the cornea are particularly prone to develop coincidentally with long-term applications of steroid. The possibility of fungal invasion must be considered in any persistent corneal ulceration where steroid treatment has been used.

Secondary bacterial ocular infection following suppression of host responses also occurs.

Dosage and Administration: Instill one drop into the conjunctival sac two to four times daily. During the initial 24 to 48 hours, the dosing frequency may be increased if necessary. Care should be taken not to discontinue therapy prematurely.

Not more than 20 milliliters should be prescribed initially and the prescription should not be refilled without further evaluation as outlined in **Precautions** above.

How Supplied: PRED-G® (prednisolone acetate 1.0%, gentamicin sulfate—0.3% base) Liquifilm® sterile ophthalmic suspension is supplied in plastic dropper bottles in the following sizes:

2 mL—NDC 0023-0106-02
5 mL—NDC 0023-0106-05
10 mL—NDC 0023-0106-10

Note: Store at room temperature. Avoid excessive heat, 40° C (104° F) and above. Protect from freezing. Shake well before using.

Caution: Federal (U.S.A.) law prohibits dispensing without prescription.

PRED–G® ℞
(prednisolone acetate, gentamicin sulfate)
S.O.P.®
sterile ophthalmic ointment

Description: PRED-G S.O.P. sterile ophthalmic ointment is a topical anti-inflammatory/anti-infective combination product for ophthalmic use.

Chemical Names: Prednisolone acetate: 11β,17,21-Trihydroxypregna-1,4-diene-3, 20-dione 21-acetate.

Gentamicin sulfate is the sulfate salt of gentamicin C_1, gentamicin C_2, and gentamicin C_{1A} which are produced by the growth of *Micromonospora purpurea.*

Contains: prednisolone acetate 0.6%
gentamicin sulfate ....equivalent to 0.3% gentamicin base
with: chlorobutanol (chloral derivative) 0.5%; white petrolatum; mineral oil; petrolatum (and) lanolin alcohol; and purified water.

Clinical Pharmacology: Corticosteroids suppress the inflammatory response to a variety of agents and they probably delay or slow healing. Since corticosteroids may inhibit the body's defense mechanism against infection, a concomitant antimicrobial drug may be used when this inhibition is considered to be clinically significant in a particular case.

The anti-infective component in PRED-G is included to provide action against specific organisms susceptible to it. Gentamicin sulfate is active *in vitro* against susceptible strains of the following microorganisms: *Staphylococcus aureus, Streptococcus pyogenes, Streptococcus pneumoniae, Enterobacter aerogenes, Escherichia coli, Hemophilus influenzae, Klebsiella pneumoniae, Neisseria gonorrhoeae, Pseudomonas aeruginosa,* and *Serratia marcescens.*

When a decision to administer both a corticosteroid and an antimicrobial is made, the administration of such drugs in combination has the advantage of greater patient compliance and convenience, with the added assurance that the appropriate dosage of both drugs is administered. When both types of drugs are in the same formulation, compatibility of ingredients is assured and the correct volume of drug is delivered and retained.

The relative potency of corticosteroids depends on the molecular structure, concentration, and release from the vehicle.

Indications and Usage: PRED-G S.O.P. is indicated for steroid-responsive inflammatory ocular conditions for which a corticosteroid is indicated and where superficial bacterial ocular infection or a risk of bacterial ocular infection exists.

Ocular steroids are indicated in inflammatory conditions of the palpebral and bulbar conjunctiva, cornea, and anterior segment of the globe where the inherent risk of steroid use in certain infective conjunctivitides is accepted to obtain a diminution in edema and inflammation. They are also indicated in chronic anterior uveitis and corneal injury from chemical, radiation, or thermal burns or penetration of foreign bodies.

The use of a combination drug with an anti-infective component is indicated where the risk of superficial ocular infection is high or where there is an expectation that potentially dangerous numbers of bacteria will be present in the eye.

The particular anti-infective drug in this product is active against the following common bacterial eye pathogens: *Staphylococcus aureus, Streptococcus pyogenes, Streptococcus pneumoniae, Enterobacter aerogenes, Escherichia coli, Hemophilus influenzae, Klebsiella pneumoniae, Neisseria gonorrhoeae, Pseudomonas aeruginosa,* and *Serratia marcescens.*

Contraindications: Epithelial herpes simplex keratitis (dendritic keratitis), vaccinia, varicella, and many other viral diseases of the cornea and conjunctiva. Mycobacterial infection of the eye. Fungal diseases of the ocular structures. Hypersensitivity to a component of the medication. (Hypersensitivity to the antibiotic component occurs at a higher rate than for other components.)

PRED-G® S.O.P.® is always contraindicated after uncomplicated removal of a corneal foreign body.

Warnings: Prolonged use may result in glaucoma, with damage to the optic nerve, defects in visual acuity and fields of vision, and in posterior subcapsular cataract formation. Prolonged use may suppress the host immune response and thus increase the hazard of secondary ocular infections. In those diseases causing thinning of the cornea or sclera, perforations have been known to occur with the use of topical steroids. In acute purulent conditions of the eye, steroids may mask infection or enhance existing infection. If these products are used for 10 days or longer, intraocular pressure should be routinely monitored even though it may be difficult in children and uncooperative patients.

Employment of a steroid medication in the treatment of patients with a history of herpes simplex requires great caution. PRED-G is contraindicated in patients with active herpes simplex keratitis.

Precautions: General: Ocular irritation and punctate keratitis have been associated with the use of Pred-G. The initial prescription and renewal of the medication order beyond 8 grams should be made by a physician only after examination of the patient's intraocular pressure, examination of the patient with the aid of magnification, such as slit lamp biomicroscopy and, where appropriate, fluorescein staining. The possibility of fungal infections of the cornea should be considered after prolonged steroid dosing.

Carcinogenesis, mutagenesis, impairment of fertility: There are no published carcinogenicity or impairment of fertility studies on gentamicin. Aminoglycoside antibiotics have been found to be non-mutagenic.

There are no published mutagenicity or impairment of fertility studies on prednisolone. Prednisolone has been reported to be non-carcinogenic.

Pregnancy: Pregnancy Category C: Gentamicin has been shown to depress newborn body weights, kidney weights, nephron counts and shows evidence of glomeruli and proximal tubule nephrotoxicity in rats when administered systemically in daily doses of approximately 500 times the maximum recommended ophthalmic dose in humans.

Prednisolone has been shown to be teratogenic in mice when given in doses 1–10 times the human dose. Dexamethasone, hydrocortisone and prednisolone were ocularly applied to both eyes of pregnant mice five times per day on days 10 through 13 of gestation. A significant increase in the incidence of cleft palate was observed in the fetuses of the treated mice. There are no adequate well-controlled studies in pregnant women. PRED-G should be used during pregnancy only if the potential benefit justifies the potential risk to the fetus.

Nursing Mothers: It is not known whether topical administration of corticosteroids could

Continued on next page

Allergan Pharm—Cont.

result in sufficient systemic absorption to produce detectable quantities in breast milk. Systemically administered corticosteroids appear in breast milk and could suppress growth, interfere with endogenous corticosteroid production, or cause other untoward effects. Because of the potential for serious adverse reactions in nursing infants from PRED-G a decision should be made whether to discontinue nursing or to discontinue the medication.

Pediatric Use: Safety and effectiveness in children have not been established.

Adverse Reactions: Adverse reactions have occurred with steroid/anti-infective combination drugs which can be attributed to the steroid component, the anti-infective component, or the combination. Exact incidence figures are not available since no denominator of treated patients is available.

The most frequent reactions observed include ocular discomfort, irritation upon instillation of the medication and punctate keratitis. These reactions have resolved upon discontinuation of the medication.

Reactions occurring most often from the presence of the anti-infective ingredient are allergic sensitizations. The reactions due to the steroid component in decreasing order of frequency are: elevation of intraocular pressure (IOP) with possible development of glaucoma, and infrequent optic nerve damage; posterior subcapsular cataract formation; and delayed wound healing.

Secondary Infection: The development of secondary infection has occurred after use of combinations containing steroids and antimicrobials. Fungal infections of the cornea are particularly prone to develop coincidentally with long-term applications of steroid. The possibility of fungal invasion must be considered in any persistent corneal ulceration where steroid treatment has been used.

Secondary bacterial ocular infection following suppression of host responses also occurs.

Dosage and Administration: A small amount (½ inch ribbon) of ointment should be applied in the conjunctival sac one to three times daily. Care should be taken not to discontinue therapy prematurely.

Not more than 8 grams should be prescribed initially and the prescription should not be refilled without further evaluation as outlined in **Precautions** above.

How Supplied: PRED-G® (prednisolone acetate 0.6%, gentamicin sulfate-0.3% base) S.O.P.® sterile ophthalmic ointment is supplied in ophthalmic ointment tubes of the following size:

3.5 g—NDC 0023-0066-04

Note: Store at controlled room temperature between 15°–30°C (59°–86°F).

Caution: Federal (U.S.A.) law prohibits dispensing without prescription.

PRED MILD® ℞

(prednisolone acetate) 0.12%
sterile ophthalmic suspension

Description: PRED MILD® (prednisolone acetate) 0.12% sterile ophthalmic suspension is a topical anti-inflammatory agent for ophthalmic use.

Chemical Name: 11β,17,21-Trihydroxypregna-1,4-diene-3,20-dione 21-acetate.

Contains:

prednisolone acetate (microfine suspension) 0.12%

with: benzalkonium chloride; polysorbate 80; boric acid; sodium citrate; sodium bisulfite; sodium chloride; edetate disodium; hydroxypropyl methylcellulose; and purified water.

Clinical Pharmacology: Prednisolone acetate is a glucocorticoid that, on the basis of weight, has 3 to 5 times the anti-inflammatory potency of hydrocortisone. Glucocorticoids inhibit the edema, fibrin deposition, capillary dilation and phagocytic migration of the acute inflammatory response as well as capillary proliferation, deposition of collagen and scar formation.

Indications and Usage: PRED MILD® is indicated for the treatment of mild to moderate noninfectious allergic and inflammatory disorders of the lid, conjunctiva, cornea and sclera (including chemical and thermal burns).

Contraindications: PRED MILD is contraindicated in acute untreated purulent ocular infections, acute superficial herpes simplex (dendritic keratitis), vaccinia, varicella and most other viral diseases of the cornea and conjunctiva, ocular tuberculosis, and fungal diseases of the eye. It is also contraindicated for individuals sensitive to any components of the formulation.

Warnings: In those diseases causing thinning of the cornea, perforation has been reported with the use of topical steroids.

Since PRED MILD contains no antimicrobial, if infection is present, appropriate measures must be taken to counteract the organism involved.

Acute purulent infections of the eye may be masked or enhanced by the use of topical steroids.

Use of steroid medication in the presence of stromal herpes simplex requires caution and should be followed by frequent mandatory slit-lamp microscopy.

As fungal infections of the cornea have been reported coincidentally with long-term local steroid applications, fungal invasion may be suspected in any persistent corneal ulceration where a steroid has been used, or is in use.

Use of topical corticosteroids may cause increased intraocular pressure in certain individuals. This may result in damage to the optic nerve with defects in the visual fields. It is advisable that the intraocular pressure be checked frequently. Posterior subcapsular cataract formation has been reported after heavy or protracted use of topical ophthalmic corticosteroids.

Contains sodium bisulfite, a sulfite that may cause allergic-type reactions including anaphylactic symptoms and life-threatening or less severe asthmatic episodes in certain susceptible people. The overall prevalence of sulfite sensitivity in the general population is unknown and probably low. Sulfite sensitivity is seen more frequently in asthmatic than in non-asthmatic people.

Precautions:

General: Patients with histories of herpes simplex keratitis should be treated with caution.

Carcinogenesis, mutagenesis, impairment of fertility: No studies have been conducted in animals or in humans to evaluate the potential of these effects.

Pregnancy Category C: Prednisolone has been shown to be teratogenic in mice when given in doses 1–10 times the human dose. There are no adequate well-controlled studies in pregnant women. Prednisolone should be used during pregnancy only if the potential benefit justifies the potential risk to the fetus. Dexamethasone, hydrocortisone and prednisolone were ocularly applied to both eyes of pregnant mice five times per day on days 10 through 13 of gestation. A significant increase in the incidence of cleft palate was observed in the fetuses of the treated mice.

Nursing Mothers: It is not known whether topical administration of corticosteroids could result in sufficient systemic absorption to produce detectable quantities in breast milk. Systemically administered corticosteroids are secreted into breast milk in quantities not likely to have a deleterious effect on the infant. Nevertheless, caution should be exercised when topical corticosteroids are administered to a nursing woman.

Pediatric use: Safety and effectiveness in children have not been established.

Adverse Reactions: Adverse reactions include increased intraocular pressure which may be associated with optic nerve damage and defects in the visual fields, posterior subcapsular cataract formation, secondary ocular infections from fungi or viruses liberated from ocular tissues and perforation of the globe when used in conditions where there is thinning of the cornea or sclera. Systemic side effects may occur rarely with extensive use of topical steroids.

Overdosage: Overdosage will not ordinarily cause acute problems. If accidentally ingested, drink fluids to dilute.

Dosage and Administration: Shake well before using. Instill 1 to 2 drops into the conjunctival sac two to four times daily. During the initial 24 to 48 hours the dosing frequency may be safely increased if necessary. Care should be taken not to discontinue therapy prematurely.

Note: Keep this and all medications out of the reach of children.

How Supplied: PRED MILD® (prednisolone acetate) 0.12% sterile ophthalmic suspension is supplied in plastic dropper bottles in the following sizes:

5 mL—NDC 11980-174-05
10 mL—NDC 11980-174-10

Note: Store at controlled room temperature 15°–30°C (59°–86°F). Protect from freezing.

Caution: Federal (U.S.A.) law prohibits dispensing without prescription.

PREFRIN® LIQUIFILM® OTC

(phenylephrine HCl 0.12%, polyvinyl alcohol 1.4%)
Vasoconstrictor (Redness Reliever) and Lubricant Eye Drops

Contains: Actives: Phenylephrine HCl 0.12%, LIQUIFILM® (polyvinyl alcohol) 1.4%. Inactives: benzalkonium chloride, edetate disodium, mono- and dibasic sodium phosphates, purified water, sodium acetate and sodium thiosulfate. pH may be adjusted with hydrochloric acid or sodium hydroxide.

FDA APPROVED USES

Indications: RELIEVES REDNESS OF THE EYE DUE TO MINOR EYE IRRITATION. FOR USE AS A LUBRICANT TO PREVENT FURTHER IRRITATION OR TO RELIEVE DRYNESS OF THE EYE.

Directions: Instill 1 to 2 drops in the affected eye(s) up to four times daily.

Warnings: If you have glaucoma, do not use this product except under the advice and supervision of a doctor. If you experience eye pain, changes in vision, continued redness or irritation of the eye, or if the condition worsens or persists for more than 72 hours, discontinue use and consult a doctor. Overuse of this product may produce increased redness of the eye. To avoid contamination, do not touch tip of container to any surface. Replace cap after using. If the solution changes color or becomes cloudy, do not use. Pupils may dilate in some individuals. Keep this and all drugs out of the reach of children. In case of accidental ingestion, seek professional assistance or contact a poison control center immediately.

Note: Not for use while wearing soft contact lenses.

PREFRIN-A™ ℞
sterile ophthalmic solution

Description:
Contains:
pyrilamine maleate.....0.1%
phenylephrine HCl 0.12%
with: benzalkonium chloride, antipyrine (0.1%), sodium bisulfite, sodium citrate, boric acid, edetate disodium, and purified water.

Indications
Based on a review of this drug by the National Academy of Sciences—National Research Council and/or other information, FDA has classified the indications as follows: "Possibly" effective: PREFRIN-A™ is useful in bringing symptomatic relief to eyes affected with allergy/inflammation/ irritation of a mild to moderate degree ... particularly when the allergic insult results from air pollutants or airborne pollens.
Final classification of the less-than-effective indications requires further investigation.

Contraindications: Should not be used in the presence of narrow-angle glaucoma. Do not use if hypersensitive to any ingredient.
Warnings: PREFRIN-A™ contains sodium bisulfite, a sulfite that may cause allergic-type reactions including anaphylactic symptoms and life-threatening or less severe asthmatic episodes in certain susceptible people. The overall prevalence of sulfite sensitivity in the general population is unknown and probably low. Sulfite sensitivity is seen more frequently in asthmatic than in nonasthmatic people.
Topical antihistamines are potential sensitizers and use may produce a local sensitivity reaction.
Because topical antihistamines may produce angle closure, this product should be used with caution in persons with a narrow angle or a history of glaucoma.
This product should not be used in the presence of infections, foreign bodies, or where irritation is severe.
Precautions: Should sensitivity or other untoward reactions occur, discontinue medication and consult with physician. Pupillary dilation may occur in some individuals.
Dosage and Administration: 1 to 2 drops in the eye(s) every 3 to 4 hours.
Note: Keep this and all medications out of the reach of children.
How Supplied: 15 mL plastic dropper bottles. NDC 11980-006-15
Caution: Federal (U.S.A) law prohibits dispensing without a prescription.

PROPINE® ℞
(dipivefrin HCl)
ophthalmic solution, USP, 0.1% sterile with C Cap™ Compliance Cap B.I.D.

Description: PROPINE® contains dipivefrin hydrochloride in a sterile, isotonic solution. Dipivefrin HCl is a white, crystalline powder, freely soluble in water.
Empirical Formula: $C_{19}H_{29}O_5N \cdot HCl$
Chemical Name: (±)-3,4-Dihydroxy-α-[(methylamino)methyl]benzyl alcohol 3,4-dipivalate hydrochloride.
Contains:
Dipivefrin HCl* 0.1%
with: benzalkonium chloride 0.005%; edetate disodium; sodium chloride; hydrochloric acid to adjust pH; and purified water.
*Licensed under U.S. Patent Nos. 3,839,584 and 3,809,714.
Clinical Pharmacology: PROPINE® (dipivefrin HCl) is a member of a class of drugs known as prodrugs. Prodrugs are usually not active in themselves and require biotransformation to the parent compound before therapeutic activity is seen. These modifications are undertaken to enhance absorption, decrease side effects and enhance stability and comfort, thus making the parent compound a more useful drug. Enhanced absorption makes the prodrug a more efficient delivery system for the parent drug because less drug will be needed to produce the desired therapeutic response.
PROPINE is a prodrug of epinephrine formed by the diesterification of epinephrine and pivalic acid. The addition of pivaloyl groups to the epinephrine molecule enhances its lipophilic character and, as a consequence, its penetration into the anterior chamber.
PROPINE is converted to epinephrine inside the human eye by enzyme hydrolysis. The liberated epinephrine, an adrenergic agonist, appears to exert its action by decreasing aqueous production and by enhancing outflow facility. The PROPINE prodrug delivery system is a more efficient way of delivering the therapeutic effects of epinephrine, with fewer side effects than are associated with conventional epinephrine therapy.
The onset of action with one drop of PROPINE occurs about 30 minutes after treatment, with maximum effect seen at about one hour.
Using a prodrug means that less drug is needed for therapeutic effect since absorption is enhanced with the prodrug. PROPINE at 0.1% dipivefrin was judged less irritating than a 1% solution of epinephrine hydrochloride or bitartrate. In addition, only 8 of 455 patients (1.8%) treated with PROPINE reported discomfort due to photophobia, glare or light sensitivity.
Indications: PROPINE (dipivefrin HCl) is indicated as initial therapy for the control of intraocular pressure in chronic open-angle glaucoma. Patients responding inadequately to other antiglaucoma therapy may respond to addition of PROPINE.
In controlled and open-label studies of glaucoma, PROPINE demonstrated a statistically significant intraocular pressure-lowering effect. Patients using PROPINE twice daily in studies with mean durations of 76–146 days experienced mean pressure reductions ranging from 20–24%.
Therapeutic response to PROPINE twice-daily is somewhat less than 2% epinephrine twice daily. Controlled studies showed statistically significant differences in lowering of intraocular pressure between PROPINE and 2% epinephrine. In controlled studies in patients with a history of epinephrine intolerance, only 3% of patients treated with PROPINE exhibited intolerance, while 55% of those treated with epinephrine again developed an intolerance.
Therapeutic response to PROPINE twice-daily therapy is comparable to 2% pilocarpine 4 times daily. In controlled clinical studies comparing PROPINE and 2% pilocarpine, there were no statistically significant differences in the maintenance of IOP levels for the two medications. PROPINE does not produce miosis or accommodative spasm which cholinergic agents are known to produce. The blurred vision and night blindness often associated with miotic agents are not present with PROPINE therapy. Patients with cataracts avoid the inability to see around lenticular opacities caused by constricted pupil.
Contraindications: PROPINE should not be used in patients with narrow angles since any dilation of the pupil may predispose the patient to an attack of angle-closure glaucoma. This product is contraindicated in patients who are hypersensitive to any of its components.
Precautions:
Aphakic Patients. Macular edema has been shown to occur in up to 30% of aphakic patients treated with epinephrine. Discontinuation of epinephrine generally results in reversal of the maculopathy.
Pregnancy: Pregnancy Category B. Reproduction studies have been performed in rats and rabbits at daily oral doses up to 10 mg/kg body weight (5 mg/kg in teratogenicity studies), and have revealed no evidence of impaired fertility or harm to the fetus due to dipivefrin HCl. There are, however, no adequate and well-controlled studies in pregnant women. Because animal reproduction studies are not always predictive of human response, this drug should be used during pregnancy only if clearly needed.
Nursing Mothers. It is not known whether this drug is excreted in human milk. Because many drugs are excreted in human milk, caution should be exercised when PROPINE is administered to a nursing woman.
Usage in Children. Clinical studies for safety and efficacy in children have not been done.
Animal Studies. Rabbit studies indicated a dose-related incidence of meibomian gland retention cysts following topical administration of both dipivefrin hydrochloride and epinephrine.
Adverse Reactions:
Cardiovascular Effects. Tachycardia, arrhythmias and hypertension have been reported with ocular administration of epinephrine.
Local Effects. The most frequent side effects reported with PROPINE alone were injection in 6.5% of patients and burning and stinging in 6%. Follicular conjunctivitis, mydriasis and allergic reactions to PROPINE have been reported infrequently. Epinephrine therapy can lead to adrenochrome deposits in the conjunctiva and cornea.
Dosage and Administration:
Initial Glaucoma Therapy. The usual dosage of PROPINE is one drop in the eye(s) every 12 hours.
Replacement with PROPINE. When patients are being transferred to PROPINE from antiglaucoma agents other than epinephrine, on the first day continue the previous medication and add one drop of PROPINE in each eye every 12 hours. On the following day, discontinue the previously used antiglaucoma agent and continue with PROPINE.
In transferring patients from conventional epinephrine therapy to PROPINE, simply discontinue the epinephrine medication and institute the PROPINE regimen.
Addition of PROPINE. When patients on other antiglaucoma agents require additional therapy, add one drop of PROPINE every 12 hours.
Concomitant Therapy. For difficult to control patients, the addition of PROPINE to other agents such as pilocarpine, carbachol, echothiophate iodide or acetazolamide has been shown to be effective.
Note: Not for injection.
How Supplied: PROPINE® (dipivefrin HCl) ophthalmic solution, USP, 0.1%, is supplied sterile in plastic dropper bottles as follows:
C Cap™ Compliance Cap B.I.D. (twice daily)
5 mL—NDC 11980-260-25
10 mL—NDC 11980-260-20
15 mL—NDC 11980-260-21
Note: Store in tight, light-resistant containers.
Caution: Federal (U.S.A.) law prohibits dispensing without prescription.
C Cap™ Compliance Cap Patient Instructions
Instructions for use:
1. On the first usage, make sure the number "1" appears in the window. If not, click the cap to the right station.
2. Remove the cap and apply medication.
3. Replace the cap. Hold the C Cap between your thumb and forefinger. Now rotate the bottle until the cap clicks to the next station.

Continued on next page

Allergan Pharm—Cont.

4. When it's time to take your next dose, repeat steps 2 and 3.

Important Notes: Don't try to catch up on missed doses by applying more than one dose at a time.

Each time you replace the cap, turn it until you hear the click.

The number in the window specifies your *next* dosage.

REFRESH® OTC
(polyvinyl alcohol 1.4%, povidone 0.6%)
Lubricant Ophthalmic Solution

Contains: Actives: Polyvinyl alcohol 1.4% and Povidone 0.6%. Inactives: purified water and sodium chloride. May also contain hydrochloric acid or sodium hydroxide to adjust pH.

FDA APPROVED USES

Indications: FOR USE AS A LUBRICANT TO PREVENT FURTHER IRRITATION OR TO RELIEVE DRYNESS OF THE EYE.

Warnings: To avoid contamination, do not touch tip of container to any surface. Do not reuse. Once opened, discard. If you experience eye pain, changes in vision, continued redness or irritation of the eye or if the condition worsens or persists for more than 72 hours, discontinue use and consult a doctor. If solution changes color or becomes cloudy, do not use. Keep this and all drugs out of the reach of children. In case of accidental ingestion, seek professional assistance or contact a poison control center immediately.

Directions: Instill 1 or 2 drops in the affected eye(s) as needed.

Note: Do not touch unit-dose tip to eye.

How Supplied: REFRESH® (polyvinyl alcohol 1.4%, povidone 0.6%) Lubricant Ophthalmic Solution is supplied in sterile, preservative-free, disposable, single-use containers of 0.01 fluid ounces each, in the following sizes:

30 SINGLE-USE CONTAINERS—NDC 0023-0506-01

50 SINGLE-USE CONTAINERS—NDC 0023-0506-50

REFRESH® PM OTC
(white petrolatum 56.8%, mineral oil 41.5%)
Lubricant Ophthalmic Ointment

Contains: Actives: white petrolatum 56.8%, mineral oil 41.5%; Inactives: lanolin alcohols; purified water and sodium chloride.

FDA APPROVED USES

Indications: FOR USE AS A LUBRICANT TO PREVENT FURTHER IRRITATION OR TO RELIEVE DRYNESS OF THE EYE.

Warnings: To avoid contamination, do not touch tip of container to any surface. Replace cap after using. If you experience eye pain, changes in vision, continued redness or irritation of the eye, or if the condition worsens or persists for more than 72 hours, discontinue use and consult a doctor. Keep this and all drugs out of the reach of children. In case of accidental ingestion, seek professional assistance or contact a poison control center immediately.

Directions: Pull down the lower lid of the affected eye and apply a small amount (one-fourth inch) of ointment to the inside of the eyelid.

Note: Store away from heat. Protect from freezing.

How Supplied: As a sterile eye lubricant in 3.5 g tube.

NDC 0023-0667-04

RELIEF® OTC
(phenylephrine HCl 0.12%, polyvinyl alcohol 1.4%)
Vasoconstrictor (Redness Reliever) and Lubricant Eye Drops

Contains: Actives: Phenylephrine HCl 0.12%, Liquifilm (polyvinyl alcohol) 1.4%. Inactives: edetate disodium mono- and dibasic sodium phosphates, purified water, sodium acetate, and sodium thiosulfate. pH adjusted with hydrochloric acid or sodium hydroxide.

FDA APPROVED USES

Indications: RELIEVES REDNESS OF THE EYE DUE TO MINOR EYE IRRITATIONS. FOR USE AS A LUBRICANT TO PREVENT FURTHER IRRITATION OR TO RELIEVE DRYNESS OF THE EYE.

Warnings: To avoid contamination, do not touch tip of container to any surface. Do not reuse. Once opened, discard. If you have glaucoma, do not use this product except under the advice and supervision of a doctor. Pupils may dilate in some individuals. If you experience eye pain, changes in vision, continued redness or irritation of the eye, or if the condition worsens or persists for more than 72 hours, discontinue use and consult a doctor. Overuse of this product may produce increased redness of the eye. If solution changes color or becomes cloudy, do not use. Keep this and all drugs out of the reach of children. In case of accidental ingestion, seek professional assistance or contact a poison control center immediately.

Directions: Instill 1 to 2 drops in the affected eye(s) up to four (4) times daily.

Note: Do not touch unit-dose tip to eye. Not for use while wearing soft contact lenses.

How Supplied: RELIEF® (phenylephrine HCl 0.12%, polyvinyl alcohol 1.4%) Vasoconstrictor (Redness Reliever) and Lubricant Eye Drops is supplied in sterile, preservative-free, disposable, single-use containers of 0.01 fluid ounces each, in the following sizes:

30 SINGLE-USE CONTAINERS—NDC 0023-0507-01

TEARS PLUS® OTC
(polyvinyl alcohol 1.4%, povidone 0.6%)
Lubricant Ophthalmic Solution

Contains: Actives: Polyvinyl alcohol 1.4% and povidone 0.6% Inactives: chlorobutanol (chloral deriv.) 0.5% purified water and sodium chloride. May also contain hydrochloric acid or sodium hydroxide to adjust pH.

FDA APPROVED USES

Indications: FOR USE AS A LUBRICANT TO PREVENT FURTHER IRRITATION OR TO RELIEVE DRYNESS OF THE EYE.

Warnings: To avoid contamination, do not touch tip of container to any surface. Replace cap after using. If you experience eye pain, changes in vision, continued redness or irritation of the eye, or if the condition worsens or persists for more than 72 hours, dicontinue use and consult a doctor. If solution changes color or becomes cloudy, do not use. Keep this and all drugs out of the reach of children. In case of accidental ingestion, seek professional assistance or contact a poison control center immediately.

Directions: Instill 1 or 2 drops in the affected eye(s) as needed.

Note: Not for use while wearing soft contact lenses.

How Supplied: TEARS PLUS® (polyvinyl alcohol 1.4%, povidone 0.6%) Lubricant Ophthalmic Solution is supplied in sterile, plastic dropper bottles in the following sizes:

½ fl oz—NDC 11980-165-15
1 fl oz—NDC 11980-165-30

Alza Corporation
PALO ALTO, CA 94303-0802

OCUSERT® Pilo-20 ℞
[*ok "u-sert*]
(pilocarpine)
Ocular Therapeutic System
20 μg/hr. for one week
and
OCUSERT® Pilo-40 ℞
(pilocarpine)
Ocular Therapeutic System
40 μg/hr. for one week

DESCRIPTION: OCUSERT® pilocarpine system is an elliptically shaped unit designed for continuous release of pilocarpine following placement in the cul-de-sac of the eye. Clinical evaluation in appropriate patients has demonstrated therapeutic efficacy of the system in the eye for one week. Two strengths are available, Pilo-20 and Pilo-40.

OCUSERT® systems contain a core reservoir consisting of pilocarpine and alginic acid. Pilocarpine is designated chemically as 2 (3H)-Furanone,3-ethyldihydro-4(1-methyl-1H-imidazol-5-yl) methyl]-, (3S-cis)-and has the following structural formula:

The core is surrounded by a hydrophobic ethylene/vinyl acetate (EVA) copolymer membrane which controls the diffusion of pilocarpine from the OCUSERT® system into the eye. The Pilo-40 membrane contains di(2-ethylhexyl) phthalate, which increases the rate of diffusion of pilocarpine across the EVA membrane. Of the total content of pilocarpine in the Pilo-20 or Pilo-40 system (5 mg or 11 mg, respectively), a portion serves as the thermodynamic diffusional energy source to release the drug and remains in the unit at the end of the week's use. The alginic acid component of the core is not released from the system. The readily visible white margin around the system contains titanium dioxide. The Pilo-20 system is 5.7 × 13.4 mm on its axes and 0.3 mm thick; the Pilo-40 system is 5.5 × 13 mm on its axes and 0.5 mm thick.

Release Rate Concept: With the OCUSERT® system form of therapy, the particular strength is described by the rated release, the mean release rate of drug from the system over seven days, in micrograms per hour. To cover the range of drug therapy needed to control the increased intraocular pressure associated with the glaucomas, two rated releases of pilocarpine from the OCUSERT® system are available, 20 and 40 micrograms per hour, for one week.

During the first few hours of the seven day time course, the release rate is higher than that prevailing over the remainder of the one-week period. The system releases drug at three times the rated value in the first hours and drops to the rated value in approximately six hours. A total of 0.3 mg to 0.7 mg pilocarpine (Pilo-20 or Pilo-40, respectively) is released during this initial six-hour period (one drop of 2% pilocarpine ophthalmic solution contains 1 mg pilocarpine). During the remainder of the seven day period the release rate is within ±20% of the rated value.

CLINICAL PHARMACOLOGY: Pilocarpine is released from the OCUSERT® system as soon as it is placed in contact with the conjunctival surfaces. Pilocarpine is a direct acting parasympathomimetic drug which produces pupillary constriction, stimulates the ciliary muscle, and increases aqueous humor outflow facility. Because of its action on ciliary muscle, pilocarpine induces transient myopia, generally more pronounced in younger patients. In association with the increase in outflow facility, there is a decrease in intraocular pressure.

Preclinical Results: The levels of ^{14}C- pilocarpine in the ocular tissues of rabbits following OCUSERT® system and eyedrop administration have been determined. The OCUSERT® system produces constant low pilocarpine levels in the ciliary body and iris. Following ^{14}C-pilocarpine eyedrop treatment, the initial levels of pilocarpine in the cornea, aqueous humor, ciliary body and iris are 3 to 5 times higher than the corresponding levels with the OCUSERT® system, declining over the next six hours to approximately the tissue concentrations maintained by the OCUSERT® system. In contrast, in the conjunctiva, lens, and vitreous the ^{14}C-pilocarpine concentrations remain consistently high from eyedrops and do not return to the constant low levels maintained by the OCUSERT® system. Pilocarpine does not accumulate in ocular tissues during OCUSERT® system use. These studies in rabbits have not been done in humans.

Clinical Results: The ocular hypotensive effect of both the Pilo-20 and Pilo-40 systems is fully developed within 1½ to 2 hours after placement in the cul-de-sac. A satisfactory ocular hypotensive response is maintained around-the-clock. Intraocular pressure reduction for an entire week is achieved with the OCUSERT® system from either 3.4 mg or 6.7 mg pilocarpine (20 or 40 μg/hour times 24 hours/day times 7 days, respectively), as compared with 28 mg administered as a 2% ophthalmic solution four times a day.

During the first several hours after insertion of an OCUSERT® pilocarpine system into the conjunctival cul-de-sac, induced myopia may occur. In contrast to the fluctuating and high levels of induced myopia typical of pilocarpine administration by eyedrop, the amount of induced myopia with OCUSERT® systems decreases after the first several hours to a low baseline level, approximately 0.5 diopters or less, which persists for the therapeutic life of the OCUSERT® system. Pilocarpine-induced miosis approximately parallels the induced myopia.

Of the 302 patients who used the OCUSERT® system in clinical studies for more than two weeks, 229 (75%) preferred it to previously used pilocarpine eyedrops. This percentage increased with further wearing experience.

INDICATIONS AND USAGE: OCUSERT® pilocarpine system is indicated for control of elevated intraocular pressure in pilocarpine responsive patients. Clinical studies have demonstrated OCUSERT® system efficacy in certain glaucomatous patients.

The patient should be instructed on the use of the OCUSERT® system and should read the package insert instructions for use. The patient should demonstrate to the ophthalmologist his ability to place, adjust and remove the units.

Concurrent Therapy: OCUSERT® systems have been used concomitantly with various opthalmic medications. The release rate of pilocarpine from the OCUSERT® system is not influenced by carbonic anhydrase inhibitors, epinephrine or timolol ophthalmic solutions, fluorescein, or anesthetic, antibiotic, or anti-inflammatory steroid ophthalmic solutions. Systemic reactions consistent with an increased rate of absorption from the eye of an autonomic drug, such as epinephrine, have been observed. The occurrence of mild bulbar conjunctival edema, which is frequently present with epinephrine ophthalmic solutions, is not influenced by the OCUSERT® pilocarpine system.

CONTRAINDICATIONS: OCUSERT® pilocarpine system is contraindicated where pupillary constriction is undesirable, such as for glaucomas associated with acute inflammatory disease of the anterior segment of the eye, and glaucomas occurring or persisting after extracapsular cataract extraction where posterior synechiae may occur.

WARNINGS: Patients with acute infectious conjunctivitis or keratitis should be given special consideration and evaluation prior to the use of the OCUSERT® pilocarpine system. Damaged or deformed systems should not be placed or retained in the eye. Systems believed to be associated with an unexpected increase in drug action should be removed and replaced with a new system.

PRECAUTIONS:

General

OCUSERT® pilocarpine system safety in retinal detachment patients and in patients with filtration blebs has not been established. The conjunctival erythema and edema associated with epinephrine ophthalmic solutions are not substantially altered by concomitant OCUSERT® pilocarpine system therapy. The use of pilocarpine drops should be considered when intense miosis is desired in certain ocular conditions.

Drug Interactions

Although ophthalmic solutions have been used effectively in conjunction with the OCUSERT® system, systemic reactions consistent with an increased rate of absorption from the eye of an autonomic drug, such as epinephrine, have been observed. In rare instances, reactions of this type can be severe.

Carcinogenesis, Mutagenesis, Impairment of Fertility

No long-term carcinogenicity and reproduction studies in animals have been conducted with the OCUSERT® system.

Pregnancy Category C

Although the use of the OCUSERT® pilocarpine system has not been reported to have adverse effect on pregnancy, the safety of its use in pregnant women has not been absolutely established. While systemic absorption of pilocarpine from the OCUSERT® system is highly unlikely, pregnant women should use it only if clearly needed.

Nursing Mothers

It is not known whether pilocarpine is excreted in human milk. Because many drugs are excreted in human milk, caution should be exercised when the OCUSERT® system is used by a nursing woman.

Pediatric Use

Safety and effectiveness in children have not been established.

ADVERSE REACTIONS: Ciliary spasm is encountered with pilocarpine usage but is not a contraindication to continued therapy unless the induced myopia is debilitating to the patient. Irritation from pilocarpine has been infrequently encountered and may require cessation of therapy depending on the judgement of the physician. True allergic reactions are uncommon but require discontinuation of therapy should they occur.

Although withdrawal of the peripheral iris from the anterior chamber angle by miosis may reduce the tendency for narrow angle closure, miotics can occasionally precipitate angle closure by increasing the resistance to aqueous flow from posterior to anterior chamber. Miotic agents may also cause retinal detachment; thus, care should be exercised with all miotic therapy especially in young myopic patients.

Corneal abrasion and visual impairment have been reported with use of the OCUSERT® system.

Some patients may notice signs of conjunctival irritation, including mild erythema with or without a slight increase in mucous secretion when they first use OCUSERT® pilocarpine systems. These symptoms tend to lessen or disappear after the first week of therapy. In rare instances a sudden increase in pilocarpine effects has been reported during system use.

DOSAGE AND ADMINISTRATION:

Initiation of Therapy: A patient whose intraocular pressure has been controlled by 1% or 2% pilocarpine eyedrop solution has a higher probability of pressure control with the Pilo-20 system than a patient who has used a higher strength pilocarpine solution and might require Pilo-40 therapy. However, there is no direct correlation between the OCUSERT® system (Pilo-20 or Pilo-40) and the strength of pilocarpine eyedrop solutions required to achieve a given level of pressure lowering. The OCUSERT® system reduces the amount of drug necessary to achieve adequate medical control; therefore, therapy may be started with the OCUSERT® Pilo-20 system irrespective of the strength of pilocarpine solution the patient previously required. Because of the patient's age, family history, and disease status or progression, however, the ophthalmologist may elect to begin therapy with the Pilo-40. The patient should then return during the first week of therapy for evaluation of his intraocular pressure, and as often therafter as the ophthalmologist deems necessary.

If the pressure is satisfactorily reduced with the OCUSERT® Pilo-20 system the patient should continue its use, replacing each unit every 7 days. If the physician desires intraocular pressure reduction greater than that achieved by the Pilo-20 system, the patient should be transferred to the Pilo-40 system. If necessary, an epinephrine ophthalmic solution or a carbonic anhydrase inhibitor may be used concurrently with OCUSERT® system.

After a satisfactory therapeutic regimen has been established with the OCUSERT® pilocarpine system, the frequency of follow-up should be determined by the ophthalmologist according to the status of the patient's disease process.

Placement and Removal of the OCUSERT® System: The OCUSERT® system is readily placed in the eye by the patient, according to patient instructions provided in the package. The instructions also describe procedures for removal of the system. It is strongly recommended that the patient's ability to manage the placement and removal of the system be reviewed at the first patient visit after initiation of therapy.

Since the pilocarpine-induced myopia from the OCUSERT® systems may occur during the first several hours of therapy (average of 1.4 diopters in a group of young subjects), the patient should be advised to place the system into the conjunctial cul-de-sac at bedtime. By morning the induced myopia is at a stable level (about 0.5 diopters or less in young subjects).

Sanitary Handling: Patients should be instructed to wash their hands thoroughly with soap and water before touching or manipulating the OCUSERT® system. In the event a displaced unit contacts unclean surfaces, rinsing with cool tap water before replacing is advisable. Obviously bacteriologically contaminated units should be discarded and replaced with a fresh unit.

OCUSERT® System Retention in the Eye: During the initial adaptation period, the OCUSERT® unit may slip out of the conjunctival cul-de-sac onto the cheek. The patient is usually aware of such movement and can replace the unit without difficulty.

In those patients in whom retention of the OCUSERT® unit is a problem, superior cul-de-sac placement is often more desirable. The OCUSERT® unit can be manipulated from the lower to the upper conjunctival cul-de-sac by a gentle digital massage through the lid, a technique readily learned by the patient. If possible the unit should be moved before sleep to the

Continued on next page

Alza—Cont.

upper conjunctival cul-de-sac for best retention. Should the unit slip out of the conjunctival cul-de-sac during sleep, its ocular hypotensive effect following loss continues for a period of time comparable to that following instillation of eyedrops. The patient should be instructed to check for the presence of the OCUSERT® unit before retiring at night and upon arising.
HOW SUPPLIED: OCUSERT® Pilo-20 and Pilo-40 systems are available in packages containing eight individual sterile systems.
STORAGE AND HANDLING: Store under refrigeration (36°–46°F).
CAUTION: ***Federal law prohibits dispensing without prescription.***
ALZA Corp.,
Palo Alto, CA 94304
Printed in USA, 1991

Ayerst Laboratories
Division of American Home Products Corporation
685 THIRD AVE.
NEW YORK, NY 10017-4071

As a result of a merger of Wyeth Laboratories and Ayerst Laboratories, all prescription products formerly of Ayerst are products of Wyeth-Ayerst Laboratories. All nonprescription products formerly of Ayerst are products of Whitehall Laboratories.

Bausch & Lomb Personal Products Division
1400 N GOODMAN ST.
ROCHESTER, NY 14692-0450

ALLERGY DROPS OTC
Lubricant/Redness Reliever Eye Drops

Description: BAUSCH & LOMB Allergy Drops is a sterile lubricating eye drop that relieves minor irritation caused by allergens—pollen, dust, animal hair, air pollutants, and other common eye irritants. It relieves redness and keeps on working to protect eyes against further irritation.
Unlike other eye drops, BAUSCH & LOMB Allergy Drops contains a special ingredient that provides longer lasting relief from itching, burning, dry, irritated eyes.
Ingredients: Polyethylene glycol 300 (0.2%), naphazoline hydrochloride (0.012%). Also contains: boric acid, disodium edetate, sodium borate, sodium chloride; preserved with benzalkonium chloride (0.01%).
Indications: Relieves redness of the eye due to minor eye irritations. For the temporary relief of burning and irritation due to dryness of the eye and for use as a protectant against further irritation, or to relieve dryness of the eye.
Warnings: To avoid contamination, do not touch tip of container to any surface. Replace cap after using. If solution changes color or becomes cloudy, do not use. If you experience eye pain, changes in vision, continued redness or irritation of the eye, or if the condition worsens or persists for more than 72 hours, discontinue use and consult a doctor. If you have glaucoma, do not use this product except under the advice and supervision of a doctor. Overuse of this product may produce increased redness of the eye.
Keep this and all medication out of the reach of children.
REMOVE CONTACT LENSES BEFORE USING.
Directions: Instill 1 or 2 drops in the affected eye(s) up to four times daily.
Store at room temperature.
How Supplied: In plastic bottles of 0.5 fl oz.

DRY EYE THERAPY™ OTC
Lubricating Eye Drops
Preservative Free

Ingredients: Glycerin 0.3%, with: calcium chloride, magnesium chloride, purified water, potassium chloride, sodium chloride, sodium citrate, sodium phosphate, and zinc chloride.
Indications: For the temporary relief of burning and irritation due to dryness of the eye and for use as a lubricant to prevent further irritation. For the temporary relief of discomfort due to minor irritations of the eye or to exposure to wind or sun.
Description: Bausch & Lomb Dry Eye Therapy, like natural tears, contains a lubricant and four essential nutrients: calcium, zinc, potassium, and magnesium. It provides soothing relief for dry eyes.
Warnings: To avoid contamination, do not touch tip of container to any surface. Do not re-use. Once opened, discard. If you experience eye pain, changes in vision, continued redness or irritation of the eye, or if the condition worsens or persists for more than 72 hours, discontinue use and consult a doctor. If solution changes color or becomes cloudy, do not use.
Use only if single-use container is intact.
Keep this and all drugs out of the reach of children.
Store at room temperature.
Directions:
- Make sure single-use container is intact before use.
- Separate one container from the strip of four.
- Open the single-use container by completely twisting off the top tab.
- Place thumb and forefinger on the marks on the center of the bubble.
- Gently squeeze 1 to 2 drops in the affected eye(s).
- After placing the drops in eye(s), throw away the container. Do not re-use.

Dry Eye Therapy may be used as often as needed.
How Supplied: 32 sterile, single-use containers, each 0.01 fl. oz.

DUOLUBE OTC
Sterile Lubricant Eye Ointment

Description: White petrolatum 80% and mineral oil 20%. Contains no preservatives.
Indications: For use as a lubricant to prevent further irritation or to relieve dryness of the eye.
Directions: Pull down the lower lid of the affected eye and apply a small amount (one-fourth inch) of Duolube ointment to the inside of the eyelid.
Warnings: To avoid contamination, do not touch tip of container to any surface. Replace cap after using. If you experience eye pain, changes in vision, continued redness, irritation of the eye, or if the condition worsens or persists for more than 72 hours, discontinue use and consult a doctor. KEEP OUT OF REACH OF CHILDREN. NOT FOR USE WITH CONTACT LENSES.
DO NOT USE IF BOTTOM RIDGE OF CAP IS EXPOSED PRIOR TO INITIAL USE.
Store at room temperature.
How Supplied: In ⅛-oz (NDC 10119-020-13) tube.

EYE WASH OTC
Sterile Isotonic Buffered Solution

Description: A sterile, isotonic solution that contains boric acid, purified water, sodium borate and sodium chloride; preserved with disodium edetate 0.025% and sorbic acid 0.1%. CONTAINS NO THIMEROSAL (MERCURY).
Indications: For cleansing the eye to help relieve irritation, burning, stinging and itching by removing loose, foreign material, air pollutants (smog or pollen) or chlorinated water.
Warnings: To avoid contamination, do not touch tip of container to any surface. Replace cap after using. If you experience eye pain, changes in vision, continued redness or irritation of the eye, or if the condition worsens or persists, consult a doctor. Obtain immediate medical treatment for all open wounds in or near the eyes. If solution changes color or becomes cloudy, do not use.
Use only as directed. If you experience any chemical burns, consult a doctor immediately. KEEP OUT OF REACH OF CHILDREN.
Directions: With Eye Cup—Rinse cup with BAUSCH & LOMB® Eye Wash immediately before and after each use. Avoid contamination of rim and inside surfaces of cup. Fill cup one-half full with BAUSCH & LOMB Eye Wash. Apply cup tightly to the affected eye to prevent spillage and tilt head backward. Open eyelids wide and rotate eyeball to thoroughly wash the eye.
NOTE: Enclosed eye cup is sterile if packaging intact.
Directions: Without Eye Cup—Flush the affected eye as needed, controlling the rate of flow of solution by pressure on the bottle.
How Supplied: In plastic dropper bottles of 4 fl oz, packaged with sterile eye cup.

MOISTURE DROPS® OTC
Artificial Tears

Description: BAUSCH & LOMB MOISTURE DROPS Artificial Tears quickly provides soothing relief to dry, itchy, burning, irritated eyes. Its unique triple-action formula keeps on working, so your eyes stay moist, healthy, protected against further irritation. And unlike some eye drops, MOISTURE DROPS can be used as often as needed.
Ingredients: Hydroxypropyl methylcellulose (0.5%), dextran 70 (0.1%) and glycerin (0.2%). Also contains: boric acid, disodium edetate, potassium chloride, sodium borate, sodium chloride; preserved with benzalkonium chloride (0.01%).
Indications: For the temporary relief of burning and irritation due to dryness of the eye and for use as a protectant against further irritation, or to relieve dryness of the eye.
Warnings: To avoid contamination, do not touch tip of container to any surface. Replace cap after using. If you experience eye pain, changes in vision, continued redness or irritation of the eye, or if the condition worsens or persists for more than 72 hours, discontinue use and consult a doctor. If solution changes color or becomes cloudy, do not use.
Keep this and all medication out of the reach of children.
REMOVE CONTACT LENSES BEFORE USING.
Directions: Instill 1 or 2 drops in the affected eye(s) as needed.
Store at room temperature.
How Supplied: In plastic bottles of 0.5 and 1.0 fl oz.

Bausch & Lomb Pharmaceutical Division

8500 HIDDEN RIVER PARKWAY
TAMPA, FL 33637

NDC 24208	PRODUCT	
825-55	**ATROPINE SULFATE OPHTHALMIC OINTMENT, 1%-STERILE** ⅛ oz. (3.5 gram) tubes	℞
750-	**ATROPINE SULFATE OPHTHALMIC SOLUTION, 1%-STERILE** 5ml: -60 15ml: -06	℞
565-55	**BACITRACIN OPHTHALMIC OINTMENT-STERILE** (500 units/gram) ⅛ oz. (3.5 gram) tubes	℞
605-	**BALANCED SALT SOLUTION** 15ml plastic squeeze bottle -64 500ml glass bottle -99	℞
550-55	**CHLORAMPHENICOL OPHTHALMIC OINTMENT, 1%-STERILE** ⅛ oz. (3.5 gram) tubes	℞
690-03	**CHLORAMPHENICOL OPHTHALMIC SOLUTION, 0.5% STERILE** 7.5ml	℞
640-55	**DEXAMETHASONE SODIUM PHOSPHATE OPHTHALMIC OINTMENT, 0.05%, USP-STERILE** ⅛ oz. (3.5 gram) tubes	℞
720-02	**DEXAMETHASONE SODIUM PHOSPHATE OPHTHALMIC SOLUTION, 0.1%, USP-STERILE** 5ml	℞
795-55	**DEXASPORIN® OINTMENT** Neomycin and Polymyxin B Sulfates and Dexamethasone 0.1% Ophthalmic Ointment-Sterile ⅛ oz. (3.5 gram) tubes	℞
830-60	**DEXASPORIN® SUSPENSION** Neomycin and Polymyxin B Sulfates and Dexamethasone 0.1% Ophthalmic Suspension-Sterile 5ml	℞
740-	**PHENYLEPHRINE HYDROCHLORIDE OPHTHALMIC SOLUTION, 2.5%-STERILE** 2ml: -59 5ml: -02 15ml: -06	℞
910-	**ERYTHROMYCIN OPHTHALMIC OINTMENT-STERILE** ⅛ oz. (3.5 gram) tubes -55 1g: U/D 50's -19	℞
595-73	**EYE DROPS** Tetrahydrozoline Hydrochloride Ophthalmic Solution-Sterile ½ oz. (15 ml)	OTC
835-80	**EYE WASH** Eye Irrigating Solution-Sterile 4 fl. oz. (120 ml)	OTC
575-55	**GENTAMICIN OINTMENT** Gentamicin Sulfate Ophthalmic Ointment-Sterile ⅛ oz. (3.5 gram) tubes	℞
580-	**GENTAMICIN SOLUTION** Gentamicin Sulfate Ophthalmic Solution-Sterile USP 5ml: -60 15ml: -64	℞
-730-	**PROPARACAINE HYDROCHLORIDE OPHTHALMIC SOLUTION, 0.5%, USP-STERILE** 2ml: -01 15ml: -06	℞
-733-60	**PROPARACAINE, FLUORESCEIN** Proparacaine HCl and Fluorescein Sodium Ophthalmic Solution, 0.5% and 0.25%, USP, Sterile 5 ml	℞
-480-55	**LUBRITEARS OINTMENT** White petrolatum, Mineral Oil, Anhydrous Lanolin, Lubricant Eye Ointment (Sterile) ⅛ oz. (3.5 gram) tube	OTC
-840-64	**LUBRITEARS SOLUTION** Hydroxypropyl Methylcellulose 2906, 0.3%, Dextran 70, 0.1% Lubricant Eye Drops (Sterile) ½ fl oz (15ml)	OTC
-585-	**TROPICAMIDE OPHTHALMIC SOLUTION, 1%, USP-STERILE** 2ml: -59 15ml: -64	℞
-590-64	**TROPICAMIDE OPHTHALMIC SOLUTION, 0.5%, USP-STERILE** 15ml	℞
-279-15	**OPCON®** Naphazoline Hydrocholoride Ophthalmic Solution, 0.1% USP-Sterile 15ml	℞
-781-15	**OPCON A®** Naphazoline Hydrochloride, 0.025% and Pheniramine maleate 0.3% Ophthalmic Solution, Sterile 15ml	℞
-278-	**MUROCOLL® 2** Phenylephrine Hydrochloride, 10% Scopolamine Hydrobromide, 0.3% 5 mL: -05	℞
-280-	**MUROCEL® SOLUTION** Methylcellulose, 1% 15 mL: -15	℞
-955-60	**NEO-DEXAIR®** Neomycin Sulfate and Dexamethasone Sodium Phosphate Ophthalmic Solution-Sterile 5ml	℞
-555-55	**OCUMYCIN™** Bacitracin Zinc and Polymyxin B Sulfate Ophthalmic Ointment-Sterile ⅛ oz. (3.5 gram) tubes	℞
-780-55	**OCUTRICIN® OINTMENT** Neomycin and Polymyxin B Sulfates and Bacitracin Zinc Ophthalmic Ointment-Sterile ⅛ oz. (3.5 gram) tubes	℞
-785-55	**OCUTRICIN® HC OINTMENT** Neomycin and Polymyxin B Sulfates, Bacitracin Zinc, and Hydrocortisone Ophthalmic Ointment-Sterile ⅛ oz. (3.5 gram) tubes	℞
-790-	**OCUTRICIN® SOLUTION** Neomycin and Polymyxin B Sulfates and Gramicidin Ophthalmic Solution-Sterile 2ml: -59 10ml: -62	℞
-526-61	**OCUTRICIN® HC SUSPENSION** Neomycin and Polymyxin B Sulfates and Hydrocortisone Ophthalmic Suspension 7.5ml	℞
-735-	**PENTOLAIR SOLUTION** Cyclopentolate Hydrochloride Ophthalmic Solution, 1%, USP -Sterile 2ml: -01 5ml: -60 15ml: -06	℞
-870-55	**PETROLATUM OINTMENT** White Petrolatum and Mineral Oil Lubricant Eye Ointment (Sterile) ⅛ oz. (3.5 gram) tube	OTC
-805-64	**PILOSTAT™ 0.5%** Pilocarpine Hydrochloride Ophthalmic Solution, 0.5%-sterile 15ml	℞
-675-06	**PILOSTAT™ 1%** Pilocarpine Hydrochloride Ophthalmic Solution, 1%-Sterile 15ml: -06 TWIN PAK 2×15 ml: -30	℞
-680-	**PIOLSTAT™ 2%** Pilocarpine Hydrochloride Ophthalmic Solution, 2%-Sterile 15ml: -06 TWIN PAK 2×15 ml: -30	℞
-810-64	**PILOSTAT™ 3%** Pilocarpine Hydrochloride Ophthalmic Solution, 3%-Sterile 15ml	℞
-685-	**PILOSTAT™ 4%** Pilocarpine Hydrochloride Ophthalmic Solution, 4%-Sterile 15ml: -06 TWIN PAK 2×15 ml: -30	℞
-820-64	**PILOSTAT™ 6%** Pilocarpine Hydrochloride Ophthalmic Solution, 6%-Sterile 15ml	℞
-715-	**PREDNISOLONE SODIUM PHOSPHATE OPHTHALMIC SOLUTION, 1% USP-STERILE** 5ml: -02 15ml: -06	℞
-645-55	**SULPHRIN® OINTMENT** Sulfacetamide Sodium 10% and Prednisolone Acetate 0.5% Ophthalmic Ointment-Sterile ⅛ oz. (3.5 gram) tubes	℞
-775-	**SULPHRIN®** Sulfacetamide Sodium 10% and Prednisolone Acetate 0.5% Ophthalmic Suspension-Sterile 5ml: -60 15ml: -64	℞
-770-02	**SODIUM SULFACETAMIDE OPHTHALMIC OINTMENT, 10%, USP STERILE** ⅛ oz. (3.5 gram) tubes	℞
-915-	**SULPRED® SUSPENSION** Sulfacetamide Sodium 10% and Prednisolone Acetate 0.2% Suspension-Sterile 5ml -60 10ml -62	℞
-670	**SULFACETAMIDE SODIUM OPHTHALMIC SOLUTION, 10%, USP-STERILE** 2ml: -59 15ml: -04	℞
-665-64	**SULFACETAMIDE SODIUM OPHTHALMIC SOLUTION 15% USP, STERILE** 15 ml	℞
-695-64	**SULFACETAMIDE SODIUM OPHTHALMIC SOLUTION, 30% USP-STERILE** 15ml	℞

Continued on next page

Bausch & Lomb—Cont.

-760-	**DRY EYES OINTMENT** White Petrolatum Mineral Oil Anhydrous Lanolin Lubricant Eye Ointment-Sterile 0.7 g: U/D 24's-07 ⅛ oz. (3.5 gram) tubes: -02	OTC
-755-04	**DRY EYES SOLUTION** Polyvinyl Alcohol 1.4% Lubricant Eye Drops-Sterile 15ml	OTC
-920-64	**TETRACAINE HYDRO-CHLORIDE OPHTHALMIC SOLUTION 0.5%-STERILE** 15ml	℞
-275-	**OPTIPRANOLOL™ SOLUTION** Metipranolol Hydrochloride Ophthalmic Solution, 0.3%-Sterile 2 ml: -03 5 ml: -07 10 ml: -10	℞
-276-	**MURO® 128 2% SOLUTION** Sodium Chloride Ophthalmic Solution, 2%-Sterile 15 ml: -15	OTC
-277-	**MURO® 128 5% SOLUTION** Sodium Chloride Ophthalmic Solution, 5%-Sterile 15 ml: -15 30 ml: -30	OTC
-385-55	**MURO® 128 5% OINTMENT** Sodium Chloride Ophthalmic Ointment, 5%-Sterile	OTC

BIO-COR® 12 Collagen Corneal Shield ℞
BIO-COR® 24 Collagen Corneal Shield ℞
BIO-COR® 72 Collagen Corneal Shield ℞

PRODUCT OVERVIEW

Key Facts
BIO-COR® Collagen Corneal Shields are fabricated from porcine scleral tissue. Porcine scleral tissue has a high percentage of collagen and its collagen closely resembles the collagen molecules of the human eye.

Major Uses
BIO-COR® Collagen Corneal Shields are used for the relief of discomfort from post-surgical, traumatic, and non-traumatic corneal conditions.

Safety Information
Patients should be screened for any known allergies to collagen or porcine derived products.

PRESCRIBING INFORMATION

BIO-COR® 12 Collagen Corneal Shield ℞
BIO-COR® 24 Collagen Corneal Shield ℞
BIO-COR® 72 Collagen Corneal Shield ℞

Description: The BIO-COR® Collagen Corneal Shields are clear, pliable, thin films fabricated from porcine scleral tissue. Porcine scleral tissue has a high percentage of collagen and its collagen closely resembles the collagen molecules of the human eye.
The BIO-COR® 12 Collagen Corneal Shield is made of a non-crosslinked collagen and is 0.0127–0.071 mm thick in a spherical shell shape with a diameter of 14.5 mm and a base curve of 9.0 mm. The shield promotes corneal epithelial healing. The shield also provides protection for corneal wounds and/or incisions, lubricating them as it gradually dissolves within approximately 12 hours.
Indication for Use: The BIO-COR® 12 HR Collagen Corneal Shield is indicated for relief of discomfort and to promote corneal epithelial wound healing following surgery, traumatic, and nontraumatic corneal conditions.
The BIO-COR® 24 Collagen Corneal Shield is made of crosslinked collagen and is 0.0127–0.071 mm thick in a spherical shell shape with a diameter of 14.5 mm and a base curve of 9.0 mm. The shield promotes corneal epithelial healing. The shield also provides protection for corneal wounds and/or incisions, lubricating them as it gradually dissolves within approximately 24 hours.
Indication for Use: The BIO-COR® 24 HR Collagen Corneal Shield is indicated for relief of discomfort and to promote corneal epithelial wound healing following surgery, traumatic, and nontraumatic corneal conditions.
The BIO-COR® 72 Collagen Corneal Shield is made of crosslinked collagen and is 0.0127–0.071 mm thick in a spherical shell shape with a diameter of 14.5 mm and a base curve of 9.0 mm. The shield provides protection for corneal wounds and/or incisions, lubricating them as it gradually dissolves within approximately 72 hours.
Indication for Use: The BIO-COR® 72 HR Collagen Corneal Shield is indicated for relief of discomfort from post-surgical, traumatic, and nontraumatic corneal conditions.
Because of their shape, the shields are easily applied to the eye. Once applied, they absorb the ocular fluids on the eye, begin to dissolve, and conform to the cornea. The BIO-COR® Collagen Corneal Shields are based on technology developed by Professor Svyatoslav Fyodorov.
Contraindication: Professional judgement must be used by the practitioners in using the BIO-COR® Collagen Corneal Shield on patients who demonstrate the following conditions:
—evidence of acute external ocular infections
—intraocular infection
—blepharitis
—chalazion
—allergic reaction to collagen
—allergic reaction to porcine derived products
Precautions: Avoid heat above 40°C (104°F), or temperatures at or below freezing. Physicians should use care in screening their patients for any known allergies to collagen or porcine derived products. In addition, patients should be monitored for reactions to the corneal collagen shield, (i.e. conjunctival hyperemia and edema, erythema, lacrimation and pruritus).
Do not resterilize. Discard all open and unused Shields.
Recommended Instructions for Use: Anesthetize the eye, remove the BIO-COR® Collagen Corneal Shield from its protective case using a pair of blunt forceps, fill the protective case well with lubricating fluid, and immerse the shield until saturated, (approximately three minutes). Using a pair of blunt forceps, place the lubricated shield over the wound or injury and hydrate the shield and eye thorougly. The eye may be patched.
The Physician should use professional judgement in using the BIO-COR® Collagen Corneal Shield for repeated application.
Storage: Store at Controlled Room Temperature 15°–30°C (59°–86°F).
How Supplied: Each shield with tweezers is supplied in a sterile pouch. The pouch is marked with the lot number and expiration date.
CAUTION: Federal law (U.S.A.) prohibits dispensing without prescription.
Rev. 1/90

Shown in Product Identification Section, page 103

MURO 128® OTC
[*mŭ 'rō 128*]
Sodium Chloride 2% and 5% Hypertonicity Ophthalmic Solution

Ingredients: Each mL Contains: Sodium Chloride 2% or 5%, Propylene Glycol, Hydroxypropyl Methycellulose 2910, Sodium Borate, Boric Acid, Purified Water.
Preservatives: Methylparaben 0.023%, Propylparaben 0.01%.
Indication: For the temporary relief of corneal edema.
Warnings: Do not use this product except under the advice and supervision of a doctor. If you experience eye pain, changes in vision, continued redness or irritation of the eye, or if the condition worsens or persists, consult a doctor. To avoid contamination of the product do not touch the tip of the container to any surface. Replace cap after using. This product may cause temporary burning and irritation on being instilled into the eye.
If the solution changes color or becomes cloudy, do not use.
KEEP THIS AND ALL DRUGS OUT OF THE REACH OF CHILDREN.
In case of accidental ingestion, seek professional assistance or contact a Poison Control Center immediately.
Directions: Instill 1 or 2 drops in the affected eye(s) every 3 or 4 hours, or as directed by a physician.
How Supplied: Muro 128 2% soltion is supplied in ½ Fl. Oz. (15 mL) plastic controlled dropper tip bottles.
15 mL—NDC 24208-276-15
Muro 128 5% solution is supplied in ½ or 1 *Fl. Oz. (15 or 30 mL) plastic controlled dropper tip bottles.*
15 mL—NDC 24208-277-15
30 mL—NDC 24208-277-30
KEEP TIGHTLY CLOSED. STORE AT ROOM TEMPERATURE.
USE ONLY IF IMPRINTED NECKBAND IS INTACT.
MURO is a trademark of MURO Pharmaceutical, Inc.

Shown in Product Identification Section, page 103

MURO 128® OINTMENT OTC
[*mŭ 'rō 128*]
Sodium Chloride 5%

Description: Sodium Chloride Ophthalmic Ointment is used to draw water out of the cornea of the eye.
Each Gram Contains: ACTIVE: Sodium Chloride, 5% (50mg); INACTIVES: White Petrolatum, Mineral Oil, Anhydrous Lanolin, Purified Water.
Indication: For the temporary relief of corneal edema.
Directions: Pull down the lower lid of the affected eye(s) and apply a small amount (one-fourth inch) of the ointment to the inside of the eyelid, one or more times daily, or as directed by a doctor.
Warnings: To avoid contamination, do not touch tip of container to any surface. Replace cap after using. Do not use this product except under the advice and supervision of a doctor. If you experience eye pain, changes in vision, continued redness or irritation of the eye, or if the condition worsens or persists, consult a doctor. This product may cause temporary burning and irritation on being instilled into the eye.
KEEP THIS AND ALL DRUGS OUT OF THE REACH OF CHILDREN.
In case of accidental ingestion, seek professional assistance or contact a Poison Control Center immediately.

DO NOT USE IF IMPRINTED SEAL ON BOX IS BROKEN OR MISSING

FOR USE IN THE EYES ONLY
How Supplied: Sodium Chloride Ophthalmic Ointment is supplied in a ⅛ oz. (3.5g) tube.
NDC 24208-385-55

Shown in Product Identification Section, page 103

MUROCOLL® 2 ℞
Phenylephrine Hydrochloride 10% and Scopolamine HBr 0.3% Ophthalmic Solution
STERILE OPHTHALMIC SOLUTION

Each mL Contains: ACTIVES: Phenylephrine HCl 10%; Scopolamine HBr 0.3% INACTIVES: Disodium Phosphate, Citric Acid, Sodium Metabisulfite, Edetate Disodium, Purified Water PRESERVATIVE: Benzalkonium Chloride, 0.01%. The active ingredients are represented by the chemical structures:

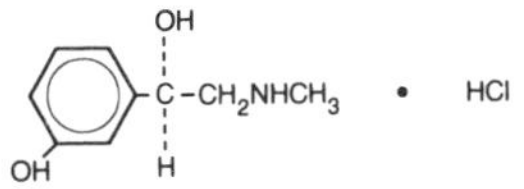

OH | C-CH2NHCH3 • HCl | H, OH

Established Name: Phenylephrine Hydrochloride
Chemical Name: Benzenemethanol, 3-hydroxy-[α]-[(methylamino)methyl]-, hydrochloride(S).

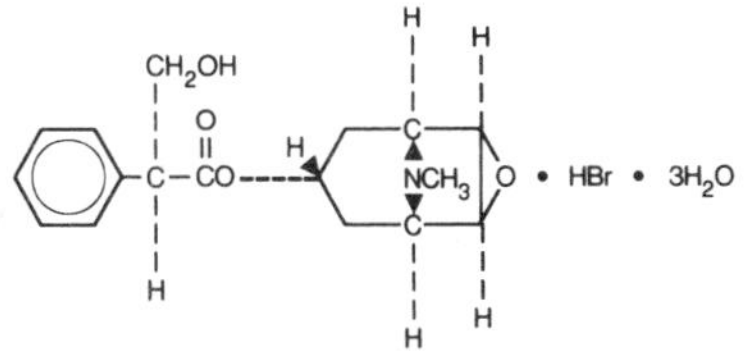

CH2OH, O, C-CO, H, NCH3, O • HBr • 3H2O

Established Name: Scopolamine Hydrobromide
Chemical Name: Benzeneacetic acid, [α]-(hydroxymethyl)-, 9-methyl-3-oxa-9-azatricyclo [3.3.1.0^{2,4}]non-7-yl ester, hydrobromide, trihydrate, [7(S)-[1 α,2 β, 4 β, 5 α,7 β]]
Clinical Pharmacology: Phenylephrine produces pupil dilation and vasoconstriction [alpha adrenergic effects]. Scopolamine produces dilation of the pupil and paralysis of accommodation [anticholinergic effects].
Indications and Usage: Murocoll® 2 is indicated for mydriasis, cycloplegia and treatment of iritis to prevent formation of posterior synechiae.
Contraindications: Narrow angle glaucoma, a tendency toward glaucoma or hypersensitivity to any ingredient.
Warnings: For topical ophthalmic use only. This product may increase IOP in the normal eye. Use with extreme caution in infants and small children. Contains sodium metabisulfite, a sulfite that may cause allergic-type reactions including anaphylactic symptoms and life-threatening or less severe asthmatic episodes in certain susceptible people. The overall prevalence of sulfite sensitivity in the general population is unknown and probably low. Sulfite sensitivity is seen more frequently in asthmatic than in nonasthmatic poeple.
Precautions: Murocoll® 2 should be used with caution in patients with marked hypertension or advanced arteriosclerotic changes and insulin dependent diabetics. To avoid excessive absorption, the lacrimal puncta should be occluded with digital pressure for 1 to 2 minutes after instillation.
To avoid inducing angular glaucoma, an estimation of the depth of the angle of the anterior chamber should be made.
Drug Interactions: The pressor effect of sympathomimetic amines is markedly potentiated by monoamine oxidase (MAO) inhibitors. Excessive elevation of blood pressure and hypertensive crisis may occur if used concomitantly.
Patient Warning: Patients should be advised not to drive or engage in other hazardous activities when drowsy or while pupils are dilated. Patients may experience sensitivity to light and should protect eyes in bright illumination during dilation. Patients should be warned not to get this preparation in their child's mouth and to wash their hands and the child's hands following administration.
Adverse Reactions: Transitory stinging on initial instillation may be expected. Redness usually occurs which is a normal therapeutic response. Headache or browache frequently occurs but will usually diminish on continued treatment. Conjunctival allergy rarely occurs. Pigmentary deposits in the lids, conjunctiva or cornea may occur after prolonged use. Systemic effects have occasionally been reported such as anxiety, fear, palpitation, tachycardia extrasystoles, cardiac arrythmia, hypertension, trembling, sweating and pallor.
Dosage and Administration: Mydriasis: Initially, instill 1 or 2 drops in eye(s). Repeat in 5 minutes if necessary to produce mydriasis in highly pigmented irides. Post-op: instill 1 to 2 drops in eye(s) 3 to 4 times a day when desirable to maintain dilation and rest ciliary body.

USE ONLY IF IMPRINTED NECKBAND IS INTACT.

How Supplied: Murocoll® 2 is supplied in 5 mL plastic controlled dropper tip bottles. 5 mL [NDC-24208-278-05]
Note: DO NOT USE IF BROWNISH COLOR APPEARS.
Storage: Store At Controlled Room Temperature 15°-30°C [59°-86°F]. PROTECT FROM LIGHT
KEEP OUT OF REACH OF CHILDREN.
Caution: Federal law prohibits dispensing without prescription.

OPTIPRANOLOL™ ℞
Metipranolol Hydrochloride 0.3%
Sterile Ophthalmic Solution

Description: OPTIPRANOLOL™ (metipranolol hydrochloride 0.3%) Sterile Ophthalmic Solution contains metipranolol, a non-selective beta-adrenergic receptor blocking agent. Metipranolol is a white, odorless, crystalline powder. The hydrochloride is soluble in water. The molecular weight is 309.38.
The empiric chemical formula of metipranolol is $C_{17}H_{27}NO_4$.
The chemical name of metipranolol is (±)-1-(4-Hydroxyl-2, 3, 5-trimethylphenoxyl)-3-(isopropylamino)-2-propanol-4-acetate.
The chemical structure of metipranolol is:

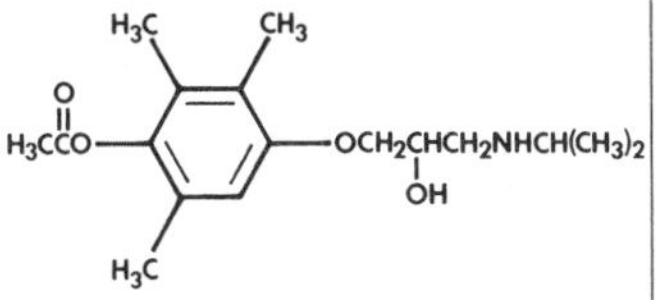

H3C, CH3, O, H3CCO, OCH2CHCH2NHCH(CH3)2, OH, H3C

Each mL of OPTIPRANOLOL™ Ophthalmic Solution 0.3% contains 3 mg of metripranolol. The inactive ingredients are: benzalkonium chloride 0.004% (as a preservative), glycerol, sodium chloride, edetate disodium, povidone, hydrochloric acid and/or sodium hydroxide (to adjust pH), and purified water.
Clinical Pharmacology: Metipranolol blocks beta$_1$ and beta$_2$ (non-selective) adrenergic receptors. It does not have significant intrinsic sympathomimetic activity, and has only weak local anesthetic (membrane-stabilizing) and myocardial depressant activity.
Orally administered beta-adrenergic blocking agents reduce cardiac output in both healthy subjects and patients with heart disease. In patients with severe impairment of myocardial function, beta-adrenergic receptor antagonists may inhibit the sympathetic stimulatory effect necessary to maintain adequate cardiac output.
Beta-adrenergic receptor blockade in the bronchi and bronchioles may result in significantly increased airway resistance from unopposed para-sympathetic activity. Such an effect is potentially dangerous in patients with asthma or other bronchospastic conditions (see CONTRAINDICATIONS and WARNINGS).
OPTIPRANOLOL™ Ophthalmic Solution, when applied topically in the eye, has the action of reducing elevated as well as normal intraocular pressure (IOP), whether or not accompanied by glaucoma. Elevated intraocular pressure is a major risk factor in the pathogenesis of glaucomatous visual field loss. The higher the level of intraocular pressure, the greater the likelihood of glaucomatous visual field loss and optic nerve damage.
The primary mechanism of the ocular hypotensive action of metipranolol is most likely due to a reduction in aqueous humor production. A slight increase in outflow may be an additional mechanism. OPTIPRANOLOL™ Ophthalmic Solution reduces IOP with little or no effect on pupil size or accommodation.
Animal Pharmacology: In rabbits administered metipranolol in one eye at 2 to 4 fold increased concentrations, multi-focal interstitial nephritis was observed in male animals, and lympho-hystiocytic and heterophilic interstitial pneumonia was observed in female animals. The clinical relevance of these findings is unknown.
Indications and Usage: OPTIPRANOLOL™ Ophthalmic Solution is indicated in the treatment of ocular conditions where lowering intraocular pressure is likely to be of therapeutic benefit; including patients with ocular hypertension, and patients with chronic open angle glaucoma.
In controlled studies of patients with intraocular pressure greater than 24 mmHg at baseline, OPTIPRANOLOL™ Ophthalmic Solution reduced the average intraocular pressure approximately 20–26%.
The onset of action of OPTIPRANOLOL™ Ophthalmic Solution, as measured by a reduction in intraocular pressure, occurs within 30 minutes after a single administration. The maximum effect occurs at about 2 hours. A reduction in intraocular pressure can be demonstrated 24 hours after a single dose. Clinical studies in patients with glaucoma treated for up to two years indicate that an intraocular pressure lowering effect is maintained.
In clinical trials, OPTIPRANOLOL™ Ophthalmic Solution was safely used during concommitant therapy with pilocarpine, epinephrine or acetazolamide.
Contraindications: Hypersensitivity to any component of this product.
OPTIPRANOLOL™ Ophthalmic Solution is contraindicated in patients with bronchial asthma or a history of bronchial asthma, or severe chronic obstructive pulmonary disease; symptomatic sinus bradycardia; greater than a first degree atrioventricular block; cardiogenic shock; or overt cardiac failure.
Warnings: As with other topically applied ophthalmic drugs, this drug may be absorbed systemically. Thus, the same adverse reactions found with systemic administration of beta-adrenergic blocking agents may occur with topical administration. For example, severe respiratory reactions and cardiac reactions, including death due to bronchospasm in patients with asthma, and rarely, death in association with cardiac failure, have been reported following topical application of beta-adrenergic blocking agents (see CONTRAINDICATIONS).
Since OPTIPRANOLOL™ Ophthalmic Solution had a minor effect on heart rate and blood pressure in clinical studies, caution should be observed in treating patients with a history of cardiac failure. Treatment with OPTIPRANOLOL™ Ophthalmic Solution should be

Continued on next page

Bausch & Lomb—Cont.

discontinued at the first evidence of cardiac failure.

OPTIPRANOLOL™ Ophthalmic Solution, or other beta blockers, should not, in general, be administered to patients with chronic obstructive pulmonary disease (e.g., chronic bronchitis, emphysema) of mild or moderate severity (see CONTRAINDICATIONS). However, if the drug is necessary in such patients, then it should be administered with caution since it may block bronchodilation produced by endrogenous and exogenous catecholamine stimulation of $beta_2$ receptors.

Precautions:

General: Because of potential effects of beta-adrenergic receptor blocking agents relative to blood pressure and pulse, these agents should be used with caution in patients with cerebrovascular insufficiency. If signs or symptoms suggesting reduced cerebral blood flow develop following initiation of therapy with OPTIPRANOLOL™ Ophthalmic Solution, alternative therapy should be considered.

Some authorities recommend gradual withdrawal of beta-adrenergic receptor blocking agents in patients undergoing elective surgery. If necessary during surgery, the effects of beta-adrenergic receptor blocking agents may be reversed by sufficient doses of such agonists as isoproterenol, dopamine, dobutamine or levarterenol.

While OPTIPRANOLOL™ Ophthalmic Solution has demonstrated a low potential for systemic effect, it should be used with caution in patients with diabetes (especially labile diabetes) because of possible masking of signs and symptoms of acute hypoglycemia.

Beta-adrenergic receptor blocking agents may mask certain signs and symptoms of hyperthyroidism, and their abrupt withdrawal might precipitate a thyroid storm.

Beta-adrenergic blockade has been reported to potentiate muscle weakness consistent with certain myasthenic symptoms (e.g., diplopia, ptosis, and generalized weakness).

Risk of anaphylactic reaction: While taking beta-blockers, patients with a history of severe anaphylactic reaction to a variety of allergens may be more reactive to repeated challenge, either accidental, diagnostic, or therapeutic. Such patients may be unresponsive to the usual doses of epinephrine used to treat allergic reaction.

Drug Interactions: OPTIPRANOLOL™ Ophthalmic Solution should be used with caution in patients who are receiving a beta-adrenergic blocking agent orally, because of the potential for additive effects on systemic beta-blockade. Close observation of the patient is recommended when a beta-blocker is administered to patients receiving catecholamine-depleting drugs such as reserpine, because of possible additive effects and the production of hypotension and/or bradycardia.

Caution should be used in the coadministration of beta-adrenergic receptor blocking agents, such as metipranolol, and oral or intravenous calcium channel antagonists, because of possible precipitation of left ventricular failure, and hypotension. In patients with impaired cardiac function, who are receiving calcium channel antagonists, coadministration should be avoided.

The concomitant use of beta-adrenergic receptor blocking agents with digitalis and calcium channel antagonists may have additive effects, prolonging arterioventricular conduction time.

Caution should be used in patients using concomitant adrenergic psychotropic drugs.

Ocular: In patients with angle-closure glaucoma, the immediate treatment objective is to re-open the angle by constriction of the pupil with a miotic agent. OPTIPRANOLOL™ Ophthalmic Solution has little or no effect on the pupil, therefore, when it is used to reduce intraocular pressure in angle-closure glaucoma, it should be used only with concomitant administration of a miotic agent.

Carcinogenesis, Mutagenesis, Impairment of Fertility: Lifetime studies with metipranolol have been conducted in mice at oral doses of 5, 50 and 100 mg/kg/day and in rats at oral doses of up to 70 mg/kg/day. Metipranolol demonstrated no carcinogenic effect. In the mouse study, female animals receiving the low, but not the intermediate or high dose had an increased number of pulmonary adenomas. The significance of this observation is unknown. In a variety of *in vitro* and *in vivo* bacterial and mammalian cell assays, metipranolol was nonmutagenic.

Reproduction and fertility studies of metipranolol in rats and mice showed no adverse effect on male fertility at oral doses of up to 50 mg/kg/day, and female fertility at oral doses of up to 25 mg/kg/day.

Pregnancy:

Pregnancy Category C. No drug related effects were reported for the segment II teratology study in fetal rats after administration, during organogenesis, to dams of up to 50 mg/kg/day. OPTIPRANOLOL™ Ophthalmic Solution has been shown to increase fetal resorption, fetal death, and delayed development when administered orally to rabbits at 50 mg/kg during organogenesis.

There are no adequate and well-controlled studies in pregnant women. OPTIPRANOLOL™ Ophthalmic Solution should be used during pregnancy only if the potential benefit justifies the potential risk to the fetus.

Nursing Mothers: It is not known whether OPTIPRANOLOL™ Ophthalmic Solution is excreted in human milk. Because many drugs are excreted in human milk, caution should be exercised when OPTIPRANOLOL™ Ophthalmic Solution is administered to nursing women.

Pediatric Use: Safety and effectiveness in children have not been established.

Adverse Reactions: In clinical trials, the use of OPTIPRANOLOL™ Ophthalmic Solution has been associated with transient local discomfort.

Other ocular adverse reactions, such as conjunctivitis, eyelid dermatitis, blepharitis, blurred vision, tearing, browache, abnormal vision, photophobia, and edema have been reported in small numbers of patients, either in U.S. clinical trials or from post-marketing experience in Europe.

Other systemic adverse reactions, such as allergic reaction, headache, asthenia, hypertension, myocardial infarct, atrial fibrillation, angina, papitation, bradycardia, nausea, rhinitis, dyspnea, epistaxis, bronchitis, coughing, dizziness, anxiety, depression, somnolence, nervousness, arthritis, myalgia, and rash have also been reported in small numbers of patients.

Overdosage No information is available on overdosage of OPTIPRANOLOL™ Ophthalmic Solution in humans. The symptoms which might be expected with an overdose of a systemically administered beta-adrenergic receptor blocking agent are bradycardia, hypotension and acute cardiac failure.

Dosage and Administration: The recommended dose is one drop of OPTIPRANOLOL™ Ophthalmic Solution in the affected eye(s) twice a day.

If the patient's IOP is not at a satisfactory level on this regimen, use of more frequent administration or a larger dose of OPTIPRANOLOL™ Ophthalmic Solution is not known to be of benefit. Concomitant therapy to lower intraocular pressure can be instituted.

How Supplied: OPTIPRANOLOL™ Ophthalmic Solution is a sterile, isotonic, aqueous solution which is clear and colorless. It is supplied in white 5 mL or 10 mL size, opaque, plastic ophthalmic bottle dispensers with a controlled drop tip and a white plastic screw-top cap as follows:

2 mL: NDC 24208-275-03
5 mL: NDC 24208-275-07
10 mL: NDC 24208-275-09

Storage: Store at controlled room temperature, 15°- *30°C (59°-86°F).*

FOR OPHTHALMIC USE ONLY

Bausch & Lomb
Pharmaceutical Division
Tampa, FL 33637

Shown in Product Identification Section, page 103

OPCON-A® ℞

Naphazoline Hydrochloride 0.025%
Pheniramine Maleate 0.3%
Ophthalmic Solution
STERILE OPHTHALMIC SOLUTION

Description: A sterile ophthalmic solution.
Each mL Contains: ACTIVES: Naphazoline HCl 0.025% [0.25 mg], Pheniramine Maleate 0.3% [3.0 mg]; INACTIVES: Boric Acid, Hydroxypropyl Methylcellulose 2910, Sodium Chloride, Sodium Borate, Edetate Disodium, Purified Water. Sodium Hydroxide and/or Hydrochloric Acid may be added to adjust pH. PRESERVATIVE: Benzalkonium Chloride 0.01%

Established Name: Naphazoline Hydrochloride

Chemical Name: 1-H-Imidazole, 4,5-dihydro 2-[1-naphthalenylmethyl]-,monohydrochloride

Established Name: Pheniramine Maleate

Chemical Name: N, N-Dimethyl-gamma-phenyl-2-pyridine-propanamine, [Z]-Butenedioic acid.

Clinical Pharmacology: Opcon-A® combines the effects of the antihistamine, pheniramine maleate, and the decongestant naphazoline.

Indications and Usage: Based on a review of a related combination of drugs by the National Academy of Sciences National Research Council and/or other information, FDA has classified the indications as follows: "Possibly" effective: For relief of ocular irritation and/or congestion or for the treatment of allergic or inflammatory ocular conditions. Final classification of the less-than-effective indication requires further investigation.

Contraindications: Hypersensitivity to one or more of the ingredients. Do not use in the presence of narrow angle glaucoma.

Warnings: A severe hypertensive crisis may ensue in patients under MAO inhibitor medication from use of a sympathomimetic drug. Safety and effectiveness in children have not been established. Use in infants and children may result in CNS depression leading to coma and marked reduction in body temperature.

Precautions: Use with caution in elderly patients with severe cardiovascular disease including cardiac arrhythmias, patients with poorly controlled hypertension, patients with diabetes especially those with a tendency toward diabetic ketoacidosis. To prevent contaminating the dropper tip and solution, do not touch eyelids or surrounding area with the dropper tip of the bottle. For ophthalmic use.
Adverse Reactions: Pupillary dilation, increase in intraocular pressure, systemic effects due to absorption [i.e. hypertension, cardiac irregularities, hyperglycemia]. Drowsiness may be experienced in some patients.
Dosage and Administration: Instill 1 or 2 drops into each eye 3 or 4 times daily.
FOR OPHTHALMIC USE ONLY

USE ONLY IF IMPRINTED NECKBAND IS INTACT.

How Supplied: Opcon-A® is supplied in 15 mL plastic controlled dropper tip bottles.
15 mL—[NDC 24208-781-15]
Storage: Store At Controlled Room Temperature 15°–30° C [59°–86°F].
KEEP TIGHTLY CLOSED
PROTECT FROM LIGHT
KEEP OUT OF REACH OF CHILDREN.
Caution: Federal law prohibits dispensing without prescription.

PILOSTAT™ ℞
PILOCARPINE HYDROCHLORIDE
Sterile Ophthalmic Solution

Description: Pilostat™ is a cholinergic prepared as a sterile topical ophthalmic solution. The active ingredient is represented by the chemical structural formula:

$C_{11}H_{16}N_2O_2 \cdot HCl$ Mol.Wt. 244.70
2 (3*H*)-Furanone, 3-ethyldihydro-4-[(1-methyl-1*H*-imidazol-5-yl) methyl]·monohydrochloride, (3*S*-*cis*)

Pilocarpine HCl 0.5%
Each mL contains:
Active: Pilocarpine Hydrochloride 0.5% (5 mg)
Inactives: Anydrous Monobasic Sodium Phosphate, Hydroxypropyl Methylcellulose 2906, Sodium Chloride, Edetate Disodium, Anhydrous Dibasic Sodium Phosphate, Purified Water.
Preservative: Benzalkonium Chloride 0.01%
Pilocarpine HCl 3%
Each mL Contains:
Active: Pilocarpine Hydrochloride 3% (30 mg)
Inactives: Hydroxypropyl Methylcellulose 2906, Anhydrous Monobasic Sodium Phosphate, Edetate Disodium, Purified Water.
Preservative: Benzalkonium Chloride 0.01%
Pilocarpine HCl 1%, 2% and 4%
Each mL contains:
Active: Pilocarpine Hydrochloride 1% (10 mg), 2% (20 mg) or 4% (40 mg)
Inactives: Anhydrous Monobasic Sodium Phosphate, Hydroxypropyl Methylcellulose 2906, Edetate Disodium, Anhydrous Dibasic Sodium Phosphate, Purified Water. Sodium Hydroxide and/or Hydrochloric Acid may be added to adjust pH.
Preservative: Benzalkonium Chloride 0.01%
Pilocarpine HCl 6%
Each mL Contains:
Active: Pilocarpine Hydrochloride 6% (60 mg)
Inactives: Hydroxypropyl Methylcellulose 2906, Anyhydrous Monobasic Sodium Phosphate, Edetate Disodium, Anhydrous Dibasic Sodium Phosphate, Purified Water.
Preservative: Benzalkonium Chloride 0.01%

Clinical Pharmacology: The actions of pilocarpine hydrochloride are those of pilocarpine, a cholinergic substance. Its penetration, following topical application to the eye, results in parasympathomimetic reactions by responsive tissues.

Indications and Usage: Pilocarpine hydrochloride can be used in the medical management of glaucoma, especially open-angle glaucoma, in those cases in which the intraocular pressure can be controlled adequately by the topical administration of pilocarpine. In acute (closed-angle) glaucoma, pilocarpine hydrochloride may be used alone, or in combination with other cholinergic agents or carbonic anhydrase inhibitors, to relieve tension prior to emergency surgery. Patients may be maintained on pilocarpine hydrochloride as long as intraocular pressure is controlled and there is no deterioration in the visual fields. The choice of concentration should be determined by the severity of the condition and the response of the patient. Pilocarpine hydrochloride is also indicated to counter the effects of cycloplegics and mydriatics following surgery or ophthalmoscopic examination.

Contraindications: Parasympathomimetics are contraindicated where miosis is undesirable such as acute iritis or pupillary block glaucoma. This product is also contraindicated in persons hypersensitive to one or more of the components of this preparation.

Warnings: Not for internal use. To prevent contaminating the dropper tip and solution, care should be taken not to touch the eyelids or surrounding areas with the dropper tip of the bottle.

Precautions: This pilocarpine-induced miosis may cause difficulty in dark adaptation. The patient should exercise caution when involved in night driving or other hazardous activities in poor light.

Carcinogenesis, Mutagenesis, Impairment of Fertility: There have been no long-term studies done using pilocarpine in animals to evaluate carcinogenic potential.

Pregnancy Category C: Animal studies have not been conducted with pilocarpine. It is also not known whether pilocarpine can cause fetal harm when administered to a pregnant woman or can affect reproduction capacity. Pilocarpine should be given to a pregnant woman only if clearly needed.

Nursing Mothers: It is not known whether the drug is excreted in human milk. Because many drugs are excreted in human milk, caution should be exercised when pilocarpine is administered to a nursing woman.

Adverse Reactions:
OCULAR: Ciliary spasm, conjunctival vascular congestion, temporal or supraorbital headache, lacrimation and induced myopia may occur. This is especially true in younger individuals who have recently started administration. Reduced visual acuity in poor illumination is frequently experienced by older individuals and individuals with lens opacity. Miotic agents may also cause *retinal detachment:* thus, care should be exercised with all miotic therapy especially in young myopic patients. Lens opacity may occur with prolonged use of pilocarpine.
SYSTEMIC: Systemic reactions following topical administration, although extremely rare, have included hypertension, tachycardia, bronchiolar spasm, pulmonary edema, salivation, sweating, nausea, vomiting, and diarrhea.

Dosage and Administration: The initial dose is one or two drops in the affected eye(s). This may be repeated up to three or four times daily or as directed by a physician. The frequency of instillation and concentration of pilocarpine hydrochloride ophthalmic solution are determined by the severity of the glaucoma and miotic response of the patient. Individuals with heavily pigmented irides may require higher strengths. During acute phases, the miotic must be instilled into the unaffected eye to prevent an attack of angle-closure glaucoma.

USE ONLY IF IMPRINTED NECKBAND IS INTACT.

How Supplied: Pilocarpine Hydrochloride Ophthalmic Solution, USP, Sterile, is supplied in a plastic squeeze bottle with a controlled tip applicator in the following strengths and sizes:
Pilostat 0.5%
15mL (NDC 24208-806-64)
Pilostat 1%
15mL (NDC 24208-675-06)
TWIN-PACK: 2 × 15mL (NDC 24208-675-30)
Pilostat 2%
15mL (NDC 24208-680-06)
TWIN PACK: 2 ×15mL (NDC 24208-680-30)
Pilostat 3%
15mL (NDC 24208-820-64
Pilostat 4%
15mL (NDC 24208-685-06)
TWIN PACK: 2 × 15mL (NDC 24208-685-30)
Pilostat 6%
15mL (NDC 24208-820-64)
Storage: Store at 8°–27°C (46° —80°F).
KEEP OUT OF REACH OF CHILDREN
FOR OPHTHALMIC USE ONLY.
Caution: Federal law prohibits dispensing without prescription.
REV. 6/90

Burroughs Wellcome Co.
3030 CORNWALLIS ROAD
RESEARCH TRIANGLE PARK,
NC 27709

LITERATURE AVAILABLE: Folders, package inserts, and file cards.

CORTISPORIN® ℞
[*kor 'tĭ-spor "ĭn*]
OPHTHALMIC OINTMENT Sterile
(Polymyxin B Sulfate-Bacitracin Zinc-Neomycin Sulfate-Hydrocortisone)

Description: Cortisporin® Ophthalmic Ointment (polymyxin B sulfate-bacitracin zinc-neomycin sulfate-hydrocortisone) is a sterile antimicrobial and anti-inflammatory ointment for ophthalmic use. Each gram contains: Aerosporin® (polymyxin B sulfate) 10,000 units, bacitracin zinc 400 units, neomycin sulfate equivalent to 3.5 mg neomycin base, hydrocortisone 10 mg (1%) and special white petrolatum, qs.
Polymyxin B sulfate is the sulfate salt of polymyxin B_1 and B_2, which are produced by the growth of *Bacillus polymyxa* (Prazmowski) Migula (Fam. Bacillaceae). It has a potency of not less than 6,000 polymyxin B units per mg, calculated on an anhydrous basis.
Bacitracin zinc is the zinc salt of bacitracin, a mixture of related cyclic polypeptides (mainly bacitracin A) produced by the growth of an organism of the *licheniformis* group of *Bacillus subtilis* (Fam. Bacillaceae). It has a potency of not less than 40 bacitracin units per mg.
Neomycin sulfate is the sulfate salt of neomycin B and C, which are produced by the growth of *Streptomyces fradiae* Waksman (Fam. Streptomycetaceae). It has a potency equivalent of not less than 600 μg of neomycin standard per mg, calculated on an anhydrous basis.
Hydrocortisone, 11β, 17, 21-trihydroxypregn-4-ene-3, 20-dione, is an anti-inflammatory hormone.

Continued on next page

Burroughs Wellcome—Cont.

Clinical Pharmacology: Corticoids suppress the inflammatory response to a variety of agents and they may delay healing. Since corticoids may inhibit the body's defense mechanism against infection, a concomitant antimicrobial drug may be used when this inhibition is considered to be clinically significant in a particular case.
The anti-infective components in the combination are included to provide action against specific organisms susceptible to them.
Polymyxin B sulfate, bacitracin zinc and neomycin sulfate together are considered active against the following microorganisms: *Staphylococcus aureus*, streptococci, including *Streptococcus pneumoniae, Escherichia coli, Haemophilus influenzae, Klebsiella-Enterobacter* species, *Neisseria* species and *Pseudomonas aeruginosa.*
When used topically, polymyxin B, bacitracin and neomycin are rarely irritating, and absorption from the intact skin or mucous membrane is insignificant. The incidence of skin sensitization to this combination has been shown to be low on normal skin.[1,2] Since these antibiotics are seldom used systemically, the patient is spared sensitization to those antibiotics which might later be required systemically.
When a decision to administer both a corticoid and antimicrobials is made, the administration of such drugs in combination has the advantage of greater patient compliance and convenience, with the added assurance that the intended dosage of both drugs is administered, plus assured compatibility of ingredients when both types of drug are in the same formulation and particularly that the intended volume of each drug is delivered simultaneously, thereby avoiding dilution of either medication by successive applications.
The relative potency of corticosteroids depends on the molecular structure, concentration and release from the vehicle.
Indications and Usage: For steroid-responsive inflammatory ocular conditions for which a corticosteroid is indicated and where bacterial infection or a risk of bacterial ocular infection exists.
Ocular steroids are indicated in inflammatory conditions of the palpebral and bulbar conjunctiva, cornea and anterior segment of the globe where the inherent risk of steroid use in certain infective conjunctivitides is accepted to obtain a diminution in edema and inflammation. They are also indicated in chronic anterior uveitis and corneal injury from chemical, radiation, or thermal burns, or penetration of foreign bodies.
The use of a combination drug with an anti-infective component is indicated where the risk of infection is high or where there is an expectation that potentially dangerous numbers of bacteria will be present in the eye.
The particular anti-infective drugs in this product are active against the following common bacterial eye pathogens: *Staphylococcus aureus,* streptococci, including *Streptococcus pneumoniae, Escherichia coli, Haemophilus influenzae, Klebsiella-Enterobacter* species, *Neisseria* species and *Pseudomonas aeruginosa.*
The product does not provide adequate coverage against *Serratia marcescens.*
Contraindications: Epithelial herpes simplex keratitis (dendritic keratitis), vaccinia, varicella, and many other viral diseases of the cornea and conjunctiva. Mycobacterial infection of the eye. Fungal diseases of ocular structures. Hypersensitivity to a component of the medication. (Hypersensitivity to the antibiotic component occurs at a higher rate than for other components.)
The use of these combinations is always contraindicated after uncomplicated removal of a corneal foreign body.
Warnings: Prolonged use may result in glaucoma, with damage to the optic nerve, defects in visual acuity and fields of vision, and posterior subcapsular cataract formation. Prolonged use may suppress the host response and thus increase the hazard of secondary ocular infections. In those diseases causing thinning of the cornea or sclera, perforations have been known to occur with the use of topical steroids. In acute purulent conditions of the eye, steroids may mask infection or enhance existing infection. If these products are used for 10 days or longer, intraocular pressure should be routinely monitored even though it may be difficult in children and uncooperative patients.
Employment of steroid medication in the treatment of herpes simplex requires great caution.
Neomycin sulfate may cause cutaneous sensitization. A precise incidence of hypersensitivity reactions (primarily skin rash) due to topical neomycin is not known.
The manifestations of sensitization to neomycin are usually itching, reddening and edema of the conjunctiva and eyelid. It may be manifest simply as a failure to heal. During long-term use of neomycin-containing products, periodic examination for such signs is advisable, and the patient should be told to discontinue the product if they are observed. These symptoms subside quickly on withdrawing the medication. Neomycin-containing applications should be avoided for the patient thereafter.
Precautions:
General: The initial prescription and renewal of the medication order beyond 8 grams should be made by a physician only after examination of the patient with the aid of magnification, such as slit lamp biomicroscopy and, where appropriate, fluorescein staining.
The possibility of persistent fungal infections of the cornea should be considered after prolonged steroid dosing.
Allergic cross-reactions may occur which could prevent the use of any or all of the following antibiotics for the treatment of future infections: kanamycin, paromomycin, streptomycin, and possibly gentamicin.
Carcinogenesis, Mutagenesis, Impairment of Fertility: Long-term studies in animals (rats, rabbits, mice) showed no evidence of carcinogenicity attributable to oral administration of corticosteroids.
Pregnancy: ***Teratogenic Effects:*** Pregnancy Category C. Corticosteroids have been shown to be teratogenic in rabbits when applied topically at concentrations of 0.5% on days 6–18 of gestation and in mice when applied topically at a concentration of 15% on days 10–13 of gestation. There are no adequate and well-controlled studies in pregnant women. Corticosteroids should be used during pregnancy only if the potential benefit justifies the potential risk to the fetus.
Nursing Mothers: Hydrocortisone appears in human milk following oral administration of the drug. Since systemic absorption of hydrocortisone may occur when applied topically, caution should be exercised when Cortisporin Ophthalmic Ointment is used by a nursing woman.
Adverse Reactions: Adverse reactions have occurred with steroid/anti-infective combination drugs which can be attributed to the steroid component, the anti-infective component, or the combination. Reactions occurring most often from the presence of the anti-infective ingredient are localized hypersensitivity, including itching, swelling and conjunctival erythema. Local irritation on instillation has also been reported. Exact incidence figures are not available since no denominator of treated patients is available.
The reactions due to the steroid component in decreasing order of frequency are: elevation of intraocular pressure (IOP) with possible development of glaucoma, and infrequent optic nerve damage; posterior subcapsular cataract formation; and delayed wound healing.
Secondary Infection: The development of secondary infection has occurred after use of combinations containing steroids and antimicrobials. Fungal infections of the cornea are particularly prone to develop coincidentally with long-term applications of steroid. The possibility of fungal invasion must be considered in any persistent corneal ulceration where steroid treatment has been used.
Secondary bacterial ocular infection following suppression of host responses also occurs.
Dosage and Administration: Apply the ointment in the affected eye every 3 or 4 hours, depending on the severity of the condition.
Not more than 8 grams should be prescribed initially and the prescription should not be refilled without further evaluation as outlined in PRECAUTIONS above.
How Supplied: Tube of ⅛ oz with ophthalmic tip (NDC-0081-0197-86).
Store at 15°–25°C (59°–77°F).
References:

1. Leyden JJ and Kligman AM. Contact Dermatitis to Neomycin Sulfate. *JAMA* 242 (12):1276–1278, 1979.
2. Prystowsky SD, Allen AM, Smith RW, Nonomura JH, Odom RB and Akers WA. Allergic Contact Hypersensitivity to Nickel, Neomycin, Ethylenediamine, and Benzocaine. *Arch Dermatol* 115:959–962, 1979.

CORTISPORIN® ℞

[*kor 'tĭ spor "ĭn*]
OPHTHALMIC SUSPENSION Sterile
(Polymyxin B Sulfate-Neomycin Sulfate-Hydrocortisone)

Description: Cortisporin® Ophthalmic Suspension (polymyxin B sulfate-neomycin sulfate-hydrocortisone) is a sterile antimicrobial and anti-inflammatory suspension for ophthalmic use. Each ml contains: Aerosporin® (polymyxin B sulfate) 10,000 units, neomycin sulfate equivalent to 3.5 mg neomycin base and hydrocortisone 10 mg (1%). The vehicle contains thimerosal 0.001% (added as a preservative) and the inactive ingredients cetyl alcohol, glyceryl monostearate, mineral oil, polyoxyl 40 stearate, propylene glycol and water for injection. Sulfuric acid may be added to adjust pH.
Polymyxin B sulfate is the sulfate salt of polymyxin B_1 and B_2, which are produced by the growth of *Bacillus polymyxa* (Prazmowski) Migula (Fam. Bacillaceae). It has a potency of not less than 6,000 polymyxin B units per mg, calculated on an anhydrous basis.
Neomycin sulfate is the sulfate salt of neomycin B and C, which are produced by the growth of *Streptomyces fradiae* Waksman (Fam. Streptomycetaceae). It has a potency equivalent of not less than 600 μg of neomycin standard per mg, calculated on an anhydrous basis.
Hydrocortisone, 11β, 17, 21-trihydroxypregn 4- ene-3,20-dione, is an anti-inflammatory hormone.
Clinical Pharmacology: Corticoids suppress the inflammatory response to a variety of agents and they may delay healing. Since corticoids may inhibit the body's defense mechanism against infection, a concomitant antimicrobial drug may be used when this inhibition is considered to be clinically significant in a particular case.
The anti-infective components in the combination are included to provide action against specific organisms susceptible to them. Polymyxin B sulfate and neomycin sulfate together are considered active against the following microorganisms: *Staphylococcus aureus, Esherichia coli, Haemophilus influenzae, Klebsiella-En*

robacter species, *Neisseria* species and *Pseu-* omonas aeruginosa.

hen used topically, polymyxin B and neomy- n are rarely irritating, and absorption from ne intact skin or mucous membrane is insig- ificant. The incidence of skin sensitization to his combination has been shown to be low on ormal skin.[1,2] Since these antibiotics are sel- om used systemically, the patient is spared ensitization to those antibiotics which might ter be required systemically.

hen a decision to administer both a corticoid nd antimicrobials is made, the administration such drugs in combination has the advan- ge of greater patient compliance and conven- nce, with the added assurance that the in- nded dosage of both drugs is administered, us assured compatibility of ingredients when oth types of drug are in the same formulation nd, particularly that the intended volume of ach drug is delivered simultaneously, thereby voiding dilution of either medication by suc- essive instillations.

he relative potency of corticosteroids depends n the molecular structure, concentration, and elease from the vehicle.

ndications and Usage: For steroid-respon- ve inflammatory ocular conditions for which corticosteroid is indicated and where bacte- al infection or a risk of bacterial ocular infec- on exists.

cular steroids are indicated in inflammatory onditions of the palpebral and bulbar con- nctiva, cornea and anterior segment of the lobe where the inherent risk of steroid use in ertain infective conjunctivitides is accepted to btain a diminution in edema and inflamma- on. They are also indicated in chronic ante- ior uveitis and corneal injury from chemical, adiation, or thermal burns, or penetration of reign bodies.

he use of a combination drug with an anti- fective component is indicated where the sk of infection is high or where there is an xpectation that potentially dangerous num- ers of bacteria will be present in the eye.

he particular anti-infective drugs in this roduct are active against the following com- on bacterial eye pathogens: *Staphylococcus ureus, Escherichia coli, Haemophilus influen- ae, Klebsiella-Enterobacter* species, *Neisseria* pecies, and *Pseudomonas aeruginosa.*

he product does not provide adequate cover- ge against *Serratia marcescens* and strepto- occi, including *Streptococcus pneumoniae.*

ontraindications: Epithelial herpes sim- lex keratitis (dendritic keratitis), vaccinia, aricella, and many other viral diseases of the ornea and conjunctiva. Mycobacterial infec- on of the eye. Fungal diseases of ocular struc- ures. Hypersensitivity to a component of the edication. (Hypersensitivity to the antibiotic omponent occurs at a higher rate than for ther components.)

he use of these combinations is always contra- dicated after uncomplicated removal of a orneal foreign body.

arnings: Prolonged use may result in glau- oma, with damage to the optic nerve, defects n visual acuity and fields of vision, and poste- ior subcapsular cataract formation. Pro- nged use may suppress the host response and hus increase the hazard of secondary ocular nfections. In those diseases causing thinning the cornea or sclera, perforations have been nown to occur with the use of topical steroids. n acute purulent conditions of the eye, ster- ids may mask infection or enhance existing nfection. If these products are used for 10 days r longer, intraocular pressure should be rou- nely monitored even though it may be diffi- ult in children and uncooperative patients.

mployment of steroid medication in the treat- ent of herpes simplex requires great caution.

eomycin sulfate may cause cutaneous sensiti- ation. A precise incidence of hypersensitivity reactions (primarily skin rash) due to topical neomycin is not known.

The manifestations of sensitization to neomycin are usually itching, reddening and edema of the conjunctiva and eyelid. It may be manifest simply as a failure to heal. During long-term use of neomycin-containing products, periodic examination for such signs is advisable, and the patient should be told to discontinue the product if they are observed. These symptoms subside quickly on withdrawing the medication. Neomycin-containing applications should be avoided for the patient thereafter.

Precautions:

General: The initial prescription and renewal of the medication order beyond 20 milliliters should be made by a physician only after examination of the patient with the aid of magnification, such as slit lamp biomicroscopy and, where appropriate, fluorescein staining.

The possibility of persistent fungal infections of the cornea should be considered after prolonged steroid dosing.

Allergic cross-reactions may occur which could prevent the use of any or all of the following antibiotics for the treatment of future infections: kanamycin, paromomycin, streptomycin, and possibly gentamicin.

Carcinogenesis, Mutagenesis, Impairment of Fertility: Long-term studies in animals (rats, rabbits, mice) showed no evidence of carcinogenicity attributable to oral administration of corticosteroids.

Pregnancy: *Teratogenic Effects:* Pregnancy Category C. Corticosteroids have been shown to be teratogenic in rabbits when applied topically at concentrations of 0.5% on days 6–18 of gestation and in mice when applied topically at a concentration of 15% on days 10–13 of gestation. There are no adequate and well-controlled studies in pregnant women. Corticosteroids should be used during pregnancy only if the potential benefit justifies the potential risk to the fetus.

Nursing Mothers: Hydrocortisone appears in human milk following oral administration of the drug. Since systemic absorption of hydrocortisone may occur when applied topically, caution should be exercised when Cortisporin Ophthalmic Suspension is used by a nursing woman.

Adverse Reactions: Adverse reactions have occurred with steroid/anti-infective combination drugs which can be attributed to the steroid component, the anti-infective component, or the combination. Reactions occurring most often from the presence of the anti-infective ingredient are localized hypersensitivity, including itching, swelling and conjunctival erythema. Local irritation on instillation has also been reported. Exact incidence figures are not available since no denominator of treated patients is available.

The reactions due to the steroid component in decreasing order of frequency are: elevation of intraocular pressure (IOP) with possible development of glaucoma, and infrequent optic nerve damage; posterior subcapsular cataract formation; and delayed wound healing.

Secondary Infection: The development of secondary infection has occurred after use of combinations containing steroids and antimicrobials. Fungal infections of the cornea are particularly prone to develop coincidentally with long-term applications of steroid. The possibility of fungal invasion must be considered in any persistent corneal ulceration where steroid treatment has been used.

Secondary bacterial ocular infection following suppression of host responses also occurs.

Dosage and Administration: One or two drops in the affected eye every 3 or 4 hours, depending on the severity of the condition. The suspension may be used more frequently if necessary.

Not more than 20 milliliters should be prescribed initially and the prescription should not be refilled without further evaluation as outlined in PRECAUTIONS above.

SHAKE WELL BEFORE USING.

How Supplied: Plastic DROP DOSE® dispenser bottle of 7.5 ml (NDC-0081-0193-02). Store at 15°–25°C (59°–77°F).

References:

1. Leyden JJ and Kligman AM. Contact Dermatitis to Neomycin Sulfate. *JAMA* 242 (12):1276–1278, 1979.
2. Prystowsky SD, Allen AM, Smith RW, Nonomura JH, Odom RB and Akers WA. Allergic Contact Hypersensitivity to Nickel, Neomycin, Ethylenediamine, and Benzocaine. *Arch Dermatol* 115:959–962, 1979.

NEOSPORIN® ℞

[*nē″ō-spor′ĭn*]

OPHTHALMIC OINTMENT Sterile
(Polymyxin B Sulfate-Bacitracin Zinc-Neomycin Sulfate)

Description: Neosporin Ophthalmic Ointment (polymyxin B sulfate-bacitracin zinc-neomycin sulfate) is a sterile antimicrobial ointment for ophthalmic use. Each gram contains: Aerosporin® (polymyxin B sulfate) 10,000 units, bacitracin zinc 400 units, neomycin sulfate equivalent to 3.5 mg neomycin base and special white petrolatum, qs.

Polymyxin B sulfate is the sulfate salt of polymyxin B_1 and B_2 which are produced by the growth of *Bacillus polymyxa* (Prazmowski) Migula (Fam. Bacillaceae). It has a potency of not less than 6,000 polymyxin B units per mg, calculated on an anhydrous basis.

Bacitracin zinc is the zinc salt of bacitracin, a mixture of related cyclic polypeptides (mainly bacitracin A) produced by the growth of an organism of the *licheniformis* group of *Bacillus subtilis* (Fam. Bacillaceae). It has a potency of not less than 40 bacitracin units per mg.

Neomycin sulfate is the sulfate salt of neomycin B and C, which are produced by the growth of *Streptomyces fradiae* Waksman (Fam. Streptomycetaceae). It has a potency equivalent of not less than 600 μg of neomycin standard per mg, calculated on an anhydrous basis.

Clinical Pharmacology: A wide range of antibacterial action is provided by the overlapping spectra of polymyxin B sulfate, bacitracin and neomycin. The spectrum of action encompasses most bacterial pathogens capable of causing external infections of the eye and its adnexa.

Polymyxin B is bactericidal for a variety of gram-negative organisms. It increases the permeability of the bacterial cell membrane by interacting with the phospholipid components of the membrane.

Bacitracin is bactericidal for a variety of gram-positive and gram-negative organisms. It interferes with bacterial cell wall synthesis by inhibition of the regeneration of phospholipid receptors involved in peptidoglycan synthesis.

Neomycin is bactericidal for many gram-positive and gram-negative organisms. It is an aminoglycoside antibiotic which inhibits protein synthesis by binding with ribosomal RNA and causing misreading of the bacterial genetic code.

When used topically, polymyxin B, bacitracin and neomycin are rarely irritating, and absorption from the intact skin or mucous membrane is insignificant. The incidence of skin sensitization to this combination has been shown to be low on normal skin.[1,2] Since these antibiotics are seldom used systemically, the patient is spared sensitization to those antibiotics which might later be required systemically.

Continued on next page

Burroughs Wellcome—Cont.

Microbiology: Polymyxin B sulfate, bacitracin zinc and neomycin sulfate together are considered active against the following microorganisms: *Staphylococcus aureus,* streptococci, including *Streptococcus pneumoniae, Escherichia coli, Haemophilus influenzae, Klebsiella-Enterobacter* species, *Neisseria* species and *Pseudomonas aeruginosa.* The product does not provide adequate coverage against *Serratia marcescens.*

Indications and Usage: Neosporin Ophthalmic Ointment is indicated in the short-term treatment of superficial external ocular infections caused by organisms susceptible to one or more of the antibiotics contained therein.

Contraindications: This product is contraindicated in those individuals who have shown hypersensitivity to any of its components.

Warnings: The manifestations of sensitization to neomycin are usually itching, reddening and edema of the conjunctiva and eyelid. It may be manifest simply as a failure to heal. During long-term use of neomycin-containing products, periodic examination for such signs is advisable, and the patient should be told to discontinue the product if they are observed. These symptoms subside quickly on withdrawing the medication. Neomycin-containing applications should be avoided for the patient thereafter.

Precautions:

General: As with other antibiotic preparations, prolonged use may result in overgrowth of nonsusceptible organisms including fungi. Appropriate measures should be taken if this occurs.

Allergic cross-reactions may occur which could prevent the use of any or all of the following antibiotics for the treatment of future infections: kanamycin, paromomycin, streptomycin, and possibly gentamicin.

Information for Patients: If redness, irritation, swelling or pain persists or increases, discontinue use and contact your physician.

Avoid contaminating the applicator tip with material from the eye, fingers, or other source. This caution is necessary if the sterility of the ointment is to be preserved.

Adverse Reactions: Neomycin Sulfate may cause cutaneous and conjunctival sensitization. A precise incidence of hypersensitivity reactions (primarily skin rash) due to topical neomycin is not known.

Dosage and Administration: Apply the ointment every 3 or 4 hours for 7 to 10 days, depending on the severity of the infection.

How Supplied: Tube of $\frac{1}{8}$ oz with ophthalmic tip (NDC-0081-0732-86).

Store at 15°-25°C (59°-77°F).

References:

1. Leyden JJ, and Kligman AM. Contact Dermatitis to Neomycin Sulfate, *JAMA* 242 (12): 1276–1278, 1979.
2. Prystowsky SD, Allen AM, Smith RW, Nonomura JH, Odom RB, and Akers WA. Allergic Contact Hypersensitivity to Nickle, Neomycin, Ethylenediamine, and Benzocaine. *Arch Dermatol* 115:959–962, 1979.

NEOSPORIN® ℞

[nē″ō-spor′ĭn]

OPHTHALMIC SOLUTION Sterile

(Polymyxin B Sulfate-Neomycin Sulfate-Gramicidin)

Description: Neosporin Ophthalmic Solution (polymyxin B sulfate-neomycin sulfate-gramicidin) is a sterile antimicrobial solution for ophthalmic use. Each ml contains: Aerosporin® (polymyxin B sulfate) 10,000 units, neomycin sulfate equivalent to 1.75 mg neomycin base and gramicidin 0.025 mg. The vehicle contains alcohol 0.5%, thimerosal 0.001% (added as a preservative) and the inactive ingredients propylene glycol, polyoxyethylene polyoxypropylene compound, sodium chloride and water for injection.

Polymyxin B sulfate is the sulfate salt of polymyxin B_1 and B_2 which are produced by the growth of *Bacillus polymyxa* (Prazmowski) Migula (Fam. Bacillaceae). It has a potency of not less than 6,000 polymyxin B units per mg, calculated on an anhydrous basis.

Neomycin sulfate is the sulfate salt of neomycin B and C, which are produced by the growth of *Streptomyces fradiae* Waksman (Fam. Streptomycetaceae). It has a potency equivalent of not less than 600 μg of neomycin standard per mg, calculated on an anhydrous basis.

Gramicidin (also called Gramicidin D) is a mixture of three pairs of antibacterial substances (Gramicidin A, B and C) produced by the growth of *Bacillus brevis* Dubos (Fam. Bacillaceae). It has a potency of not less than 900 μg of standard gramicidin per mg.

Clinical Pharmacology: A wide range of antibacterial action is provided by the overlapping spectra of polymyxin B sulfate, neomycin and gramicidin. The spectrum of action encompasses most bacterial pathogens capable of causing external infections of the eye and its adnexa.

Polymyxin B is bactericidal for a variety of gram-negative organisms. It increases the permeability of the bacterial cell membrane by interacting with the phospholipid components of the membrane.

Neomycin is bactericidal for many gram-positive and gram-negative organisms. It is an aminoglycoside antibiotic which inhibits protein synthesis by binding with ribosomal RNA and causing misreading of the bacterial genetic code.

Gramicidin is bactericidal for a variety of gram-positive organisms. It increases the permeability of the bacterial cell membrane to inorganic cations by forming a network of channels through the normal lipid bilayer of the membrane.

When used topically, polymyxin B, neomycin and gramicidin are rarely irritating, and absorption from the intact skin or mucous membrane is insignificant. The incidence of skin sensitization to this combination has been shown to be low on normal skin.[1,2] Since these antibiotics are seldom used systemically, the patient is spared sensitization to those antibiotics which might later be required systemically.

Microbiology: Polymyxin B sulfate, neomycin sulfate and gramicidin together are considered active against the following microorganisms: *Staphylococcus aureus,* streptococci, including *Streptococcus pneumoniae, Escherichia coli, Haemophilus influenzae, Klebsiella-Enterobacter* species, *Neisseria* species and *Pseudomonas aeruginosa.* The product does not provide adequate coverage against *Serratia marcescens.*

Indications and Usage: Neosporin Ophthalmic Solution is indicated in the short-term treatment of superficial external ocular infections caused by organisms susceptible to one or more of the antibiotics contained therein.

Contraindications: This product is contraindicated in those individuals who have shown hypersensitivity to any of its components.

Warnings: The manifestations of sensitization to neomycin are usually itching, reddening and edema of the conjunctiva and eyelid. It may be manifest simply as a failure to heal. During long-term use of neomycin-containing products, periodic examination for such signs is advisable, and the patient should be told to discontinue the product if they are observed. These symptoms subside quickly on withdrawing the medication. Neomycin-containing applications should be avoided for the patien thereafter.

Precautions:

General: As with other antibiotic prepara tions, prolonged use may result in overgrowt of nonsusceptible organisms including fung Appropriate measures should be taken if thi occurs.

Allergic cross-reactions may occur which coul prevent the use of any or all of the followin antibiotics for the treatment of future infec tions: kanamycin, paromomycin, streptomy cin, and possibly gentamicin.

Information for Patients: If redness, irrita tion, swelling or pain persists or increases, dis continue use and contact your physician.

Avoid contaminating the applicator tip wit material from the eye, fingers, or other source This caution is necessary if the sterility of th drops is to be preserved.

Adverse Reactions: Neomycin Sulfate ma cause cutaneous and conjunctival sensitiza tion. A precise incidence of hypersensitivit reactions (primarily skin rash) due to topica neomycin is not known.

Dosage and Administration: The sug gested dosage is one or two drops in the a fected eye two to four times daily, or more fre quently as required, for 7 to 10 days. In acut infections, initiate therapy with one or tw drops every 15 to 30 minutes, reducing the fre quency of instillation gradually as the infec tion is controlled.

How Supplied: Drop Dose® of 10 ml (plasti dispenser bottle) (NDC-0081-0728-69).

Store at 15°-25°C (59°-77°F) and protect fron light.

References:

1. Leyden JJ, and Kligman AM. Contact Der matitis to Neomycin Sulfate. *JAM* 242(12):1276–1278, 1979.
2. Prystowsky SD, Allen AM, Smith RW Nonomura JH, Odom RB and Akers WA Allergic Contact Hypersensitivity to Nicke Neomycin, Ethylenediamine, and Benzo caine. *Arch Dermatol* 115:959–962, 1979.

POLYSPORIN® ℞

[pah ″l ē-spor ′ĭn]

OPHTHALMIC OINTMENT Sterile

(Polymyxin B-Bacitracin)

Description: Each gram contains Aerosp rin® (Polymyxin B Sulfate) 10,000 units, bac tracin zinc 500 units, special white petrolatu qs.

Actions: Polymyxin B attacks gram-negativ bacilli, including virtually all strains of *Pse domonas aeruginosa* and *H influenzae* species. Bacitracin is active against most gram-positiv bacilli and cocci, including hemolytic strept cocci.

Indications: For the treatment of superficia ocular infections involving the conjunctiv and/or cornea caused by organisms susceptibl to polymyxin B sulfate and bacitracin zinc.

Contraindications: This product is contra indicated in those individuals who have show hypersensitivity to any of its components.

Warnings: Ophthalmic ointments may re tard corneal healing.

Precautions: As with other antibiotic prepa rations, prolonged use may result in ove growth of nonsusceptible organisms, includin fungi. Appropriate measures should be taken this occurs.

Dosage and Administration: Apply th ointment every 3 or 4 hours, depending on th severity of the infection.

How Supplied: Tube of $\frac{1}{8}$ oz with ophtha mic tip (NDC 0081-0797-86).

IROPTIC® ℞

ī-rŏp'tĭk"]

PHTHALMIC SOLUTION, 1% Sterile Trifluridine)

)escription: Viroptic is the brand name for rifluridine (also known as trifluorothymidine, $_3$TdR, F_3T), an antiviral drug for topical treatment of epithelial keratitis caused by Herpes implex virus. The chemical name of trifluridine is 2′-deoxy-5-(trifluoromethyl)uridine.

'iroptic sterile ophthalmic solution contains % trifluridine in an aqueous solution with cetic acid and sodium acetate (buffers), soium chloride, and thimerosal 0.001% (added s a preservative).

linical Pharmacology: Trifluridine is a uorinated pyrimidine nucleoside with *in vitro* nd *in vivo* activity against Herpes simplex irus, types 1 and 2 and vacciniavirus. Some trains of Adenovirus are also inhibited *in vitro.*

'rifluridine interferes with DNA synthesis in ultured mammalian cells. However, its antiviral mechanism of action is not completely nown.

n vitro perfusion studies on excised rabbit corneas have shown that trifluridine penetrates he intact cornea as evidenced by recovery of arental drug and its major metabolite, 5-carboxy-2′-deoxyuridine, on the endothelial side of he cornea. Absence of the corneal epithelium nhances the penetration of trifluridine approximately two-fold.

ntraocular penetration of trifluridine occurs fter topical instillation of Viroptic into human eyes. Decreased corneal integrity or stromal or uveal inflammation may enhance the enetration of trifluridine into the aqueous umor. Unlike the results of ocular penetration of trifluridine *in vitro,* 5-carboxy-2′-deoxyridine was not found in detectable concentrations within the aqueous humor of the human ye.

ystemic absorption of trifluridine following herapeutic dosing with Viroptic appears to be egligible. No detectable concentrations of rifluridine or 5-carboxy-2′-deoxyuridine were ound in the sera of adult healthy normal subects who had Viroptic instilled into their eyes even times daily for 14 consecutive days.

ndications and Usage: Viroptic (Trifluridine) Ophthalmic Solution, 1% is indicated for he treatment of primary keratoconjunctivitis nd recurrent epithelial keratitis due to Herpes simplex virus, types 1 and 2. Viroptic is lso effective in the treatment of epithelial eratitis that has not responded clinically to he topical administration of idoxuridine or hen ocular toxicity or hypersensitivity to doxuridine has occurred. In a smaller number f patients found to be resistant to topical idarabine, Viroptic was also effective.

he clinical efficacy of Viroptic in the treatment of stromal keratitis and uveitis due to Ierpes simplex virus or ophthalmic infections aused by vacciniavirus and Adenovirus has ot been established by well-controlled clinical rials. Viroptic has not been shown to be effective in the prophylaxis of Herpes simplex virus eratoconjunctivitis and epithelial keratitis by vell-controlled clinical trials. Viroptic is ot effective against bacterial, fungal or hlamydial infections of the cornea or nonviral rophic lesions.

)uring controlled multicenter clinical trials, 2 of 97 (95%) patients (78 of 81 with dendritic nd 14 of 16 with geographic ulcers) responded o Viroptic therapy as evidenced by complete orneal re-epithelialization within the 14-day herapy period. In these controlled studies, 56 f 75 (75%) patients (49 of 58 with dendritic nd 7 of 17 with geographic ulcers) responded o idoxuridine therapy. The mean time to corneal re-epithelialization for dendritic ulcers (6 ays) and geographic ulcers (7 days) was simiar for both therapies. In other clinical studies, Viroptic was evaluated in the treatment of Herpes simplex virus keratitis in patients who were unresponsive or intolerant to the topical administration of idoxuridine or vidarabine. Viroptic was effective in 138 of 150 (92%) patients (109 of 114 with dendritic and 29 of 36 with geographic ulcers) as evidenced by corneal re-epithelialization. The mean time to corneal re-epithelialization was 6 days for patients with dendritic ulcers and 12 days for patients with geographic ulcers.

Contraindications: Viroptic (Trifluridine) Ophthalmic Solution, 1%, is contraindicated for patients who develop hypersensitivity reactions or chemical intolerance to trifluridine.

Warnings:

The recommended dosage and frequency of administration should not be exceeded (see DOSAGE AND ADMINISTRATION).

Precautions:

General: Viroptic (Trifluridine) Ophthalmic Solution, 1% should be prescribed only for patients who have a clinical diagnosis of herpetic keratitis.

Viroptic may cause mild local irritation of the conjunctiva and cornea when instilled but these effects are usually transient.

Although documented *in vitro* viral resistance to trifluridine has not been reported following multiple exposure to Viroptic, the possibility exists of viral resistance development.

Drug Interactions: The following drugs have been administered topically to the eye and concurrently with Viroptic in a limited number of patients without apparent evidence of adverse interaction: antibiotics—chloramphenicol, erythromycin, polymyxin B sulfate, bacitracin, gentamicin sulfate, tetracycline HCl, sodium sulfacetamide, neomycin sulfate; steroids—dexamethasone, dexamethasone sodium phosphate, prednisolone acetate, prednisolone sodium phosphate, hydrocortisone, fluorometholone; and other ophthalmic drugs—atropine sulfate, scopolamine hydrobromide, naphazoline hydrochloride, cyclopentolate hydrochloride, homatropine hydrobromide, pilocarpine, l-epinephrine hydrochloride, sodium chloride.

Carcinogenesis, Mutagenesis, Impairment of Fertility: ***Mutagenic Potential:*** Trifluridine has been shown to exert mutagenic, DNA-damaging and cell-transforming activities in various standard *in vitro* test systems, and clastogenic activity in *Vicia faba* cells. It did not induce chromosome aberrations in bone marrow cells of male or female rats following a single subcutaneous dose of 100 mg/kg, but was weakly positive in female, but not in male, rats following daily subcutaneous administration at 700 mg/kg/day for 5 days.

Although the significance of these test results is not clear or fully understood, there exists the possibility that mutagenic agents may cause genetic damage in humans.

Oncogenic Potential. Lifetime carcinogenicity bioassays in rats and mice given daily subcutaneous doses of trifluridine have been performed. Rats tested at 1.5, 7.5 and 15 mg/kg/day had increased incidences of adenocarcinomas of the intestinal tract and mammary glands, hemangiosarcomas of the spleen and liver, carcinosarcomas of the prostate gland and granulosa-thecal cell tumors of the ovary. Mice were tested at 1, 5 and 10 mg/kg/day; those given 10 mg/kg/day trifluridine had significantly increased incidences of adenocarcinomas of the intestinal tract and uterus. Those given 10 mg/kg/day also had a significantly increased incidence of testicular atrophy as compared to vehicle control mice.

Pregnancy: The drug should not be prescribed for pregnant women unless the potential benefits outweigh the potential risks.

Teratogenic Potential. Kury and Crosby[1] found that trifluridine was teratogenic when injected directly into the yolk sac of developing chick embryos. Itoi *et al.*[2] found that topical application of 1% trifluridine ophthalmic solution to the eyes of rabbits on days 6–18 of pregnancy produced no teratogenic effects. Trifluridine was not teratogenic when given subcutaneously to rats at doses up to 5.0 mg/kg/day although drug-induced fetal toxicity (delayed ossification of portions of the skeletal system) was observed at the 2.5 mg/kg/day dose level. Trifluridine was not teratogenic when given subcutaneously to rabbits at doses up to 5.0 mg/kg/day. Drug-induced fetal toxicity (delayed ossification of portions of the skeletal system) was observed at the 2.5 mg/kg/day dose level. A 1.0 mg/kg/day dose was considered to be a no-effect level in both rats and rabbits. Based upon these findings in animals, it is unlikely that Viroptic would cause embryonic or fetal damage if given in the recommended ophthalmic dosage to pregnant women. A safe dose, however, has not been established for the human embryo or fetus.

Nursing Mothers: It is unlikely that trifluridine is excreted in human milk after ophthalmic instillation of Viroptic because of the relatively small dosage ($\leq$ 5.0 mg/day), its dilution in body fluids and its extremely short half-life (approximately 12 minutes). The drug should not be prescribed for nursing mothers unless the potential benefits outweigh the potential risks.

Adverse Reactions: The most frequent adverse reactions reported during controlled clinical trials were mild, transient burning or stinging upon instillation (4.6%) and palpebral edema (2.8%). Other adverse reactions in decreasing order of reported frequency were superficial punctate keratopathy, epithelial keratopathy, hypersensitivity reaction, stromal edema, irritation, keratitis sicca, hyperemia, and increased intraocular pressure.

Overdosage: Overdosage by ocular instillation is unlikely because any excess solution should be quickly expelled from the conjunctival sac.

Acute overdosage by accidental oral ingestion of Viroptic has not occurred. However, should such ingestion occur, the 75 mg dosage of trifluridine in a 7.5 mL bottle of Viroptic is not likely to produce adverse effects. Single intravenous doses of 15–30 mg/kg/day in children and adults with neoplastic disease produce reversible bone marrow depression as the only potentially serious toxic effect and only after 3–5 courses of therapy.[3] The acute oral LD_{50} in the mouse and rat was 4379 mg/kg or higher.

Dosage and Administration: Instill one drop of Viroptic Ophthalmic Solution, 1% onto the cornea of the affected eye every two hours while awake for a maximum daily dosage of nine drops until the corneal ulcer has completely re-epithelialized. Following re-epithelialization, treatment for an additional seven days of one drop every four hours while awake for a minimum daily dosage of five drops is recommended.

If there are no signs of improvement after seven days of therapy or complete re-epithelialization has not occurred after 14 days of therapy, other forms of therapy should be considered. Continuous administration of Viroptic for periods exceeding 21 days should be avoided because of potential ocular toxicity.

How Supplied: Viroptic Ophthalmic Solution, 1% is supplied as a sterile ophthalmic solution in a plastic Drop Dose® dispenser bottle of 7.5 mL. (NDC 0081-0968-02)

Store under refrigeration 2° to 8°C (36° to 46°F).

Animal Pharmacology and Animal Toxicology: Corneal wound healing studies in rabbits showed that Viroptic did not significantly retard closure of epithelial wounds. However, mild toxic changes such as intracellular edema of the basal cell layer, mild thin-

Continued on next page

Burroughs Wellcome—Cont.

ning of the overlying epithelium and reduced strength of stromal wounds were observed. Whereas instillation of Viroptic into rabbit eyes during a subchronic toxicity study produced some degree of corneal epithelial thinning, a 12-month chronic toxicity study in rabbits in which Viroptic was instilled into eyes in intermittent, multiple, full-therapy courses showed no drug- related changes in the cornea.

References:

1. Kury G, Crosby RJ: The teratogenic effect of 5-trifluoromethyl-2′-deoxyuridine in chicken embryos. *Toxicol Appl Pharmacol* 1967;11:72–80.
2. Itoi M, Getter JW, Kaneko N, et al: Teratogenicities of ophthalmic drugs. I. Antiviral ophthalmic drugs. *Arch Ophthalmol* 1975;93:46–51.
3. Ansfield FJ, Ramirez G: Phase I and II studies of 2′-deoxy-5-(trifluoromethyl)-uridine (NSC-75520). *Cancer Chemother Rep* 1971;55(pt 1):205–208.

CIBA Vision Ophthalmics

11460 JOHN'S CREEK PARKWAY
ATLANTA, GA 30136

VOLTAREN OPHTHALMIC™
(diclofenac sodium 0.1%)
Sterile Ophthalmic Solution

Description: Voltaren Ophthalmic (diclofenac sodium) 0.1% solution is a sterile, topical, nonsteroidal, anti-inflammatory product for ophthalmic use. Diclofenac sodium is designated chemically as 2-[(2,6-dichlorophenyl) amino] benzeneacetic acid, monosodium salt, with an empirical formula of $C_{14}H_{10}CL_2NO_2Na$. The structural formula of diclofenac sodium is

Voltaren Ophthalmic is available as a sterile solution, which contains diclofenac sodium 0.1% (1 mg/mL).

Inactive Ingredients. Boric acid, edetate disodium (1 mg/mL), polyoxyl 35 castor oil, purified water, sorbic acid (2 mg/mL), and tromethamine.

Diclofenac sodium is a faintly yellow-white to light-beige, slightly hygroscopic crystalline powder. It is freely soluble in methanol, sparingly soluble in water, very slightly soluble in acetonitrile, and insoluble in chloroform and in 0.1N hydrochloric acid. Its molecular weight is 318.14. Voltaren Ophthalmic 0.1% is an isoosmotic physiologically compatible solution with an osmolality of about 300 mOsmol/1000 g, buffered at approximately pH 7.2. Voltaren Ophthalmic solution has a faint characteristic odor of castor oil.

Clinical Pharmacology: Diclofenac sodium is one of a series of phenylacetic acids that have demonstrated anti-inflammatory and analgesic properties in pharmacological studies. It is thought to inhibit the enzyme cyclooxygenase, which is essential in the biosynthesis of prostaglandins.

Prostaglandins have been shown in many animal models to be mediators of certain kinds of intraocular inflammation. In studies performed in animal eyes, prostaglandins have been shown to produce disruption of the blood-aqueous humor barrier, vasodilation, increased vascular permeability, leukocytosis, and increased intraocular pressure. Prostaglandins also appear to play a role in the miotic response produced during ocular surgery by constricting the iris sphincter independently of cholinergic mechanisms. In clinical studies, Voltaren Ophthalmic has been shown to decrease the signs and symptoms of inflammation resulting from cataract surgery.

Results from clinical studies indicate that Voltaren Ophthalmic has no significant effect upon intraocular pressure; however, elevations in intraocular pressure may occur following cataract surgery.

Results from a bioavailability study established that plasma levels of diclofenac following ocular instillation of two drops of Voltaren Ophthalmic to each eye were below the limit of quantitation (10 ng/mL) over a 4-hour period. This study suggests that limited, if any, systemic absorption occurs with Voltaren Ophthalmic.

In two doubled-masked, controlled, efficacy studies of postoperative inflammation, a total of 206 cataract patients were treated with Voltaren Ophthalmic and 103 patients were treated with vehicle placebo. Voltaren Ophthalmic was statistically favored over vehicle placebo at all three visits over a 2-week period for the clinical assessments of inflammation (anterior chamber cells and flare, conjunctival erythema and ciliary flush). The patients in these trials were safely continued on Voltaren Ophthalmic for a period of up to 6 weeks.

In two separate, double-masked, comparative studies the effects of Voltaren Ophthalmic and prednisolone sodium phosphate 1% on the blood-aqueous humor barrier were examined by anterior chamber fluorophotometry at 1 week post surgery. Each study compared 37 patients in the Voltaren Ophthalmic group with 40 patients in the prednisolone group. Voltaren Ophthalmic was statistically more effective than prednisolone in expediting reestablishment of the blood-aqueous humor barrier disrupted by cataract extraction. However, the clinical benefit or harm in the reestablishment of the blood-aqueous barrier is unknown.

Voltaren Ophthalmic has been safely administered in conjunction with other ophthalmic medications such as antibiotics, beta blockers, carbonic anhydrase inhibitors, cycloplegics, and mydriatics.

Indications and Usage: Voltaren Ophthalmic is indicated for the treatment of postoperative inflammation in patients who have undergone cataract extraction.

Contraindications: Voltaren Ophthalmic is contraindicated in patients concurrently wearing soft contact lenses and in patients who are hypersensitive to any component of the medication. Patients wearing hydrogel soft contact lenses who have used Voltaren Ophthalmic concurrently have experienced ocular irritation manifested by redness and burning.

Warnings: There is the potential for cross-sensitivity to acetylsalicylic acid, phenylacetic acid derivatives, and other nonsteroidal anti-inflammatory agents. Therefore, caution should be used when treating individuals who have previously exhibited sensitivities to these drugs.

With some nonsteroidal anti-inflammatory drugs, there exists the potential for increased bleeding time due to interference with thrombocyte aggregation. There have been reports that ocularly applied nonsteroidal anti-inflammatory drugs may cause increased bleeding of ocular tissues (including hyphemas) in conjunction with ocular surgery.

Precautions:

General: It is recommended that Voltaren Ophthalmic be used with caution in surgical patients with known bleeding tendencies or who are receiving other medications that may prolong bleeding time.

Voltaren may slow or delay healing.

Carcinogenesis, Mutagenesis, Impairment of Fertility: Long-term carcinogenicity studies in rats given oral Voltaren up to 2 mg/kg/day (approximately the human oral dose) have revealed no significant increases in tumor incidence. There was a slight increase in benign rat mammary fibroadenomas in mid-dose females (high-dose females had excessive mortality) but the increase was not significant for this common rat tumor. A 2-year carcinogenicity study conducted in mice employing oral Voltaren up to 2 mg/kg/day did not reveal any oncogenic potential. Voltaren did not show mutagenic potential in various mutagenicity studies including the Ames test. Voltaren administered to male and female rats at 4 mg/kg/day did not affect fertility.

Pregnancy:

Teratogenic Effects:

Pregnancy Category B: Reproduction studies performed in mice at oral doses up to 5,000 times (20 mg/kg/day) and in rats and rabbits at oral doses up to 2,500 times (10 mg/kg/day) the human topical dose have revealed no evidence of teratogenicity due to Voltaren, despite the induction of maternal toxicity and fetal toxicity. In rats, maternally toxic doses were associated with dystocia, prolonged gestation, reduced fetal weights and growth, and reduced fetal survival. Voltaren has been shown to cross the placental barrier in mice and rats.

There are, however, no adequate and well-controlled studies in pregnant women. Because animal reproduction studies are not always predictive of human response, this drug should be used during pregnancy only if clearly needed.

Nonteratogenic Effects: Because of the known effects of prostaglandin-inhibiting drugs on the fetal cardiovascular system (closure of the ductus arteriosus), the use of Voltaren Ophthalmic during late pregnancy should be avoided.

Pediatric Use: Safety and effectiveness in children have not been established.

Adverse Reactions:

Ocular: Transient burning and stinging was reported in 15% of patients across all studies with the use of topical Voltaren Ophthalmic. In cataract studies, keratitis occurred in 28% of patients receiving Voltaren Ophthalmic; most of the cases of keratitis occurred prior to drug therapy. Elevated intraocular pressure was reported in 15% of patients receiving Voltaren Ophthalmic; most of these cases occurred post surgery and prior to drug administration. Other ocular medical problems included anterior chamber reaction and ocular allergy.

Systemic: Nausea and vomiting occurred in 1% of patients receiving Voltaren Ophthalmic and in 0.5% of patients receiving vehicle alone. Viral infections occurred in $\leq 1\%$ of each of the Voltaren Ophthalmic and vehicle groups.

Overdosage: Overdosage will not ordinarily cause acute problems. If accidentally ingested, fluids should be taken to dilute the medication.

Dosage and Administration: One drop of Voltaren Ophthalmic should be applied to the affected eye four times daily beginning 24 hours after cataract surgery and continuing throughout the first 2 weeks of the postoperative period.

How Supplied: Voltaren Ophthalmic 0.1% (1 mg/mL) Sterile Solution is supplied in dropper-tip, plastic squeeze bottles in the following sizes:

Bottles of 2.5 mL ....NDC 58768-100-02
Bottles of 5 mL ....NDC 58768-100-05

Store between 59°–86°F (15°–30°C). Protect from light.

Dispense in original, unopened container only.

Dist. by:
CIBA Vision Ophthalmics

A Division of Ciba Vision Corporation
Atlanta, Georgia 30136
Shown in Product Identification Section, page 103

CooperVision, Inc.
3495 WINTON PLACE
ROCHESTER, NY 14623

EYESCRUB™ Sterile Eyelid Cleanser
Lid Cleanser for Blepharitis Patients
An extra gentle, hypoallergenic sterile cleanser

Cleanser ingredients: Water for Injection USP, PEG-200 Glyceryl Tallowate, Disodium Laureth Sulfosuccinate, Cocamidopropylamine Oxide, PEG-78 Glyceryl Cocoate, Benzyl Alcohol and Disodium EDTA.
Ready to use, needs no diluting. For External Use Only. Do Not Use Directly In The Eye.
The Development of EYEscrub: Developed by a leading ophthalmologist and a pharmacist, EYEscrub Sterile Eyelid Cleanser and EYEscrub Cleansing Pads provide an easy to use system for daily eyelid hygiene. EYEscrub Cleanser is a patented, extremely mild, nonirritating, hypoallergenic solution that is pH balanced for maximum comfort.
EYEscrub Cleansing Pads are made from special, virtually lint-free non-shedding, soft fibers that do not leave foreign material around the eyes. Once the Pads are wetted with EYEscrub Cleanser, a rich, microbubble lather is produced that is remarkably safe for daily eyelid hygiene.
Preferred Cleansing Regimen
Directions for Use:

1. **The warm compress.** Apply a warm compress such as a washcloth soaked in very warm water to closed eyes for several minutes before cleansing. This is essential to loosen oily debris and scales and to soothe the area around the eye.
2. **The lather.** Wet, but do not saturate an EYEscrub Cleansing Pad with EYEscrub Cleanser, fold the pad over and rub between thumb and forefinger to work up a lather. Eyescrub's special formula creates a unique microbubble lather which helps gently loosen debris.
3. **The cleansing.** In front of a well illuminated mirror, expose the lower eyelid edge by pulling the skin down with your finger.
   Rub the pad several times along the lid at the base where the lashes grow out. Be careful not to rub the surface of the eye. Next, using your finger, pull the upper lid up towards the brow and away from the eye surface. Repeat the process on the upper lid edge at the base of the lashes, again being careful not to rub the eye surface. Close the eye and rub the pad vigorously across the eyelashes several times. Open the eye, discard the pad and leave the lather on the area you cleaned. Repeat the process on the other eye using a clean EYEscrub Cleansing Pad.
4. **The rinse.** Thoroughly rinse both eyes with clean, warm water and pat dry.

Alternative Cleansing Regimen
Directions for Use: A cotton tipped applicator may be used in place of EYEscrub Cleansing Pads according to your eyecare professional's instructions or your personal preference. When using the cotton tipped applicator, place a few drops of EYEscrub Sterile Eyelid Cleanser on the padding and keep massaging it with your fingers until a lather forms. Then follow procedure for Preferred Cleanser Regimen.
Management for Blepharitis Patients: Irritation and inflammation of eyelids are common occurrences of blepharitis. Eyelids can also become reddened, thickened, scaly and have frequent styes. In severe cases, loss of lashes, scarring, and irregularity of the lid margin may occur. Such chronic lid conditions can also affect the surface of the eye by causing burning, itching, redness, and foreign body sensation. Causes may be related to excessive bacteria or fungus on the eyelids, abnormalities of the skin glands that produce the oily layer of the tear film, and skin conditions such as seborrhea. Management of patients with this condition is directed at control of microbial growth and physical removal of residues such as scales, lid crusts and excess oil. The use of a regimen of warm compresses and mechanical massage around the eyes combined with a non-irritating surfactant cleanser to remove residual debris is the cleansing regimen most often recommended by eyecare professionals.
EYEscrub InfoLine 1-800-225-2578
If your local pharamcy does not have EYEscrub, call and we will help you find a local source.
Manufactured for:
CooperVision®
CooperVision, Inc.
Rochester, NY 14623
1-800-225-2578
EYEscrub™ is a trademark of CooperVision, Inc. Patented Formula
© CooperVision 1991

Eagle Vision, Inc.
6263 POPLAR AVENUE—SUITE 650
MEMPHIS, TN 38119 U.S.A.

Nationwide (800) 222-7584
Local (901) 682-9400
FAX (901) 761-5736

EAGLE VISION–FREEMAN™ PUNCTUM PLUG INSERTION KIT
(Silicone Punctum Plugs)

Plug can be used in the treatment of certain dry eye conditions in which a reduction of tear outflow is deemed appropriate. It is inserted by the ophthalmologist to reversibly occlude one or both punctal openings. This serves as an alternate to occulsion by cautery.
How Supplied: Each sterile packaged kit contains 2 plugs, a dilator/inserter and physician instructions. Size availability by diameter and length: Mini—.76mm × 1.6mm, Micro—.91mm × 1.6mm, Small—1.06mm × 1.6mm, Medium—1.27mm × 2.3mm, Standard—1.4mm × 2.8mm, Large—1.7mm × 2.8mm and Flow Controller, 1.4mm × 2.8mm (with open nose). Also sterile packaged in Triple-Pack containing two each of Standard, Medium and Small Plugs. Bulk packaging also available in Multi-Packs (10 Plugs) and 20-Packs (20 Plugs) in the Standard, Medium and Small.

TEMPORARY INTRACANALICULAR COLLAGEN IMPLANTS

Uses: For the diagnosis and treatment of certain dry eye conditions. Temporary Intracanalicular Collagen Implants are inserted by the eyecare practitioner in one or both lacrimal canaliculi to decrease the tear outflow temporarily. Instructions are provided in package insert.
Contraindications are tearing secondary to chronic dacryocystitis with mucopurulent discharge infections.
How Supplied: Sterile inserts 2 mm in length. Box of either 0.2mm, 0.3mm or 0.4mm dia. implants, 6 implants per pack, and 12 packs per box.

COLOR BAR™ SCHIRMER TEAR TEST

Use: A blue COLOR BAR with an FDA approved dye is imprinted on each strip that travels the tear flow and leaves a soft blue, easy to read, vignette on the millimeter scale preprinted on each strip. Each sterile sealed clear pouch contains two strips, one with "R" and one with "L", indicating right or left eye, printed at the bottom.
How Supplied: Sterile packaged, 5 pouches per envelope, 10 envelopes per box. A total of 100 strips for 50 tests.

EV™ LID-CLEANSER KIT

Use: Whenever daily hygiene is indicated. Ideal for eyelid cleaning and facial cosmetic removal. Mild and pH adjusted, EV™ Lid-Cleanser contains no irritating dyes or perfumes. Ready to use—do not dilute.
Directions: Gently cleanse skin or eyelid area with moistened pad to remove oily debris, crusted matter, and cosmetics. Rinse area after use.
How Supplied: 8 oz. Bottle with 100 cleansing pads per kit. 12 kits per case. Also, .5 oz Travel Bottle w/pads.

LACTOPLATE™
(Lactoferrin Immunological Assay Test)

The Lactoplate is a procedure to diagnose the lacrimal gland function. The test is based on the difference in tear lactoferrin concentration between normal and KCS tears. The complete items for tear sampling, room temperature immunological assay and results assessment are provided. There is no need for incubation or standard curve preparation.
How Supplied: In kits of 4, 8 or 16 Lactoplates (one kit sufficient for both eyes).

EV™ MONOCANALICULAR STENT
(Stent for the Lacrimal Canaliculus)

Use: Sterile open-bored silicone stent can be used by the ocular surgeon in the repair of selected lacerations of the lacrimal canaliculus. Trim the 35mm length tubing to desired length, insert through the punctal opening and thread into the nasal portion of the severed canaliculus. In eyes with appropriate puncta, it can be held in place without sutures. This provides a stent with a patent opening available for tear outflow and eliminates the need to thread the fellow canaliculus. The configuration of the silicone punctum plug can hold the stent in position during the healing process.
Device Description: Each stent comprises a silicone punctum plug modified to have an open central canal attached with silicone adhesive to a 35mm length of silicone tubing.
How Supplied: Individually sterile packaged in three sizes: Pediatric, .7mm dia. tubing and small plug with 1.0mm dome; Regular, .8mm dia. tubing and standard plug with 1.5mm dome; Large, .9mm dia. tubing and large plug with 1.9mm dome.

MOIST EYE™ MOISTURE PANELS
(Moisture Panels for Eyeglasses)

Uses: Designed to reduce evaporative loss of tears when deemed necessary by the eye care practitioner. Panels are fit between the lens and the frame. Assists in retaining moisture within the shielded eyeglass area.
How Supplied: Eight panels per envelope.

EV™ ROSE BENGAL

Uses: For diagnosis of dry eye conditions. Rose Bengal stains non-viable tissue observed in exposure keratitis associated with dry eye conditions.

Continued on next page

Eagle Vision—Cont.

Contents: Each ml contains 10 mg of Rose Bengal in a base containing Polyvinylpyrrolidone, Sodium Borate, Polyethylene Glycol p-isooctylphenol 10 $(CH_2)_2O$, made isotonic with Sodium Chloride. Preservative: Thimerosal 0.01%.
How Supplied: 5 ml sterile plastic dropper bottle. Sold separately or in cases of 12.

Fisons Corporation
P.O. BOX 1710
ROCHESTER, NY 14603

OPTICROM® 4% ℞
[*op "tĭ-krōm*]
Ophthalmic Solution
(cromolyn sodium ophthalmic solution, USP)

Description: Each milliliter of OPTICROM 4% Ophthalmic Solution (cromolyn sodium ophthalmic solution, USP) contains 40 mg cromolyn sodium in purified water with 0.01% benzalkonium chloride to preserve and 0.1% EDTA (edetate disodium, USP) to stabilize the solution. OPTICROM is a clear, colorless, sterile solution with a pH of 4.0–7.0. It is intended for topical administration to the eye.
Chemically, cromolyn sodium is the disodium salt of 1,3-bis(2-carboxychromon-5-yloxy)-2-hydroxypropane. Its chemical structure is:

Pharmacologic Category: Mast cell stabilizer
Clinical Pharmacology: *In vitro* and *in vivo* animal studies have shown that cromolyn sodium inhibits the degranulation of sensitized mast cells which occurs after exposure to specific antigens. Cromolyn sodium acts by inhibiting the release of histamine and SRS-A (slow-reacting substance of anaphylaxis) from the mast cell.
Another activity demonstrated *in vitro* is the capacity of cromolyn sodium to inhibit the degranulation of non-sensitized rat mast cells by phospholipase A and the subsequent release of chemical mediators. Another study showed that cromolyn sodium did not inhibit the enzymatic activity of released phospholipase A on its specific substrate.
Cromolyn sodium has no intrinsic vasoconstrictor, antihistaminic or anti-inflammatory activity.
Cromolyn sodium is poorly absorbed. When multiple doses of cromolyn sodium ophthalmic solution are instilled into normal rabbit eyes, less than 0.07% of the administered dose of cromolyn sodium is absorbed into the systemic circulation (presumably by way of the eye, nasal passages, buccal cavity and gastrointestinal tract). Trace amounts (less than 0.01%) of the cromolyn sodium dose penetrate into the aqueous humor and clearance from this chamber is virtually complete within 24 hours after treatment is stopped.
In normal volunteers, analysis of drug excretion indicates that approximately 0.03% of cromolyn sodium is absorbed following administration to the eye.
A study on corneal epithelial wound healing in albino rabbits failed to demonstrate any significant difference in the rate of corneal re-epithelialization between cromolyn sodium ophthalmic solution, sterile saline solution, no treatment and an ophthalmic corticosteroid.
Indications and Usage: OPTICROM is indicated in the treatment of vernal keratoconjunctivitis, vernal conjunctivitis, giant papillary conjunctivitis, and vernal keratitis.
Symptomatic response to therapy (decreased itching, tearing, redness and discharge) is usually evident within a few days, but longer treatment for up to six weeks is sometimes required.
Once symptomatic improvement has been established, therapy should be continued for as long as needed to sustain improvement.
If required, corticosteroids may be used concomitantly with OPTICROM.
Users of soft (hydrophilic) contact lenses should refrain from wearing lenses while under treatment with OPTICROM (see **Contraindications**). Wear can be resumed within a few hours after discontinuation of the drug.
Contraindications: OPTICROM is contraindicated in those patients who have shown hypersensitivity to cromolyn sodium or to any of the other ingredients.
As with all ophthalmic preparations containing benzalkonium chloride, patients are advised not to wear soft contact lenses during treatment with OPTICROM.
Precautions: General: Patients may experience a transient stinging or burning sensation following application of OPTICROM.
The recommended frequency of administration should not be exceeded. The dose for adults and children is 1–2 drops in each eye 4–6 times a day at regular intervals.
Carcinogenesis, Mutagenesis, and Impairment of Fertility: Long term studies in mice (12 months intraperitoneal treatment followed by six months observation), hamsters (12 months intraperitoneal treatment followed by 12 months observation), and rats (18 months subcutaneous treatment) showed no neoplastic effect of cromolyn sodium.
No evidence of chromosomal damage or cytotoxicity was obtained in various mutagenesis studies.
No evidence of impaired fertility was shown in laboratory animal reproduction studies.
Pregnancy: Pregnancy Category B. Reproduction studies with cromolyn sodium administered parenterally to pregnant mice, rats and rabbits in doses up to 338 times the human clinical doses produced no evidence of fetal malformations. Adverse fetal effects (increased resorption and decreased fetal weight) were noted only at the very high parenteral doses that produced maternal toxicity. There are, however, no adequate and well controlled studies in pregnant women. Because animal reproduction studies are not always predictive of human response, this drug should be used during pregnancy only if clearly needed.
Nursing Mothers: It is not known whether this drug is excreted in human milk. Because many drugs are excreted in human milk, caution should be exercised when OPTICROM is administered to a nursing woman.
Pediatric Use: Safety and effectiveness in children below the age of 4 years have not been established.
Adverse Reactions: The most frequently reported adverse reaction attributed to the use of OPTICROM, on the basis of reoccurrence following readministration, is transient ocular stinging or burning upon instillation.
The following adverse reactions have been reported as infrequent events. It is unclear whether they are attributable to the drug:
Conjunctival injection
Watery eyes
Itchy eyes
Dryness around the eye
Puffy eyes
Eye irritation
Styes
Dosage and Administration: The dose for adults and children is 1–2 drops in each eye 4–6 times a day at regular intervals. One drop contains approximately 1.6 mg cromolyn sodium. Patients should be advised that the effect of OPTICROM therapy is dependent upon its administration at regular intervals, as directed.
How Supplied: OPTICROM is supplied as 10 mL of solution in an opaque polyethylene eye drop bottle.
NDC 0585-0680-01 10 mL bottle
Keep tightly closed and out of the reach of children. Store below 30°C (86°F) and protect from light. Store in original carton.
Caution: Federal law prohibits dispensing without prescription.
OPTICROM and FISONS are Registered Trade Marks of FISONS plc.
Made in England Revised 2/90

Information on Fisons' products appearing in these pages is current as of 2/90. Please consult the package insert currently accompanying the product, or Fisons Pharmaceuticals, P.O. Box 1710, Rochester, NY 14603, (716) 475 9000.

RF 046A
Shown in Product Identification Section, page 103

Health Maintenance Programs, Inc.
7 WESTCHESTER PLAZA
ELMSFORD, NY 10523

OPHTHALMIC NUTRIENTS™ OTC
Contains a Range of Antioxidant Vitamins, Minerals, Calcium/Vitamin D_3 and Glutathione Nutritional Supplements.

Each Ophthalmic Nutrients™ Blister Contains Nutritional Antioxidant Supplements:

Antioxidants/Vitamins	Quantity	RDA
2 Yellow Capsules:		
Ascorbic Acid/C	1000 MG	1667%
Glutathione	100 MG	—
Niacinamide/B-3	20 MG	100%
Riboflavin/B-2	20 MG	1176%
Calcium Pantothenate/B-5	10 MG	100%
Pyridoxine HCl/B-6	2 MG	100%
Thiamine HCl/B-1	1.5 MG	100%
Cholecalciferol/D_3	125 IU	31%
Cyanocobalamin/B-12	100 MCG	1667%
Calcium (as the carbonate)	250 MG	25%
Zinc (as the oxide)	30 MG	200%
Manganese (as the sulfate)	5 MG	125%
Copper (as the oxide)	1 MG	50%
Selenium (as sodium selenate)	25 MCG	45%
1 Red Capsule		
Beta Carotene	15 MG	—
dl-Alpha Tocopheryl Acetate/E	100 IU	333%

Adult Food Supplement: Take one packet after meals or snacks twice a day or as directed by your physician, with a glass of water.
60 packets/180 capsules

Refer to contents page for information on Contact Lenses.

IOLAB Corporation Pharmaceutical Division

a Johnson & Johnson Company
500 IOLAB DRIVE
CLAREMONT, CA 91711

ARGYROL® S.S. 10% OTC
(mild silver protein)
Sterile Ophthalmic Solution
How Supplied: 0.5 and 1 fl. oz.

ATROPISOL® (atropine sulfate) 1% ℞
Sterile Ophthalmic Solution
How Supplied: 5mL, 15mL and 12×1mL DROPPERETTE®

CATARASE® 1:5000 (chymotrypsin) ℞
Sterile Ophthalmic Solution
How Supplied: 2mL univial

IOCARE® Balanced Salt Solution ℞
Sterile Ophthalmic Solution
How Supplied: 36×15mL and 6×500mL

DACRIOSE® OTC
Sterile Ophthalmic Irrigating Solution
How Supplied: 0.5, 1 and 4 fl. oz.

DEXACIDIN® ℞
(Dexamethasone, Neomycin and Polymyxin B Sulfates)
Sterile Ophthalmic Suspension
How Supplied: 5mL

DEXACIDIN® (Dexamethasone, Neomycin and Polymyxin B Sulfates) Ophthalmic Ointment ℞
Preservative Free and Lanolin Free
How Supplied: 3.5gm

DROPPERETTES® Applicator—
Sterile Package

ARGYROL® S.S. 20% (mild silver protein) ℞
Sterile Ophthalmic Solution
How Supplied: 12×1mL DROPPERETTE®

ATROPISOL® ½% (atropine sulfate) ℞
Sterile Ophthalmic Solution
How Supplied: 12×1mL DROPPERETTE®

ATROPISOL® 1% (atropine sulfate) ℞
Sterile Ophthalmic Solution
How Supplied: 12×1mL DROPPERETTE®

ATROPISOL® 2% (atropine sulfate) ℞
Sterile Ophthalmic Solution
How Supplied: 12×1mL DROPPERETTE®

Epinephrine 1:1000 (Rfg.) ℞
Sterile Ophthalmic Solution
How Supplied: 12×1mL DROPPERETTE®

Fluorescein Sodium 2% ℞
Sterile Ophthalmic Solution
How Supplied: 12×1mL DROPPERETTE®

Homatropine HBr 2% ℞
Sterile Ophthalmic Solution
How Supplied: 12×1mL DROPPERETTE®

Homatropine HBr 5% ℞
Sterile Ophthalmic Solution
How Supplied: 12×1mL DROPPERETTE®

Phenylephrine HCl 10% (Rfg.) ℞
Sterile Ophthalmic Solution
How Supplied: 12×1mL DROPPERETTE®

PILOCAR® 1% (pilocarpine HCl) ℞
Sterile Ophthalmic Solution
How Supplied: 12×1mL DROPPERETTE®

PILOCAR® 2% (pilocarpine HCl) ℞
Sterile Ophthalmic Solution
How Supplied: 12×1mL DROPPERETTE®

PILOCAR® 4% (pilocarpine HCl) ℞
Sterile Ophthalmic Solution
How Supplied: 12×1mL DROPPERETTE®

SULF-10® (sulfacetamide sodium 10%) ℞
Sterile Ophthalmic Solution
How Supplied: 12×1mL DROPPERETTE®

Tetracaine HCl ½% ℞
Sterile Ophthalmic Solution
How Supplied: 12×1mL DROPPERETTE®

E-PILO-1® ℞
(epinephrine bitartrate—pilocarpine HCl)
Sterile Ophthalmic Solution
How Supplied: 10mL

E-PILO-2® ℞
(epinephrine bitartrate—pilocarpine HCl)
Sterile Ophthalmic Solution
How Supplied: 10mL

E-PILO-3® ℞
(epinephrine bitartrate—pilocarpine HCl)
Sterile Ophthalmic Solution
How Supplied: 10mL

E-PILO-4® ℞
(epinephrine bitartrate—pilocarpine HCl)
Sterile Ophthalmic Solution
How Supplied: 10mL

E-PILO-6® ℞
(epinephrine bitartrate—pilocarpine HCl)
Sterile Ophthalmic Solution
How Supplied: 10mL

Eserine Sulfate 0.25% ℞
Sterile Ophthalmic Ointment
How Supplied: 3.5gm

FLUOR-OP® (fluorometholone 0.1%) ℞
Sterile Ophthalmic Suspension
How Supplied: 5, 10 and 15mL

FUNDUSCEIN®-10 Injection 10% ℞
(fluorescein sodium)
How Supplied: 12×5mL amps

FUNDUSCEIN®-25 Injection 25% ℞
(fluorescein sodium)
How Supplied: 12×3mL amps

GENTACIDIN® (gentamicin sulfate) ℞
Sterile Ophthalmic Solution
How Supplied: 5mL

GENTACIDIN® (gentamicin sulfate) ℞
Ophthalmic Ointment
Preservative Free and Lanolin Free
How Supplied: 3.5gm

GLUCOSE-40® (liquid glucose) ℞
Sterile Ophthalmic Ointment
How Supplied: 3.5gm

GONIOSOL® OTC
(hydroxypropyl methylcellulose 2.5%)
Sterile Ophthalmic Solution
How Supplied: 15mL

Homatropine Hydrobromide 2% ℞
Sterile Ophthalmic Solution
How Supplied: 5mL

Homatropine Hydrobromide 5% ℞
Sterile Ophthalmic Solution
How Supplied: 5mL

HYPOTEARS® Lubricating Eye Drops OTC
Sterile Ocular Lubricant
How Supplied: 0.5 and 1 fl. oz.

HYPOTEARS® PF Preservative Free Lubricating Eye Drops
Sterile Ocular Lubricant
How Supplied: 30 single-use vials per carton

HYPOTEARS® Ophthalmic Ointment OTC
Preservative Free and Lanolin Free
How Supplied: 3.5gm

INFLAMASE® MILD ⅛% ℞
(prednisolone sodium phosphate)
Sterile Ophthalmic Solution
How Supplied: 5 and 10mL

INFLAMASE® FORTE 1% ℞
(prednisolone sodium phosphate)
Sterile Ophthalmic Solution
How Supplied: 5, 10 and 15mL

MIOCHOL® (acetylcholine chloride) ℞
Intraocular with IOCARE®
Steri-Tags™
How Supplied: 2mL univial,

IOCARE® Steri-Tags™

MIOCHOL® System Pak™ ℞
Miochol Intraocular (acetylcholine chloride) 2mL univial
IOCARE® Steri-Tags™, 3mL B-D® Syringe
0.2 Micron DynaGard™ Filter

MIOCHOL® System Pak™ Plus ℞
IOCARE® Balanced Salt Solution
Miochol Intraocular (acetylcholine chloride) 2mL univial
IOCARE® Steri-Tags™, 3mL B-D® Syringe
0.2 Micron Dynagard™ Filter
2×15mL IOCARE® Balanced Salt Solution

PILOCAR® (pilocarpine HCl) ℞
Sterile Ophthalmic Solution ½%
How Supplied: 15mL, Twin Pack (2×15mL)

PILOCAR® (pilocarpine HCl) ℞
Sterile Ophthalmic Solution 1%
How Supplied: 15mL, Twin Pack (2×15mL), DROPPERETTE® (12×1mL)

PILOCAR® (pilocarpine HCl) ℞
Sterile Ophthalmic Solution 2%
How Supplied: 15mL, Twin Pack (2×15mL), DROPPERETTE® (12×1mL)

PILOCAR® (pilocarpine HCl) ℞
Sterile Ophthalmic Solution 3%
How Supplied: 15mL, Twin Pack (2×15mL)

PILOCAR® (pilocarpine HCl) ℞
Sterile Ophthalmic Solution 4%
How Supplied: 15mL, Twin Pack (2×15mL), DROPPERETTE® (12×1mL)

PILOCAR® (pilocarpine HCl) ℞
Sterile Ophthalmic Solution 6%
How Supplied: 15mL, Twin Pack (2×15mL)

SULF-10® (sodium sulfacetamide) ℞
Sterile Ophthalmic Solution 10%
How Supplied: 15mL, DROPPERETTE® (12×1mL)

TEARISOL® OTC
Sterile Ocular Eye Lubricant
How Supplied: 0.5 fl. oz.

VASOCIDIN® ℞
(sulfacetamide sodium-prednisolone sodium phosphate)
Sterile Ophthalmic Solution
How Supplied: 5 and 10mL

VASOCIDIN® ℞
(sulfacetamide sodium-prednisolone acetate)
Sterile Ophthalmic Ointment
Preservative Free and Lanolin Free
How Supplied: 3.5gm

VASOCLEAR® (0.02% naphazoline HCl) OTC
Sterile Ophthalmic Solution
How Supplied: 15mL

VASOCLEAR® A (0.02% naphazoline HCl and 0.25% zinc sulfate) OTC
Sterile Ophthalmic Solution
How Supplied: 15mL

Vasocon-A ℞
(naphazoline HCl 0.05%-antazoline phosphate 0.5%)
Sterile Ophthalmic Solution
How Supplied: 15mL

Vasocon-Regular ℞
(naphazoline HCl 0.1%)
Sterile Ophthalmic Solution
How Supplied: 15mL

VASOSULF® ℞
(sulfacetamide sodium-phenylephrine hydrochloride)
Sterile Ophthalmic Solution
How Supplied: 5 and 15mL

Continued on next page

IOLAB Pharm—Cont.

IOCARE LINE

DEXAMETHASONE SODIUM PHOSPHATE INJECTION, USP ℞
For Intravenous, Intramuscular, Intra-articular, Intralesional and Soft Tissue Injection
How Supplied: 5ml vial, 4mg/ml for injection

DEXAMETHASONE SODIUM PHOSPHATE STERILE OPHTHALMIC ℞
SOLUTION, USP 0.1%
Dexamethasone Phosphate Equivalent
How Supplied: 5ml Dropper

GENTAMICIN SULFATE INJECTION, USP
40mg per ml ℞
Each ml contains Gentamicin Sulfate, USP equivalent to 40mg Gentamicin. For Parenteral Administration
How Supplied: 2ml vial (80mg)/40mg per ml

NEOMYCIN AND POLYMYXIN B SULFATES AND GRAMICIDIN ℞
OPHTHALMIC SOLUTION
How Supplied: 10ml Dropper

NEOMYCIN AND POLYMYXIN B SULFATES AND HYDROCORTISONE ℞
OPHTHALMIC SUSPENSION
How Supplied: 7.5ml Dropper

NEOMYCIN SULFATE-DEXAMETHASONE SODIUM ℞
PHOSPHATE STERILE OPHTHALMIC SOLUTION, USP
How Supplied: 5ml Dropper

PHENYLEPHRINE HYDROCHLORIDE STERILE OPHTHALMIC ℞
SOLUTION, USP 2.5%
How Supplied: 15ml Dropper

DEXACIDIN® ℞

[deks 'a-si-din]
(Neomycin and Polymyxin B Sulfates and Dexamethasone)
Ophthalmic Suspension
Ophthalmic Ointment

Description: DEXACIDIN Ophthalmic Suspension is a multidose, anti-infective steroid combination in a sterile topical ophthalmic suspension having the following composition:
Dexamethasone.................................. 1 mg/mL
Neomycin... 3.5 mg/mL
(represented by neomycin sulfate)
Polymyxin B Sulfate............. 10,000 units/mL
in a solution containing hydroxypropyl methycellulose, sodium chloride, polysorbate 20 and purified water; preserved with benzalkonium chloride. Hydrochloric acid is added to adjust pH.
DEXACIDIN Ophthalmic Ointment is a multidose, anti-infective steroid combination in a sterile topical ophthalmic ointment having the following composition:
Dexamethasone..1 mg/g
Neomycin...3.5 mg/g
(represented by neomycin sulfate)
Polymyxin B Sulfate ....10,000 units/g
in a bland base containing white petrolatum and mineral oil.
The chemical name for dexamethasone is: Pregna-1,4-diene-3,20-dione,9-fluoro-11,17,21-trihydroxy-16-methy l-,(11β, 16α)-, which has the following chemical structure:

Clinical Pharmacology: Corticoids suppress the inflammatory response to a variety of agents and they probably delay or slow healing. Since corticoids may inhibit the body's defense mechanism against infection, a concomitant antimicrobial drug may be used when this inhibition is considered to be clinically significant in a particular case.
When a decision to administer both a corticoid and an antimicrobial is made, the administration of such drugs in combination has the advantage of greater patient compliance and convenience, with the added assurance that the appropriate dosage of both drugs is administered, plus assured compatibility of ingredients when both types of drugs are in the same formulation and, particularly, that the correct volume of drug is delivered and retained.
The relative potency of corticosteroids depends on the molecular structure, concentration and release from the vehicle.
Indications and Usage: For steroid-responsive inflammatory ocular conditions for which a corticosteroid is indicated and where bacterial infection or a risk of bacterial ocular infection exists.
Ocular steroids are indicated in inflammatory conditions of the palpebral and bulbar conjunctiva, cornea, and anterior segment of the globe where the inherent risk of steroid use in certain infective conjunctivitides is accepted to obtain a diminution in edema and inflammation. They are also indicated in chronic anterior uveitis and corneal injury from chemical, radiation, thermal burns, or penetration of foreign bodies.
The use of a combination drug with an anti-infective component is indicated where the risk of infection is high or where there is an expectation that potentially dangerous numbers of bacteria will be present in the eye.
The particular anti-infective drugs in this product are active against the following common bacterial eye pathogens: **Staphylococcus aureus, Escherichia coli, Haemophilus influenzae, Klebsiella/Enterobacter** species, **Neisseria** species, and **Pseudomonas aeruginosa.**
This product does not provide adequate coverage against: **Serratia marcescens** and Streptococci, including **Streptococcus pneumoniae.**
Contraindications: Epithelial herpes simplex keratitis (dendritic keratitis), vaccinia, varicella, and many other viral diseases of the cornea and conjunctiva. Mycobacterial infection of the eye. Fungal diseases of ocular structures. Hypersensitivity to a component of the medication. (Hypersensitivity to the antibiotic component occurs at a higher rate than for other components.)
The use of these combinations is always contraindicated after uncomplicated removal of a corneal foreign body.
Warnings: Prolonged use may result in glaucoma, with damage to the optic nerve, defects in visual acuity and fields of vision, and posterior subcapsular cataract formation. Prolonged use may suppress the host response and thus increase the hazard of secondary ocular infections. In those diseases causing thinning of the cornea or sclera, perforations have been known to occur with the use of topical steroids. In acute purulent conditions of the eye, steroids may mask infection or enhance existing infection. If these products are used for 10 days or longer, intraocular pressure should be routinely monitored even though it may be difficult in children and uncooperative patients.
Products containing neomycin sulfate may cause cutaneous sensitization.
Employment of steroid medication in the treatment of herpes simplex requires great caution.
Precautions: The initial prescription and renewal of the medication order beyond 20 mL of the suspension or 8 g of the ointment, should be made by a physician only after examination of the patient with the aid of magnification, such as slit lamp biomicroscopy and, where appropriate, fluorescein staining.
The possibility of persistent fungal infections of the cornea should be considered after prolonged steroid dosing.
Adverse Reactions: Adverse reactions have occurred with steroid/anti-infective combination drugs which can be attributed to the steroid component, the anti-infective component, or the combination. Exact incidence figures are not available since no denominator of treated patients is available.
Reactions occurring most often from the presence of the anti-infective ingredient are allergic sensitizations. The reactions due to the steroid component in decreasing order of frequency are: elevation of intraocular pressure (IOP) with possible development of glaucoma, and infrequent optic nerve damage; posterior subcapsular cataract formation; and delayed wound healing.
Secondary Infection: The development of secondary infection has occurred after use of combinations containing steroids and antimicrobials. Fungal infections of the cornea are particularly prone to develop coincidentally with long term applications of steroid. The possibility of fungal invasion must be considered in any persistent corneal ulceration where steroid treatment has been used.
Secondary bacterial ocular infection following suppression of host responses also occurs.
Dosage and Administration:
(SHAKE WELL BEFORE USING)
DEXACIDIN Ophthalmic Suspension: One to two drops topically in the conjunctival sac(s). In severe disease, drops may be used hourly being tapered to discontinuation as the inflammation subsides. In mild disease, drops may be used up to four to six times daily.
Not more than 20 mL should be prescribed initially and the prescription should not be refilled without further evaluation as outlined in PRECAUTIONS above.
DEXACIDIN Ophthalmic Ointment: Apply a small amount into the conjunctival sac(s) up to three or four times daily or apply at bedtime adjunctively with drops.
Not more than 8 g should be prescribed initially and the prescription should not be refilled without further evaluation as outlined in PRECAUTIONS above.
How Supplied: DEXACIDIN Ophthalmic Suspension: 3 mL dropper-tip plastic squeeze bottles. NDC 0058-2250-03 and 5 mL dropper tip plastic squeeze bottles. NDC 0058-2250-05
DEXACIDIN Ophthalmic Ointment: 3.5 g (1/8 oz.) tube. NDC 0058-2255-01.
KEEP CONTAINER TIGHTLY CLOSED.
Store at 15° to 30°C (59°–86°F). Keep from freezing.
Caution: Federal law prohibits dispensing without prescription.
DEXACIDIN Ophthalmic Ointment
Mfg. by:
Altana Inc.
Melville, NY 11747

FLUOR-OP® ℞

(Fluorometholone) Ophthalmic Suspension USP 0.1%

Description: FLUOR-OP (fluorometholone) ophthalmic suspension is a sterile suspension for topical ophthalmic administration having the following composition:
Fluorometholone ....1 mg/mL
with: polyvinyl alcohol 1.4%; benzalkonium chloride 0.004%; edetate disodium; sodium chloride; sodium phosphate monobasic, monohydrate; sodium phosphate dibasic, anhydrous, polysorbate 80; purified water; and sodium hydroxide to adjust the pH.
The chemical name for fluorometholone is 9-fluoro-11β,17-dihydroxy-6α-methylpregna

,4-diene-3, 20-dione. It has the following hemical structure:

Fluorometholone

'LUOROMETHOLONE is an odorless, white o slightly yellow-white powder with a melting oint in the range of 280°C, with some decomosition, an empirical formula of $C_{22}H_{29}FO_4$ nd a molecular weight of 376.47. It has a char-cteristic ultraviolet absorption maximum in nethanol at 239 millimicrons.

Clinical Pharmacology: Inhibition of the nflammatory response to inciting agents of nechanical, chemical or immunological na-ure. No generally accepted explanation of this teroid property has been advanced. Adreno-orticosteroids and their derivatives are capa-le of producing a rise in intraocular pressure. n clinical studies on patients' eyes treated vith both dexamethasone and fluorometho-one, fluorometholone demonstrated a lower ropensity to increase intraocular pressure han did dexamethasone.

ndications and Usage: For steroid respon-ive inflammation of the palpebral and bulbar onjunctiva, cornea and anterior segment of he globe.

Contraindications:

Acute superficial herpes simplex keratitis.

'ungal diseases of ocular structures.

Vaccinia, varicella and most other viral dis-ases of the cornea and conjunctiva.

Tuberculosis of the eye.

Hypersensitivity to the constituents of this nedication.

Warnings: Steroid medication in the treat-nent of herpes simplex keratitis (involving the troma) requires great caution; frequent slit-amp microscopy is mandatory.

Prolonged use may result in glaucoma, damage o the optic nerve, defects in visual acuity and ields of vision, posterior subcapsular cataract ormation, or may aid in the establishment of econdary ocular infections from fungi or viruses liberated from ocular tissue.

n those diseases causing thinning of the cor-nea or sclera, perforation has been known to occur with use of topical steroids.

Acute purulent untreated infection of the eye nay be masked or activity enhanced by pres-nce of steroid medication.

Safety and effectiveness have not been demon-trated in children of the age group 2 years or elow.

Precautions: As fungal infections of the cor-nea are particularly prone to develop coinci-lentally with long-term local steroid applica-ions, fungus invasion must be suspected in any persistent corneal ulceration where a ste-oid has been used or is in use.

ntraocular pressure should be checked fre-quently.

Use in Pregnancy: Safety of the use of topical steroids during pregnancy has not been estab-ished.

Adverse Reactions: Glaucoma with optic nerve damage, visual acuity or field defects, posterior subcapsular cataract formation, sec-ondary ocular infection from pathogens liber-ated from ocular tissues, perforation of the globe.

Dosage and Administration: 1 to 2 drops nstilled into the conjunctival sac two to four times daily (SHAKE WELL BEFORE USING). During the initial 24 to 48 hours, the dosage may be safely increased to 2 drops every hour. Care should be taken not to discontinue therapy prematurely.

How Supplied: FLUOR-OP Ophthalmic Suspension:

3 mL plastic squeeze bottle with dropper tip **NDC** 0058-2358-03

5 mL plastic squeeze bottle with dropper tip **NDC** 0058-2358-05

10 mL plastic squeeze bottle with dropper tip **NDC** 0058-2358-10

15 mL plastic squeeze bottle with dropper tip **NDC** 0058-2358-15

To be dispensed only in original, unopened container.

STORE AT 15°–30°C (59°–86°F). Protect from freezing.

Caution: Federal law prohibits dispensing without prescription.

GENTACIDIN® ℞

(gentamicin sulfate)
Ophthalmic Solution, USP—Sterile
Ophthalmic Ointment, USP—Sterile

Each gram or ml contains gentamicin sulfate, USP equivalent to 3.0 mg gentamicin.

Description: Gentamicin sulfate is a water-soluble antibiotic of the aminoglycoside group active against a wide variety of pathogenic gram-negative and gram-positive bacteria.

GENTACIDIN Ophthalmic Solution is a sterile, aqueous solution buffered to approximately pH 7 for use in the eye. Each ml contains gentamicin sulfate, USP (equivalent to 3.0 mg gentamicin), dried sodium phosphate, monobasic sodium phosphate, sodium chloride, and purified water; preserved with benzalkonium chloride.

GENTACIDIN Ophthalmic Ointment is a sterile ointment, each gram containing gentamicin sulfate, USP (equivalent to 3.0 mg gentamicin) in a bland base of white petrolatum and mineral oil.

Clinical Pharmacology: The gram-positive bacteria against which gentamicin sulfate is active include coagulase-positive and coagulase-negative staphylococci, including certain strains that are resistant to penicillin: Group A beta-hemolytic and nonhemolytic streptococci; and **Diplococcus pneumoniae.** The gram-negative bacteria against which gentamicin sulfate is active include certain strains of **Pseudomonas aeruginosa,** indole-positive and indole-negative **Proteus** species, **Escherichia coli, Klebsiella pneumoniae** (Friedlander's bacillus), **Haemophilus influenza** and **Haemophilus aegyptius** (Koch-Weeks bacillus), **Aerobacter aerogenes, Moraxella lacunata** (diplobacillus of Morax-Axenfeld), and **Neisseria** species, including **Neisseria gonorrhoea.** Organisms resistant to gentamicin have been reported, including Staphylococcus epidermidis, Pseudomonas species and other organisms.

Indications and Usage: GENTACIDIN Ophthalmic Solution and Ointment are indicated in the topical treatment of infections of the external eye and its adnexa caused by susceptible bacteria. Such infections may include conjunctivitis, keratitis and keratoconjunctivitis, corneal ulcers, blepharitis and blepharoconjunctivitis, acute meibomianitis, and dacryocystitis.

Contraindications: GENTACIDIN Ophthalmic Solution and Ointment are contraindicated in patients with known hypersensitivity to any of the components.

Warnings: GENTACIDIN Ophthalmic Solution is not for injection. It should never be injected subconjunctivally, nor should it be directly introduced into the anterior chamber of the eye.

If irritation persists or increases, discontinue use and consult a physician.

Precautions: Prolonged use of topical antibiotics may give rise to overgrowth of nonsusceptible organisms, such as fungi. Should this occur, or if irritation or hypersensitivity to any component of the drug develops, discontinue use of the preparation and institute appropriate therapy.

Ophthalmic ointments may retard corneal healing.

Do not touch container tip to any surface, since this may contaminate the drug. Keep container tightly closed.

Adverse Reactions: Transient irritation has been reported with the use of gentamicin sulfate ophthalmic solutions. Occasional burning or stinging may occur with the use of GENTACIDIN Ophthalmic Ointment.

Dosage and Administration: GENTACIDIN Ophthalmic Solution: Instill one or two drops into affected eye(s) every four hours. In severe infections, dosage may be increased to as much as two drops once every hour.

GENTACIDIN Ophthalmic Ointment: Apply a small amount to the affected eye(s) two to three times a day.

How Supplied: GENTACIDIN Ophthalmic Solution: 3 ml dropper-tip plastic squeeze bottles. (NDC 0058-2365-03) 5 ml dropper-tip plastic squeeze bottles. (NDC 0058-2365-05).

GENTACIDIN Ophthalmic Ointment: 3.5 gm (1/8 oz.) sterile tube. (NDC 0058-2370-01).

To be dispensed only in original unopened container.

Store GENTACIDIN Ophthalmic Solution and Ointment between 2°–30°C (36°–86°F).

KEEP OUT OF REACH OF CHILDREN.

Caution: Federal law prohibits dispensing without prescription.

GENTACIDIN Ophthalmic Ointment
Mfg. by:
Altana Inc.
Melville, NY 11747

HYPOTEARS® OTC

LUBRICATING EYE DROPS
HYPOTEARS® PF, Preservative-Free
Lubricating Eye Drops
HYPOTEARS® OINTMENT (eye lubricant)
Preservative & Lanolin Free

Description: HYPOTEARS Lubricating Eye Drops is a sterile, soothing hypotonic solution for use as an artificial tear and lubricant.

HYPOTEARS PF is a hypotonic and preservative-free solution, specially formulated to be a soothing artificial tear and lubricant.

HYPOTEARS Ointment is a preservative and lanolin-free eye lubricant.

Indications: For use as an ocular lubricant for the temporary relief of burning and irritation due to dryness of the eye or to exposure to wind or sun. Helps protect against further eye irritation.

Warnings: If you experience eye pain, changes in vision, continued redness or irritation of the eye, or if the condition worsens or persists for more than 72 hours, discontinue use and consult a doctor. To avoid contamination, do not touch tip of container to any surface. Keep out of reach of children.

Eye Drops: Replace cap after using.

If solution of HYPOTEARS Eye Drops changes color or becomes cloudy, do not use. Do not use these products if you are allergic to any of their ingredients.

PF: Use only if single-use container is intact. Use immediately after opening container. Do not store open container.

Ointment: Store away from heat.

Directions:

Eye Drops: Adults and Children: Instill 1 or 2 drops in the affected eye(s) as needed.

Continued on next page

IOLAB Pharm—Cont.

Ointment: Pull down the lower lid of the affected eye and apply a small amount (¼ inch) of ointment to the inside of the eyelid.
PF: To open, twist the top of the container. Apply 1–2 drop(s) in affected eye(s), as needed. Discard container immediately after use.
Contains:
Eye Drops: Polyvinyl Alcohol 1% in the Lipiden™ polymeric vehicle (polyethylene glycol 400, dextrose, edetate disodium, and purified water); preserved with benzalkonium chloride.
PF: Polyvinyl alcohol 1% in the Lipiden™ polymeric vehicle (polyethylene glycol 400, dextrose, edetate disodium, and purified water).
Ointment: White petrolatum and light mineral oil.
How Supplied:
Eye Drops: 15 mL and 30 mL plastic squeeze bottle with dropper tip.
NDC 0058-0130-15
NDC 0058-0130-30
Eye Drops (PF): 30 convenient single-use containers, 0.02 fl. oz. each.
NDC 0058-0132-30
Ointment: ⅛ oz. (3.5 g) tube
NDC 0058-0131-01
Store at 15°–30°C (59°–86°F).
Ointment mfd. by:
Altana Inc.
Melville, NY 11747
PF mfd. by:
Automatic Liquid Packaging
Woodstock, IL 60098

INFLAMASE® MILD ⅛% ℞
[*in 'fla-mās*]
(prednisolone sodium phosphate)
Ophthalmic Solution

INFLAMASE® FORTE 1%
(prednisolone sodium phosphate)
Ophthalmic Solution

Description: INFLAMASE MILD and INFLAMASE FORTE (prednisolone sodium phosphate) ophthalmic solutions are sterile solutions for ophthalmic administration having the following compositions:

INFLAMASE MILD
Prednisolone Sodium Phosphate..1.25 mg/mL
(adrenocortical steroid/anti-inflammatory)
(equivalent to Prednisolone Phosphate 1.1 mg/mL)

INFLAMASE FORTE
Prednisolone Sodium Phosphate.....10 mg/mL
(adrenocortical steroid/anti-inflammatory)
(equivalent to Prednisolone Phosphate 9.1 mg/mL)

in buffered, isotonic solutions containing sodium biphosphate, sodium phosphate anhydrous, sodium chloride, edetate disodium and purified water; preserved with benzalkonium chloride, 0.1 mg/mL.
The chemical name for prednisolone sodium phosphate, $C_{21}H_{27}Na_2O_8P$, is Pregna-1,4-diene-3,20-dione,11,17-dihydroxy-21-(phosphonooxy)-,disodium salt,(11β)-, which has the following chemical structure:

Prednisolone Sodium Phosphate

Clinical Pharmacology: Prednisolone sodium phosphate causes inhibition of the inflammatory response to inciting agents of a mechanical, chemical or immunological nature. No generally accepted explanation of this steroid property has been advanced.
Indications and Usage: INFLAMASE MILD and INFLAMASE FORTE Ophthalmic Solutions are indicated for the treatment of the following conditions: steroid responsive inflammatory conditions of the palpebral and bulbar conjunctiva, cornea, and anterior segment of the globe, such as allergic conjunctivitis, acne rosacea, superficial punctate keratitis, herpes zoster keratitis, iritis, cyclitis, selected infective conjunctivitis when the inherent hazard of steroid use is accepted to obtain an advisable diminution in edema and inflammation; corneal injury from chemical, radiation, or thermal burns, or penetration of foreign bodies.
INFLAMASE FORTE Ophthalmic Solution is recommended for moderate to severe inflammations, particularly when unusually rapid control is desired. In stubborn cases of anterior segment eye disease, systemic adrenocortical hormone therapy may be required. When the deeper ocular structures are involved, systemic therapy is necessary.
Contraindications: The use of these preparations is contraindicated in the presence of acute superficial herpes simplex keratitis, fungal diseases of ocular structures, acute infectious stages of vaccinia, varicella and most other viral diseases of the cornea and conjunctiva, tuberculosis of the eye and hypersensitivity to a component of this preparation.
The use of these preparations is always contraindicated after uncomplicated removal of a superficial corneal foreign body.
Warnings: Employment of steroid medication in the treatment of herpes simplex keratitis involving the stroma requires great caution; frequent slit-lamp microscopy is mandatory.
Prolonged use may result in elevated intraocular pressure and/or glaucoma, damage to the optic nerve, defects in visual acuity and fields of vision, posterior subcapsular cataract formation, or may result in secondary ocular infections. Viral, bacterial and fungal infections of the cornea may be exacerbated by the application of steroids. In those diseases causing thinning of the cornea or sclera, perforation has been known to occur with the use of topical steroids. Acute purulent untreated infection of the eye may be masked or activity enhanced by the presence of steroid medication.
These drugs are not effective in mustard gas keratitis and Sjögren's keratoconjunctivitis. If irritation persists or develops, the patient should be advised to discontinue use and consult prescribing physician.
Precautions: As fungal infections of the cornea are particularly prone to develop coincidentally with long-term local steroid applications, fungus invasion must be suspected in any persistent corneal ulceration where a steroid has been used or is in use.
Intraocular pressure should be checked frequently.
Pregnancy: Teratogenic Effects: Pregnancy Category C: Animal reproductive studies have not been conducted with prednisolone sodium phosphate. It is also not known whether prednisolone sodium phosphate can cause fetal harm when administered to a pregnant woman or can affect reproductive capacity. Prednisolone sodium phosphate should be given to a pregnant woman only if clearly needed.
The effect of prednisolone sodium phosphate on the later growth, development and functional maturation of the child is unknown.
Nursing Mothers: It is not known whether this drug is excreted in human milk. Because many drugs are excreted in human milk, caution should be exercised when prednisolone sodium phosphate is administered to a nursing woman.
Pediatric Use: Safety and effectiveness in children have not been established.
Adverse Reactions: The following adverse reactions have been reported: glaucoma with optic nerve damage, visual acuity and field defects, posterior subcapsular cataract formation, secondary ocular infections from pathogens including herpes simplex and fungi, and perforation of the globe.
Rarely, filtering blebs have been reported when topical steroids have been used following cataract surgery.
Rarely, stinging or burning may occur.
Dosage and Administration: Depending on the severity of inflammation, instill one or two drops of solution into the conjunctival sac up to every hour during the day and every two hours during night as necessary as initial therapy.
When a favorable response is observed, reduce dosage to one drop every four hours.
Later, further reduction in dosage to one drop three to four times daily may suffice to control symptoms.
The duration of treatment will vary with the type of lesion and may extend from a few days to several weeks, according to therapeutic responses. Relapses, more common in chronic active lesions than in self-limiting conditions usually respond to retreatment.
How Supplied:
3 mL plastic squeeze bottle with dropper tip
INFLAMASE FORTE........NDC 0058-2877-0
5 mL plastic squeeze bottle with dropper tip
INFLAMASE MILD ....NDC 0058-2875-0
INFLAMASE FORTE........NDC 0058-2877-0
10 mL plastic squeeze bottle with dropper tip
INFLAMASE MILD ....NDC 0058-2875-1
INFLAMASE FORTE........NDC 0058-2877-1
15 mL plastic squeeze bottle with dropper tip
INFLAMASE FORTE........NDC 0058-2877-1
To be dispensed only in original, unopened container.
STORE AT CONTROLLED ROOM TEMPERATURE 15°–30°C (59°–86°F).
Protect from light. Keep out of reach of children.
Caution: Federal law prohibits dispensing without prescription.

MIOCHOL® ℞
(acetylcholine chloride)
1:100 INTRAOCULAR

Description: MIOCHOL (acetylcholine chloride) is a parasympathomimetic preparation for intraocular use packaged in a vial of two compartments: the lower chamber containing acetylcholine chloride 20 mg and mannitol 60 mg; the upper chamber containing sterile water for injection 2 mL.
The reconstituted liquid will be a sterile isotonic solution containing 20 mg acetylcholine chloride (1:100 solution) and 3% mannitol. Mannitol is used in the process of lyophilizing acetylcholine chloride, and is not considered an active ingredient.
The chemical name for acetylcholine chloride $C_7H_{16}ClNO_2$, is 2-acetoxyethyltrimethyl ammonium chloride and is represented by the following chemical structure:

$$CH_3\overset{O}{\overset{\|}{C}}O(CH_2)_2N^+(CH_3)_3 \quad Cl^-$$

Clinical Pharmacology: Acetylcholine is a naturally occurring neurohormone which mediates nerve impulse transmission at all cholinergic sites involving somatic and autonomic nerves. After release from the nerve ending, acetylcholine is rapidly inactivated by the enzyme acetylcholinesterase by hydrolysis to acetic acid and choline.
Direct application of acetylcholine to the iris will cause rapid miosis of short duration. Topical ocular instillation of acetylcholine to the intact eye causes no discernible response as

cholinesterase destroys the molecule more rapidly than it can penetrate the cornea.

Indications and Usage: To obtain complete miosis of the iris in seconds after delivery of the lens in cataract surgery, in penetrating keratoplasty, iridectomy and other anterior segment surgery where rapid, complete miosis may be required.

Contraindications: There are presently no known contraindications to the use of MIOCHOL (acetylcholine chloride) Intraocular.

Warnings: If blister or peelable backing is damaged or broken, sterility of the enclosed bottle cannot be assured. Open under aseptic conditions only.

WARNING: DO NOT GAS STERILIZE

Precautions: General: In the reconstitution of the solution, as described under Directions for Using Univial, if the center rubber plug seal in the univial does not go down or is down, do not use the vial.

If miosis is to be obtained quickly and completely with MIOCHOL, obstructions to miosis, such as anterior or posterior synechiae, may require surgery prior to administration of MIOCHOL. In cataract surgery, use MIOCHOL only after delivery of the lens. **Note:** Aqueous solutions of acetylcholine chloride are unstable. Prepare solution immediately before use. Do not use solution which is not clear and colorless. Discard any solution that has not been used.

Drug Interactions: Although clinical studies with acetylcholine chloride and animal studies with acetylcholine or carbachol revealed no interference, and there is no known pharmacological basis for an interaction, there have been reports that acetylcholine chloride and carbachol have been ineffective when used in patients treated with topical nonsteroidal anti-inflammatory agents.

Pediatric Use: Safety and effectiveness in children have not been established.

Adverse Reactions: Infrequent cases of corneal edema, corneal clouding, and corneal decompensation have been reported with the use of MIOCHOL.

Adverse reactions have been reported rarely which are indicative of systemic absorption. These include bradycardia, hypotension, flushing, breathing difficulties and sweating.

Overdosage: Atropine sulfate (0.5 to 1 mg) should be given intramuscularly or intravenously and should be readily available to counteract possible overdosage. Epinephrine (0.1 to 1 mg subcutaneously) is also of value in overcoming severe cardiovascular or bronchoconstrictor responses.

Dosage and Administration: With a new needle of sturdy gauge, 18–20, draw all of the solution into a dry, sterile syringe. Replace needle with a suitable atraumatic cannula for intraocular irrigation.

The MIOCHOL solution is instilled into the anterior chamber before or after securing one or more sutures. Instillation should be gentle and parallel to the iris face and tangential to pupil border.

If there are no mechanical hindrances, the pupil is rapidly constricted and the peripheral iris drawn away from the angle of the anterior chamber. Any anatomical hindrance to miosis may require surgery to permit the desired effect of the drug. In most cases, ½ to 2 mL produces satisfactory miosis. The MIOCHOL solution need not be flushed from the chamber after miosis occurs. Since the action of acetylcholine is of short duration, pilocarpine may be applied topically before dressing to maintain miosis.

In cataract surgery, use MIOCHOL only after delivery of the lens.

Note: Aqueous solutions of acetylcholine chloride are unstable. Prepare solution immediately before use. Do not use solution which is not clear and colorless. Discard any solution that has not been used.

DIRECTIONS FOR USING THE UNIVIAL: STERILE UNLESS PACKAGE OPEN OR BROKEN

1. Inspect univial while inside unopened blister. Diluent must be in upper chamber.
2. Peel open blister.
3. Aseptically transfer univial to sterile field. Maintain sterility of outer container during preparation of solution.
4. Immediately before use, give plunger-stopper a quarter turn and press to force diluent and center plug into lower chamber.
5. Shake gently to dissolve drug.
6. Discard univial and any unused solution.

How Supplied:

2 mL sterile univial **NDC** 0058-2757-45

MIOCHOL with IOCARE® Steri-Tags™: **NDC** 0058-2757-52
- One MIOCHOL 2 mL sterile univial
- One pack IOCARE Steri-Tags sterile labels

MIOCHOL System Pak™: **NDC** 0058-2763-53
- One MIOCHOL 2 mL sterile univial
- One pack IOCARE Steri-Tags sterile labels
- One B-D® 3 mL sterile syringe
- One Dynagard™ 0.2 micron sterile filter

MIOCHOL System Pak Plus IOCARE Balanced Salt Solution: **NDC** 0058-2764-54
- One MIOCHOL 2 mL sterile univial
- One pack IOCARE Steri-Tags sterile labels
- One B-D 3 mL sterile syringe
- One Dynagard 0.2 micron sterile filter
- Two 15 mL IOCARE Balanced Salt Solution

KEEP FROM FREEZING

Store at 15°–30°C (59°–86°F)

Caution: Federal law prohibits dispensing without prescription.

Shown in Product Identification Section, page 103

PILOCAR® ℞

[*pī'lō-car"*]

(pilocarpine hydrochloride)
Ophthalmic Solution

Description: PILOCAR (pilocarpine hydrochloride) ophthalmic solution is a sterile solution for ophthalmic administration having the following composition:

Plastic Squeeze Bottle

Pilocarpine Hydrochloride ....5, 10, 20, 30, 40, or 60mg/mL

(cholinergic/parasympathomimetic)

in a buffered solution of boric acid, potassium chloride, hydroxypropylmethyl cellulose, sodium carbonate, edetate disodium and purified water, preserved with benzalkonium chloride.

Dropperettes® Applicator

Pilocarpine Hydrochloride ...10, 20 or 40mg/mL

(cholinergic/parasympathomimetic)

is an isotonic, buffered solution of boric acid, potassium chloride, sodium carbonate and purified water, preserved with benzalkonium chloride.

The chemical name is 2(3H)-Furanone, 3-ethyldihydro -4- [(1-methyl -1H- imidazol-5-yl) methyl]-, monohydrochloride, (3S-cis)-.

It has the following structure:

[Structure: pilocarpine hydrochloride — CH_3CH_2, H, H, CH_2, H, N^+–CH_3, N, O, O; Cl^-]

Clinical Pharmacology: Pilocarpine is a direct acting cholinergic (parasympathomimetic) agent causing pupillary constriction and reduction of intraocular pressure.

Indications and Usage: PILOCAR ophthalmic solution is indicated for the treatment of primary open-angle glaucoma and also to lower intraocular pressure prior to surgery for acute angle-closure glaucoma. It may be used in combination with other miotics, beta adrenergic blocking agents, carbonic anhydrase inhibitors, hyperosmotic agents, or epinephrine.

Contraindications: When constriction is undesirable such as in acute iritis and in persons hypersensitive to one or more of the components of this preparation.

Precautions: The pilocarpine-induced miosis may cause difficulty in dark adaptation. The patient should exercise caution when involved in night driving or other hazardous activities in poor light.

Not for internal use. To prevent contaminating the dropper tip and solution, care should be taken not to touch the eyelids or surrounding areas with the dropper tip of the bottle.

Carcinogenesis, Mutagenesis, Impairment of Fertility: There have been no long-term studies done using pilocarpine in animals to evaluate carcinogenic potential.

Pregnancy: Pregnancy Category C. Animal reproduction studies have not been conducted with pilocarpine. It is also not known whether pilocarpine can cause fetal harm when administered to a pregnant woman or can affect reproduction capacity. Pilocarpine should be given to a pregnant woman only if clearly needed.

Nursing Mothers: It is not known whether this drug is excreted in human milk. Because many drugs are excreted in human milk, caution should be exercised when pilocarpine is administered to a nursing woman.

Adverse Reactions: Ocular: Ciliary spasm, conjunctival vascular congestion, temporal or supraorbital headache, lacrimation, and induced myopia may occur. This is especially true in younger individuals who have recently started administration. Reduced visual acuity in poor illumination is frequently experienced by older individuals and individuals with lens opacity. Miotic agents may also cause **retinal detachment**; thus, care should be exercised with all miotic therapy especially in young myopic patients. Lens opacity may occur with prolonged use of pilocarpine.

Systemic: Systemic reactions following topical administration, although extremely rare, have included hypertension, tachycardia, bronchiolar spasm, pulmonary edema, salivation, sweating, nausea, vomiting, and diarrhea.

Dosage and Administration: The initial dose is one or two drops. This may be repeated up to six times daily. The frequency of instillation and concentration of PILOCAR ophthalmic solution are determined by the severity of the glaucoma and miotic response of the patient.

During acute phases, the miotic must be instilled into the unaffected eye to prevent an attack of angle-closure glaucoma.

How Supplied: 0.5%, 1%, 2%, 3%, 4%, and 6% solution: in 15mL plastic dropper-tip squeeze bottles.

0.5%, 1%, 2%, 3%, 4%, and 6% solution: in a Twin Pack of 2 × 15mL plastic dropper-tip squeeze bottles.

1%, 2%, 4%: 1mL DROPPERETTES® Applicators package of 12.

Keep bottle tightly closed when not in use.

Caution: Federal law prohibits dispensing without prescription.

Shown in Product Identification Section, page 103

VASOCIDIN® ℞

[*vas'o-si-din*]

(sulfacetamide sodium-prednisolone acetate)
Sterile Ophthalmic Ointment

Description: VASOCIDIN is a sterile ophthalmic ointment combining an anti-infective

Continued on next page

IOLAB Pharm—Cont.

and an adrenocortical steroid having the following composition:

Sulfacetamide Sodium .... 100 mg/g (bacteriostatic antibacterial)

Prednisolone Acetate .... 5 mg/g (adrenocortical steroid/anti-inflammatory)

in a base containing white petrolatum and mineral oil.

The chemical name for sulfacetamide sodium is Acetamide, N-[(4-aminophenyl) sulfonyl]-, monosodium salt, monohydrate.

The chemical name for prednisolone acetate is 11β, 17, 21-trihydroxy-pregna-1, 4-diene-3, 20-dione, 21-acetate.

They have the following chemical structures:

Sulfacetamide Sodium

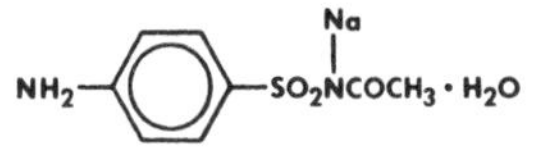

Prednisolone Acetate

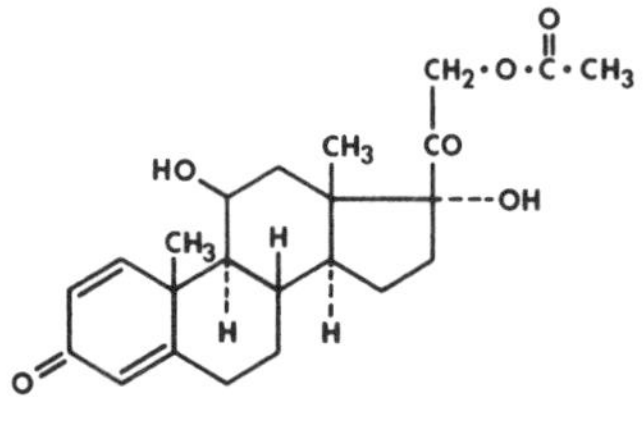

Clinical Pharmacology: Corticoids suppress the inflammatory response to a variety of agents and they probably delay or slow healing. Since corticoids may inhibit the body's defense mechanism against infection, a concomitant antimicrobial drug may be used when this inhibition is considered to be clinically significant in a particular case.

The anti-infective component in VASOCIDIN Ophthalmic Ointment is included to provide action against specific organisms susceptible to it. SEE INDICATIONS AND USAGE SECTION BELOW.

When a decision to administer both a corticoid and an antimicrobial is made, the administration of such drugs in combination has the advantage of greater patient compliance and convenience, with the added assurance that the appropriate dosage of both drugs is administered. There is assured compatibility of ingredients when both types of drugs are in the same formulation and, particularly, that the correct volume of drug is delivered and retained.

The relative potency of corticosteroids depends on the molecular structure, concentration, and release from the vehicle.

Indications and Usage: For steroid-responsive inflammatory ocular conditions for which a corticosteroid is indicated and where bacterial infection or a risk of bacterial ocular infection exists.

Ocular steroids are indicated in inflammatory conditions of the palpebral and bulbar conjunctiva, cornea, and anterior segment of the globe where the inherent risk of steroid use in certain infective conjunctivitides is accepted to obtain a diminution in edema and inflammation. They are also indicated in chronic anterior uveitis and corneal injury from chemical, radiation, or thermal burns or penetration of foreign bodies.

The use of a combination drug with an anti-infective component is indicated where the risk of infection is high or where there is an expectation that potentially dangerous numbers of bacteria will be present in that eye.

The particular anti-infective drug in this product is active against the following common bacterial eye pathogens:

Escherichia coli
Staphylococcus aureus
Streptococcus pneumonia
Streptococcus (viridans group)
Pseudomonas species
Haemophilus influenzae
Klebsiella species
Enterobacter species

This product does not provide adequate coverage against:

Neisseria species
Serratia marcescens

Contraindications: VASOCIDIN Ophthalmic Ointment is contraindicated in epithelial herpes simplex keratitis (dendritic keratitis), vaccinia, varicella and most other viral diseases of the cornea and conjunctiva. VASOCIDIN is also contraindicated in mycobacterial infection of the eye, fungal diseases of ocular structures, in individuals with known or suspected hypersensitivity to any of the ingredients of this preparation, to sulfonamides, or to corticosteroids. (Hypersensitivity to the antimicrobial components occurs at a higher rate than for other components.)

The use of this combination is always contraindicated after uncomplicated removal of a corneal foreign body.

Warnings: Prolonged use may result in glaucoma with damage to the optic nerve, defects in visual acuity and fields of vision, and in posterior subcapsular cataract formation.

Prolonged use may suppress the host response and thus increase the hazard of secondary ocular infections. In those diseases causing thinning of the cornea or sclera, perforations have been known to occur with the use of topical steroids. In acute purulent conditions of the eye, steroids may mask infection or enhance existing infection. If this product is used for 10 days or longer, intraocular pressure should be routinely monitored even though it may be difficult in children and uncooperative patients.

Employment of steroid medication in the treatment of herpes simplex requires great caution.

A significant percentage of staphylococcal isolates are completely resistant to sulfonamides.

Precautions: The initial prescription and renewal of the medication order beyond 8 gm of VASOCIDIN Ophthalmic Ointment should be made by a physician only after examination of the patient with the aid of magnification, such as slit lamp biomicroscopy and, where appropriate, fluorescein staining.

The possibility of fungal infections of the cornea should be considered after prolonged steroid dosing.

Sensitization may recur when a sulfonamide is readministered irrespective of the route of administration and cross-sensitivity among different sulfonamides may occur. (See ADVERSE REACTIONS.) Cross-allergenicity among corticosteroids has been demonstrated.

If signs of hypersensitivity or other untoward reactions occur, discontinue use of this preparation.

Ophthalmic ointments may retard corneal healing.

Adverse Reactions: Adverse reactions have occurred with steroid/anti-infective combination drugs which can be attributed to the steroid component, the anti-infective component, or the combination. Exact incidence figures are not available since no denominator of treated patients is available.

Sulfacetamide sodium may cause local irritation.

Although sensitivity reactions to sulfacetamide sodium are rare, an isolated incident of Stevens-Johnson syndrome was reported in a patient who had experienced a previous bullous drug reaction to an orally administered sulfonamide, and a single instance of local hypersensitivity was reported which progressed to a fatal syndrome resembling systemic lupus erythematosus.

Reactions occurring most from the presence of the anti-infective ingredient are allergic sensitizations. The reactions due to the steroid component in decreasing order of frequency are: elevation of intraocular pressure (IOP) with possible development of glaucoma, and infrequent optic nerve damage; posterior subcapsular cataract formation; and delayed wound healing.

Corticosteroid-containing preparations can also cause acute interior uveitis or perforation of the globe. Mydriasis, loss of accommodation and ptosis have occasionally been reported following local use of corticosteroids.

Secondary Infection: The development of secondary infection has occurred after use of combinations containing steroids and antimicrobials. Fungal infections of the cornea are particularly prone to develop coincidentally with long-term applications of steroid. The possibility of fungal invasion must be considered in any persistent corneal ulceration where steroid treatment has been used.

Secondary bacterial ocular infection following suppression of host responses also occurs.

Dosage and Administration: VASOCIDIN Ophthalmic Ointment: A small amount should be applied in the conjunctival sac three or four times daily and once or twice at night.

The initial prescription should not be more than 8 gm of the ointment and the prescription should not be refilled without further evaluation as outlined in the PRECAUTIONS SECTION.

Dosage should be adjusted according to the needs of the patient. VASOCIDIN Ophthalmic Ointment may be reduced, but care should be taken not to discontinue therapy prematurely. In chronic conditions, withdrawal of treatment should be carried out by gradually decreasing the frequency of application.

How Supplied: 3.5 gm (1/8 oz.) sterile tube: to be dispensed only in original, unopened container. Store at controlled room temperature 15°–30°C (59°–86°F).

KEEP OUT OF REACH OF CHILDREN.

Caution: Federal law prohibits dispensing without prescription.

Manufactured By:
Altana Inc.
Melville, NY 11747

VASOCIDIN® ℞

(sulfacetamide sodium-prednisolone sodium phosphate)
Ophthalmic Solution

Description: VASOCIDIN is a sterile topical ophthalmic solution combining an anti-infective and an adrenocortical steroid having the following composition:

Sulfacetamide Sodium ....100 mg/mL (bacteriostatic antibacterial)

Prednisolone Sodium Phosphate ..2.5 mg/mL (equivalent to Prednisolone Phosphate 2.3 mg/mL) (adrenocortical steroid/anti-inflammatory)

In a solution containing edetate disodium, poloxamer 407, boric acid, purified water, preserved with thimerosal 0.1 mg/mL. Hydrochloric acid and/or sodium hydroxide added to adjust pH.

The chemical name for sulfacetamide sodium is Acetamide, N-[(4-aminophenyl) sulfonyl]-, monosodium salt, monohydrate.

The chemical name for prednisolone sodium phosphate is 11β, 17, 21-trihydroxypregna-1,4-diene-3,20-dione, 21-(disodium phosphate).

They have the following chemical structures:

[See chemical formula at top of next column.]

Sulfacetamide Sodium

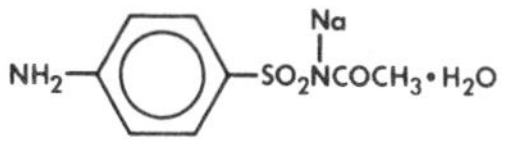

$NH_2-C_6H_4-SO_2N(Na)COCH_3 \cdot H_2O$

Prednisolone Sodium Phosphate

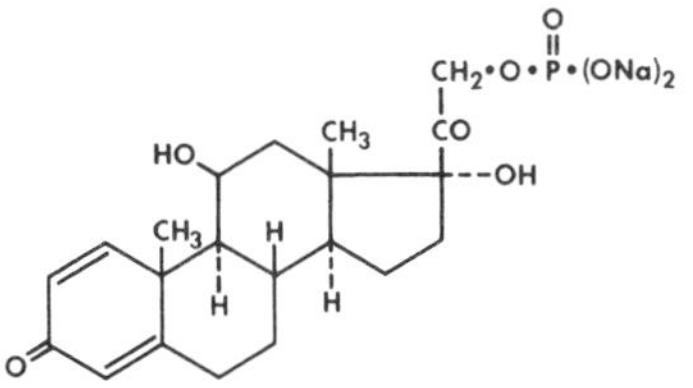

[structural formula: $CH_2 \cdot O \cdot P(O) \cdot (ONa)_2$, CO, OH, HO, CH_3, H]

Clinical Pharmacology: Corticoids suppress the inflammatory response to a variety of agents and they probably delay or slow healing. Since corticoids may inhibit the body's defense mechanism against infection, a concomitant antimicrobial drug may be used when this inhibition is considered to be clinically significant in a particular case.
The anti-infective component in VASOCIDIN Ophthalmic Solution is included to provide action against specific organisms susceptible to it. Sulfacetamide sodium is active *in-vitro* against susceptible strains of the following microorganisms: *Escherichia coli, Staphylococcus aureus, Streptococcus pneumoniae, Streptococcus (viridans group), Haemophilus influenzae, Klebsiella* species, and *Enterobacter* species. SEE INDICATIONS AND USAGE SECTION BELOW.
Sulfacetamide sodium exerts a bacteriostatic effect against susceptible bacteria by restricting the synthesis of folic acid required for growth through competition with p-aminobenzoic acid.
Some strains of bacteria may be resistant to sulfacetamide or resistant strains may emerge in vivo.
When a decision to administer both a corticoid and an antimicrobial is made, the administration of such drugs in combination has the advantage of greater patient compliance and convenience, with the added assurance that the appropriate dosage of both drugs is administered, plus assured compatibility of ingredients when both types of drugs are in the same formulation and, particularly, that the correct volume of drug is delivered and retained.
The relative potency of corticosteroids depends on the molecular structure, concentration, and release from the vehicle.
Prednisolone, applied topically to the eye, has been shown to be taken up into the anterior chamber of the eye by measurement of drug levels in rabbit eyes, and in humans, by measuring the effect on aqueous humor dynamics and intraocular pressure. Although some systemic absorption is likely, this has not been documented due to the extremely small amount of drug applied with an ophthalmic solution, and the inability at present to detect and measure extremely small concentrations of prednisolone in the blood. Although no direct studies exist demonstrating the uptake of sulfacetamide sodium into the eye, there are experiments which demonstrate significant absorption when it is applied to the skin.
Indications and Usage: VASOCIDIN is indicated for steroid-responsive inflammatory ocular conditions for which a corticosteroid is indicated and where superficial bacterial ocular infection or a risk of bacterial ocular infection exists. Ocular steroids are indicated in inflammatory conditions of the palpebral and bulbar conjunctiva, cornea, and anterior segment of the globe where the inherent risk of steroid use in certain infective conjunctivitides is accepted to obtain a diminution in edema and inflammation. They are also indicated in chronic anterior uveitis and corneal injury from chemical, radiation, or thermal burns or penetration of foreign bodies.
The use of a combination drug with an anti-infective component is indicated where the risk of superficial ocular infection is high or where there is an expectation that potentially dangerous numbers of bacteria will be present in the eye.
The particular anti-infective drug in this product is active against the following common bacterial eye pathogens:
Escherichia coli, Staphylococcus aureus, Streptococcus pneumoniae, Streptococcus (viridans group), Haemophilus influenzae, Klebsiella species, and *Enterobacter* species.
This product does not provide adequate coverage against:
Neisseria species, *Serratia marcescens*
Contraindications: VASOCIDIN Ophthalmic Solution is contraindicated in epithelial herpes simplex keratitis (dendritic keratitis), vaccinia, varicella and most other viral diseases of the cornea and conjunctiva. VASOCIDIN is also contraindicated in mycobacterial infection of the eye, fungal diseases of ocular structures, in individuals with known or suspected hypersensitivity to any of the ingredients of this preparation, to other sulfonamides, or to other corticosteroids. (Hypersensitivity to the antimicrobial components occurs at a higher rate than for other components).
The use of these combinations is always contraindicated after uncomplicated removal of a superficial corneal foreign body.
Warnings: NOT FOR INJECTION INTO THE EYE. Prolonged use may result in glaucoma with damage to the optic nerve, defects in visual acuity and fields of vision, and in posterior subcapsular cataract formation.
Acute anterior uveitis may occur in susceptible individuals, primarily Blacks.
Prolonged use may suppress the host response and thus increase the hazard of secondary ocular infections. In those diseases causing thinning of the cornea or sclera, perforations have been known to occur with the use of topical steroids. In acute purulent conditions of the eye, steroids may mask infection or enhance existing infection. If this product is used for 10 days or longer, intraocular pressure should be routinely monitored even though it may be difficult in children and uncooperative patients. Steroids should be used with caution in the presence of glaucoma. Intraocular pressure should be checked frequently.
The use of steroids after cataract surgery may delay healing and increase the incidence of filtering blebs.
Employment of steroid medication in the treatment of herpes simplex requires great caution.
A significant percentage of staphylococcal isolates are completely resistant to sulfonamides.
Topical steroids are not effective in mustard gas keratitis and Sjögren's keratoconjunctivitis.
Fatalities have occurred, although rarely, due to severe reactions to sulfonamides including Stevens-Johnson syndrome, toxic epidermal necrolysis, fulminant hepatic necrosis, agranulocytosis, aplastic anemia, and other blood dyscrasias. Sensitizations may recur when a sulfonamide is readministered irrespective of the route of administration. If signs of hypersensitivity or other serious reactions occur, discontinue use of this preparation. Cross-sensitivity among corticosteroids have been demonstrated (see ADVERSE REACTIONS).
Do not administer this product to patients who are sensitive/allergic to thimerosal or any other mercury-containing ingredient.
Precautions: The initial prescription and renewal of the medication order beyond 20 mL of VASOCIDIN Ophthalmic Solution should be made by a physician only after examination of the patient with the aid of magnification, such as slit-lamp biomicroscopy and, where appropriate, fluorescein staining. If signs and symptoms fail to improve after two weeks, the patient should return to the office for further evaluation.
The possibility of fungal infections of the cornea should be considered after prolonged steroid dosing. Fungal cultures should be taken when appropriate.
Whenever it is suspected that the infection is caused by organisms not sensitive to sulfonamides, supplemental therapy with appropriate antibiotic agents should be included.
In deep-seated infections, such as endophthalmitis, panophthalmitis, or when systemic infection is present or threatens, specific systemic (antibiotic, sulfonamide) therapy should be employed. Local treatment may be used as adjunctive therapy.
If the infection fails to respond promptly, the medication should be discontinued and other appropriate measures started.
The p-aminobenzoic acid present in purulent exudates competes with sulfonamides and can reduce their effectiveness.
Sulfonamide solutions darken on prolonged standing and exposure to heat and light. Do not use if solution has darkened. Yellowing does not affect activity.
Information to the Patient: If inflammation or pain persists longer than 48 hours or becomes aggravated, the patient should be advised to discontinue use of the medication and consult a physician.
This product is sterile when packaged. To prevent contamination, care should be taken to avoid touching dropper tip to eyelids or to any other surface. The use of this dispenser by more than one person may spread infection. Keep bottle tightly closed when not in use. Protect from light. Sulfonamide solutions darken on prolonged standing and exposure to heat and light. Do not use if solution has darkened. Yellowing does not affect activity. Keep out of the reach of children.
Laboratory Tests: Eyelid cultures and tests to determine the sensitivity of organisms to sulfacetamide may be indicated if signs and symptoms persist or recur in spite of the recommended course of treatment with VASOCIDIN Ophthalmic Solution.
Drug Interactions: VASOCIDIN Ophthalmic Solution is incompatible with silver preparations. Local anesthetics related to p-aminobenzoic acid may antagonize the action of the sulfonamides.
Carcinogenesis, Mutagenesis, and Impairment of Fertility: Long-term animal studies for carcinogenic potential have not been performed with prednisolone or sulfacetamide. One author detected chromosomal nondisjunction in the yeast *Saccharomyces cerevisiae* following application of sulfacetamide sodium. The significance of this finding to the topical ophthalmic use of sulfacetamide sodium in the human is unknown. Mutagenic studies with prednisolone have been negative. Studies on reproduction and fertility have not been performed with sulfacetamide. A long-term chronic toxicity study in dogs showed that high oral doses of prednisolone prevented estrus. A decrease in fertility was seen in male and female rats that were mated following oral dosing with another glucocorticoid.
Pregnancy Category C: Prednisolone has been shown to be teratogenic in rabbits, hamsters, and mice. In mice, a dosage administered in multiples ranging from 2.5 to 25 times the common therapeutic dose to both eyes caused a significant, dose-related increase in the incidence of cleft palate in the fetuses. There are no adequate and well-controlled studies in pregnant women dosed with corticosteroids. Animal reproduction studies have not been conducted with sulfacetamide sodium. It is not

Continued on next page

IOLAB Pharm—Cont.

known whether sulfacetamide sodium can cause fetal harm when administered to a pregnant woman or whether it can affect reproductive capacity.
VASOCIDIN Ophthalmic Solution should be used during pregnancy only if the potential benefit justifies the potential risk to the fetus.
Nursing Mothers: It is not known whether sulfacetamide is absorbed systemically from ophthalmic administration, but since prednisolone is absorbed systemically and since it is detectable in very small amounts in human milk, nursing should be temporarily discontinued while VASOCIDIN is being used.
Pediatric Use: Safety and effectiveness in children below the age of six years have not been established.
Adverse Reactions: Adverse reactions have occurred with steroid/anti-infective combination drugs which can be attributed to the steroid component, the anti-infective component, or the combination. Exact incidence figures are not available since no denominator of treated patients is available.
Reactions occurring most often from the presence of the anti-infective ingredient are allergic sensitizations. Fatalities have occurred, although rarely, due to severe reactions to sulfonamides including Stevens-Johnson syndrome, toxic epidermal necrolysis, fulminant hepatic necrosis, agranulocytosis, aplastic anemia, and other blood dyscrasias (see WARNINGS).
Sulfacetamide sodium may cause local irritation.
The reactions due to the steroid component in decreasing order of frequency are: elevation of intraocular pressure (IOP) with possible development of glaucoma, and infrequent optic nerve damage; posterior subcapsular cataract formation; and delayed wound healing.
Although systemic effects are extremely uncommon, there have been rare occurrences of systemic hypercorticoidism after use of topical steroids.
Corticosteroid-containing preparations can also cause acute anterior uveitis or perforation of the globe. Mydriasis, loss of accommodation and ptosis have occasionally been reported following local use of corticosteroids.
Secondary Infection: The development of secondary infection has occurred after use of combinations containing steroids and antimicrobials. Fungal and viral infections of the cornea are particularly prone to develop coincidentally with long-term applications of steroid. The possibility of fungal invasion must be considered in any persistent corneal ulceration where steroid treatment has been used.
Secondary bacterial ocular infection following suppression of host responses also occurs.
Overdosage: Acute overdosing with VASOCIDIN Ophthalmic Solution is not expected to lead to life-threatening situations. Large single oral doses of prednisone (> 5g/kg) in rats did not cause death (prednisone is rapidly converted to prednisolone after oral dosing and prednisolone and prednisone have equivalent glucocorticoid potency.) The oral LD_{50} of sulfacetamide in mice is 16.5 g/kg.
Dosage and Administration: Instill two drops of VASODICIN Ophthalmic Solution topically in the eye(s) every four hours.
Not more than 20 mL should be prescribed initially. If signs and symptoms fail to improve after two weeks, patients should be re-evaluated (see PRECAUTIONS).
Care should be taken not to discontinue therapy prematurely. In chronic conditions, withdrawal of treatment should be carried out by gradually decreasing the frequency of application.
How Supplied: 5 mL and 10 mL dropper-tip plastic squeeze bottles; to be dispensed only in original, unopened container. Store at controlled room temperature, 15° to 30°C (59° to 86°F). Keep from freezing. PROTECT FROM LIGHT.
Sulfonamide solutions darken on prolonged standing and exposure to heat and light. Do not use if solution has darkened. Yellowing does not affect activity.
KEEP OUT OF REACH OF CHILDREN.
Caution: Federal law prohibits dispensing without prescription.

VASOCON-A® ℞
[*vas″o-kon*]
(naphazoline hydrochloride-antazoline phosphate)
Ophthalmic Solution

Description: VASOCON-A (naphazoline hydrochloride-antazoline phosphate) is a combination of an antihistamine and a vasoconstrictor prepared as a sterile solution for ophthalmic administration having the following composition:
Naphazoline Hydrochloride ..... 0.5 mg/mL
Antazoline Phosphate .... 5 mg/mL
in a solution containing polyethylene glycol 8000, sodium chloride, polyvinyl alcohol, edetate disodium and purified water, preserved with benzalkonium chloride (0.1 mg/mL). Sodium hydroxide and/or hydrochloric acid added to adjust pH when necessary. It has a pH of 5.5-6.3 and a tonicity of 280-350 mOsm/kg.
The chemical name for naphazoline hydrochloride is 1 H-imidazole,4,5-dihydro-2-(1-naphthalenyl-methyl)-,monohydrochloride.
The chemical name for antazoline phosphate is 1 H-imidazole-2-methanamine,4,5-dihydro-N-phenyl-N-(phenylmethyl)-,phosphate (1:1).
The active ingredients have the following chemical structures:

Naphazoline Hydrochloride

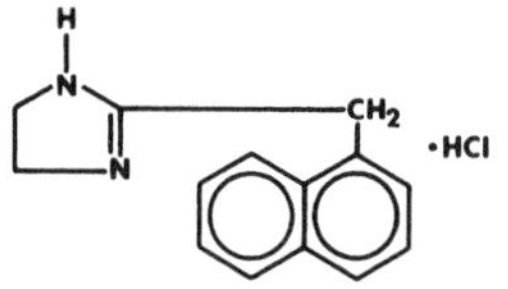

H, N, N, CH_2, •HCl

Antazoline Phosphate

H, N, N, CH_2NCH_2, • H_3PO_4

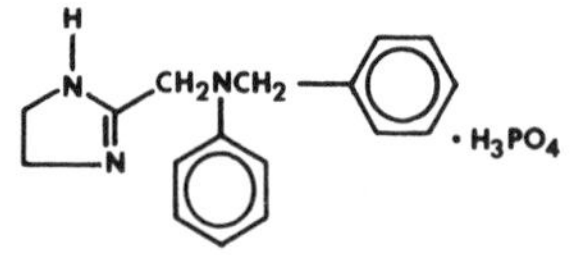

Clinical Pharmacology: VASOCON-A combines the effects of the antihistamine, antazoline, and the vasoconstrictor, naphazoline. Naphazoline hydrochloride is an alpha-sympathetic receptor agonist (sympathomimetic) producing vasoconstriction. Antazoline phosphate is an H_1-receptor antagonist producing antihistaminic effects.
Indications and Usage:
VASOCON-A Ophthalmic Solution is indicated for relief of signs and symptoms of allergic conjunctivitis.
Contraindications: Contraindicated in the presence of an anatomically narrow angle or in narrow angle glaucoma or in persons hypersensitive to one or more of the components of this preparation. VASOCON-A is contraindicated while soft contact lenses are being worn.
Warnings: Patients under therapy with monoamine oxidase (MAO) inhibitors may experience a severe hypertensive crisis if given a sympathomimetic drug. (See PRECAUTIONS)
Use of drugs in this pharmacologic class may cause CNS depression leading to unconsciousness and/or coma. Marked reduction in body temperature may occur in children, especially infants. Patients are advised not to wear contact lenses during treatment with VASOCON A.
Precautions:
General: Use with caution in the presence of hypertension, cardiovascular abnormalities, hyperglycemia (diabetes), hyperthyroidism, ocular infection or injury and when other medications are being used.
Information to the patient: For topical use only. To prevent contaminating the dropper tip and solution, care should be taken not to touch the eyelids or surrounding areas with the dropper tip of the bottle. Keep bottle tightly closed when not in use. Protect from light. Do not use if the solution has darkened. Patients should be advised to discontinue the drug and consult a physician if relief is not obtained within 48 hours of therapy; if irritation, blurring or redness persists or increases; or if symptoms of systemic absorption occur, i.e., dizziness, headache, nausea, decrease in body temperature or drowsiness.
Overuse of this product may produce increased redness/irritation of the eyes.
Drug Interactions: Concurrent use of maprotiline or tricyclic antidepressants and naphazoline may potentiate the pressor effect of naphazoline. Patients under therapy with MAO inhibitors may experience a severe hypertensive crisis if given a sympathomimetic drug. (See WARNINGS)
Carcinogenesis, Mutagenesis, Impairment of Fertility: There have been no long-term studies done using naphazoline and/or antazoline in animals to evaluate carcinogenic or mutagenic potential.
Pregnancy: Pregnancy Category C. Animal reproduction studies have not been conducted with naphazoline and/or antazoline. It is also not known whether naphazoline and/or antazoline can cause fetal harm when administered to a pregnant woman or can affect reproduction capacity. VASOCON-A Ophthalmic Solution should be given to a pregnant woman only if clearly needed. There are no available data on the effect of the drug on later growth, development, and functional maturation of the child.
Nursing Mothers: It is not known whether naphazoline and/or antazoline are excreted in human milk. Because many drugs are excreted in human milk, caution should be exercised when these drugs are administered to a nursing woman.
Pediatric Use: Safety and effectiveness in children have not been established. (See WARNINGS)
Adverse Reactions:
Ocular: The most frequent complaint with the use of VASOCON-A Ophthalmic Solution is that of mild transient stinging/burning. Other adverse experiences that have been reported with naphazoline and/or antazoline include mydriasis, increased redness, irritation, blurring, punctate keratitis, lacrimation, increased intraocular pressure.
Systemic: Dizziness, headache, nausea, sweating, nervousness, drowsiness, weakness, hypertension, cardiac irregularities and hyperglycemia.
Dosage and Administration: Instill one to two drops in the conjunctival sac(s) every two hours as needed, but not to exceed four times per day.
How Supplied: VASOCON-A Ophthalmic Solution: 15 mL plastic dropper tip squeeze bottles. Keep tightly closed when not in use. Protect from light.
NDC 0058-2880-15
Do not store above 25°C (79°F).
Caution: Federal law prohibits dispensing without prescription.

VASOSULF® ℞
[*vas "o-sulf*]
(sulfacetamide sodium–phenylephrine hydrochloride)
Ophthalmic Solution

Description: VASOSULF (sulfacetamide sodium-phenylephrine hydrochloride) ophthalmic solution is a sterile solution for ophthalmic administration having the following composition:

Sulfacetamide Sodium 150mg/mL
(bacteriostatic antibacterial)
Phenylephrine Hydrochloride 1.25mg/mL
(sympathomimetic)

in a solution of mono and dibasic sodium phosphate, sodium thiosulfate, poloxamer 188 and purified water, preserved with methylparaben and propylparaben. Hydrochloric acid added to adjust pH when necessary.
The chemical name for sulfacetamide sodium is Acetamide, N-[(4-aminophenyl)sulfonyl]-, monosodium salt, monohydrate.
The chemical name for phenylephrine hydrochloride is Benzenemethanol, 3-hydroxy-α-[(methylamino)-methyl]-, hydrochloride (R)-.
They have the following chemical structures:

Sulfacetamide Sodium

$NH_2-C_6H_4-SO_2N(Na)COCH_3 \cdot H_2O$

Phenylephrine Hydrochloride

$[HO-C_6H_4-CH(OH)-CH_2\overset{+}{N}H_2CH_3]\ Cl^-$

Clinical Pharmacology: Sulfacetamide sodium exerts a bacteriostatic effect against a wide range of gram-positive and gram-negative microorganisms by restricting through competition with p-aminobenzoic acid, the synthesis of folic acid which bacteria require for growth. Phenylephrine hydrochloride is an alpha sympathetic receptor agonist producing vasoconstriction.
Indications and Usage: VASOSULF ophthalmic solution is indicated for the treatment of conjunctivitis, corneal ulcer, and other superficial ocular infections due to susceptible microorganisms, and an adjunctive in systemic sulfonamide therapy of trachoma.
Contraindications: Contraindicated in persons hypersensitive to one or more of the components of this preparation.
Precautions: The solutions are incompatible with silver preparations. Local anesthetics related to p-aminobenzoic acid may antagonize the action of the sulfonamides. Bacteria initially sensitive to sulfonamides may acquire resistance to the drug. Nonsusceptible organisms, including fungi, may proliferate with the use of this preparation. Sulfonamides are inactivated by the p-aminobenzoic acid present in purulent exudates.
If signs of hypersensitivity or other untoward reactions occur, discontinue use of the preparation.

To prevent contaminating the dropper tip and solution, care should be taken not to touch the eyelids or surrounding area with the dropper tip of the bottle. Keep bottle tightly closed when not in use and protect from light. Do not use if the solution has darkened or contains a precipitate.
For topical use only.
Carcinogenesis, Mutagenesis, Impairment of Fertility: There have been no long-term studies done using sulfacetamide and/or phenylephrine in animals to evaluate carcinogenic potential.
Pregnancy: Pregnancy Category C. Animal reproduction studies have not been conducted with sulfacetamide and/or phenylephrine. It is also not known whether sulfacetamide and/or phenylephrine can cause fetal harm when administered to a pregnant woman or can affect reproduction capacity. Sulfacetamide and/or phenylephrine should be given to a pregnant woman only if clearly needed.
Nursing Mothers: It is not known whether these drugs are excreted in human milk. Because many drugs are excreted in human milk, caution should be exercised when sulfacetamide and/or phenylephrine is administered to a nursing woman.
Pediatric Use: Safety and effectiveness in children have not been established.
Adverse Reactions: Headache or browache, blurred vision, local irritation, burning, transient stinging, transient epithelial keratitis, and reactive hyperemia. Sensitization reactions to sulfacetamide sodium may occur, although rarely. Reactions occurring most often from the presence of the anti-infective ingredient are allergic sensitizations. Although hypersensitivity reactions to sulfacetamide sodium are rare, instances of Stevens-Johnson syndrome, systemic lupus erythematosus (in one case producing a fatal outcome), exfoliative dermatitis, toxic epidermal necrolysis, and photosensitivity have been reported following the use of sulfonamide preparations.
Dosage and Administration: Instill one or two drops into lower conjunctival sac every two or three hours during the day, less often at night.
How Supplied: 5mL and 15mL plastic dropper tip squeeze bottles.
NDC 0058-2883-05
NDC 0058-2883-15
Keep tightly closed when not in use. Protect from light.
Store at 15° to 30°C (59° to 86°F).
Caution: Federal law prohibits dispensing without prescription.

Kabi Pharmacia Ophthalmics Inc.
605 E. HUNTINGTON DRIVE
MONROVIA, CA 91017

HEALON® ℞
(sodium hyaluronate)

Description: Healon® is a sterile, nonpyrogenic, viscoelastic preparation of a highly purified, noninflammatory, high molecular weight fraction of sodium hyaluronate.
Healon® contains 10 mg/ml of sodium hyaluronate, dissolved in physiological sodium chloride phosphate buffer (pH 7.0–7.5). This high molecular weight polymer is made up of repeating disaccharide units of N-acetylglucosamine and sodium glucuronate linked by β 1–3 and β 1–4 glycosidic bonds.
Characteristics: Sodium hyaluronate is a physiological substance that is widely distributed in the extracellular matrix of connective tissues in both animals and man. For example, it is present in the vitreous and aqueous humor of the eye, the synovial fluid, the skin and the umbilical cord. Sodium hyaluronates prepared from various human and animal tissues are not chemically different from each other.
Healon® is a specific fraction of sodium hyaluronate developed as an ophthalmo-surgical aid for use in anterior segment and vitreous procedures. It is specific in that:

1. It has a high molecular weight;
2. It is reported to be nonantigenic[1,6].
3. It does not cause inflammatory[2] or foreign body reactions;
4. It has a high viscosity.

Furthermore, the 1% solution of Healon® is transparent, is reported to remain in the anterior chamber for less than 6 days[3] and protects corneal endothelial cells[4,5] and other ocular structures. Healon® does not interfere with epithelialization and normal wound healing.
Uses: Healon® is indicated for use as a surgical aid in cataract extraction (intra- and extracapsular), IOL implantation, corneal transplant, glaucoma filtration and retinal attachment surgery.
In surgical procedures in the anterior segment of the eye, instillation of Healon® serves to maintain a deep anterior chamber during surgery, allowing for efficient manipulation with less trauma to the corneal endothelium and other surrounding tissues.
Furthermore, its viscoelasticity helps to push back the vitreous face and prevent formation of a post-operative flat chamber.
In posterior segment surgery Healon® serves as a surgical aid to gently separate, maneuver and hold tissues. Healon® creates a clear field of vision thereby facilitating intra- and postoperative inspection of the retina and photocoagulation.
Contraindications: At present there are no known contraindications to the use of Healon® when used as recommended.
Precautions: Those normally associated with the surgical procedure being performed.
Overfilling the anterior or posterior segment of the eye with Healon® may cause increased intraocular pressure, glaucoma, or other ocular damage.
Postoperative intraocular pressure may also be elevated as a result of pre-existing glaucoma, compromised outflow, and by operative procedures and sequelae thereto, including enzymatic zonulysis, absence of an iridectomy, trauma to filtration structures, and by blood and lenticular remnants in the anterior chamber. Since the exact role of these factors is difficult to predict in any individual case, the following precautions are recommended:

- Don't overfill the eye chambers with Healon® (except in glaucoma surgery—see Application section).
- In posterior segment procedures in aphakic diabetic patients special care should be exercised to avoid using large amounts of Healon®.
- Remove some of the Healon® by irrigation and/or aspiration at the close of surgery (except in glaucoma surgery—see Application section).
- Carefully monitor intraocular pressure, especially during the immediate postoperative period. If significant rises are observed, treat with appropriate therapy.

Care should be taken to avoid trapping air bubbles behind Healon®.
Because Healon® is a highly purified fraction extracted from avian tissues and is known to contain minute amounts of protein, the physician should be aware of potential risks of the type that can occur with the injection of any biological material.
Because of reports of an occasional release of minute rubber particles, presumably formed when the diaphragm is punctured, the physician should be aware of this potential problem. Express a small amount of Healon® from the syringe prior to use and carefully examine the remainder as it is injected.
Avoid reuse of cannulas. If reuse becomes necessary, rinse cannula thoroughly with sterile distilled water.
Sporadic reports have been received indicating that Healon® may become "cloudy" or form a slight precipitate following instillation into the eye. The clinical significance of these reports, if any, is not known since the majority received

Continued on next page

Kabi Pharmacia—Cont.

to date do not indicate any harmful effects on ocular tissues. The physician should be aware of this phenomenon and, should it be observed, remove the cloudy or precipitated material by irrigation and/or aspiration.
In vitro laboratory studies suggest that this phenomenon may be related to interactions with certain concomitantly adminstered ophthalmic medications.
Use only if solution is clear.
Adverse Reactions: Healon® is extremely well tolerated after injection into human eyes. A transient rise of intraocular pressure postoperatively has been reported in some cases.
In posterior segment surgery intraocular pressure rises have been reported in some patients, especially in aphakic diabetics, after injection of large amount of Healon®.
Rarely, postoperative inflammatory reactions (iritis, hypopyon) as well as incidents of corneal edema and corneal decompensation have been reported. Their relationship to Healon® has not been established.
Applications
Cataract surgery—IOL implantation
A sufficient amount of Healon® is slowly, and carefully introduced (using a cannula or needle) into the anterior chamber.
Injection of Healon® can be performed either before or after delivery of the lens. Injection prior to lens delivery will, however, have the additional advantage of protecting the corneal endothelium from possible damage arising from the removal of the cataractous lens[5]. Healon® may also be used to coat surgical instruments and the IOL prior to insertion.
Additional Healon® can be injected during surgery to replace any Healon® lost during surgical manipulation (see Precautions section).
Glaucoma filtration surgery
In conjunction with performing of the trabeculectomy, Healon® is injected slowly and carefully through a corneal paracentesis to reconstitute the anterior chamber. Further injection of Healon® can be continued allowing it to extrude into the subconjunctival filtration site and through and around the sutured outer scleral flap.
Corneal transplant surgery
After removal of the corneal button, the anterior chamber is filled with Healon®. The donor graft can then be placed on top of the bed of Healon® and sutured in place. Additional Healon® may be injected to replace the Healon® lost as a result of surgical manipulation (see Precautions section). Healon® has also been used in the anterior chamber of the donor eye prior to trepanation to protect the corneal endothelial cells of the graft[5].
Retinal attachment surgery
Healon® is slowly introduced into the vitreous cavity. By directing the injection, Healon® can be used to separate membranes (e.g., epiretinal membranes) away from the retina for safe excision and release of traction. Healon® also serves to maneuver tissues into the desired position, e.g., to gently push back a detached retina or unroll a retinal flap, and aids in holding the retina against the sclera for reattachment.
How Supplied: Healon® is a sterile, nonpyrogenic, viscoelastic preparation supplied in disposable glass syringes, delivering 0.85 ml, 0.55 ml or 0.4 ml sodium hyaluronate (10 mg/ml) dissolved in physiological sodium chloride-phosphate buffer (pH 7.0–7.5). Each ml of Healon® contains 10 mg of sodium hyaluronate, 8.5 mg sodium chloride, 0.28 mg of disodium hydrogen phosphate dihydrate, 0.04 mg of sodium dihydrogen phosphate hydrate and q.s. water for injection U.S.P. Healon® syringes are terminally sterilized and aseptically packaged.
A sterile single-use 27 G cannula is enclosed in the 0.4 ml, 0.55 ml and 0.85 ml boxes.
Refrigerated Healon® should be allowed to attain room temperature (approximately 30 minutes) prior to use.
For intraocular use.
Store at 2–8°C.
Protect from freezing.
Protect from light.
Caution: Federal law restricts this device to sale by or on the order of a physician.

References:

1. *Richter, W., Ryde, M. & Zetterström, O.:* Nonimmunogenicity of a purified sodium hyaluronate preparation in man. Int Arch Appl Immun 59:45–48 (1979).
2. *Balazs, E. A.:* Ultrapure hyaluronic acid and the use thereof. U.S. Patent 4,141,973 (1979).
3. *Balazs, E. A., Miller, D. & Stegmann, R.:* Viscosurgery and the use of Na-hyaluronate in intraocular lens implantation. Lecture , Cannes, France (1979).
4. *Miller, D. & Stegmann, R.:* Use of Na-hyaluronate in anterior segment eye surgery. Am Intra-Ocular Implant Soc J 6 (1980b) p 13–15.
5. *Pape, L. G. & Balazs, E. A.:* The use of sodium hyaluronate (Healon®) in human anterior segment surgery. Ophthalmol 87 (1980) p 699–705.
6. *Richter, W.:* Non-immunogenicity of purified hyaluronic acid preparations tested by passive cutaneous anaphylaxis. Int Arch All 47 (1974) p211–217.

MANUFACTURED BY
Kabi Pharmacia AB
Uppsala, Sweden
For Kabi Pharmacia Ophthalmics Inc.
Monrovia, CA 91017-7136
Revised: July 1991
Healon is covered by
U.S. patent 4,141,973, 1979

HEALON® YELLOW ℞
(sodium hyaluronate)

Information listed for Healon® also applies to Healon® Yellow with the following exceptions.
Description: Healon® Yellow Sodium hyaluronate is a sterile, nonpyrogenic, yellow viscoelastic preparation of a highly purified, noninflammatory, high molecular weight fraction of sodium hyaluronate and fluorescein sodium. Healon® Yellow contains 10 mg/ml of sodium hyaluronate and 0.005 mg/ml of fluorescein sodium, dissolved in physiological sodium chloride-phosphate buffer (pH 7.0–7.5). This high molecular weight polymer is made up of repeating disaccharide units of N-acetylglucosamine and sodium glucuronate linked by β1–3 and β1–4 glycosidic bonds.
It is yellow and transparent.
The fluorescein sodium in Healon® Yellow facilitates the visualization of the product during the surgical procedure.
How Supplied: Healon® Yellow is a sterile, nonpyrogenic viscoelastic preparation supplied in disposable glass syringes, delivering either 0.55 ml or 0.85 ml sodium hyaluronate (10 mg/ml) and fluorescein sodium (0.005 mg/ml) dissolved in physiological sodium chloride-phosphate buffer (pH 7.0–7.5). Each ml of Healon® Yellow contains 10 mg of sodium hyaluronate, 0.005 mg of fluorescein sodium, 8.5 mg sodium chloride, 0.28 mg of disodium hydrogen phosphate dihydrate, 0.04 mg of sodium dihydrogen phosphate hydrate and q.s. water for injection USP.
A sterile single-use 27G cannula is enclosed in each box.

La Haye Laboratories, Inc.
2205 152ND AVENUE, N.E.
REDMOND, WA 98052

ICAPS PLUS® OTC

[See table below.]
Vitamins
Beta Carotene (Pro Vitamin A): A water soluble relative of Vitamine A that is a potent antioxidant
Vitamin C: Vitamin C is a well known water soluble antioxidant nutrient that works synergistically along with other antioxidants. Humans cannot make their own Vitamin C.
Vitamin E: Vitamin E is an important lipid soluble antioxidant. It helps protect fats, especially cell membranes, in our bodies from uncontrolled oxidation and free radicals.
Vitamin B-2: Vitamin B-2 is necessary for the production of the enzyme glutathione reductase, which recycles oxidized glutathione back into its reduced form.
Minerals
Zinc Acetate: Zinc is an extremely important antioxidant mineral and is necessary for the production of 200 enzymes in addition to DNA synthesis and cell division.
Copper: Copper is included for two reasons: 1. When supplementing the diet with Zinc, it is critical to also include Copper in order to negate the chance of Zinc created Copper deficiency anemia. 2. Copper is a constituent of intracellular superoxide dismutase, an important antioxidant.
Selenium: Selenium is an antioxidant mineral necessary for the production of glutathione peroxidase, which breaks down hydrogen peroxide in the body.
Manganese: Manganese is a constituent of mitochondrial superoxide dismutase which in turn converts free radicals into less dangerous chemical entities.
L-Cysteine: The Amino Acid. A component of the Amino Acid Glutathione, an antioxidant.
Description: Each ICAPS Plus® to be taken orally contains the above.
Indications: ICAPS Plus is specifically formulated as an Antioxidant Vitamin and Mineral Supplement. ICAPS Plus is an OTC nutritional supplement and is indicated to provide

Vitamin/ Mineral	Source	Amount	Adults-US RDA
Vitamin A	Beta Carotene	5000 I.U.	(100%)
Vitamin C	Ascorbic Acid	250mg	(420%)
Vitamin B-2	Riboflavin	10mg	(590%)
Vitamin E	d-alph tocopheryl Succinate	50 I.U.	170%
Zinc	Zinc Acetate	20mg	130%
Copper	Copper Amino Acid Chelate	1mg	50%
Manganese	Manganese Amino Acid Chelate	5 mg	—
Selenium	Selenomethionine	20mcg.	—
L-Cysteine	L-Cysteine	25 mg	—

—No US RDA Established

vitamins and minerals either missing from the diet or for deficiencies associated with restricted diets, improper food intake and decreased absorbtion, or as a general nutritional supplement.

Recommended Intake: Two or Four tablets per day to be taken after meals. Intake should be divided between two meals.

How Supplied: 120 Golden Oval film coated tablets per bottle. Keep tightly closed in a dry place at controlled room temperature.

Lacrimedics, Inc.

9008 NEWBY STREET
ROSEMEAD, CA 91770

"HERRICK LACRIMAL PLUG"™

Instructions For Use:

FOR LONG TERM NASO-LACRIMAL OCCLUSION IN PATIENTS WITH "DRY EYE", TEARING DISORDERS, CONTACT LENS INTOLERANCE OR DISCOMFORT, AND RELATED EAR, NOSE, AND THROAT AND SINUS CONDITIONS.

Use of the "HERRICK LACRIMAL PLUG"™ is indicated in patients who respond favorably to the "Lacrimal Efficiency Test"™ with dissolvable COLLAGEN IMPLANTS (from Lacrimedics, Inc.).

Symptoms that may benefit include: Conjunctivitis, corneal ulcer, keratitis, recurrent corneal erosion, filamentary keratitis, pterygium, pinguecula, corneal abrasion or perforation, persistant wound defects, stingy mucous discharge, light sensitivity, blepharitis, blepharospasm, chalazia, sties, and other external eye conditions.

Secondary non-ocular symptoms that may respond include sinusitis, rhinitis, hay fever and allergy symptoms, runny nose, post nasal drip, chronic cough, chronic bronchitis, sinus pressure, headaches, middle ear congestion, toothaches, sneezing, snoring and other conditions.

Naso-lacrimal occlusion is known to:

—Enhance the lubricating pre-corneal tear film.

—Reduce tear drainage into the nose, throat, and sinus which might cause nasal congestions, sinusitis, chronic cough, post-nasal drip, headaches, sneezing, middle ear congestion, and toothaches.

—Reduce eye irritation, burning, and redness.

—Maximize the pre-corneal concentration of natural antibacterial factors such as lysozyme, lactoferrin and IgA.

—Maximize the therapeutic index of topical ocular medications by increasing the focal concentration and reducing drainage away from the eye.

—Enchance the tear lake necessary for comfortable contact lens wear, reduce surface drying, contact lens decentration, protein deposits, light sensitivity, solutions sensitivity, and chronic infections of the eye and lid.

—Provide long-term symptomatic relief from "Dry Eye" symptoms not available from eyedrops.

—Minimize drying of the cornea thus reducing corneal abrasions, poor wound healing, and the risk of corneal ulcers.

—Cause the cornea to become compact (desirable before invasive corneal procedures).

—Reduce the risk of Exposure Keratitis during surgical procedures.

—Reduce glare and photosensitivity caused from diffraction of light as it passes through the tear film and cornea.

—Reduce excess tearing and watery eyes caused from eye irritation and resultant reflex tearing.

—Optimize the refractive surface through which light passes.

The "Herrick Lacrimal Plug"™ was introduced in 1990. Its design allows for ease of insertion, comfort after placement, and dependability after insertion.

The "HERRICK LACRIMAL PLUG"™ is provided in sterile packets contaiing two (2) plug each. Each plug is pre-assembled on an insertion stilette. A sliding styrafoam guide is mounted on the stilette to facilitate insertion.

The "HERRICK LACRIMAL PLUG"™ is available in .3mm, and .5mm diameter (descriptive of the long thin "shaft" of the plug). A radio opaque material (Bismuth Trioxide) is added to allow for X-ray of the device. A 5mm "tail" is available in the larger diameter to facilitate removal via the punctum.

Dilation of the punctum and topical anesthetic is not required for insertion of the "HERRICK LACRIMAL PLUG"™. Because the plug works in the horizontal canaliculus (away from the lid margin) it will not touch the cornea, nor will it fall out of the punctum.

Insertion:

1. Place a sterile sealed packet of "HERRICK LACRIMAL PLUG"™ on a table or tray.
2. Peel back the tyvek lid to expose the two (2) insertion assemblies of the "HERRICK LACRIMAL PLUG"™. Each insertion assembly includes: one (1) "HERRICK LACRIMAL PLUG"™, one (1) insertion stilette (wire), and one (1) sliding styrafoam guide.
3. Remove one insertion assembly and position in your hand between your thumb, and index finger (with the "HERRICK LACRIMAL PLUG"™ in an inferior position).
4. While visualizing the punctum under high magnification (a slit lamp, operating microscope, or high power "loops" may be used) place the long thin portion of the "HERRICK LACRIMAL PLUG"™ into the punctum.
5. While positioning the insertion assembly directly above the punctum advance the thin tip of the "HERRICK LACRIMAL PLUG"™ down into the punctum until the large upper portion of the plug rests on the punctal opening.
6. While maintaining the thin tip of the "HERRICK LACRIMAL PLUG"™ down within the punctum, "tilt" the upper portion of the insertion assembly laterally (the stilette should be pointed somewhat inferiorly down toward the nose).
   This places lateral traction of the eyelid and straightens out the angle between the vertical and horizontal canaliculus thus clearing the way for advancement of the "HERRICK LACRIMAL PLUG"™ down into the horizontal canaliculus.
7. Advance the plug down out of sight. As the plug passes the punctum the large hollow end will fold in upon itself. After placement it re-opens and gains its original shape.
8. Once the plug is down out of sight within the horizontal canaliculus reverse the direction of the insertion stilette. The friction from the walls of the canaliculus should cause the plug to detach from the stilette and remain within the canaliculus.
9. (Optional) Should the plug remain fixed on the end of the insertion stilette after retrieving the stilette from the punctum, reposition the plug into the punctum and advance the sliding styrafoam guide down the length of the stilette so as to force the plug off the tip into the punctum.
   After the "HERRICK LACRIMAL PLUG"™ is released within the canaliculus the force of the blink mechanism and the direction of tear flow through the tear drainage system will cause the plug to migrate into the distal end of the horizontal canaliculus (5 to 7 MM below the punctum).
   While maintaining the thin tip of the "HERRICK LACRIMAL PLUG"™ down within the punctum, "tilt" the upper portion of the insertion assembly laterally (the stilette should be pointed somewhat inferiorly down toward the nose).

BE CAREFUL NOT TO PUNCTURE THE CANALICULUS DURING INSERTION. The canaliculus may be punctured if the plug is forced too hard, or in the wrong direction (see diagram of anatomy). Puncture will cause pain, and will increase the risk of infection.

Should puncture occur remove the "HERRICK LACRIMAL PLUG"™ until such time as the wound heals and no swelling or redness persists.

Use of the "HERRICK LACRIMAL PLUG"™ is contra-indicated in patients with tearing secondary to chronic dacryocystitis with mucopurulent discharge.

Patients experiencing epiphora (constant tearing) prior to insertion of the "HERRICK LACRIMAL PLUG"™ should be carefully evaualated for obstruction of the tear drinage pathway (e.g. as with irrigation, or probing).

REMOVAL OF THE "HERRICK LACRIMAL PLUG"™ FROM THE CANALICULUS MAY BE AFFECTED BY THE USE OF IRRIGATION, OR PROBING. This may be required should the patient experience epiphora, irritation, or infection after placement of the plug. These procedures force the plug down into the nasolacrimal sac where it then flushes out into the nose or throat.

LACRIMEDICS, INC. REQUIRES THAT ALL PATIENTS BEING TREATED WITH THE "HERRICK LACRIMAL PLUG"™:

1) Be given complete (written) information describing the benefits and drawbacks of this and other methods of naso-lacrimal occlusion.
2) Be informed about alternatives to naso-lacrimal occlusion (such as eyedrops, ointments, humidifiers, protective goggles, etc.) which might be used to manage dry eye symptoms, and . . .
3) **SIGN A WRITTEN DOCUMENT WHICH ACKNOWLEDGES THE RECEIPT OF THIS INFORAMTION, AND WHICH EXPRESSES CONSENT (IN ADVANCE) OF THE INSERTION OF THE "HERRICK LACRIMAL PLUG"™.**

The "HERRICK LACRIMAL PLUG"™ is an altenative to other methods of naso-lacrimal occlusion which include argon laser canaliculoplasty, electric cautery, and the "Freeman Punctum Plug"™.

For more information on non-dissolvable "HERRICK LACRIMAL PLUG"™, DISSOLVABLE COLLEGEN IMPLANTS, dry eye brochures, videos, forceps, patient evaluation forms, billing forms, or other products from Lacrimedics, Inc. contact:

Lacrimedics, Inc.
250 N. Linden Ave., #287
Rialto, CA 92376
(800) 367-8327

Direct all product performance reports and clinical observations to the attention of the Product Supervisor.

(Patent #4,550,546, Robert S. Herrick, M.D.)

THE "LACRIMAL EFFICIENCY TEST"™ WITH COLLAGEN IMPLANTS

Instructions for Use:

FOR TEMPORARY ENHANCEMENT OF THE PRE-CORNEAL TEAR FILM BY OCCULSION OF THE HORIZONTAL CANALICULUS

- **To diagnose Dry Eye, tearing disorders, and related conditions involving the nose, throat, sinus, and middle ear.**
- **To evaluate benefits of long term naso-lacrimal occlusion** (e.g.: laser canaliculoplasty, electric cautery, plastic punctum plugs, or

Continued on next page

Lacrimedics—Cont.

the new silicone "Herrick Lacrimal Plug"™ by Lacrimedics).

- **To increase eye lubrication without the use of eye drops.**
- **To increase the therapeutic index of ocular medications.**
- **To reduce complications and systemic side effects of topical medications** (e.g.: beta blockers).
- **To prepare corneal tissue for surgery.**
- **To optimize post-operative healing conditions.**
- **To elevate antibacterial factors in the precorneal tear film** (lactoferrin, lysozyme, lgA).
- **To reduce eye irritation and resultant reflex tearing** (watery or occasionally tearing eyes, mostly saline).
- **To identify dry contact lens conditions that may benefit from naso-lacrimal occulusion** (e.g.: surface drying, lens discomfort or intolerance, protein deposits, lens decentration, solution sensitivity, light sensitivity, and chronic infections of the eye and lid).

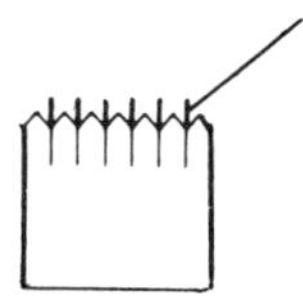

COLLAGEN IMPLANTS are provided in sterile boxes containing 12 packets each, with 6 plugs per packet (72 plugs/box). COLLAGEN IMPLANTS are .2mm, .3mm, .4mm, .5mm, and .6mm diameters, all 2mm long.
Standard JEWELER'S FORCEPS are used to insert COLLAGEN IMPLANTS while DILATION of the punctum and TOPICAL ANESTHETIC are optional.

Insertion:

1. Place the patient at a slip lamp or use magnifying loops so as to visualize the punctum. Determine what size COLLAGEN IMPLANT to use (.2mm, .3mm, .4mm, .5mm, or .6mm diameter).
2. Remove a sterile packet from a box of COLLAGEN IMPLANTS and peel back the lid to expose the blue styrofoam holder.
3. Remove the blue holder from the packet and use jewelers forceps to grasp one of the plugs from between the grooves.
4. Visualize the punctum under magnification and place the lower end of the plug into the punctum and then release the forceps. The sides of the punctum should stabilize the plug in a vertical position.
5. While holding the forceps tangential to the globe open the tips and use one point (or use the closed tips) to advance the plug below the punctum (out of sight) into the horizontal canaliculus.
6. Should difficulty be experienced in inserting the plugs all the way apply lateral traction to the lid to help straighten out the angle between the vertical and the horizontal canaliculus. This may help clear the way for insertion.
7. After pushing the plug down out of sight withdraw the forceps and repeat the procedure for all test puncta.
8. Insertion into upper and lower canaliculus, and the use of the largest diameter plug possible will help maximize the test response and minimize any false negative response.
9. After insertion reinspect all puncta to ensure that the plugs have not begun to "slip out". This may result from shallow placement and can result in irritation or corneal abrasions.

Tearing Patients:
CONSTANT TEARING (epiphora) may be caused by obstruction of the tear drain and should be evaluated accordingly (irrigation, probing, or more advanced procedures may be used).
OCCASIONAL TEARING or WATERY EYES may be caused from eye irritation and resultant REFLEX TEARING. Dilution of the basal tear secretion by reflex tears can decrease antibacterial factors in the tear film and may elevate the patients chance of infection.
Once placed within the horizontal canaliculus COLLAGEN IMPLANTS absorb the tear fluid and become very soft. After ten to fifteen minutes COLLAGEN IMPLANTS double in size and begin to block 60% to 80% of tear drainage (if placed in the upper and lower lids of the test eye).
After four to seven days COLLAGEN IMPLANTS dissolve requiring no removal. Should patients experience symptomatic improvement during testing with COLLAGEN IMPLANTS permanent naso-lacrimal occulsion may be indicated (as with the "Herrick Lacrimal Plug"™ from Lacrimedics).

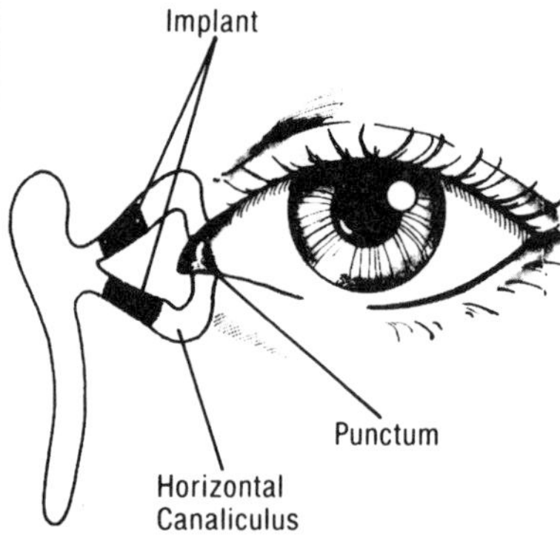

Indications for Use:
Conjunctivitis, corneal ulcer, keratitis, recurrent corneal erosion, filamentary keratitis, pterygium, pinguecula, corneal abrasion or perforation, persistant wound defects, stringy mucous discharge, light sensitivity, blepharitis, blepharospasm, chalazia, sties, and other external eye conditions.
Secondary conditions include sinusitis, rhinitis, hay fever and allergy type symptoms, runny nose, post nasal drip, chronic cough, chronic bronchitis, sinus pressure, headaches, middle ear congestion, toothaches, sneezing, snoring, and other conditions.

Contraindications:
Tearing secondary to chronic dacryocystitis with mucopurulent discharge.
Patients with obvious dry eye symptoms failing to respond to COLLAGEN IMPLANTS may require advanced testing with the "Herrick Stitch Test"™ (approximately 100% occlusion). A 9/0 or 10/0 nylon suture is used to temporarily sew the puncta closed.
For more information on COLLAGEN IMPLANTS, the HERRICK LACRIMAL PLUG™ the Herrick Stitch Test™, dry eye brochures, dry eye videos, jewelers forceps, or other related material, or to place an order contact:

LACRIMEDICS, INC.
250 N. Linden Ave. #287
Rialto, CA 92376
or Call (800) 367-8327
USA and Canada

Patent No. 4,660,546 (Robert S. Herrick, M.D.)

Lederle Laboratories

A Division of American Cyanamid Co.
ONE CYANAMID PLAZA
WAYNE, NJ 07470

see Storz Ophthalmics, Inc. page 307

Merck Sharp & Dohme

DIVISION OF MERCK & CO., INC.
WEST POINT, PA 19486

CHIBROXIN™ ℞
(Norfloxacin, MSD)
Sterile Ophthalmic Solution

Description
CHIBROXIN* (Norfloxacin, MSD) Ophthalmic Solution is a synthetic broad-spectrum antibacterial agent supplied as a sterile isotonic solution for topical ophthalmic use. Norfloxacin, a fluoroquinolone, is 1-ethyl-6-fluoro-1,4-dihydro-4-oxo-7-(1-piperazinyl) -3- quinolinecarboxylic acid. Its empirical formula is $C_{16}H_{18}FN_3O_3$ and the structural formula is:

Norfloxacin is a white to pale yellow crystalline powder with a molecular weight of 319.34 and a melting point of about 221°C. It is freely soluble in glacial acetic acid and very slightly soluble in ethanol, methanol and water.
CHIBROXIN Ophthalmic Solution 0.3% is supplied as a sterile isotonic solution. Each mL contains 3 mg norfloxacin. Inactive ingredients: disodium edetate, sodium acetate, sodium chloride, hydrochloric acid (to adjust pH) and water for injection. Benzalkonium chloride 0.0025% is added as preservative. The pH of CHIBROXIN is approximately 5.2 and the osmolarity is approximately 285 mOsmol/liter.
Norfloxacin, a fluoroquinolone, differs from quinolones by having a fluorine atom at the 6 position and a piperazine moiety at the 7 position.

Clinical Pharmacology
Microbiology
Norfloxacin has *in vitro* activity against a broad spectrum of gram-positive and gram-negative aerobic bacteria. The fluorine atom at the 6 position provides increased potency against gram-negative organisms and the piperazine moiety at the 7 position is responsible for anti-pseudomonal activity.
Norfloxacin inhibits bacterial deoxyribonucleic acid synthesis and is bactericidal. At the molecular level three specific events are attributed to CHIBROXIN in *E. coli* cells:

1) inhibition of the ATP-dependent DNA supercoiling reaction catalyzed by DNA gyrase;
2) inhibition of the relaxation of supercoiled DNA;
3) promotion of double-stranded DNA breakage.

There is generally no cross-resistance between norfloxacin and other classes of antibacterial agents. Therefore, norfloxacin generally demonstrates activity against indicated organisms resistant to some other antimicrobial agents. When such cross-resistance does occur, it is probably due to decreased entry of the drugs into the bacterial cells. Antagonism has been demonstrated *in vitro* between norfloxacin and nitrofurantoin.
Norfloxacin has been shown to be active against most strains of the following organisms

*Trademark of MERCK & CO., INC.

both *in vitro* and clinically in ophthalmic infections (see INDICATIONS AND USAGE):

Gram-positive bacteria including:
Staphylococcus aureus
(including both penicillinase-producing and methicillin-resistant strains)
Staphylococcus epidermidis
Staphylococcus warnerii
Streptococcus pneumoniae

Gram-negative bacteria including:
Acinetobacter calcoaceticus
Aeromonas hydrophila
Haemophilus influenzae
Proteus mirabilis
Serratia marcescens

Norfloxacin has been shown to be active *in vitro* against most strains of the following organisms; however, *the clinical significance of these data in ophthalmic infections is unknown.*

Gram-positive bacteria:
Bacillus cereus
Enterococcus faecalis (formerly *Streptococcus faecalis*)
Staphylococcus saprophyticus

Gram-negative bacteria:
Citrobacter diversus
Citrobacter freundii
Edwardsiella tarda
Enterobacter aerogenes
Enterobacter cloacae
Escherichia coli
Hafnia alvei
Haemophilus aegyptius (Koch-Weeks bacillus)
Klebsiella oxytoca
Klebsiella pneumoniae
Klebsiella rhinoscleromatis
Morganella morganii
Neisseria gonorrhoeae
Proteus vulgaris
Providencia alcalifaciens
Providencia rettgeri
Providencia stuartii
Pseudomonas aeruginosa
Salmonella typhi
Vibrio cholerae
Vibrio parahemolyticus
Yersinia enterocolitica

Other:
Ureaplasma urealyticum

Norfloxacin is not active against obligate anaerobes.

Clinical Studies

Clinical studies were conducted comparing CHIBROXIN Ophthalmic Solution (n=152) with ophthalmic solutions of tobramycin, gentamicin, and chloramphenicol (n=158) in patients with conjunctivitis and positive bacterial cultures. After seven days of therapy with CHIBROXIN Ophthalmic Solution, 72 percent of patients were clinically cured. Of those cured, 85 percent had all their pathogens eradicated. Eradication was also achieved in 62 percent (23/37) of patients whose clinical outcome was not completely cured by day seven. These results were similar among all treatment groups.

Another clinical study compared CHIBROXIN Ophthalmic Solution with placebo in patients with conjunctivitis and positive bacterial cultures. Placebo in this study was the liquid vehicle for CHIBROXIN Ophthalmic Solution and contained the preservative. After five days of therapy, 64 percent (36/56) of patients on CHIBROXIN Ophthalmic Solution were clinically cured compared to 50 percent (23/46) of patients receiving placebo. Of those cured, 78 percent had all their pathogens eradicated. Eradication was also achieved in 50 percent (10/20) of patients whose clinical outcome was not completely cured. The response to CHIBROXIN Ophthalmic Solution was statistically significantly better than the response to placebo.

Indications and Usage

CHIBROXIN Ophthalmic Solution is indicated for the treatment of conjunctivitis when caused by susceptible strains of the following bacteria:
*Acinetobacter calcoaceticus**
*Aeromonas hydrophila**
Haemophilus influenzae
*Proteus mirabilis**
*Serratia marcescens**
Staphylococcus aureus
Staphylococcus epidermidis
*Staphylococcus warnerii**
Streptococcus pneumoniae

Appropriate monitoring of bacterial response to topical antibiotic therapy should accompany the use of CHIBROXIN Ophthalmic Solution.

Contraindications

CHIBROXIN Ophthalmic Solution is contraindicated in patients with a history of hypersensitivity to norfloxacin, or the other members of the quinolone group of antibacterial agents or any other component of this medication.

Warnings

NOT FOR INJECTION INTO THE EYE.

Serious and occasionally fatal hypersensitivity (anaphylactoid or anaphylactic) reactions, some following the first dose, have been reported in patients receiving systemic quinolone therapy. Some reactions were accompanied by cardiovascular collapse, loss of consciousness, tingling, pharyngeal or facial edema, dyspnea, urticaria, and itching. Only a few patients had a history of hypersensitivity reactions. Serious anaphylactoid or anaphylactic reactions require immediate emergency treatment with epinephrine. Oxygen, intravenous steroids and airway management, including intubation, should be administered as indicated.

Precautions

General

As with other antibiotic preparations, prolonged use may result in overgrowth of nonsusceptible organisms, including fungi. If superinfection occurs, appropriate measures should be initiated. Whenever clinical judgment dictates, the patient should be examined with the aid of magnification, such as slit lamp biomicroscopy and, where appropriate, fluorescein staining.

Information For Patients

Patients should be instructed to avoid allowing the tip of the dispensing container to contact the eye or surrounding structures.

Patients should be advised that norfloxacin may be associated with hypersensitivity reactions, even following a single dose, and to discontinue the drug at the first sign of a skin rash or other allergic reaction.

Drug Interactions

Specific drug interaction studies have not been conducted with norfloxacin ophthalmic solution. However, the systemic administration of some quinolones has been shown to elevate plasma concentrations of theophylline, interfere with the metabolism of caffeine, and enhance the effects of the oral anticoagulant warfarin and its derivatives. Elevated serum levels of cyclosporine have been reported with concomitant use of cyclosporine with norfloxacin. Therefore, cyclosporine serum levels should be monitored and appropriate cyclosporine dosage adjustments made when these drugs are used concomitantly.

Carcinogenesis, Mutagenesis, Impairment of Fertility

No increase in neoplastic changes was observed with norfloxacin as compared to controls in a study in rats, lasting up to 96 weeks at doses eight to nine times the usual human oral dose*.

*Efficacy for this organism was studied in fewer than 10 infections.

Norfloxacin was tested for mutagenic activity in a number of *in vivo* and *in vitro* tests. Norfloxacin had no mutagenic effect in the dominant lethal test in mice and did not cause chromosomal aberrations in hamsters or rats at doses 30 to 60 times and usual oral dose*. Norfloxacin had no mutagenic activity *in vitro* in the Ames microbial mutagen test, Chinese hamster fibroblasts and V-79 mammalian cell assay. Although norfloxacin was weakly positive in the Rec-assay for DNA repair, all other mutagenic assays were negative including a more sensitive test (V-79).

Norfloxacin did not adversely affect the fertility of male and female mice at oral doses up to 33 times the usual human oral dose*.

Pregnancy

Pregnancy Category C: Norfloxacin has been shown to produce embryonic loss in monkeys when given in doses 10 times the maximum human oral dose* (400 mg b.i.d.), with peak plasma levels that are two to three times those obtained in humans. There has been no evidence of a teratogenic effect in any of the animal species tested (rat, rabbit, mouse, monkey) at 6 to 50 times the human oral dose. There are no adequate and well-controlled studies in pregnant women. CHIBROXIN Ophthalmic Solution should be used during pregnancy only if the potential benefit justifies the potential risk to the fetus.

Nursing Mothers

It is not known whether norfloxacin is excreted in human milk following ocular administration. Because many drugs are excreted in human milk, and because of the potential for serious adverse reactions in nursing infants from norfloxacin, a decision should be made to discontinue nursing or to discontinue the drug, taking into account the importance of the drug to the mother (see ANIMAL PHARMACOLOGY).

Pediatric Use

Safety and effectiveness in infants below the age of one year have not been established.

Although quinolones including norfloxacin have been shown to cause arthropathy in immature animals after oral administration, topical ocular administration of other quinolones to immature animals has not shown any arthropathy and there is no evidence that the ophthalmic dosage form of those quinolones has any effects on the weight-bearing joints.

Adverse Reactions

In clinical trials, the most frequently reported drug-related adverse reaction was local burning or discomfort. Other drug-related adverse reactions were conjunctival hyperemia, chemosis, photophobia and a bitter taste following instillation.

Dosage and Administration

The recommended dose in adults and pediatric patients (one year and older) is one or two drops of CHIBROXIN Ophthalmic Solution applied topically to the affected eye(s) four times daily for up to seven days. Depending on the severity of the infection, the dosage for the first day of therapy may be one or two drops every two hours during the waking hours.

How Supplied

CHIBROXIN Ophthalmic Solution is a clear, colorless to light yellow solution.

*All factors are based on a standard patient weight of 50 kg. The usual oral dose of norfloxacin is 800 mg daily. One drop of CHIBROXIN Ophthalmic Solution 0.3% contains about 1/6,666 of this dose (0.12 mg).

Continued on next page

Information on the Merck Sharp & Dohme products listed on these pages is the full prescribing information from product circulars in effect August 31, 1991.

Merck Sharp & Dohme—Cont.

No. 3526—CHIBROXIN Ophthalmic Solution 0.3% is supplied in a white, opaque, plastic OCUMETER* ophthalmic dispenser with a controlled drop tip as follows:
NDC 0006-3526-03, 5 mL.

Storage

Store CHIBROXIN Ophthalmic Solution at room temperature, 15°–30°C (59°–86°F). Protect from light.

Animal Pharmacology

The oral administration of single doses of norfloxacin, six times the recommended human oral dose**, caused lameness in immature dogs. Histologic examination of the weight-bearing joints of these dogs revealed permanent lesions of the cartilage. Related drugs also produced erosions of the cartilage in weight-bearing joints and other signs of arthropathy in immature animals of various species.

Additional Cautionary Information

Norfloxacin is available as an oral dosage form in addition to the ophthalmic dosage form. The following adverse effects, while they have not been reported with the ophthalmic dosage form, have been reported with the oral dosage form. However, it should be noted that the usual dosage of oral norfloxacin (800 mg/day) contains 6,666 times the amount in one drop of CHIBROXIN Ophthalmic Solution 0.3% (0.12 mg).

Convulsions have been reported in patients receiving oral norfloxacin. Convulsions, increased intracranial pressure, and toxic psychoses have been reported with other drugs in this class. Orally administered quinolones may also cause central nervous system (CNS) stimulation which may lead to tremors, restlessness, lightheadedness, confusion and hallucinations. If these reactions occur in patients receiving norfloxacin, the drug should be discontinued and appropriate measures instituted.

The effects of norfloxacin on brain function or on the electrical activity of the brain have not been tested. Therefore, as with all quinolones, norfloxacin should be used with caution in patients with known or suspected CNS disorders, such as severe cerebral arteriosclerosis, epilepsy, and other factors which predispose to seizures.

The following adverse effects have been reported with Tablets NOROXIN* (Norfloxacin, MSD). *Hypersensitivity Reactions:* Hypersensitivity reactions including anaphylactoid reactions, angioedema, dyspnea, urticaria, arthritis, arthralgia, myalgia; *Gastrointestinal:* Pseudomembranous colitis, hepatitis, pancreatitis; *Hematologic:* Neutropenia, leukopenia, thrombocytopenia; *Nervous System/Psychiatric:* CNS effects characterized as generalized seizures and myoclonus; psychic disturbances including psychotic reactions and confusion, depression; *Skin:* Toxic epidermal necrolysis, Stevens-Johnson syndrome and erythema multiforme, exfoliative dermatitis, rash, photosensitivity; *Special Senses:* Transient hearing loss.

Abnormal laboratory values observed with oral norfloxacin included elevation of ALT (SGPT) and AST (SGOT), alkaline phosphatase, BUN, serum creatinine, and LDH.

Please consult the package circular for Tablets NOROXIN (Norfloxacin, MSD) for additional information concerning these and other adverse effects and other cautionary information.

---

*Registered trademark of MERCK & CO., INC.

**All factors are based on a standard patient weight of 50 kg. The usual oral dose of norfloxacin is 800 mg daily. One drop of CHIBROXIN Ophthalmic Solution 0.3% contains about 1/6,666 of this dose (0.12 mg).

A.H.F.S. Category: 52:04
DC 7679101 Issued June 1991

Shown in Product Identification Section, page 103

DARANIDE® ℞
(Dichlorphenamide, MSD), U.S.P. Tablets

Description

DARANIDE® (Dichlorphenamide, MSD) is an oral carbonic anhydrase inhibitor. Dichlorphenamide, a dichlorinated benzenedisulfonamide, is known chemically as 4,5-dichloro-1,3-benzenedisulfonamide. Its empirical formula is $C_6H_6Cl_2N_2O_4S_2$ and its structural formula is:

Dichlorphenamide is a white or practically white, crystalline compound with a molecular weight of 305.16. It is very slightly soluble in water but soluble in dilute solutions of sodium carbonate and sodium hydroxide. Dilute alkaline solutions of dichlorphenamide are stable at room temperature.

DARANIDE is supplied as tablets, for oral administration, each containing 50 mg dichlorphenamide. Inactive ingredients are D&C Yellow 10, lactose, magnesium stearate, and starch.

Clinical Pharmacology

Carbonic anhydrase inhibitors reduce intraocular pressure by partially suppressing the secretion of aqueous humor (inflow), although the mechanism by which they do this is not fully understood. Evidence suggests that HCO_3^- ions are produced in the ciliary body by hydration of carbon dioxide under the influence of carbonic anhydrase and diffuse into the posterior chamber with $Na+$ ions. The aqueous fluid contains more $Na+$ and HCO_3^- ions than does plasma and consequently is hypertonic. Water is attracted to the posterior chamber by osmosis. Systemic administration of a carbonic anhydrase inhibitor has been shown to inactivate carbonic anhydrase in the ciliary body of the rabbit's eye and to reduce the high concentration of HCO_3^- ions in ocular fluids. As is the case with all carbonic anhydrase inhibitors, DARANIDE in high doses causes some decrease in renal blood flow and glomerular filtration rate.

In man, DARANIDE begins to act within an hour and maximal effect is observed in two to four hours. The lowered intraocular tension may be maintained for approximately 6 to 12 hours.

Indications and Usage

For adjunctive treatment of: chronic simple (open-angle) glaucoma, secondary glaucoma, and preoperatively in acute angle-closure glaucoma where delay of surgery is desired in order to lower intraocular pressure.

Contraindications

DARANIDE is contraindicated in hepatic insufficiency, renal failure, adrenocortical insufficiency, hyperchloremic acidosis, or in conditions in which serum levels of sodium or potassium are depressed. DARANIDE should not be used in patients with severe pulmonary obstruction who are unable to increase their alveolar ventilation since their acidosis may be increased.

DARANIDE is contraindicated in patients who are hypersensitive to this product.

Precautions

General

Potassium excretion is increased by DARANIDE and hypokalemia may develop with brisk diuresis, when severe cirrhosis is present, or during concomitant use of steroids or ACTH. Interference with adequate oral electrolyte intake will also contribute to hypokalemia. Hypokalemia can sensitize or exaggerate the response of the heart to the toxic effects of digitalis (e.g., increased ventricular irritability). Hypokalemia may be avoided or treated by use of potassium supplements such as foods with a high potassium content. DARANIDE should be used with caution in patients with respiratory acidosis.

Drug Interactions

Caution is advised in patients receiving concomitant high-dose aspirin and carbonic anhydrase inhibitors, as anorexia, tachypnea, lethargy and coma have been rarely reported due to a possible drug interaction.

Carcinogenesis, Mutagenesis, Impairment of Fertility

Long-term studies in animals have not been performed to evaluate the effects upon fertility or carcinogenic potential of DARANIDE.

Pregnancy

Pregnancy Category C. Dichlorphenamide has been shown to be teratogenic in the rat (skeletal anomalies) when given in doses 100 times the human dose. There are no adequate and well-controlled studies in pregnant women. DARANIDE should not be used in women of childbearing age or in pregnancy, especially during the first trimester, unless the potential benefits outweigh the potential risks.

Nursing Mothers

It is not known whether dichlorphenamide is excreted in human milk. Because many drugs are excreted in human milk, caution should be exercised when dichlorphenamide is administered to a nursing woman.

Pediatric Use

Safety and effectiveness in children have not been established.

Adverse Reactions

Certain side effects characteristic of carbonic anhydrase inhibitors may occur with DARANIDE, particularly with increasing doses. The most common effects include gastrointestinal disturbances (anorexia, nausea, and vomiting), drowsiness and paresthesias.

Included in the listing which follows are some adverse reactions which have not been reported with DARANIDE. However, pharmacological similarities among the carbonic anhydrase inhibitors make it advisable to consider the following reactions when dichlorphenamide is administered. *Central Nervous System/Psychiatric:* ataxia, tremor, tinnitus, headache, weakness, nervousness, globus hystericus, lassitude, depression, confusion, disorientation, dizziness; *Gastrointestinal:* constipation, hepatic insufficiency; *Metabolic:* loss of weight, metabolic acidosis, electrolyte imbalance (hypokalemia, hyperchloremia), hyperuricemia; *Hypersensitivity:* skin eruptions, pruritus, fever; *Hematologic:* leukopenia, agranulocytosis, thrombocytopenia; *Genitourinary:* urinary frequency, renal colic, renal calculi, phosphaturia.

Overdosage

The oral LD_{50} of DARANIDE is 1710 and 2600 mg/kg in the mouse and rat respectively.

Symptoms of overdosage or toxicity may include drowsiness, anorexia, nausea, vomiting, dizziness, paresthesias, ataxia, tremor and tinnitus.

In the event of overdosage, induce emesis or perform gastric lavage. The electrolyte disturbance most likely to be encountered from overdosage is hyperchloremic acidosis that may respond to bicarbonate administration. Potassium supplementation may be required. The patient should be carefully observed and given supportive treatment.

Dosage and Administration

DARANIDE is usually given in conjunction with topical ocular hypotensive agents. In acute angle-closure glaucoma, it may be used together with miotics and osmotic agents in an attempt to reduce intraocular tension rapidly. If this is not quickly relieved, surgery may be mandatory.

Dosage must be adjusted carefully to meet the requirements of the individual patient. A priming dose of 100 to 200 mg of DARANIDE (2 to 4 tablets) is suggested for adults, followed by 100 mg (2 tablets) every 12 hours until the desired response has been obtained. The recommended maintenance dosage for adults is 25 to 50 mg (½ to 1 tablet) once to three times daily.

How Supplied

No. 3256—Tablets DARANIDE, 50 mg each, are yellow, round, scored, compressed tablets, coded MSD 49. They are supplied as follows:

NDC 0006-0049-68 bottles of 100.

A.H.F.S. Category: 52:10

DC 7412517 Issued November 1986

Shown in Product Identification Section, page 103

DECADRON® Phosphate ℞

(Dexamethasone Sodium Phosphate, MSD), U.S.P.
0.05% Dexamethasone Phosphate Equivalent
Sterile Ophthalmic Ointment

Description

Dexamethasone sodium phosphate is 9-fluoro-11β, 17-dihydroxy-16α-methyl-21-(phosphonooxy)pregna-1,4-diene-3,20-dione disodium salt. Its empirical formula is $C_{22}H_{28}FNa_2O_8P$ and its structural formula is:

[structural formula]

Glucocorticoids are adrenocortical steroids, both naturally occurring and synthetic. Dexamethasone is a synthetic analog of naturally occurring glucocorticoids (hydrocortisone and cortisone). Dexamethasone sodium phosphate is a water soluble, inorganic ester of dexamethasone. Its molecular weight is 516.41.

Sterile Ophthalmic Ointment DECADRON® Phosphate (Dexamethasone Sodium Phosphate, MSD) is a topical steroid ointment containing dexamethasone sodium phosphate equivalent to 0.5 mg (0.05%) dexamethasone phosphate in each gram. Inactive ingredients: white petrolatum and mineral oil.

Dexamethasone sodium phosphate is an inorganic ester of dexamethasone.

Clinical Pharmacology

Dexamethasone sodium phosphate suppresses the inflammatory response to a variety of agents and it probably delays or slows healing. No generally accepted explanation of these steroid properties have been advanced.

Indications and Usage

For the treatment of the following conditions: Steroid responsive inflammatory conditions of the palpebral and bulbar conjunctiva, cornea, and anterior segment of the globe, such as allergic conjunctivitis, acne rosacea, superficial punctate keratitis, herpes zoster keratitis, iritis, cyclitis, selected infective conjunctivitis when the inherent hazard of steroid use is accepted to obtain an advisable diminution in edema and inflammation; corneal injury from chemical or thermal burns, or penetration of foreign bodies.

Contraindications

Epithelial herpes simplex keratitis (dendritic keratitis).

Acute infectious stages of vaccinia, varicella, and many other viral diseases of the cornea and conjunctiva.

Mycobacterial infection of the eye.

Fungal diseases of ocular structures.

Hypersensitivity to a component of the medication.

Warnings

Prolonged use may result in ocular hypertension and/or glaucoma, with damage to the optic nerve, defects in visual acuity and fields of vision, and posterior subcapsular cataract formation. Prolonged use may suppress the host response and thus increase the hazard of secondary ocular infections. In those diseases causing thinning of the cornea or sclera, perforations have been known to occur with the use of topical corticosteroids. In acute purulent conditions of the eye, corticosteroids may mask infection or enhance existing infection. If these products are used for 10 days or longer, intraocular pressure should be routinely monitored even though it may be difficult in children and uncooperative patients.

Employment of corticosteroid medication in the treatment of herpes simplex other than epithelial herpes simplex keratitis, in which it is contraindicated, requires great caution; periodic slit-lamp microscopy is essential.

Precautions

General

The possibility of persistent fungal infections of the cornea should be considered after prolonged corticosteroid dosing.

Carcinogenesis, Mutagenesis, Impairment of Fertility

Long-term animal studies have not been performed to evaluate the carcinogenic potential or the effect on fertility of Ophthalmic Ointment DECADRON Phosphate.

Pregnancy

Pregnancy Category C. Dexamethasone has been shown to be teratogenic in mice and rabbits following topical ophthalmic application in multiples of the therapeutic dose.

In the mouse, corticosteroids produce fetal resorptions and a specific abnormality, cleft palate. In the rabbit, corticosteroids have produced fetal resorptions and multiple abnormalities involving the head, ears, limbs, palate, etc.

There are no adequate or well-controlled studies in pregnant women. Ophthalmic Ointment DECADRON Phosphate should be used during pregnancy only if the potential benefit to the mother justifies the potential risk to the embryo or fetus. Infants born of mothers who have received substantial doses of corticosteroids during pregnancy should be observed carefully for signs of hypoadrenalism.

Nursing Mothers

Topically applied steroids are absorbed systemically. Therefore, because of the potential for serious adverse reactions in nursing infants from dexamethasone sodium phosphate, a decision should be made whether to discontinue nursing or discontinue the drug, taking into account the importance of the drug to the mother.

Pediatric Use

Safety and effectiveness in children have not been established.

Adverse Reactions

Glaucoma with optic nerve damage, visual acuity and field defects, posterior subcapsular cataract formation, secondary ocular infection from pathogens including herpes simplex, perforation of the globe.

Rarely, filtering blebs have been reported when topical steroids have been used following cataract surgery.

Rarely, stinging or burning may occur.

Dosage and Administration

The duration of treatment will vary with the type of lesion and may extend from a few days to several weeks, according to therapeutic response. Relapses, more common in chronic active lesions than in self-limited conditions, usually respond to retreatment.

Apply a thin coating of ointment three or four times a day. When a favorable response is observed, reduce the number of daily applications to two, and later to one a day as a maintenance dose if this is sufficient to control symptoms.

Ophthalmic Ointment DECADRON Phosphate is particularly convenient when an eye pad is used. It may also be the preparation of choice for patients in whom therapeutic benefit depends on prolonged contact of the active ingredients with ocular tissues.

How Supplied

No. 7615—0.05% Sterile Ophthalmic Ointment DECADRON Phosphate is a clear unctuous ointment and is supplied as follows:

NDC 0006-7615-04 in 3.5 g tubes
(6505-00-961-5508 0.05% 3.5 g).

A.H.F.S. Category: 52:08

DC 6033127 Issued July 1986

Shown in Product Identification Section, page 103

DECADRON® Phosphate ℞

(Dexamethasone Sodium Phosphate, MSD), U.S.P.
0.1% Dexamethasone Phosphate Equivalent
Sterile Ophthalmic Solution

Description

Dexamethasone sodium phosphate is 9-fluoro-11β, 17-dihydroxy-16α-methyl-21-(phosphonooxy)pregna-1,4-diene-3,20-dione disodium salt. Its empirical formula is $C_{22}H_{28}FNa_2O_8P$ and its structural formula is:

[structural formula]

Glucocorticoids are adrenocortical steroids, both naturally occurring and synthetic. Dexamethasone is a synthetic analog of naturally occurring glucocorticoids (hydrocortisone and cortisone). Dexamethasone sodium phosphate is a water soluble, inorganic ester of dexamethasone. It is approximately three thousand times more soluble in water at 25°C than hydrocortisone. Its molecular weight is 516.41.

Ophthalmic Solution DECADRON® Phosphate (Dexamethasone Sodium Phosphate, MSD) in the 5 mL OCUMETER® ophthalmic dispenser is a topical steroid solution containing dexamethasone sodium phosphate equivalent to 1 mg (0.1%) dexamethasone phosphate in each milliliter of buffered solution. Inactive ingredients: creatinine, sodium citrate, sodium borate, polysorbate 80, disodium edetate, hydrochloric acid to adjust pH, and water for injection. Sodium bisulfite 0.1%, phenylethanol 0.25% and benzalkonium chloride 0.02% added as preservatives.

Continued on next page

Information on the Merck Sharp & Dohme products listed on these pages is the full prescribing information from product circulars in effect August 31, 1991.

Merck Sharp & Dohme—Cont.

Clinical Pharmacology
Dexamethasone sodium phosphate suppresses the inflammatory response to a variety of agents and it probably delays or slows healing. No generally accepted explanation of these steroid properties have been advanced.
Indications and Usage
For the treatment of the following conditions:
Ophthalmic:
Steroid responsive inflammatory conditions of the palpebral and bulbar conjunctiva, cornea, and anterior segment of the globe, such as allergic conjunctivitis, acne rosacea, superficial punctate keratitis, herpes zoster keratitis, iritis, cyclitis, selected infective conjunctivitis when the inherent hazard of steroid use is accepted to obtain an advisable diminution in edema and inflammation; corneal injury from chemical or thermal burns, or penetration of foreign bodies.
Otic:
Steroid responsive inflammatory conditions of the external auditory meatus, such as allergic otitis externa, selected purulent and nonpurulent infective otitis externa when the hazard of steroid use is accepted to obtain an advisable diminution in edema and inflammation.
Contraindications
Epithelial herpes simplex keratitis (dendritic keratitis).
Acute infectious stages of vaccinia, varicella, and many other viral diseases of the cornea and conjunctiva.
Mycobacterial infection of the eye.
Fungal diseases of ocular or auricular structures.
Hypersensitivity to any component of this product, including sulfites (see WARNINGS).
Perforation of a drum membrane.
Warnings
Prolonged use may result in ocular hypertension and/or glaucoma, with damage to the optic nerve, defects in visual acuity and fields of vision, and posterior subcapsular cataract formation. Prolonged use may suppress the host response and thus increase the hazard of secondary ocular infections. In those diseases causing thinning of the cornea or sclera, perforations have been known to occur with the use of topical corticosteroids. In acute purulent conditions of the eye or ear, corticosteroids may mask infection or enhance existing infection. If these products are used for 10 days or longer, intraocular pressure should be routinely monitored even though it may be difficult in children and uncooperative patients.
Employment of corticosteroid medication in the treatment of herpes simplex other than epithelial herpes simplex keratitis, in which it is contraindicated, requires great caution; periodic slit-lamp microscopy is essential.
Ophthalmic Solution DECADRON Phosphate contains sodium bisulfite, a sulfite that may cause allergic-type reactions including anaphylactic symptoms and life-threatening or less severe asthmatic episodes in certain susceptible people. The overall prevalence of sulfite sensitivity in the general population is unknown and probably low. Sulfite sensitivity is seen more frequently in asthmatic than in nonasthmatic people.
Precautions
General
The possibility of persistent fungal infections of the cornea should be considered after prolonged corticosteroid dosing.
Carcinogenesis, Mutagenesis, Impairment of Fertility
Long-term animal studies have not been performed to evaluate the carcinogenic potential or the effect on fertility of Ophthalmic Solution DECADRON Phosphate.
Pregnancy
Pregnancy Category C. Dexamethasone has been shown to be teratogenic in mice and rabbits following topical ophthalmic application in multiples of the therapeutic dose.
In the mouse, corticosteroids produce fetal resorptions and a specific abnormality, cleft palate. In the rabbit, corticosteroids have produced fetal resorptions and multiple abnormalities involving the head, ears, limbs, palate, etc.
There are no adequate or well-controlled studies in pregnant women. Ophthalmic Solution DECADRON Phosphate should be used during pregnancy only if the potential benefit to the mother justifies the potential risk to the embryo or fetus. Infants born of mothers who have received substantial doses of corticosteroids during pregnancy should be observed carefully for signs of hypoadrenalism.
Nursing Mothers
Topically applied steroids are absorbed systemically. Therefore, because of the potential for serious adverse reactions in nursing infants from dexamethasone sodium phosphate, a decision should be made whether to discontinue nursing or discontinue the drug, taking into account the importance of the drug to the mother.
Pediatric Use
Safety and effectiveness in children have not been established.
Adverse Reactions
Glaucoma with optic nerve damage, visual acuity and field defects, posterior subcapsular cataract formation, secondary ocular infection from pathogens including herpes simplex, perforation of the globe.
Rarely, filtering blebs have been reported when topical steroids have been used following cataract surgery.
Rarely, stinging or burning may occur.
Dosage and Administration
The duration of treatment will vary with the type of lesion and may extend from a few days to several weeks, according to therapeutic response. Relapses, more common in chronic active lesions than in self-limited conditions, usually respond to retreatment.
Eye—Instill one or two drops of solution into the conjunctival sac every hour during the day and every two hours during the night as initial therapy. When a favorable response is observed, reduce dosage to one drop every four hours. Later, further reduction in dosage to one drop three or four times daily may suffice to control symptoms.
Ear—Clean the aural canal thoroughly and sponge dry. Instill the solution directly into the aural canal. A suggested initial dosage is three or four drops two or three times a day. When a favorable response is obtained, reduce dosage gradually and eventually discontinue.
If preferred, the aural canal may be packed with a gauze wick saturated with solution. Keep the wick moist with the preparation and remove from the ear after 12 to 24 hours. Treatment may be repeated as often as necessary at the discretion of the physician.
How Supplied
Sterile Ophthalmic Solution DECADRON Phosphate is a clear, colorless to pale yellow solution.
No. 7643—Ophthalmic Solution DECADRON Phosphate is supplied as follows:
NDC 0006-7643-03 in 5 mL white, opaque, plastic OCUMETER ophthalmic dispenser with a controlled drop tip.
(6505-00-007-4536 0.1% 5 mL)
A.H.F.S. Category: 52:08
DC 7261515 Issued February 1987
Shown in Product Identification Section, page 103

FLOROPRYL® ℞
(Isoflurophate, MSD), U.S.P.
Sterile Ophthalmic Ointment
For Topical Application into the Conjunctival Sac Only

Description
FLOROPRYL® (Isoflurophate, MSD) is available as 0.025% sterile ophthalmic ointment in polyethylene mineral oil gel. Isoflurophate has a molecular weight of 184.15 and is known chemically as bis (1-methylethyl) phosphorofluoridate. Its empirical formula is $C_6H_{14}FO_3P$ and its structural formula is:

$$(CH_3)_2CH{-}O{-}\overset{\overset{\displaystyle F}{|}}{\underset{\underset{\displaystyle O}{\|}}{P}}{-}O{-}CH(CH_3)_2$$

Clinical Pharmacology
FLOROPRYL is a cholinesterase inhibitor with sustained activity. Application to the eye produces intense miosis and ciliary muscle contraction due to inhibition of cholinesterase, allowing acetylcholine to accumulate at sites of cholinergic transmission.
FLOROPRYL *irreversibly* inactivates cholinesterase. Thus, following use of FLOROPRYL in the eye, cholinesterase must be either regenerated or supplied from depots elsewhere in the body before ophthalmic action dependent on cholinesterase returns.
If given systemically in sufficient amounts, FLOROPRYL reduces plasma cholinesterase to zero. However, when applied locally to the eye, plasma cholinesterase is usually reduced only slightly.
Indications and Usage
Open-angle glaucoma (FLOROPRYL should be used in glaucoma only when shorter-acting miotics have proved inadequate.)
Conditions obstructing aqueous outflow, such as synechial formation, that are amenable to miotic therapy
Following iridectomy
Accommodative esotropia (accommodative convergent strabismus)
Contraindications
Hypersensitivity to any component of this product.
Because of the toxicity of cholinesterase inhibitors in general, FLOROPRYL is contraindicated in women who are or who may become pregnant. If this drug is used during pregnancy, or if the patient becomes pregnant while taking this drug, the patient should be apprised of the potential hazard to the fetus.
Because miotics may aggravate inflammation, FLOROPRYL should not be used in active uveal inflammation and/or glaucoma associated with iridocyclitis.
Warnings
In patients receiving cholinesterase inhibitors such as FLOROPRYL, succinylcholine should be administered with extreme caution before and during general anesthesia because of possible respiratory and cardiovascular collapse.
Because of possible adverse additive effects, FLOROPRYL should be administered only with extreme caution to patients with myasthenia gravis who are receiving systemic anticholinesterase therapy; conversely, extreme caution should be exercised in the use of an anticholinesterase drug for the treatment of myasthenia gravis patients who are already undergoing topical therapy with cholinesterase inhibitors.
Precautions
General
FLOROPRYL should be used with caution in patients with chronic angle-closure (narrow-angle) glaucoma or in patients with narrow angles, because of the possibility of producing pupillary block and increasing angle blockage. Gonioscopy is recommended prior to medication with FLOROPRYL.

When an intraocular inflammatory process is present, the intensity and persistence of miosis and ciliary muscle contraction that result from anticholinesterase therapy require abstention from, or cautious use of, FLOROPRYL.
Systemic effects are infrequent when FLOROPRYL is applied carefully. The hands should be washed immediately following application.
Discontinue FLOROPRYL if salivation, urinary incontinence, diarrhea, profuse sweating, muscle weakness, respiratory difficulties, shock, or cardiac irregularities occur.
Persons receiving cholinesterase inhibitors who are exposed to organophosphate-type insecticides and pesticides (gardeners, organophosphate plant or warehouse workers, farmers, residents of communities which are undergoing insecticide spraying or dusting, etc.) should be warned of the added systemic effects possible from absorption through the respiratory tract or skin. Wearing of respiratory masks, frequent washing, and clothing changes may be advisable.
Anticholinesterase drugs should be used with extreme caution, if at all, in patients with marked vagotonia, bronchial asthma, spastic gastrointestinal disturbances, peptic ulcer, pronounced bradycardia and hypotension, recent myocardial infarction, epilepsy, parkinsonism, and other disorders that may respond adversely to vagotonic effects.
After long-term use of FLOROPRYL, dilation of blood vessels and resulting greater permeability increase the possibility of hyphema during ophthalmic surgery. Therefore, this drug should be discontinued before surgery.
Despite observance of all precautions and the use of only the recommended dose, there is some evidence that repeated administration may cause depression of the concentration of cholinesterase in the serum and erythrocytes, with resultant systemic effects.

Drug Interactions

See WARNINGS regarding possible drug interactions of FLOROPRYL with succinylcholine or with other anticholinesterase agents.

Carcinogenesis, Mutagenesis, Impairment of Fertility

Long-term studies in animals have not been performed to evaluate the effects of FLOROPRYL on fertility or carcinogenic potential.

Pregnancy

Pregnancy Category X: See CONTRAINDICATIONS.

Nursing Mothers

It is not known whether this drug is excreted in human milk. Because of the potential for serious adverse reactions in nursing infants from FLOROPRYL, a decision should be made whether to discontinue nursing or to discontinue the drug, taking into account the importance of the drug to the mother.

Pediatric Use

The occurrence of iris cysts is more frequent in children. (See ADVERSE REACTIONS and DOSAGE AND ADMINISTRATION.)
Extreme caution should be exercised in children receiving FLOROPRYL who may require general anesthesia (see WARNINGS).
Since FLOROPRYL is a potent cholinesterase inhibitor it should be kept out of the reach of children.

Adverse Reactions

Stinging, burning, lacrimation, lid muscle twitching, conjunctival and ciliary redness, brow ache, headache, and induced myopia with visual blurring may occur.
As with all miotic therapy, retinal detachment has been reported occasionally.
Activation of latent iritis or uveitis may occur.
Iris cysts may form, enlarge, and obscure vision. Occurrence is more frequent in children. The iris cyst usually shrinks upon discontinuance of the miotic. Rarely, the cyst may rupture or break free into the aqueous. Frequent examination for this occurrence is advised.
Prolonged use may cause conjunctival thickening and obstruction of nasolacrimal canals.
Systemic effects, which occur rarely, are suggestive of increased cholinergic activity. Such effects may include nausea, vomiting, abdominal cramps, diarrhea, urinary incontinence, salivation, sweating, difficulty in breathing, bradycardia, or cardiac irregularities. Medical management of systemic effects may be indicated (see TREATMENT OF ADVERSE EFFECTS).
Lens opacities have been reported in patients on miotic therapy. Routine slit-lamp examinations, including the lens, should accompany prolonged use.
Paradoxical increase in intraocular pressure may follow anticholinesterase application. This may be alleviated by pupil-dilating medication.

Treatment of Adverse Effects

If FLOROPRYL is taken systemically by accident, or if systemic effects occur after topical application in the eye or from accidental skin contact, atropine sulfate in a dose (for adults) of 0.4 to 0.6 mg or more should be given parenterally (intravenously if necessary). The recommended dosage of atropine in infants and children up to 12 years of age is 0.01 mg/kg repeated every two hours as needed until the desired effect is obtained, or adverse effects of atropine preclude further usage. The maximum single dose should not exceed 0.4 mg.
The use of much larger doses of atropine in treating anticholinesterase intoxication in adults has been reported in the literature. Initially 2 to 6 mg may be given followed by 2 mg every hour or more often, as long as muscarinic effects continue. The greater possibility of atropinization with large doses, particularly in sensitive individuals, should be borne in mind.
Pralidoxime* chloride has been reported to be useful in treatment of systemic effects due to cholinesterase inhibitors. However, its use is recommended in addition to and not as a substitute for atropine.
A short-acting barbiturate is indicated if convulsions occur that are not entirely relieved by atropine. Barbiturate dosage should be carefully adjusted to avoid central respiratory depression. Marked weakness or paralysis of muscles of respiration should be treated promptly by artificial respiration and maintenance of a clear airway.
The oral LD_{50} of FLOROPRYL is 37 mg/kg in the mouse, 5–10 mg/kg in the rat, and 4–10 mg/kg in the rabbit.

Dosage and Administration

FLOROPRYL *is intended solely for topical use in the conjunctival sac.*
Isoflurophate hydrolyzes in the presence of water to form hydrofluoric acid. To prevent absorption of moisture and loss of potency, the ointment tube should be kept tightly closed; the tip of the tube should not be washed or allowed to touch the eyelid or other moist surface.
Whenever possible, FLOROPRYL should be applied at night before retiring to lessen blurring of vision. As it is an extremely potent drug, it should be used with great care and only by those familiar with its use and thoroughly indoctrinated in the technic of application.
The required dose is applied in the conjunctival sac, with the patient supine, care being taken not to touch the cornea with the tip of the tube. *Wash the hands immediately after administration.*
FLOROPRYL *should not be used more often than directed. Caution is necessary to avoid overdosage.*
Keep frequency of use to a minimum in all patients, but especially in children, to reduce the chance of iris cyst development (see ADVERSE REACTIONS). If tolerance develops, another miotic should be used. FLOROPRYL may be resumed later.

Glaucoma

For initial therapy ¼ inch strip of ophthalmic ointment FLOROPRYL 0.025 per cent is placed in the glaucomatous eye every 8 to 72 hours. A decrease in intraocular pressure should occur within a few hours. During this period, keep the patient under supervision and make tonometric examinations at least hourly for 3 or 4 hours to be sure that no immediate rise in pressure occurs (see ADVERSE REACTIONS).

Strabismus

Essentially equal visual acuity of both eyes is a prerequisite to successful treatment. For initial evaluation FLOROPRYL may be used as a diagnostic aid to determine if an accommodative factor exists. This is especially useful preoperatively in young children and in patients with normal hypermetropic refractive errors.
Not more than ¼ inch strip of ointment is administered every night for 2 weeks. If the eyes become straighter, an accommodative factor is demonstrated. This technic may supplement or complement standard testing with atropine and trial with glasses for the accommodative factor.
In esotropia uncomplicated by amblyopia or anisometropia, ophthalmic ointment FLOROPRYL may be used in both eyes, not more than ¼ inch strip at a time every night for 2 weeks, as too severe a degree of miosis may interfere with vision. The dosage is then reduced to from ¼ inch strip every other day to ¼ inch strip once a week for 2 months, after which the patient's status should be re-evaluated.
If benefit can not be maintained with a dosage interval of at least 48 hours, therapy with FLOROPRYL should be stopped. Frequency of administration and duration of maintenance therapy depend on how long the eyes remain straight without medication. Intervals between administration should be gradually increased to the greatest length compatible with good results. Therapy may need to be continued for many years in some patients; in others, it has been possible to discontinue therapy after several months.

How Supplied

No. 7742—Sterile ophthalmic ointment FLOROPRYL 0.025 per cent is an opaque white, smooth, unctuous ointment and is supplied as follows:
NDC 0006-7742-04 in a 3.5 g tube.

Storage

Protect from moisture, freezing and excessive heat.

A.H.F.S. Category: 52:20
DC 7413720 Issued October 1987

*PROTOPAM® Chloride (Pralidoxime Chloride), Ayerst Laboratories.

Shown in Product Identification Section, page 103

HUMORSOL® ℞

(Demecarium Bromide, MSD), U.S.P.
Sterile Ophthalmic Solution
For Topical Application into the Conjunctival Sac Only

Description

Ophthalmic Solution HUMORSOL® (Demecarium Bromide, MSD) is a sterile solution supplied in two dosage strengths: 0.125 percent and 0.25 percent. The inactive ingredients are sodium chloride and water for injection; benz-

Continued on next page

Information on the Merck Sharp & Dohme products listed on these pages is the full prescribing information from product circulars in effect August 31, 1991.

Merck Sharp & Dohme—Cont.

alkonium chloride 1:5000 is added as preservative. Demecarium bromide is a quaternary ammonium compound with a molecular weight of 716.60. Its chemical name is 3,3'-[1,10-decanediylbis [(methylimino)carbonyloxy]] bis [*N,N,N*-trimethylbenzenaminium] dibromide. Its empirical formula is $C_{32}H_{52}Br_2N_4O_4$ and its structural formula is:

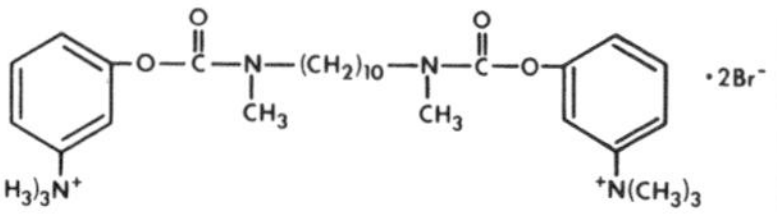

Clinical Pharmacology

HUMORSOL is a cholinesterase inhibitor with sustained activity. It acts mainly on true (erythrocyte) cholinesterase. Application of HUMORSOL to the eye produces intense miosis and ciliary muscle contraction due to inhibition of cholinesterase, allowing acetylcholine to accumulate at sites of cholinergic transmission. These effects are accompanied by increased capillary permeability of the ciliary body and iris, increased permeability of the blood-aqueous barrier, and vasodilation. Myopia may be induced or, if present, may be augmented by the increased refractive power of the lens that results from the accommodative effect of the drug. HUMORSOL indirectly produces some of the muscarinic and nicotinic effects of acetylcholine as quantities of the latter accumulate.

Indications and Usage

Open-angle glaucoma (HUMORSOL should be used in glaucoma only when shorter-acting miotics have proved inadequate).

Conditions obstructing aqueous outflow, such as synechial formation, that are amenable to miotic therapy

Following iridectomy

Accommodative esotropia (accommodative convergent strabismus)

Contraindications

Hypersensitivity to any component of this product.

Because of the toxicity of cholinesterase inhibitors in general, HUMORSOL is contraindicated in women who are or who may become pregnant. If this drug is used during pregnancy, or if the patient becomes pregnant while taking this drug, the patient should be apprised of the potential hazard to the fetus.

Because miotics may aggravate inflammation, HUMORSOL should not be used in active uveal inflammation and/or glaucoma associated with iridocyclitis.

Warnings

In patients receiving cholinesterase inhibitors such as HUMORSOL, succinylcholine should be administered with extreme caution before and during general anesthesia.

Because of possible adverse additive effects, HUMORSOL should be administered only with extreme caution to patients with myasthenia gravis who are receiving systemic anticholinesterase therapy; conversely, extreme caution should be exercised in the use of an anticholinesterase drug for the treatment of myasthenia gravis patients who are already undergoing topical therapy with cholinesterase inhibitors.

Precautions

General

Gonioscopy is recommended prior to medication with HUMORSOL.

HUMORSOL should be used with caution in patients with chronic angle-closure (narrow-angle) glaucoma or in patients with narrow angles, because of the possibility of producing pupillary block and increasing angle blockage.

When an intraocular inflammatory process is present, the intensity and persistence of miosis and ciliary muscle contraction that result from anticholinesterase therapy require abstention from, or cautious use of, HUMORSOL.

Systemic effects are infrequent when HUMORSOL is instilled carefully. Compression of the lacrimal duct for several seconds immediately following instillation minimizes drainage into the nasal chamber with its extensive absorption surface. Wash the hands immediately after instillation.

Discontinue HUMORSOL if salivation, urinary incontinence, diarrhea, profuse sweating, muscle weakness, respiratory difficulties, shock, or cardiac irregularities occur.

Persons receiving cholinesterase inhibitors who are exposed to organophosphate-type insecticides and pesticides (gardeners, organophosphate plant or warehouse workers, farmers, residents of communities which are undergoing insecticide spraying or dusting, etc.) should be warned of the added systemic effects possible from absorption through the respiratory tract or skin. Wearing of respiratory masks, frequent washing, and clothing changes may be advisable.

Anticholinesterase drugs should be used with extreme caution, if at all, in patients with marked vagotonia, bronchial asthma, spastic gastrointestinal disturbances, peptic ulcer, pronounced bradycardia and hypotension, recent myocardial infarction, epilepsy, parkinsonism, and other disorders that may respond adversely to vagotonic effects.

After long-term use of HUMORSOL, dilation of blood vessels and resulting greater permeability increase the possibility of hyphema during ophthalmic surgery. Therefore, this drug should be discontinued before surgery.

Despite observance of all precautions and the use of only the recommended dose, there is some evidence that repeated administration may cause depression of the concentration of cholinesterase in the serum and erythrocytes, with resultant systemic effects.

Drug Interactions

See WARNINGS regarding possible drug interactions of HUMORSOL with succinylcholine or with other anticholinesterase agents.

Carcinogenesis, Mutagenesis, Impairment of Fertility

Long-term studies in animals have not been performed to evaluate the effects of HUMORSOL on fertility or carcinogenic potential.

Pregnancy

Pregnancy Category X: See CONTRAINDICATIONS.

Nursing Mothers

It is not known whether this drug is excreted in human milk. Because of the potential for serious adverse reactions in nursing infants from HUMORSOL, a decision should be made whether to discontinue nursing or to discontinue the drug, taking into account the importance of the drug to the mother.

Pediatric Use

The occurrence of iris cysts is more frequent in children. (See ADVERSE REACTIONS and DOSAGE AND ADMINISTRATION.)

Extreme caution should be exercised in children receiving HUMORSOL who may require general anesthesia (see WARNINGS).

Since HUMORSOL is a potent cholinesterase inhibitor it should be kept out of the reach of children.

Adverse Reactions

Stinging, burning, lacrimation, lid muscle twitching, conjunctival and ciliary redness, brow ache, headache, and induced myopia with visual blurring may occur.

Activation of latent iritis or uveitis may occur.

As with all miotic therapy, retinal detachment has been reported occasionally.

Iris cysts may form, enlarge, and obscure vision. Occurrence is more frequent in children. The iris cyst usually shrinks upon discontinuance of the miotic. Rarely, the cyst may rupture or break free into the aqueous. Frequent examination for this occurrence is advised.

Lens opacities have been reported in patients on miotic therapy. Routine slit-lamp examinations, including the lens, should accompany prolonged use.

Paradoxical increase in intraocular pressure may follow anticholinesterase instillation. This may be alleviated by pupil-dilating medication.

Prolonged use may cause conjunctival thickening and obstruction of nasolacrimal canals.

Systemic effects, which occur rarely, are suggestive of increased cholinergic activity. Such effects may include nausea, vomiting, abdominal cramps, diarrhea, urinary incontinence, salivation, sweating, difficulty in breathing, bradycardia, or cardiac irregularities. Medical management of systemic effects may be indicated (see TREATMENT OF ADVERSE EFFECTS).

Treatment of Adverse Effects

If HUMORSOL is taken systemically by accident, or if systemic effects occur after topical application in the eye or from accidental skin contact, administer atropine sulfate parenterally (intravenously if necessary) in a dose (for adults) of 0.4 to 0.6 mg or more. The recommended dosage of atropine in infants and children up to 12 years of age is 0.01 mg/kg repeated every two hours as needed until the desired effect is obtained, or adverse effects of atropine preclude further usage. The maximum single dose should not exceed 0.4 mg.

The use of much larger doses of atropine in treating anticholinesterase intoxication in adults has been reported in the literature. Initially 2 to 6 mg may be given followed by 2 mg every hour or more often, as long as muscarinic effects continue. The greater possibility of atropinization with large doses, particularly in sensitive individuals, should be borne in mind.

Pralidoxime* chloride has been reported to be useful in treating systemic effects due to cholinesterase inhibitors. However, its use is recommended in addition to and not as a substitute for atropine.

A short-acting barbiturate is indicated if convulsions occur that are not entirely relieved by atropine. Barbiturate dosage should be carefully adjusted to avoid central respiratory depression. Marked weakness or paralysis of muscles of respiration should be treated promptly by artificial respiration and maintenance of a clear airway.

The oral LD_{50} of HUMORSOL is 2.96 mg/kg in the mouse.

Dosage and Administration

HUMORSOL *is intended solely for topical use in the conjunctival sac.*

As HUMORSOL is an extremely potent drug, the physician should thoroughly familiarize himself with its use and the technic of instillation.

The required dose is applied in the conjunctival sac, with the patient supine, care being taken not to touch the cornea with the tip of the OCUMETER® ophthalmic dispenser. *The patient or person administering the medication should apply continuous gentle pressure on the lacrimal duct with the index finger for several seconds immediately following instillation of the drops. This is to prevent drainage overflow of solution into the nasal and pharyngeal spaces, which might cause systemic absorption. Wash the hands immediately after administration.* HUMORSOL *should not be used more often than directed. Caution is necessary to avoid overdosage.*

Initial titration and dosage adjustments with HUMORSOL must be individualized to obtain maximal therapeutic effect. The patient must be closely observed during the initial period. If the response is not adequate within the first 24 hours, other measures should be considered. Keep frequency of use to a minimum in all patients, but especially in children, to reduce the chance of iris cyst development (see ADVERSE REACTIONS).

Glaucoma

For initial therapy with HUMORSOL (0.125 percent or 0.25 percent) place 1 drop (children) or 1 or 2 drops (adults) in the glaucomatous eye. A decrease in intraocular pressure should occur within a few hours. During this period, keep the patient under supervision and make tonometric examinations at least hourly for 3 or 4 hours to be sure that no immediate rise in pressure occurs (see ADVERSE REACTIONS). Duration of effect varies with the individual. The usual dosage can vary from as much as 1 or 2 drops twice a day to as little as 1 or 2 drops twice a week. The 0.125 percent strength used twice a day usually results in smooth control of the physiologic diurnal variation in intraocular pressure. This is probably the preferred dosage for most wide (open) angle glaucoma patients.

Strabismus

Essentially equal visual acuity of both eyes is a prerequisite to the successful treatment of esotropia with HUMORSOL. For initial evaluation it may be used as a diagnostic aid to determine if an accommodative factor exists. This is especially useful preoperatively in young children and in patients with normal hypermetropic refractive errors. One drop is given daily for 2 weeks, then 1 drop every 2 days for 2 to 3 weeks. If the eyes become straighter, an accommodative factor is demonstrated. This technic may supplement or complement standard testing with atropine and trial with glasses for the accommodative factor.

In esotropia uncomplicated by amblyopia or anisometropia, HUMORSOL may be instilled in both eyes, *not more than 1 drop at a time every day for 2 to 3 weeks,* as too severe a degree of miosis may interfere with vision. Then reduce the dosage to 1 drop every other day for 3 to 4 weeks and reevaluate the patient's status. HUMORSOL may be continued in a dosage of 1 drop every 2 days to 1 drop twice a week. (The latter dosage may be maintained for several months.) Evaluate the patient's condition every 4 to 12 weeks. If improvement continues, change the schedule to 1 drop once a week and eventually to a trial without medication. However, if after 4 months, control of the condition still requires 1 drop every 2 days, therapy with HUMORSOL should be stopped.

How Supplied

Sterile Ophthalmic Solution HUMORSOL is a clear, colorless, aqueous solution and is supplied in a 5 mL white, opaque, plastic OCUMETER ophthalmic dispenser with a controlled-drop tip:

No. 3255—0.125 percent solution.
NDC 0006-3255-03.

No. 3267—0.25 percent solution.
NDC 0006-3267-03.

Storage

Protect from freezing and excessive heat.

A.H.F.S. Category: 52:20

DC 7414311 Issued October 1987

*PROTOPAM® Chloride (Pralidoxime Chloride), Ayerst Laboratories

Shown in Product Identification Section, page 103

LACRISERT® Sterile Ophthalmic Insert ℞
(Hydroxypropyl Cellulose, MSD)

Description: LACRISERT® (Hydroxypropyl Cellulose, MSD) is a sterile, translucent, rod-shaped, water soluble, ophthalmic insert made of hydroxypropyl cellulose, for administration into the inferior cul-de-sac of the eye. The chemical name for hydroxypropyl cellulose is cellulose, 2-hydroxypropyl ether. It is an ether of cellulose in which hydroxypropyl groups ($-CH_2CHOHCH_3$) are attached to the hydroxyls present in the anhydroglucose rings of cellulose by ether linkages. A representative structure of the monomer is:

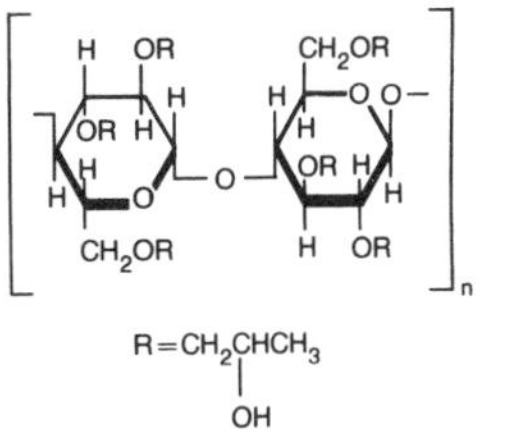

[Structure: anhydroglucose dimer with OR and CH_2OR substituents, repeating unit $]_n$]

$R = CH_2CHCH_3$ (with OH on the central carbon)

The molecular weight is typically 1×10^6. Hydroxypropyl cellulose is an off-white, odorless, tasteless powder. It is soluble in water below 38°C, and in many polar organic solvents such as ethanol, propylene glycol, dioxane, methanol, isopropyl alcohol (95%), dimethyl sulfoxide, and dimethyl formamide.

Each LACRISERT is 5 mg of hydroxypropyl cellulose. LACRISERT contains no preservatives or other ingredients. It is about 1.27 mm in diameter by about 3.5 mm long.

LACRISERT is supplied in packages of 60 units, together with illustrated instructions and a special applicator for removing LACRISERT from the unit dose blister and inserting it into the eye. A spare applicator is included in each package.

Clinical Pharmacology

Pharmacodynamics

LACRISERT acts to stabilize and thicken the precorneal tear film and prolong the tear film breakup time which is usually accelerated in patients with dry eye states. LACRISERT also acts to lubricate and protect the eye.

LACRISERT usually reduces the signs and symptoms resulting from moderate to severe dry eye syndromes, such as conjunctival hyperemia, corneal and conjunctival staining with rose bengal, exudation, itching, burning, foreign body sensation, smarting, photophobia, dryness and blurred or cloudy vision. Progressive visual deterioration which occurs in some patients may be retarded, halted, or sometimes reversed.

In a multicenter crossover study the 5 mg LACRISERT administered once a day during the waking hours was compared to artificial tears used four or more times daily. There was a prolongation of tear film breakup time and a decrease in foreign body sensation associated with dry eye syndrome in patients during treatment with inserts as compared to artificial tears; these findings were statistically significantly different between the treatment groups. Improvement, as measured by amelioration of symptoms, by slit lamp examination and by rose bengal staining of the cornea and conjunctiva, was greater in most patients with moderate to severe symptoms during treatment with LACRISERT. Patient comfort was usually better with LACRISERT than with artificial tears solution, and most patients preferred LACRISERT.

In most patients treated with LACRISERT for over one year, improvement was observed as evidenced by amelioration of symptoms generally associated with keratoconjunctivitis sicca such as burning, tearing, foreign body sensation, itching, photophobia and blurred or cloudy vision.

During studies in healthy volunteers, a thickened precorneal tear film was usually observed through the slit-lamp while LACRISERT was present in the conjunctival sac.

Pharmacokinetics and Metabolism

Hydroxypropyl cellulose is a physiologically inert substance. In a study of rats fed hydroxypropyl cellulose or unmodified cellulose at levels up to 5% of their diet, it was found that the two were biologically equivalent in that neither was metabolized.

Studies conducted in rats fed ^{14}C-labeled hydroxypropyl cellulose demonstrated that when orally administered, hydroxypropyl cellulose is not absorbed from the gastrointestinal tract and is quantitatively excreted in the feces.

Dissolution studies in rabbits showed that hydroxypropyl cellulose inserts became softer within 1 hour after they were placed in the conjunctival sac. Most of the inserts dissolved completely in 14 to 18 hours; with a single exception, all had disappeared by 24 hours after insertion. Similar dissolution of the inserts was observed during prolonged administration (up to 54 weeks).

Indications and Usage: LACRISERT is indicated in patients with moderate to severe dry eye syndromes, including keratoconjunctivitis sicca. LACRISERT is indicated especially in patients who remain symptomatic after an adequate trial of therapy with artifical tear solutions.

LACRISERT is also indicated for patients with:

Exposure keratitis
Decreased corneal sensitivity
Recurrent corneal erosions

Contraindications: LACRISERT is contraindicated in patients who are hypersensitive to hydroxypropyl cellulose.

Warnings: Instructions for inserting and removing LACRISERT should be carefully followed.

Precautions

General

If improperly placed, LACRISERT may result in corneal abrasion (see DOSAGE AND ADMINISTRATION).

Information for Patients

Patients should be advised to follow the instructions for using LACRISERT which accompany the package.

Because this product may produce transient blurring of vision, patients should be instructed to exercise caution when operating hazardous machinery or driving a motor vehicle.

Drug Interactions

Application of hydroxypropyl cellulose inserts to the eyes of unanesthetized rabbits immediately prior to or two hours before instilling pilocarpine, proparacaine HCl (0.5%), or phenylephrine (5%) did not markedly alter the magnitude and/or duration of the miotic, local corneal anesthetic, or mydriatic activity, respectively, of these agents.

Under various treatment schedules, the antiinflammatory effect of ocularly instilled dexamethasone (0.1%) in unanesthetized rabbits with primary uveitis was not affected by the presence of hydroxypropyl cellulose inserts.

Carcinogenesis, Mutagenesis, Impairment of Fertility

Feeding of hydroxypropyl cellulose to rats at levels up to 5% of their diet produced no gross or histopathologic changes or other deleterious effects.

Adverse Reactions: The following adverse reactions have been reported in patients

Continued on next page

Information on the Merck Sharp & Dohme products listed on these pages is the full prescribing information from product circulars in effect August 31, 1991.

Merck Sharp & Dohme—Cont.

treated with LACRISERT, but were in most instances mild and transient:

Transient blurring of vision
(See PRECAUTIONS)
Ocular discomfort or irritation
Matting or stickiness of eyelashes
Photophobia
Hypersensitivity
Edema of the eyelids
Hyperemia

Dosage and Administration: One LACRISERT ophthalmic insert in each eye once daily is usually sufficient to relieve the symptoms associated with moderate to severe dry eye syndromes. Individual patients may require more flexibility in the use of LACRISERT; some patients may require twice daily use for optimal results.

Clinical experience with LACRISERT indicates that in some patients several weeks may be required before satisfactory improvement of symptoms is achieved.

LACRISERT is inserted into the inferior cul-de-sac of the eye beneath the base of the tarsus, not in apposition to the cornea, nor beneath the eyelid at the level of the tarsal plate. If not properly positioned, it will be expelled into the interpalpebral fissure, and may cause symptoms of a foreign body. Illustrated instructions are included in each package. While in the licensed practitioner's office, the patient should read the instructions, then practice insertion and removal of LACRISERT until proficiency is achieved.

NOTE: Occasionally LACRISERT is inadvertently expelled from the eye, especially in patients with shallow conjunctival fornices. The patient should be cautioned against rubbing the eye(s) containing LACRISERT, especially upon awakening, so as not to dislodge or expel the insert. If required, another LACRISERT ophthalmic insert may be inserted. If experience indicates that transient blurred vision develops in an individual patient, the patient may want to remove LACRISERT a few hours after insertion to avoid this. Another LACRISERT ophthalmic insert may be inserted if needed.

If LACRISERT causes worsening of symptoms, the patient should be instructed to inspect the conjunctival sac to make certain LACRISERT is in the proper location, deep in the inferior cul-de-sac of the eye beneath the base of the tarsus. If these symptoms persist, LACRISERT should be removed and the patient should contact the practitioner.

How Supplied

No. 3380—LACRISERT, a sterile, translucent, rod-shaped, water soluble, ophthalmic insert made of hydroxypropyl cellulose, 5 mg, is supplied as follows:

NDC 0006-3380-60 in packages containing 60 unit doses, two reusable applicators and a storage container
(6505-01-153-4360, 5 mg 60's).

Storage

Store below 30°C (86°F).

DC 7415108 Issued August 1989

Shown in Product Identification Section, page 104

NEODECADRON® ℞

(Neomycin Sulfate-Dexamethasone Sodium Phosphate, MSD), U.S.P.
Sterile Ophthalmic Ointment

Description

Sterile ophthalmic ointment NEODECADRON® (Neomycin Sulfate-Dexamethasone Sodium Phosphate, MSD) is a topical corticosteroid-antibiotic ointment for use in certain disorders of the anterior segment of the eye.

Ophthalmic ointment NEODECADRON contains in each gram: dexamethasone sodium phosphate equivalent to 0.5 mg (0.05%) dexamethasone phosphate and neomycin sulfate equivalent to 3.5 mg neomycin base. Inactive ingredients: white petrolatum and mineral oil.

Dexamethasone sodium phosphate is an inorganic ester of dexamethasone. Its empirical formula is $C_{22}H_{28}FNa_2O_8P$.

Neomycin sulfate is the sulfate salt of neomycin, an antibacterial substance produced by the growth of *Streptomyces fradiae* Waksman (Fam. Streptomycetaceae).

Clinical Pharmacology

Dexamethasone sodium phosphate, a corticosteroid, suppresses the inflammatory response to a variety of agents, and it probably delays or slows healing. Since corticosteroids may inhibit the body's defense mechanism against infection, a concomitant antimicrobial drug may be used when this inhibition is considered to be clinically significant in a particular case.

Neomycin sulfate, the anti-infective component in the combination, is included to provide action against specific organisms susceptible to it. Neomycin sulfate is considered active mainly against gram-negative organisms, except *Bacteroides* spp. and *Pseudomonas aeruginosa*, which are resistant. Gram-positive organisms except for *Staphylococcus aureus* are usually resistant.

When a decision to administer both a corticosteroid and an antimicrobial is made, the administration of such drugs in combination has the advantage of greater patient compliance and convenience, with the added assurance that the appropriate dosage of both drugs is administered, plus assured compatibility of ingredient when both types of drug are in the same formulation and, particularly, that the correct volume of drug is delivered and retained.

The relative potency of corticosteroids depends on the molecular structure, concentration, and release from the vehicle.

Indications and Usage

For steroid-responsive inflammatory ocular conditions for which a corticosteroid is indicated and where bacterial infection or a risk of bacterial ocular infection exists.

Ocular steroids are indicated in inflammatory conditions of the palpebral and bulbar conjunctiva, cornea, and anterior segment of the globe where the inherent risk of steroid use in certain infective conjunctivitides is accepted to obtain a diminution in edema and inflammation. They are also indicated in chronic anterior uveitis and corneal injury from chemical, radiation, or thermal burns, or penetration of foreign bodies.

The use of a combination drug with an anti-infective component is indicated where the risk of infection is high or where there is an expectation that potentially dangerous numbers of bacteria will be present in the eye.

The particular anti-infective drug in this product is active against the following common bacterial eye pathogens:

Staphylococcus aureus
Escherichia coli
Haemophilus influenzae
Klebsiella/Enterobacter species
Neisseria species

The product does not provide adequate coverage against:

Pseudomonas aeruginosa
Serratia marcescens
Streptococci, including *Streptococcus pneumoniae*

Contraindications

Epithelial herpes simplex keratitis (dendritic keratitis), acute infectious stages of vaccinia, varicella, and many other viral diseases of the cornea and conjunctiva. Mycobacterial infection of the eye. Fungal diseases of ocular structures. Hypersensitivity to a component of the medication (hypersensitivity to the antibiotic component occurs at a higher rate than for other components).

The use of these combinations is always contraindicated after uncomplicated removal of a corneal foreign body.

Warnings

Prolonged use may result in glaucoma, with damage to the optic nerve, defects in visual acuity and fields of vision, and posterior subcapsular cataract formation. Prolonged use may suppress the host response and thus increase the hazard of secondary ocular infections. In those diseases causing thinning of the cornea or sclera, perforations have been known to occur with the use of topical corticosteroids. In acute purulent conditions of the eye, corticosteroids may mask infection or enhance existing infection. If these products are used for 10 days or longer, intraocular pressure should be routinely monitored even though it may be difficult in children and uncooperative patients.

Employment of corticosteroid medication in the treatment of herpes simplex requires great caution: periodic slit-lamp microscopy is recommended.

Any substance (e.g. neomycin sulfate) may occasionally cause cutaneous sensitization. If any reaction indicating such sensitivity is observed, discontinue use.

Precautions

The initial prescriptions and renewal of the medication order beyond 8 grams should be made by a physician only after examination of the patient with the aid of magnification, such as slit-lamp biomicroscopy and, where appropriate, fluorescein staining.

The possibility of persistent fungal infections of the cornea should be considered after prolonged corticosteroid dosing.

Usage in Pregnancy

Safety of intensive or protracted use of topical corticosteroids during pregnancy has not been substantiated.

Adverse Reactions

Adverse reactions have occurred with corticosteroid/anti-infective combination drugs which can be attributed to the corticosteroid component, the anti-infective component, or the combination. Exact incidence figures are not available since no denominator of treated patients is available.

Reactions occurring most often from the presence of the anti-infective ingredient are allergic sensitizations. The reactions due to the corticosteroid component in decreasing order of frequency are: elevation of intraocular pressure (IOP) with possible development of glaucoma, and infrequent optic nerve damage; posterior subcapsular cataract formation; and delayed wound healing.

Secondary Infection: The development of secondary infection has occurred after use of combinations containing corticosteroids and antimicrobials. Fungal infections of the cornea are particularly prone to develop coincidentally with long-term applications of corticosteroid. The possibility of fungal invasion must be considered in any persistent corneal ulceration where corticosteroid treatment has been used.

Secondary bacterial ocular infection following suppression of host responses also occurs.

Dosage and Administration

The duration of treatment will vary with the type of lesion and may extend from a few days to several weeks, according to therapeutic response. Relapses, more common in chronic active lesions than in self-limited conditions, usually respond to retreatment.

Apply a thin coating of ophthalmic ointment NEODECADRON three or four times a day. When a favorable response is observed, reduce the number of daily applications to two, and later to one a day as maintenance dose if this is sufficient to control symptoms.

Not more than 8 grams should be prescribed initially and the prescription should not be refilled without further evaluation as outlined in PRECAUTIONS above.

Ophthalmic ointment NEODECADRON is particularly convenient when an eye pad is used. It may also be the preparation of choice for patients in whom therapeutic benefit depends on prolonged contact of the active ingredients with ocular tissues.

How Supplied

No. 7617—Sterile Ophthalmic Ointment NEODECADRON is a clear, unctuous ointment, and is supplied as follows:

NDC 0006-7617-04 in 3.5 g tubes
(6505-00-823-7956 0.05% 3.5 g)

A.H.F.S. Category: 52:08
DC 6167722 Issued June 1982
Shown in Product Identification Section, page 104

NEODECADRON® ℞
(Neomycin Sulfate-Dexamethasone Sodium Phosphate, MSD), U.S.P.
Sterile Ophthalmic Solution

Description

Ophthalmic solution NEODECADRON® (Neomycin Sulfate-Dexamethasone Sodium Phosphate, MSD) is a topical corticosteroid-antibiotic solution for use in certain disorders of the anterior segment of the eye.

Each milliliter of buffered ophthalmic solution NEODECADRON in the OCUMETER® ophthalmic dispenser contains: dexamethasone sodium phosphate equivalent to 1 mg (0.1%) dexamethasone phosphate, and neomycin sulfate equivalent to 3.5 mg neomycin base. Inactive ingredients: creatinine, sodium citrate, sodium borate, polysorbate 80, disodium edetate, hydrochloric acid to adjust pH to 6.6–7.2, and water for injection. Benzalkonium chloride 0.02% and sodium bisulfite 0.1% added as preservatives.

Dexamethasone sodium phosphate is a water soluble, inorganic ester of dexamethasone. Its empirical formula is $C_{22}H_{28}FNa_2O_8P$. It is approximately three thousand times more soluble in water at 25°C than hydrocortisone.

Neomycin sulfate is the sulfate salt of neomycin, an antibacterial substance produced by the growth of *Streptomyces fradiae* Waksman (Fam. Streptomycetaceae).

Clinical Pharmacology

Dexamethasone sodium phosphate, a corticosteroid, suppresses the inflammatory response to a variety of agents, and it probably delays or slows healing. Since corticosteroids may inhibit the body's defense mechanism against infection, a concomitant antimicrobial drug may be used when this inhibition is considered to be clinically significant in a particular case.

Neomycin sulfate, the anti-infective component in the combination, is included to provide action against specific organisms susceptible to it. Neomycin sulfate is considered active mainly against gram-negative organisms, except *Bacteroides* spp. and *Pseudomonas aeruginosa*, which are resistant. Gram-positive organisms except for *Staphylococcus aureus* are usually resistant.

When a decision to administer both a corticosteroid and an anti-microbial is made, the administration of such drugs in combination has the advantage of greater patient compliance and convenience, with the added assurance that the appropriate dosage of both drugs is administered, plus assured compatibility of ingredients when both types of drug are in the same formulation and, particularly, that the correct volume of drug is delivered and retained.

The relative potency of corticosteroids depends on the molecular structure, concentration, and release from the vehicle.

Indications and Usage

For steroid-responsive inflammatory ocular conditions for which a corticosteroid is indicated and where bacterial infection or a risk of bacterial ocular infection exists.

Ocular steroids are indicated in inflammatory conditions of the palpebral and bulbar conjunctiva, cornea, and anterior segment of the globe where the inherent risk of steroid use in certain infective conjunctivitides is accepted to obtain a diminution in edema and inflammation. They are also indicated in chronic anterior uveitis and corneal injury from chemical, radiation, or thermal burns, or penetration of foreign bodies.

The use of a combination drug with an anti-infective component is indicated where the risk of infection is high or where there is an expectation that potentially dangerous numbers of bacteria will be present in the eye.

The particular anti-infective drug in this product is active against the following common bacterial eye pathogens:

Staphylococcus aureus
Escherichia coli
Haemophilus influenzae
Klebsiella/Enterobacter species
Neisseria species

The product does not provide adequate coverage against:

Pseudomonas aeruginosa
Serratia marcescens
Streptococci, including *Streptococcus pneumoniae*

Contraindications

Epithelial herpes simplex keratitis (dendritic keratitis), acute infectious stages of vaccinia, varicella, and many other viral diseases of the cornea and conjunctiva. Mycobacterial infection of the eye. Fungal diseases of ocular structures. Hypersensitivity to any component of this product, including sulfites (see WARNINGS). (Hypersensitivity to the antibiotic component occurs at a higher rate than for other components.)

The use of these combinations is always contraindicated after uncomplicated removal of a corneal foreign body.

Warnings

Prolonged use may result in glaucoma, with damage to the optic nerve, defects in visual acuity and fields of vision, and posterior subcapsular cataract formation. Prolonged use may suppress the host response and thus increase the hazard of secondary ocular infections. In those diseases causing thinning of the cornea or sclera, perforations have been known to occur with the use of topical corticosteroids. In acute purulent conditions of the eye, corticosteroids may mask infection or enhance existing infection. If these products are used for 10 days or longer, intraocular pressure should be routinely monitored even though it may be difficult in children and uncooperative patients.

Employment of corticosteroid medication in the treatment of herpes simplex requires great caution: periodic slit-lamp microscopy is recommended.

Any substance (e.g., neomycin sulfate) may occasionally cause cutaneous sensitization. If any reaction indicating such sensitivity is observed, discontinue use.

Ophthalmic Solution NEODECADRON contains sodium bisulfite, a sulfite that may cause allergic-type reactions including anaphylactic symptoms and life-threatening or less severe asthmatic episodes in certain susceptible people. The overall prevalence of sulfite sensitivity in the general population is unknown and probably low. Sulfite sensitivity is seen more frequently in asthmatic than in nonasthmatic people.

Precautions

The initial prescription and renewal of the medication order beyond 20 milliliters should be made by a physician only after examination of the patient with the aid of magnification, such as slit-lamp biomicroscopy and, where appropriate, fluorescein staining.

The possibility of persistent fungal infections of the cornea should be considered after prolonged corticosteroid dosing.

Usage in Pregnancy

Safety of intensive or protracted use of topical corticosteroids during pregnancy has not been substantiated.

Adverse Reactions

Adverse reactions have occurred with corticosteroid/anti-infective combination drugs which can be attributed to the corticosteroid component, the anti-infective component, the combination, or any other component of the product. Exact incidence figures are not available since no denominator of treated patients is available.

Reactions occurring most often from the presence of the anti-infective ingredient are allergic sensitizations. The reactions due to the corticosteroid component in decreasing order of frequency are: elevation of intraocular pressure (IOP) with possible development of glaucoma, and infrequent optic nerve damage; posterior subcapsular cataract formation; and delayed wound healing.

Secondary Infection: The development of secondary infection has occurred after use of combinations containing corticosteroids and antimicrobials. Fungal infections of the cornea are particularly prone to develop coincidentally with long-term applications of corticosteroid. The possibility of fungal invasion must be considered in any persistent corneal ulceration where corticosteroid treatment has been used. Secondary bacterial ocular infection following suppression of host responses also occurs.

Dosage and Administration

The duration of treatment will vary with the type of lesion and may extend from a few days to several weeks, according to therapeutic response. Relapses, more common in chronic active lesions than in self-limited conditions, usually respond to retreatment.

Instill one or two drops of ophthalmic solution NEODECADRON into the conjunctival sac every hour during the day and every two hours during the night as initial therapy. When a favorable response is observed, reduce dosage to one drop every four hours. Later, further reduction in dosage to one drop three or four times daily may suffice to control symptoms.

Not more than 20 milliliters should be prescribed initially and the prescription should not be refilled without further evaluation as outlined in PRECAUTIONS above.

How Supplied

Sterile ophthalmic solution NEODECADRON is a clear, colorless to pale yellow solution.

No. 7639—Ophthalmic solution NEODECADRON is supplied as follows:

NDC 0006-7639-03 in 5 mL white opaque, plastic OCUMETER ophthalmic dispenser with a controlled drop tip.
(6505-01-039-4352 0.1% 5 mL).

A.H.F.S. Category: 52:08
DC 7261319 Issued February 1987
Shown in Product Identification Section, page 104

Continued on next page

Information on the Merck Sharp & Dohme products listed on these pages is the full prescribing information from product circulars in effect August 31, 1991.

Merck Sharp & Dohme—Cont.

TIMOPTIC® ℞
(Timolol Maleate, MSD), U.S.P.
Sterile Ophthalmic Solution

Description
TIMOPTIC® (Timolol Maleate, MSD) Ophthalmic Solution is a non-selective beta-adrenergic receptor blocking agent. Its chemical name is (S)-1-[(1,1-dimethylethyl)amino]-3-[[4-(4-morpholinyl)-1,2,5-thiadiazol-3-yl]oxy]-2-propanol, (Z)-butenedioate (1:1) salt. Timolol maleate possesses an asymmetric carbon atom in its structure and is provided as the levo isomer. The nominal optical rotation of timolol maleate is:

$$[\alpha]^{25°}_{405\ nm} \text{ in 0.1N HCl (C = 5\%)} = -12.2°.$$

Its empirical formula is $C_{13}H_{24}N_4O_3S \cdot C_4H_4O_4$ and its structural formula is:

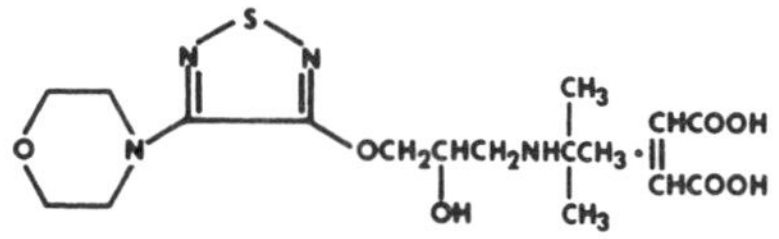

Timolol maleate has a molecular weight of 432.49. It is a white, odorless, crystalline powder which is soluble in water, methanol, and alcohol. TIMOPTIC is stable at room temperature.
TIMOPTIC Ophthalmic Solution is supplied as a sterile, isotonic, buffered, aqueous solution of timolol maleate in two dosage strengths: Each mL of TIMOPTIC 0.25% contains 2.5 mg of timolol (3.4 mg of timolol maleate). Each mL of TIMOPTIC 0.5% contains 5.0 mg of timolol (6.8 mg of timolol maleate). Inactive ingredients: monobasic and dibasic sodium phosphate, sodium hydroxide to adjust pH, and water for injection. Benzalkonium chloride 0.01% is added as preservative.

Clinical Pharmacology
Timolol maleate is a $beta_1$ and $beta_2$ (non-selective) adrenergic receptor blocking agent that does not have significant intrinsic sympathomimetic, direct myocardial depressant, or local anesthetic (membrane-stabilizing) activity.
Beta-adrenergic receptor blockade reduces cardiac output in both healthy subjects and patients with heart disease. In patients with severe impairment of myocardial function beta-adrenergic receptor blockade may inhibit the stimulatory effect of the sympathetic nervous system necessary to maintain adequate cardiac function.
Beta-adrenergic receptor blockade in the bronchi and bronchioles results in increased airway resistance from unopposed para-sympathetic activity. Such an effect in patients with asthma or other bronchospastic conditions is potentially dangerous.
TIMOPTIC Ophthalmic Solution, when applied topically in the eye, has the action of reducing elevated as well as normal intraocular pressure, whether or not accompanied by glaucoma. Elevated intraocular pressure is a major risk factor in the pathogenesis of glaucomatous visual field loss. The higher the level of intraocular pressure, the greater the likelihood of glaucomatous visual field loss and optic nerve damage.
The onset of reduction in intraocular pressure following administration of TIMOPTIC can usually be detected within one-half hour after a single dose. The maximum effect usually occurs in one to two hours and significant lowering of intraocular pressure can be maintained for periods as long as 24 hours with a single dose. Repeated observations over a period of one year indicate that the intraocular pressure-lowering effect of TIMOPTIC is well maintained.
The precise mechanism of the ocular hypotensive action of TIMOPTIC is not clearly established at this time. Tonography and fluorophotometry studies in man suggest that its predominant action may be related to reduced aqueous formation. However, in some studies a slight increase in outflow facility was also observed. Unlike miotics, TIMOPTIC reduces intraocular pressure with little or no effect on accommodation or pupil size. Thus, changes in visual acuity due to increased accommodation are uncommon, and dim or blurred vision and night blindness produced by miotics are not evident. In addition, in patients with cataracts the inability to see around lenticular opacities when the pupil is constricted is avoided.
In the clinical studies which are reported below, ocular pressure reductions to less than 22 mmHg were used as a reasonable reference point to allow comparisons between treatments. Reduction of ocular pressure to just below 22 mmHg may not be optimal for all patients; therapy should be individualized.
In controlled multiclinic studies in patients with untreated intraocular pressures of 22 mmHg or greater, TIMOPTIC 0.25 percent or 0.5 percent administered twice a day produced a greater reduction in intraocular pressure than 1, 2, 3, or 4 percent pilocarpine solution administered four times a day or 0.5, 1, or 2 percent epinephrine hydrochloride solution administered twice a day.
In the multiclinic studies comparing TIMOPTIC with pilocarpine, 61 percent of patients treated with TIMOPTIC had intraocular pressure reduced to less than 22 mmHg compared to 32 percent of patients treated with pilocarpine. For patients completing these studies, the mean reduction in pressure at the end of the study from pretreatment was 30.7 percent for patients treated with TIMOPTIC and 21.7 percent for patients treated with pilocarpine.
In the multiclinic studies comparing TIMOPTIC with epinephrine, 69 percent of patients treated with TIMOPTIC had intraocular pressure reduced to less than 22 mmHg compared to 42 percent of patients treated with epinephrine. For patients completing these studies, the mean reduction in pressure at the end of the study from pretreatment was 33.2 percent for patients treated with TIMOPTIC and 28.1 percent for patients treated with epinephrine.
In these studies, TIMOPTIC was generally well tolerated and produced fewer and less severe side effects than either pilocarpine or epinephrine. A slight reduction of resting heart rate in some patients receiving TIMOPTIC (mean reduction 2.9 beats/minute standard deviation 10.2) was observed.
TIMOPTIC has also been used in patients with glaucoma wearing conventional (PMMA) hard contact lenses, and has generally been well tolerated. TIMOPTIC has not been studied in patients wearing lenses made with materials other than PMMA.

Indications and Usage
TIMOPTIC Ophthalmic Solution has been shown to be effective in lowering intraocular pressure and may be used in:
Patients with chronic open-angle glaucoma
Patients with aphakic glaucoma
Some patients with secondary glaucoma
Other patients with elevated intraocular pressure who are at sufficient risk to require lowering of the ocular pressure.
Clinical trials have also shown that in patients who respond inadequately to multiple antiglaucoma drug therapy the addition of TIMOPTIC may produce a further reduction of intraocular pressure.

Contraindications
TIMOPTIC is contraindicated in patients with bronchial asthma or with a history of bronchial asthma, or severe chronic obstructive pulmonary disease (see WARNINGS); sinus bradycardia; second and third degree atrioventricular block; overt cardiac failure (see WARNINGS); cardiogenic shock; hypersensitivity to any component of this product.

Warnings
As with other topically applied ophthalmic drugs, this drug may be absorbed systemically. **The same adverse reactions found with systemic administration of beta-adrenergic blocking agents may occur with topical administration. For example, severe respiratory reactions and cardiac reactions, including death due to bronchospasm in patients with asthma, and rarely death in association with cardiac failure, have been reported following administration of TIMOPTIC (Timolol Maleate, MSD) (see CONTRAINDICATIONS).**
Cardiac Failure
Sympathetic stimulation may be essential for support of the circulation in individuals with diminished myocardial contractility, and its inhibition by beta-adrenergic receptor blockade may precipitate more severe failure.
In Patients Without a History of Cardiac Failure continued depression of the myocardium with beta-blocking agents over a period of time can, in some cases, lead to cardiac failure. At the first sign or symptom of cardiac failure TIMOPTIC should be discontinued.
Obstructive Pulmonary Disease
PATIENTS WITH CHRONIC OBSTRUCTIVE PULMONARY DISEASE (e.g., CHRONIC BRONCHITIS, EMPHYSEMA) OF MILD OR MODERATE SEVERITY, BRONCHOSPASTIC DISEASE OR A HISTORY OF BRONCHOSPASTIC DISEASE (OTHER THAN BRONCHIAL ASTHMA OR A HISTORY OF BRONCHIAL ASTHMA, IN WHICH 'TIMOPTIC' IS CONTRAINDICATED, see CONTRAINDICATIONS), SHOULD IN GENERAL NOT RECEIVE BETA BLOCKERS, INCLUDING 'TIMOPTIC'. However, if TIMOPTIC is necessary in such patients, then the drug should be administered with caution since it may block bronchodilation produced by endogenous and exogenous catecholamine stimulation of $beta_2$ receptors.
Major Surgery
The necessity or desirability of withdrawal of beta-adrenergic blocking agents prior to major surgery is controversial. Beta-adrenergic receptor blockade impairs the ability of the heart to respond to beta-adrenergically mediated reflex stimuli. This may augment the risk of general anesthesia in surgical procedures. Some patients receiving beta-adrenergic receptor blocking agents have been subject to protracted severe hypotension during anesthesia. Difficulty in restarting and maintaining the heartbeat has also been reported. For these reasons, in patients undergoing elective surgery, some authorities recommend gradual withdrawal of beta-adrenergic receptor blocking agents.
If necessary during surgery, the effects of beta-adrenergic blocking agents may be reversed by sufficient doses of such agonists as isoproterenol, dopamine, dobutamine or levarterenol (see OVERDOSAGE).
Diabetes Mellitus
Beta-adrenergic blocking agents should be administered with caution in patients subject to spontaneous hypoglycemia or to diabetic patients (especially those with labile diabetes) who are receiving insulin or oral hypoglycemic agents. Beta-adrenergic receptor blocking agents may mask the signs and symptoms of acute hypoglycemia.
Thyrotoxicosis
Beta-adrenergic blocking agents may mask certain clinical signs (e.g., tachycardia) of hyperthyroidism. Patients suspected of developing thyrotoxicosis should be managed carefully to avoid abrupt withdrawal of beta-adrenergic

blocking agents which might precipitate a thyroid storm.

Precautions

General

Patients who are receiving a beta-adrenergic blocking agent orally and TIMOPTIC should be observed for a potential additive effect either on the intraocular pressure or on the known systemic effects of beta blockade.

Patients should not receive two topical ophthalmic beta-adrenergic blocking agents concurrently (see DOSAGE AND ADMINISTRATION).

Because of potential effects of beta-adrenergic blocking agents relative to blood pressure and pulse, these agents should be used with caution in patients with cerebrovascular insufficiency. If signs or symptoms suggesting reduced cerebral blood flow develop following initiation of therapy with TIMOPTIC, alternative therapy should be considered.

Muscle Weakness: Beta-adrenergic blockade has been reported to potentiate muscle weakness consistent with certain myasthenic symptoms (e.g., diplopia, ptosis, and generalized weakness). Timolol has been reported rarely to increase muscle weakness in some patients with myasthenia gravis or myasthenic symptoms.

In patients with angle-closure glaucoma, the immediate objective of treatment is to reopen the angle. This requires constricting the pupil with a miotic. TIMOPTIC has little or no effect on the pupil. When TIMOPTIC is used to reduce elevated intraocular pressure in angle-closure glaucoma, it should be used with a miotic and not alone.

As with the use of other antiglaucoma drugs, diminished responsiveness to TIMOPTIC after prolonged therapy has been reported in some patients. However, in one long-term study in which 96 patients have been followed for at least 3 years, no significant difference in mean intraocular pressure has been observed after initial stabilization.

Drug Interactions

Although TIMOPTIC used alone has little or no effect on pupil size, mydriasis resulting from concomitant therapy with TIMOPTIC and epinephrine has been reported occasionally.

Close observation of the patient is recommended when a beta blocker is administered to patients receiving catecholamine-depleting drugs such as reserpine, because of possible additive effects and the production of hypotension and/or marked bradycardia, which may produce vertigo, syncope, or postural hypotension.

Caution should be used in the coadministration of beta-adrenergic blocking agents, such as TIMOPTIC, and oral or intravenous calcium antagonists, because of possible atrioventricular conduction disturbances, left ventricular failure, and hypotension. In patients with impaired cardiac function, coadministration should be avoided.

The concomitant use of beta-adrenergic blocking agents with digitalis and calcium antagonists may have additive effects in prolonging atrioventricular conduction time.

Animal Studies

No adverse ocular effects were observed in rabbits and dogs administered TIMOPTIC topically in studies lasting one and two years respectively.

Carcinogenesis, Mutagenesis, Impairment of Fertility

In a two-year oral study of timolol maleate in rats, there was a statistically significant ($P \leq 0.05$) increase in the incidence of adrenal pheochromocytomas in male rats administered 300 times the maximum recommended human oral dose* (1 mg/kg/day). Similar differences were not observed in rats administered oral doses equivalent to 25 or 100 times the maximum recommended human oral dose. In a lifetime oral study in mice, there were statistically significant ($P \leq 0.05$) increases in the incidence of benign and malignant pulmonary tumors and benign uterine polyps in female mice at 500 mg/kg/day, but not at 5 or 50 mg/kg/day. There was also a significant increase in mammary adenocarcinomas at the 500 mg/kg/day dose. This was associated with elevations in serum prolactin which occurred in female mice administered timolol at 500 mg/kg, but not at doses of 5 or 50 mg/kg/day. An increased incidence of mammary adenocarcinomas in rodents has been associated with administration of several other therapeutic agents which elevate serum prolactin, but no correlation between serum prolactin levels and mammary tumors has been established in man. Furthermore, in adult human female subjects who received oral dosages of up to 60 mg of timolol maleate, the maximum recommended human oral dosage, there were no clinically meaningful changes in serum prolactin.

There was a statistically significant increase ($P \leq 0.05$) in the overall incidence of neoplasms in female mice at the 500 mg/kg/day dosage level.

Timolol maleate was devoid of mutagenic potential when evaluated *in vivo* (mouse) in the micronucleus test and cytogenetic assay (doses up to 800 mg/kg) and *in vitro* in a neoplastic cell transformation assay (up to 100 μg/mL). In Ames tests the highest concentrations of timolol employed, 5000 or 10,000 μg/plate, were associated with statistically significant elevations ($P \leq 0.05$) of revertants observed with tester strain TA100 (in seven replicate assays), but not in the remaining three strains. In the assays with tester strain TA100, no consistent dose response relationship was observed, nor did the ratio of test to control revertants reach 2. A ratio of 2 is usually considered the criterion for a positive Ames test.

Reproduction and fertility studies in rats showed no adverse effect on male or female fertility at doses up to 150 times the maximum recommended human oral dose.

Pregnancy

Pregnancy Category C. Teratogenicity studies with timolol in mice and rabbits at doses up to 50 mg/kg/day (50 times the maximum recommended human oral dose) showed no evidence of fetal malformations. Although delayed fetal ossification was observed at this dose in rats, there were no adverse effects on postnatal development of offspring. Doses of 1000 mg/kg/day (1,000 times the maximum recommended human oral dose) were maternotoxic in mice and resulted in an increased number of fetal resorptions. Increased fetal resorptions were also seen in rabbits at doses of 100 times the maximum recommended human oral dose, in this case without apparent maternotoxicity. There are no adequate and well-controlled studies in pregnant women. TIMOPTIC should be used during pregnancy only if the potential benefit justifies the potential risk to the fetus.

Nursing Mothers

Because of the potential for serious adverse reactions from timolol in nursing infants, a decision should be made whether to discontinue nursing or to discontinue the drug, taking into account the importance of the drug to the mother.

Pediatric Use

Safety and effectiveness in children have not been established by adequate and well-controlled studies.

Adverse Reactions

TIMOPTIC Ophthalmic Solution is usually well tolerated. The following adverse reactions have been reported either in clinical trials of up to 3 years duration prior to release in 1978 or since the drug has been marketed:

BODY AS A WHOLE

Headache, asthenia, chest pain.

CARDIOVASCULAR

Bradycardia, arrhythmia, hypotension, syncope, heart block, cerebral vascular accident, cerebral ischemia, cardiac failure, palpitation, cardiac arrest.

DIGESTIVE

Nausea, diarrhea.

NERVOUS SYSTEM/PSYCHIATRIC

Dizziness, depression, increase in signs and symptoms of myasthenia gravis, paresthesia.

SKIN

Hypersensitivity, including localized and generalized rash; urticaria, alopecia.

RESPIRATORY

Bronchospasm (predominantly in patients with pre-existing bronchospastic disease), respiratory failure, dyspnea, nasal congestion, cough.

ENDOCRINE

Masked symptoms of hypoglycemia in insulin-dependent diabetics (see WARNINGS).

SPECIAL SENSES

Signs and symptoms of ocular irritation, including conjunctivitis, blepharitis, keratitis, blepharoptosis, decreased corneal sensitivity, visual disturbances including refractive changes (due to withdrawal of miotic therapy in some cases), diplopia, ptosis.

Causal Relationship Unknown: The following adverse effects have been reported, and a causal relationship to therapy with TIMOPTIC has not been established: *Body as a Whole:* Fatigue; *Cardiovascular:* Hypertension, pulmonary edema, worsening of angina pectoris; *Digestive:* Dyspepsia, anorexia, dry mouth; *Nervous System/Psychiatric:* Behavioral changes including confusion, hallucinations, anxiety, disorientation, nervousness, somnolence, and other psychic disturbances; *Special Senses:* Aphakic cystoid macular edema; *Urogenital:* Retroperitoneal fibrosis, impotence.

The following additional adverse effects have been reported in clinical experience with oral timolol maleate, and may be considered potential effects of ophthalmic timolol maleate: *Body as a Whole:* Extremity pain, decreased exercise tolerance, weight loss; *Cardiovascular:* Edema, worsening of arterial insufficiency, Raynaud's phenomenon, vasodilatation; *Digestive:* Gastrointestinal pain, hepatomegaly, vomiting; *Hematologic:* Nonthrombocytopenic purpura; *Endocrine:* Hyperglycemia, hypoglycemia; *Skin:* Pruritus, skin irritation, increased pigmentation, sweating, cold hands and feet; *Musculoskeletal:* Arthralgia, claudication; *Nervous System/Psychiatric:* Vertigo, local weakness, decreased libido, nightmares, insomnia, diminished concentration; *Respiratory:* Rales, bronchial obstruction; *Special Senses:* Tinnitus, dry eyes; *Urogenital:* Urination difficulties.

Potential Adverse Effects: In addition, a variety of adverse effects have been reported with other beta-adrenergic blocking agents and may be considered potential effects of ophthalmic timolol maleate: *Digestive:* Mesenteric arterial thrombosis, ischemic colitis; *Hematologic:* Agranulocytosis, thrombocytopenic purpura; *Nervous System:* Reversible mental depression progressing to catatonia; an acute reversible syndrome characterized by disorientation for time and place, short-term memory loss, emotional lability, slightly clouded sensorium, and

Continued on next page

* The maximum recommended single oral dose is 30 mg of timolol. One drop of TIMOPTIC 0.5% contains about 1/150 of this dose which is about 0.2 mg.

Information on the Merck Sharp & Dohme products listed on these pages is the full prescribing information from product circulars in effect August 31, 1991.

Merck Sharp & Dohme—Cont.

decreased performance on neuropsychometrics; *Allergic:* Erythematous rash, fever combined with aching and sore throat, laryngospasm with respiratory distress; *Urogenital:* Peyronie's disease.

There have been reports of a syndrome comprising psoriasiform skin rash, conjunctivitis sicca, otitis and sclerosing serositis attributed to the beta-adrenergic receptor blocking agent, practolol. This syndrome has not been reported with timolol maleate.

Overdosage

No data are available in regard to overdosage in humans.

The oral LD_{50} of the drug is 1190 and 900 mg/kg in female mice and female rats, respectively.

An *in vitro* hemodialysis study, using ^{14}C timolol added to human plasma or whole blood, showed that timolol was readily dialyzed from these fluids; however, a study of patients with renal failure showed that timolol did not dialyze readily.

The most common signs and symptoms to be expected with overdosage with administration of a systemic beta-adrenergic receptor blocking agent are symptomatic bradycardia, hypotension, bronchospasm, and acute cardiac failure. The following therapeutic measures should be considered:

(1) *Gastric lavage:* If ingested.

(2) *Symptomatic bradycardia:* Use atropine sulfate intravenously in a dosage of 0.25 mg to 2 mg to induce vagal blockade. If bradycardia persists, intravenous isoproterenol hydrochloride should be administered cautiously. In refractory cases the use of a transvenous cardiac pacemaker may be considered.

(3) *Hypotension:* Use sympathomimetic pressor drug therapy, such as dopamine, dobutamine or levarterenol. In refractory cases the use of glucagon hydrochloride has been reported to be useful.

(4) *Bronchospasm:* Use isoproterenol hydrochloride. Additional therapy with aminophylline may be considered.

(5) *Acute cardiac failure:* Conventional therapy with digitalis, diuretics, and oxygen should be instituted immediately. In refractory cases the use of intravenous aminophylline is suggested. This may be followed if necessary by glucagon hydrochloride which has been reported to be useful.

(6) *Heart block (second or third degree):* Use isoproterenol hydrochloride or a transvenous cardiac pacemaker.

Dosage and Administration

TIMOPTIC Ophthalmic Solution is available in concentrations of 0.25 and 0.5 percent. The usual starting dose is one drop of 0.25 percent TIMOPTIC in the affected eye(s) twice a day. If the clinical response is not adequate, the dosage may be changed to one drop of 0.5 percent solution in the affected eye(s) twice a day.

Since in some patients the pressure-lowering response to TIMOPTIC may require a few weeks to stabilize, evaluation should include a determination of intraocular pressure after approximately 4 weeks of treatment with TIMOPTIC.

If the intraocular pressure is maintained at satisfactory levels, the dosage schedule may be changed to one drop once a day in the affected eye(s). Because of diurnal variations in intraocular pressure, satisfactory response to the once-a-day dose is best determined by measuring the intraocular pressure at different times during the day.

Dosages above one drop of 0.5 percent TIMOPTIC twice a day generally have not been shown to produce further reduction in intraocular pressure. If the patient's intraocular pressure is still not at a satisfactory level on this regimen, concomitant therapy with pilocarpine and other miotics, and/or epinephrine, and/or systemically administered carbonic anhydrase inhibitors, such as acetazolamide, can be instituted.

When a patient is transferred from another topical ophthalmic beta-adrenergic blocking agent, that agent should be discontinued after proper dosing on one day and treatment with TIMOPTIC started on the following day with 1 drop of 0.25 percent TIMOPTIC in the affected eye(s) twice a day. The dose may be increased to one drop of 0.5 percent TIMOPTIC twice a day if the clinical response is not adequate.

When a patient is transferred from a single antiglaucoma agent, other than a topical ophthalmic beta-adrenergic blocking agent, continue the agent already being used and add one drop of 0.25 percent TIMOPTIC in the affected eye(s) twice a day. On the following day, discontinue the previously used antiglaucoma agent completely and continue with TIMOPTIC. If a higher dosage of TIMOPTIC is required, substitute one drop of 0.5 percent solution in the affected eye(s) twice a day.

When a patient is transferred from several concomitantly administered antiglaucoma agents, individualization is required. If any of the agents is an ophthalmic beta-adrenergic blocker, it should be discontinued before starting TIMOPTIC. Additional adjustments should involve one agent at a time and usually should be made at intervals of not less than one week. A recommended approach is to continue the agents being used and to add one drop of 0.25 percent TIMOPTIC in the affected eye(s) twice a day. On the following day, discontinue one of the other antiglaucoma agents. The remaining antiglaucoma agents may be decreased or discontinued according to the patient's response to treatment. If a higher dosage of TIMOPTIC is required, substitute one drop of 0.5 percent solution in the affected eye(s) twice a day. The physician may be able to discontinue some or all of the other antiglaucoma agents.

How Supplied

Sterile Ophthalmic Solution TIMOPTIC is a clear, colorless to light yellow solution.

No. 3366—TIMOPTIC Ophthalmic Solution, 0.25% timolol equivalent, is supplied in a white, opaque, plastic OCUMETER® ophthalmic dispenser with a controlled drop tip as follows:

NDC 0006-3366-32, 2.5 mL
NDC 0006-3366-03, 5 mL
(6505-01-069-6518, 0.25% 5 mL)
NDC 0006-3366-10, 10 mL
(6505-01-093-5458, 0.25% 10 mL)
NDC 0006-3366-12, 15 mL.

No. 3367—TIMOPTIC Ophthalmic Solution, 0.5% timolol equivalent, is supplied in a white, opaque, plastic OCUMETER ophthalmic dispenser with a controlled drop tip as follows:

NDC 0006-3367-32, 2.5 mL
NDC 0006-3367-03, 5 mL
(6505-01-069-6519, 0.5% 5 mL)
NDC 0006-3367-10, 10 mL
(6505-01-092-0422, 0.5% 10 mL)
NDC 0006-3367-12, 15 mL.

Storage

Protect from light. Store at room temperature.

A.H.F.S. Category: 52:36

DC 7115427 Issued August 1990

Shown in Product Identification Section, page 104

TIMOPTIC® ℞
(Timolol Maleate, MSD)
in OCUDOSE® (Dispenser)
Preservative-Free Sterile Ophthalmic Solution in a Sterile Ophthalmic Unit Dose Dispenser

Description

Timolol maleate is a non-selective beta-adrenergic receptor blocking agent. Its chemical name is (S)-1-[(1,1-dimethylethyl)amino]-3-[[4-(4-morpholinyl)-1, 2, 5-thiadiazol-3-yl]oxy]-2-propanol, (Z)-butenedioate (1:1) salt. Timolol maleate possesses an asymmetric carbon atom in its structure and is provided as the levo isomer. The nominal optical rotation of timolol maleate is

$$[\alpha]^{25°}_{405\ nm} \text{ in 0.1N HCl } (C = 5\%) = -12.2°.$$

Its empirical formula is $C_{13}H_{24}N_4O_3S \cdot C_4H_4O_4$ and its structural formula is:

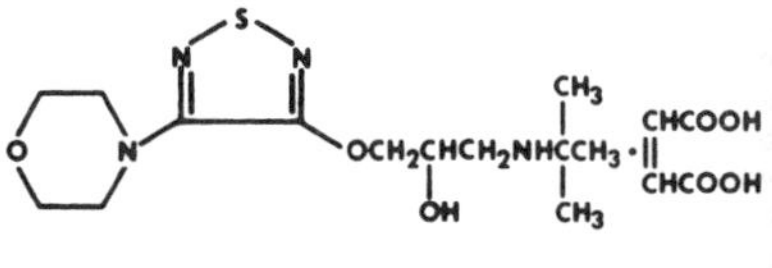

Timolol maleate has a molecular weight of 432.49. It is a white, odorless, crystalline powder which is soluble in water, methanol, and alcohol. Timolol maleate is stable at room temperature.

Timolol maleate ophthalmic solution is supplied in two formulations: Ophthalmic Solution TIMOPTIC® (Timolol Maleate, MSD), which contains the preservative, benzalkonium chloride; and Ophthalmic Solution TIMOPTIC® (Timolol Maleate, MSD), the preservative-free formulation.

Preservative-free Ophthalmic Solution TIMOPTIC is supplied in OCUDOSE®, a unit dose container as a sterile, isotonic, buffered, aqueous solution of timolol maleate in two dosage strengths: Each mL of Preservative-free TIMOPTIC in OCUDOSE 0.25% contains 2.5 mg of timolol (3.4 mg of timolol maleate). Each mL of Preservative-free TIMOPTIC in OCUDOSE 0.5% contains 5.0 mg of timolol (6.8 mg of timolol maleate). Inactive ingredients: monobasic and dibasic sodium phosphate, sodium hydroxide to adjust pH, and water for injection.

Clinical Pharmacology

Timolol maleate is a $beta_1$ and $beta_2$ (non-selective) adrenergic receptor blocking agent that does not have significant intrinsic sympathomimetic, direct myocardial depressant, or local anesthetic (membrane-stabilizing) activity.

Beta-adrenergic receptor blockade reduces cardiac output in both healthy subjects and patients with heart disease. In patients with severe impairment of myocardial function beta-adrenergic receptor blockade may inhibit the stimulatory effect of the sympathetic nervous system necessary to maintain adequate cardiac function.

Beta-adrenergic receptor blockade in the bronchi and bronchioles results in increased airway resistance from unopposed parasympathetic activity. Such an effect in patients with asthma or other bronchospastic conditions is potentially dangerous.

TIMOPTIC (Timolol Maleate, MSD), when applied topically in the eye, has the action of reducing elevated as well as normal intraocular pressure, whether or not accompanied by glaucoma. Elevated intraocular pressure is a major risk factor in the pathogenesis of glaucomatous visual field loss. The higher the level of intraocular pressure, the greater the likelihood of glaucomatous visual field loss and optic nerve damage.

The onset of reduction in intraocular pressure following administration of TIMOPTIC (Timolol Maleate, MSD) can usually be detected within one-half hour after a single dose. The maximum effect usually occurs in one to two hours and significant lowering of intraocular pressure can be maintained for periods as long as 24 hours with a single dose. Repeated observations over a period of one year indicate that the intraocular pressure-lowering effect of TIMOPTIC (Timolol Maleate, MSD) is well maintained.

The precise mechanism of the ocular hypotensive action of TIMOPTIC (Timolol Maleate, MSD) is not clearly established at this time. Tonography and fluorophotometry studies in man suggest that its predominant action may be related to reduced aqueous formation. However, in some studies a slight increase in outflow facility was also observed. Unlike miotics, TIMOPTIC (Timolol Maleate, MSD) reduces intraocular pressure with little or no effect on accommodation or pupil size. Thus, changes in visual acuity due to increased accommodation are uncommon, and dim or blurred vision and night blindness produced by miotics are not evident. In addition, in patients with cataracts the inability to see around lenticular opacities when the pupil is constricted is avoided.

Clinical studies have shown that the mean percent reductions in intraocular pressure with Preservative-free TIMOPTIC and TIMOPTIC (Timolol Maleate, MSD) were similar. Preservative-free TIMOPTIC was generally well tolerated.

In the clinical studies which are reported below, ocular pressure reductions to less than 22 mmHg were used as a reasonable reference point to allow comparisons between treatments. Reduction of ocular pressure to just below 22 mmHg may not be optimal for all patients; therapy should be individualized.

In controlled multiclinic studies in patients with untreated intraocular pressures of 22 mmHg or greater, TIMOPTIC (Timolol Maleate, MSD) 0.25 percent or 0.5 percent administered twice a day produced a greater reduction in intraocular pressure than 1, 2, 3, or 4 percent pilocarpine solution administered four times a day or 0.5, 1, or 2 percent epinephrine hydrochloride solution administered twice a day.

In the multiclinic studies comparing TIMOPTIC (Timolol Maleate, MSD) with pilocarpine, 61 percent of patients treated with TIMOPTIC (Timolol Maleate, MSD) had intraocular pressure reduced to less than 22 mmHg compared to 32 percent of patients treated with pilocarpine. For patients completing these studies, the mean reduction in pressure at the end of the study from pretreatment was 30.7 percent for patients treated with TIMOPTIC (Timolol Maleate, MSD) and 21.7 percent for patients treated with pilocarpine.

In the multiclinic studies comparing TIMOPTIC (Timolol Maleate, MSD) with epinephrine, 69 percent of patients treated with TIMOPTIC (Timolol Maleate, MSD) had intraocular pressure reduced to less than 22 mmHg compared to 42 percent of patients treated with epinephrine. For patients completing these studies, the mean reduction in pressure at the end of the study from pretreatment was 33.2 percent for patients treated with TIMOPTIC (Timolol Maleate, MSD) and 28.1 percent for patients treated with epinephrine.

In these studies, TIMOPTIC (Timolol Maleate, MSD) was generally well tolerated and produced fewer and less severe side effects than either pilocarpine or epinephrine. A slight reduction of resting heart rate in some patients receiving TIMOPTIC (Timolol Maleate, MSD) (mean reduction 2.9 beats/minute standard deviation 10.2) was observed.

TIMOPTIC (Timolol Maleate, MSD) has also been used in patients with glaucoma wearing conventional (PMMA) hard contact lenses, and has generally been well tolerated. TIMOPTIC (Timolol Maleate, MSD) has not been studied in patients wearing lenses made with materials other than PMMA.

Indications and Usage

TIMOPTIC (Timolol Maleate, MSD) has been shown to be effective in lowering intraocular pressure. Clinical studies have shown that the mean percent reductions in intraocular pressure with Preservative-free TIMOPTIC and TIMOPTIC (Timolol Maleate, MSD) are similar. When a patient is sensitive to the preservative, benzalkonium chloride, or when use of a preservative-free topical medication is advisable, Preservative-free TIMOPTIC may be used in:

Patients with chronic open-angle glaucoma
Patients with aphakic glaucoma
Some patients with secondary glaucoma
Other patients with elevated intraocular pressure who are at sufficient risk to require lowering of the ocular pressure.

Clinical trials have also shown that in patients who respond inadequately to multiple antiglaucoma drug therapy the addition of TIMOPTIC (Timolol Maleate, MSD) may produce a further reduction of intraocular pressure.

Contraindications

Preservative-free TIMOPTIC in OCUDOSE is contraindicated in patients with bronchial asthma or with a history of bronchial asthma, or severe chronic obstructive pulmonary disease (see WARNINGS); sinus bradycardia; second and third degree atrioventricular block; overt cardiac failure (see WARNINGS); cardiogenic shock; hypersensitivity to any component of this product.

Warnings

As with other topically applied ophthalmic drugs, this drug may be absorbed systemically. **The same adverse reactions found with systemic administration of beta-adrenergic blocking agents may occur with topical administration. For example, severe respiratory reactions and cardiac reactions, including death due to bronchospasm in patients with asthma, and rarely death in association with cardiac failure, have been reported following administration of TIMOPTIC (Timolol Maleate, MSD) (see CONTRAINDICATIONS).**

Cardiac Failure

Sympathetic stimulation may be essential for support of the circulation in individuals with diminished myocardial contractility, and its inhibition by beta-adrenergic receptor blockade may precipitate more severe failure.

In Patients Without a History of Cardiac Failure continued depression of the myocardium with beta-blocking agents over a period of time can, in some cases, lead to cardiac failure. At the first sign or symptom of cardiac failure Preservative-free TIMOPTIC in OCUDOSE should be discontinued.

Obstructive Pulmonary Disease

PATIENTS WITH CHRONIC OBSTRUCTIVE PULMONARY DISEASE (e.g., CHRONIC BRONCHITIS, EMPHYSEMA) OF MILD OR MODERATE SEVERITY, BRONCHOSPASTIC DISEASE OR A HISTORY OF BRONCHOSPASTIC DISEASE (OTHER THAN BRONCHIAL ASTHMA OR A HISTORY OF BRONCHIAL ASTHMA, IN WHICH 'Preservative-free TIMOPTIC in OCUDOSE' IS CONTRAINDICATED, see CONTRAINDICATIONS), SHOULD IN GENERAL NOT RECEIVE BETA BLOCKERS, INCLUDING 'Preservative-free TIMOPTIC in OCUDOSE'. However, if Preservative-free TIMOPTIC in OCUDOSE is necessary in such patients, then the drug should be administered with caution since it may block bronchodilation produced by endogenous and exogenous catecholamine stimulation of $beta_2$ receptors.

Major Surgery

The necessity or desirability of withdrawal of beta-adrenergic blocking agents prior to major surgery is controversial. Beta-adrenergic receptor blockade impairs the ability of the heart to respond to beta-adrenergically mediated reflex stimuli. This may augment the risk of general anesthesia in surgical procedures. Some patients receiving beta-adrenergic receptor blocking agents have been subject to protracted severe hypotension during anesthesia. Difficulty in restarting and maintaining the heartbeat has also been reported. For these reasons, in patients undergoing elective surgery, some authorities recommend gradual withdrawal of beta-adrenergic receptor blocking agents.

If necessary during surgery, the effects of beta-adrenergic blocking agents may be reversed by sufficient doses of such agonists as isoproterenol, dopamine, dobutamine or levarterenol (see OVERDOSAGE).

Diabetes Mellitus

Beta-adrenergic blocking agents should be administered with caution in patients subject to spontaneous hypoglycemia or to diabetic patients (especially those with labile diabetes) who are receiving insulin or oral hypoglycemic agents. Beta-adrenergic receptor blocking agents may mask the signs and symptoms of acute hypoglycemia.

Thyrotoxicosis

Beta-adrenergic blocking agents may mask certain clinical signs (e.g., tachycardia) of hyperthyroidism. Patients suspected of developing thyrotoxicosis should be managed carefully to avoid abrupt withdrawal of beta-adrenergic blocking agents which might precipitate a thyroid storm.

Precautions

General

Patients who are receiving a beta-adrenergic blocking agent orally and Preservative-free TIMOPTIC in OCUDOSE should be observed for a potential additive effect either on the intraocular pressure or on the known systemic effects of beta blockade.

Patients should not receive two topical ophthalmic beta-adrenergic blocking agents concurrently (see DOSAGE AND ADMINISTRATION).

Because of potential effects of beta-adrenergic blocking agents relative to blood pressure and pulse, these agents should be used with caution in patients with cerebrovascular insufficiency. If signs or symptoms suggesting reduced cerebral blood flow develop following initiation of therapy with Preservative-free TIMOPTIC in OCUDOSE, alternative therapy should be considered.

Muscle Weakness: Beta-adrenergic blockade has been reported to potentiate muscle weakness consistent with certain myasthenic symptoms (e.g., diplopia, ptosis, and generalized weakness). Timolol has been reported rarely to increase muscle weakness in some patients with myasthenia gravis or myasthenic symptoms.

In patients with angle-closure glaucoma, the immediate objective of treatment is to reopen the angle. This requires constricting the pupil with a miotic. TIMOPTIC (Timolol Maleate, MSD) has little or no effect on the pupil. When Preservative-free TIMOPTIC in OCUDOSE is used to reduce elevated intraocular pressure in angle-closure glaucoma, it should be used with a miotic and not alone.

As with the use of other antiglaucoma drugs, diminished responsiveness to TIMOPTIC (Timolol Maleate, MSD) after prolonged therapy has been reported in some patients. However, in one long-term study in which 96 patients have been followed for at least 3 years,

Continued on next page

Information on the Merck Sharp & Dohme products listed on these pages is the full prescribing information from product circulars in effect August 31, 1991.

Merck Sharp & Dohme—Cont.

no significant difference in mean intraocular pressure has been observed after initial stabilization.

Information for Patients

Patients should be instructed about the use of Preservative-free TIMOPTIC in OCUDOSE. Since sterility cannot be maintained after the individual unit is opened, patients should be instructed to use the product immediately after opening, and to discard the individual unit and any remaining contents immediately after use.

Drug Interactions

Although TIMOPTIC (Timolol Maleate, MSD) used alone has little or no effect on pupil size, mydriasis resulting from concomitant therapy with TIMOPTIC (Timolol Maleate, MSD) and epinephrine has been reported occasionally.

Close observation of the patient is recommended when a beta blocker is administered to patients receiving catecholamine-depleting drugs such as reserpine, because of possible additive effects and the production of hypotension and/or marked bradycardia, which may produce vertigo, syncope, or postural hypotension.

Caution should be used in the coadministration of beta-adrenergic blocking agents, such as Preservative-free TIMOPTIC in OCUDOSE, and oral or intravenous calcium antagonists, because of possible atrioventricular conduction disturbances, left ventricular failure, and hypotension. In patients with impaired cardiac function, coadministration should be avoided.

The concomitant use of beta-adrenergic blocking agents with digitalis and calcium antagonists may have additive effects in prolonging atrioventricular conduction time.

Animal Studies

No adverse ocular effects were observed in rabbits and dogs administered TIMOPTIC (Timolol Maleate, MSD) topically in studies lasting one and two years respectively.

Carcinogenesis, Mutagenesis, Impairment of Fertility

In a two-year oral study of timolol maleate in rats, there was a statistically significant ($P \leq 0.05$) increase in the incidence of adrenal pheochromocytomas in male rats administered 300 times the maximum recommended human oral dose* (1 mg/kg/day). Similar differences were not observed in rats administered oral doses equivalent to 25 or 100 times the maximum recommended human oral dose. In a lifetime oral study in mice, there were statistically significant ($P \leq 0.05$) increases in the incidence of benign and malignant pulmonary tumors and benign uterine polyps in female mice at 500 mg/kg/day, but not at 5 or 50 mg/kg/day. There was also a significant increase in mammary adenocarcinomas at the 500 mg/kg/day dose. This was associated with elevations in serum prolactin which occurred in female mice administered timolol at 500 mg/kg, but not at doses of 5 or 50 mg/kg/day. An increased incidence of mammary adenocarcinomas in rodents has been associated with administration of several other therapeutic agents which elevate serum prolactin, but no correlation between serum prolactin levels and mammary tumors has been established in man. Furthermore, in adult human female subjects who received oral dosages of up to 60 mg of timolol maleate, the maximum recommended human oral dosage, there were no clinically meaningful changes in serum prolactin.

*The maximum recommended single oral dose is 30 mg of timolol. One drop of Preservative-free TIMOPTIC in OCUDOSE 0.5% contains about 1/150 of this dose which is about 0.2 mg.

There was a statistically significant increase ($P \leq 0.05$) in the overall incidence of neoplasms in female mice at the 500 mg/kg/day dosage level.

Timolol maleate was devoid of mutagenic potential when evaluated *in vivo* (mouse) in the micronucleus test and cytogenetic assay (doses up to 800 mg/kg) and *in vitro* in a neoplastic cell transformation assay (up to 100 μg/mL). In Ames tests the highest concentrations of timolol employed, 5000 or 10,000 μg/plate, were associated with statistically significant elevations ($P \leq 0.05$) of revertants observed with tester strain TA 100 (in seven replicate assays), but not in the remaining three strains. In the assays with tester strain TA 100, no consistent dose response relationship was observed, nor did the ratio of test to control revertants reach 2. A ratio of 2 is usually considered the criterion for a positive Ames test.

Reproduction and fertility studies in rats showed no adverse effect on male or female fertility at doses up to 150 times the maximum recommended human oral dose.

Pregnancy

Pregnancy Category C. Teratogenicity studies with timolol in mice and rabbits at doses up to 50 mg/kg/day (50 times the maximum recommended human oral dose) showed no evidence of fetal malformations. Although delayed fetal ossification was observed at this dose in rats, there were no adverse effects on postnatal development of offspring. Doses of 1000 mg/kg/day (1,000 times the maximum recommended human oral dose) were maternotoxic in mice and resulted in an increased number of fetal resorptions. Increased fetal resorptions were also seen in rabbits at doses of 100 times the maximum recommended human oral dose, in this case without apparent maternotoxicity. There are no adequate and well-controlled studies in pregnant women. Preservative-free TIMOPTIC in OCUDOSE should be used during pregnancy only if the potential benefit justifies the potential risk to the fetus.

Nursing Mothers

Because of the potential for serious adverse reactions from timolol in nursing infants, a decision should be made whether to discontinue nursing or to discontinue the drug, taking into account the importance of the drug to the mother.

Pediatric Use

Safety and effectiveness in children have not been established by adequate and well-controlled studies.

Adverse Reactions

Preservative-free TIMOPTIC in OCUDOSE Ophthalmic Solution is usually well tolerated. The following adverse reactions have been reported with TIMOPTIC (Timolol Maleate, MSD), either in clinical trials of up to 3 years duration prior to release in 1978 or since the drug has been marketed, and may be expected to occur with Preservative-free TIMOPTIC.

BODY AS A WHOLE

Headache, asthenia, chest pain.

CARDIOVASCULAR

Bradycardia, arrhythmia, hypotension, syncope, heart block, cerebral vascular accident, cerebral ischemia, cardiac failure, palpitation, cardiac arrest.

DIGESTIVE

Nausea, diarrhea.

NERVOUS SYSTEM/PSYCHIATRIC

Dizziness, depression, increase in signs and symptoms of myasthenia gravis, paresthesia.

SKIN

Hypersensitivity, including localized and generalized rash; urticaria, alopecia.

RESPIRATORY

Bronchospasm (predominantly in patients with pre-existing bronchospastic disease), respiratory failure, dyspnea, nasal congestion, cough.

ENDOCRINE

Masked symptoms of hypoglycemia in insulin-dependent diabetics (see WARNINGS).

SPECIAL SENSES

Signs and symptoms of ocular irritation, including conjunctivitis, blepharitis, keratitis blepharoptosis, decreased corneal sensitivity, visual disturbances including refractive changes (due to withdrawal of miotic therapy in some cases), diplopia, ptosis.

Causal Relationship Unknown: The following adverse effects have been reported, and a causal relationship to therapy with ophthalmic timolol maleate has not been established: *Body as a Whole:* Fatigue; *Cardiovascular:* Hypertension, pulmonary edema, worsening of angina pectoris; *Digestive:* Dyspepsia, anorexia, dry mouth; *Nervous System/Psychiatric:* Behavioral changes including confusion, hallucinations, anxiety, disorientation, nervousness, somnolence, and other psychic disturbances; *Special Senses:* Aphakic cystoid macular edema; *Urogenital:* Retroperitoneal fibrosis, impotence.

The following additional adverse effects have been reported in clinical experience with oral timolol maleate, and may be considered potential effects of ophthalmic timolol maleate: *Body as a Whole:* Extremity pain, decreased exercise tolerance, weight loss; *Cardiovascular:* Edema, worsening of arterial insufficiency, Raynaud's phenomenon, vasodilatation; *Digestive:* Gastrointestinal pain, hepatomegaly, vomiting; *Hematologic:* Nonthrombocytopenic purpura; *Endocrine:* Hyperglycemia, hypoglycemia; *Skin:* Pruritus, skin irritation, increased pigmentation, sweating, cold hands and feet; *Musculoskeletal:* Arthralgia, claudication; *Nervous System/Psychiatric:* Vertigo, local weakness, decreased libido, nightmares, insomnia, diminished concentration; *Respiratory:* Rales, bronchial obstruction; *Special Senses:* Tinnitus, dry eyes; *Urogenital:* Urination difficulties.

Potential Adverse Effects: In addition, a variety of adverse effects have been reported with other beta-adrenergic blocking agents and may be considered potential effects of ophthalmic timolol maleate: *Digestive:* Mesenteric arterial thrombosis, ischemic colitis; *Hematologic:* Agranulocytosis, thrombocytopenic purpura; *Nervous System:* Reversible mental depression progressing to catatonia; an acute reversible syndrome characterized by disorientation for time and place, short-term memory loss, emotional lability, slightly clouded sensorium, and decreased performance on neuropsychometrics; *Allergic:* Erythematous rash, fever combined with aching and sore throat, laryngospasm with respiratory distress; *Urogenital:* Peyronie's disease.

There have been reports of a syndrome comprising psoriasiform skin rash, conjunctivitis sicca, otitis and sclerosing serositis attributed to the beta-adrenergic receptor blocking agent, practolol. This syndrome has not been reported with timolol maleate.

Overdosage

No data are available in regard to overdosage in humans.

The oral LD_{50} of timolol maleate is 1190 and 900 mg/kg in female mice and female rats, respectively.

An *in vitro* hemodialysis study, using ^{14}C timolol added to human plasma or whole blood, showed that timolol was readily dialyzed from these fluids; however, a study of patients with renal failure showed that timolol did not dialyze readily.

The most common signs and symptoms to be expected with overdosage with administration of a systemic beta-adrenergic receptor blocking agent are symptomatic bradycardia, hypotension, bronchospasm, and acute cardiac failure. The following additional therapeutic measures should be considered:

4) *Gastric lavage:* If ingested.
2) *Symptomatic bradycardia:* Use atropine sulfate intravenously in a dosage of 0.25 mg to 2 mg to induce vagal blockade. If bradycardia persists, intravenous isoproterenol hydrochloride should be administered cautiously. In refractory cases the use of a transvenous cardiac pacemaker may be considered.
3) *Hypotension:* Use sympathomimetic pressor drug therapy, such as dopamine, dobutamine or levarterenol. In refractory cases the use of glucagon hydrochloride has been reported to be useful.
4) *Bronchospasm:* Use isoproterenol hydrochloride. Additional therapy with aminophylline may be considered.
5) *Acute cardiac failure:* Conventional therapy with digitalis, diuretics, and oxygen should be instituted immediately. In refractory cases the use of intravenous aminophylline is suggested. This may be followed if necessary by glucagon hydrochloride which has been reported to be useful.
6) *Heart block (second or third degree):* Use isoproterenol hydrochloride or a transvenous cardiac pacemaker.

Dosage and Administration

Preservative-free TIMOPTIC in OCUDOSE is a sterile solution that does not contain a preservative. The solution from one individual unit is to be used immediately after opening for administration to one or both eyes. Since sterility cannot be guaranteed after the individual unit is opened, the remaining contents should be discarded immediately after administration.

Preservative-free TIMOPTIC in OCUDOSE is available in concentrations of 0.25 and 0.5 percent. The usual starting dose is one drop of 0.25 percent Preservative-free TIMOPTIC in OCUDOSE in the affected eye(s) administered twice a day. Apply enough gentle pressure on the individual container to obtain a single drop of solution. If the clinical response is not adequate, the dosage may be changed to one drop of 0.5 percent solution in the affected eye(s) administered twice a day.

Since in some patients the pressure-lowering response to Preservative-free TIMOPTIC in OCUDOSE may require a few weeks to stabilize, evaluation should include a determination of intraocular pressure after approximately 4 weeks of treatment with Preservative-free TIMOPTIC in OCUDOSE.

If the intraocular pressure is maintained at satisfactory levels, the dosage schedule may be changed to one drop once a day in the affected eye(s). Because of diurnal variations in intraocular pressure, satisfactory response to the once-a-day dose is best determined by measuring the intraocular pressure at different times during the day.

Dosages above one drop of 0.5 percent TIMOPTIC (Timolol Maleate, MSD) twice a day generally have not been shown to produce further reduction in intraocular pressure. If the patient's intraocular pressure is not at a satisfactory level during treatment with Preservative-free TIMOPTIC in OCUDOSE 0.5 percent, concomitant therapy with pilocarpine and other miotics, and/or epinephrine, and/or systemically administered carbonic anhydrase inhibitors, such as acetazolamide, can be instituted taking into consideration that the preparation(s) used concomitantly may contain one or more preservatives.

When a patient is transferred from another topical ophthalmic beta-adrenergic blocking agent, that agent should be discontinued after proper dosing on one day and treatment with Preservative-free TIMOPTIC in OCUDOSE started on the following day with 1 drop of 0.25 percent Preservative-free TIMOPTIC in OCUDOSE in the affected eye(s) twice a day. The dose may be increased to one drop of 0.5 percent Preservative-free TIMOPTIC in OCUDOSE twice a day if the clinical response is not adequate.

When a patient is transferred from a single antiglaucoma agent, other than a topical ophthalmic beta-adrenergic blocking agent, continue the agent already being used and add one drop of 0.25 percent Preservative-free TIMOPTIC in OCUDOSE in the affected eye(s) twice a day. On the following day, discontinue the previously used antiglaucoma agent completely and continue with Preservative-free TIMOPTIC in OCUDOSE. If a higher dosage of Preservative-free TIMOPTIC in OCUDOSE is required, substitute one drop of 0.5 percent solution in the affected eye(s) twice a day.

When a patient is transferred from several concomitantly administered antiglaucoma agents, individualization is required. If any of the agents is an ophthalmic beta-adrenergic blocker, it should be discontinued before starting Preservative-free TIMOPTIC in OCUDOSE. Additional adjustments should involve one agent at a time and usually should be made at intervals of not less than one week. A recommended approach is to continue the agents being used and to add one drop of 0.25 percent Preservative-free TIMOPTIC in OCUDOSE in the affected eye(s) twice a day. On the following day, discontinue one of the other antiglaucoma agents. The remaining antiglaucoma agents may be decreased or discontinued according to the patient's response to treatment. If a higher dosage of Preservative-free TIMOPTIC in OCUDOSE is required, substitute one drop of 0.5 percent solution in the affected eye(s) twice a day. The physician may be able to discontinue some or all of the other antiglaucoma agents.

How Supplied

Preservative-free Sterile Ophthalmic Solution TIMOPTIC in OCUDOSE is a clear, colorless to light yellow solution.

No. 3542—Preservative-free TIMOPTIC, 0.25% timolol equivalent, is supplied in OCUDOSE, a clear polyethylene unit dose container. Each individual unit contains 0.45 mL of solution, and is available in a foil laminate overwrapped pouch as follows:

NDC 0006-3542-60; 60 Individual Unit Doses (6505-01-316-8791, 0.25% 60 Individual Unit Doses).

No. 3543—Preservative-free TIMOPTIC, 0.5% timolol equivalent, is supplied in OCUDOSE, a clear polyethylene unit dose container. Each individual unit contains 0.45 mL of solution, and is available in a foil laminate overwrapped pouch as follows:

NDC 0006-3543-60; 60 Individual Unit Doses (6505-01-284-5154, 0.5% 60 Individual Unit Doses).

Storage

Store Preservative-free TIMOPTIC in OCUDOSE at room temperature.

Because evaporation can occur through the unprotected polyethylene unit dose container and prolonged exposure to direct light can modify the product, the unit dose container should be kept in the protective foil overwrap and used within one month after the foil package has been opened.

A.H.F.S. Category: 52:36

DC 7475304 Issued August 1990

Shown in Product Identification Section, page 104

Information on the Merck Sharp & Dohme products listed on these pages is the full prescribing information from product circulars in effect August 31, 1991.

Ocumed, Inc.

119 HARRISON AVENUE
ROSELAND, NJ 07068

(UNIT DOSE) PRODUCTS

OCU-TEARS PF™
in Ophtha-Dose™ unit dispenser Preservative Free, (Polyvinyl Alcohol ocular lubricant), Sterile Ophthalmic Solution.
How supplied: 60 Ophtha-Dose™ Single Use Container NDC #51944-4485-01
120 Ophtha-Dose™ Single Use Container NDC #51944-4485-02

(MULTI-DOSE) PRODUCTS

BASOL-S ℞
(balanced salt solutiion)
Sterile Surgical Solution
How Supplied: In 15 ml dropper bottle and in a 500 ml bottle.

EYE-ZINE
(tetrahydrozoline hydrochloride 0.05%)
Sterile eye drops
How Supplied: In 0.5 fl. oz. plastic dropper bottle.

IRI-SOL
(irrigating eye wash)
Sterile isotonic buffered solution
How Supplied: In 0.5 fl. oz., 1 fl. oz. and 4 fl. oz. plastic dispenser bottle.

OCU-CAINE ℞
(proparacaine hydrochloride 0.5%)
Sterile Ophthalmic Solution
How Supplied: In 2 ml and 15 ml plastic dropper bottle.

OCU-CARPINE ℞
(pilocarpine hydrochloride)
(0.5%, 1%, 2%, 3%, 4%. 5% and 6%)
Sterile Ophthalmic Solution
How Supplied: 15 ml Plastic Dropper Bottles.

OCU-CHLOR ℞
(chloramphenicol 1%)
Sterile Ophthalmic Ointment
How Supplied: In 3.5 g tubes with ophthalmic tip.

OCU-CHLOR ℞
(chloramphenicol 0.5%)
Sterile Ophthalmic Solution
How Supplied: In 7.5 ml and 15 ml plastic dropper bottle.

OCU-CORT ℞
(polymyxin B sulfate 10,000 u/g)
(neomycin sulfate-equiv. 3.5 mg/g)
(zinc bacitracin 400 u/g)
(hydrocortisone 1%)
Sterile Ophthalmic Ointment
How Supplied: In 3.5 g tubes with ophthalmic tip.

OCU-DEX ℞
(dexamethasone sodium phosphate 0.05%)
Sterile Ophthalmic Ointment
How Supplied: In 3.5 g tube with ophthalmic tip.

OCU-DEX ℞
(dexamethasone sodium phosphate 0.1%)
Sterile Ophthalmic Solution
How Supplied: In 5 ml plastic dropper bottle

OCU-LONE-C ℞
(sulfacetamide sodium 100 mg)
(prednisolone acetate 5 mg.)
Sterile Ophthalmic ointment
How Supplied: In 3.5 g tube with ophthalmic tip.

Continued on next page

Ocumed—Cont.

OCU-LONE-C ℞
(sulfacetamide sodium 100 mg)
prednisolone acetate 5 mg)
Sterile Ophthalmic Suspension
How Supplied: In 5 ml amd 15 ml plastic dropper bottle.

OCU-LUBE
(white petrolatum base ocular lubricant)
Sterile ophthalmic Ointment
How Supplied: In 3.5 g tube with ophthalmic tip.

OCU-MYCIN ℞
(gentamicin sulfate—equiv. 3.0 mg)
Sterile Ophthalmic Ointment
How Supplied: In 3.5 g tubes with ophthalmic tip.

OCU-MYCIN ℞
(gentamicin sulfate—equiv. 3.0 mg.)
Sterile Ophthalmic Solution
How Supplied: In 5 ml and 15 ml plastic dropper bottle.

OCU-PENTOLATE ℞
(cyclopentolate hydrochloride 1%)
Sterile Ophthalmic Solution
How Supplied: In 2 ml, 5 ml and 15 ml plastic dropper bottle.

OCU-PHRIN
(phenylephrine hydrochloride 0.12%)
Sterile Eye Drops
How Supplied: In 0.5 fl. oz. plastic dropper bottle.

OCU-PHRIN ℞
(phenylephrine hydrochloride 2.5% and 10%)
Sterile Ophthalmic Solution
How Supplied: In 5 ml and 15 ml plastic dropper bottle.

OCU-PRED ℞
(prednisolone sodium phosphate 0.125%)
Sterile Ophthalmic Solution
How Supplied: In 5 ml and 15 ml plastic dropper bottle.

OCU-PRED FORTE ℞
(prednisolone sodium phosphate 1%)
Sterile Ophthalmic Solution
How Supplied: In 5 ml and 15 ml plastic dropper bottle.

OCU-PRED-A ℞
(prednisolone acetate 1%)
Sterile Ophthalmic Suspension
How Supplied: In 5 ml and 10 ml plastic dropper bottle.

OCU-SOL
(hard contact lens solution)
Sterile antiseptic wetting and lubricating solution
How Supplied: In 2 oz. plastic dispenser bottle.

OCU-SPOR-B ℞
(polymyxin B sulfate—10,000 u/cc)
(neomycin sulfate—equiv. 3.5 mg/g)
(zinc bacitracin 400 u/g)
Sterile Ophthalmic Ointment
How Supplied: In 3.5 g tubes with ophthalmic tip.

OCU-SPOR-G ℞
(polymyxin B sulfate—10,000 u/cc)
(neomycin sulfate—equiv. 1.75 mg/cc)
(gramicidin 0.025%)
Sterile Ophthalmic Solution
How Supplied: In 10 cc plastic dropper bottle.

OCU-SUL-10 ℞
(sodium sulfacetamide 10%)
Sterile Ophthalmic Ointment
How Supplied: In 3.5 g tubes with ophthalmic tip.

OCU-SUL-10 ℞
(sodium sulfacetamide 10%)
Sterile Ophthalmic Solution
How Supplied: In 15 ml plastic bottles.

OCU-SUL-15 ℞
(sodium sulfacetamide 15%)
Sterile Ophthalmic Solution
How Supplied: In 15 ml plastic bottles.

OCU-SUL-30 ℞
(sodium sulfacetamide 30%)
Sterile Ophthalmic Solution
How Supplied: In 15 ml plastic bottles.

OCU-TEARS
(polyvinyl alcohol ocular lubricant)
Sterile Ophthalmic Solution
How Supplied: In 0.5 fl. oz. plastic dropper bottle.

OCU-TROL ℞
(polymyxin B sulfate 10,000 u/g)
(neomycin sulfate—equiv. 3.5 mg/g)
(dexamethasone 0.1%)
Sterile Ophthalmic Ointment
How Supplied: In 3.5 g tube with ophthalmic tip.

OCU-TROL ℞
(polymyxin B sulfate 10,000 u/g)
(neomycin sulfate—equiv. 3.5 mg/g)
dexamethesone 0.1%)
Sterile Ophthalmic Suspension
How Supplied: In 5 ml plastic dropper bottle.

OCU-TROPIC ℞
(tropicamide 0.5% and 1.0%)
Sterile Ophthalmic Solution
How Supplied: In 15 ml plastic dropper bottle.

OCU-TROPINE ℞
(atropine sulfate 1%)
Sterile Ophthalmic Ointment
How Supplied: In 3.5 g tubes with ophthalmic tip.

OCU-TROPINE ℞
(atropine sulfate 1%)
Sterile Ophthalmic Solution
How Supplied: In 15 ml plastic dropper bottle.

OCU-ZOLINE ℞
(naphazoline hydrochloride 0.1%)
Sterile Ophthalmic Solution
How Supplied: In 15 ml plastic dropper bottle.

Parke-Davis
Division of Warner-Lambert Company
MORRIS PLAINS, NEW JERSEY
07950

CHLOROMYCETIN® ℞
[*klo "ro-mi-se 'tin*]
HYDROCORTISONE OPHTHALMIC
(Chloramphenicol and Hydrocortisone Acetate for Suspension, USP)

> **WARNING**
> Bone marrow hypoplasia including aplastic anemia and death has been reported following the local application of chloramphenicol. Chloramphenicol should not be used when less potentially dangerous agents would be expected to provide effective treatment.

Description: Chloromycetin® Hydrocortisone Ophthalmic (Chloramphenicol and Hydrocortisone Acetate for Suspension, USP) is a sterile, buffered antibiotic/antiinflammatory dry mixture for suspension for ophthalmic administration. Each vial of Chloromycetin Hydrocortisone Ophthalmic contains 12.5 mg chloramphenicol and 25 mg hydrocortisone acetate with boric acid-sodium borate buffer, cholesterol, methylcellulose, sodium chloride, and Phemerol® (benzethonium chloride), 0.1 mg per ml, in the suspension when prepared as directed. A 5-mL vial of Sterile Distilled Water is included in each package for use as a diluent in the preparation of a suspension of Chloromycetin Hydrocortisone suitable for ophthalmic use.

The chemical names for chloramphenicol are:
(1) Acetamide,2,2-dichloro-N-[2-hydroxy-1-(hydroxymethyl)-2-(4-nitrophenyl) ethyl]-, and
(2) D-*threo* -(–)-2,2-Dichloro-N-[β-hydroxy-α-(hydroxymethyl)-*p* -nitrophenethyl] acetamide

Chloramphenicol has the following empirical and structural formulas:

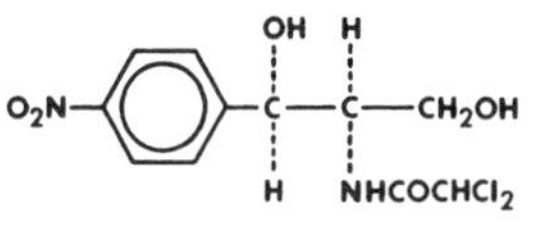

$C_{11}H_{12}Cl_2N_2O_5$ Mol Wt 323.13

The chemical names for hydrocortisone acetate are:
(1) Pregn-4-ene-3,20-dione,21-(acetyloxy)-11,17-dihydroxy-,(11β)-, and
(2) 17-Hydroxycorticosterone 21-acetate

Hydrocortisone acetate has the following empirical and structural formulas:

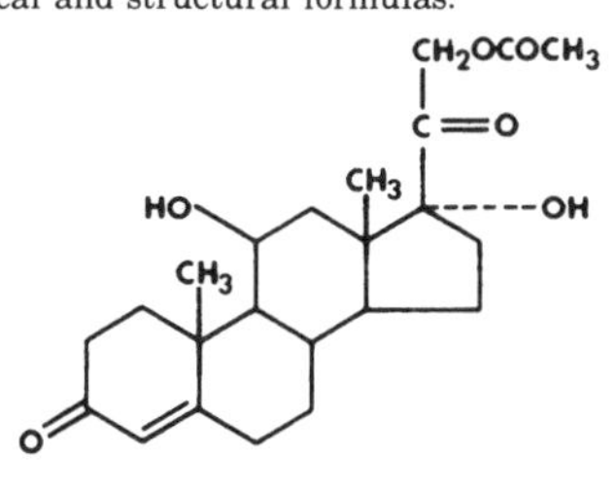

$C_{23}H_{32}O_6$ Mol Wt 404.50

Clinical Pharmacology: Corticoids suppress the inflammatory response to a variety of agents and they probably delay or slow healing. Since corticoids may inhibit the body's defense mechanism against infection, a concomitant antimicrobial drug may be used when this inhibition is considered to be clinically significant in a particular case.

The antiinfective component in this combination is included to provide action against specific organisms susceptible to it. Chloramphenicol is considered active against a wide spectrum of gram-negative and gram-positive organisms such as *Escherichia coli, Haemophilus influenzae, Staphylococcus aureus, Streptococcus hemolyticus,* and *Moraxella lacunata* (Morax-Axenfeld bacillus). Development of resistance to chloramphenicol can be regarded as minimal for staphylococci and many other species of bacteria. Chloramphenicol is primarily bacteriostatic and acts by inhibition of protein synthesis by interfering with the transfer of activated amino acids from soluble RNA to ribosomes. It has been noted that chloramphenicol is found in measurable amounts in the aqueous humor following local application to the eye.

When a decision to administer both a corticoid and an antimicrobial is made, the administration of such drugs in combination has the advantage of greater patient compliance and convenience, with the added assurance that the appropriate dosage of both drugs is administered, plus assured compatibility of ingredients when both types of drug are in the same formulation and, particularly, that the correct volume of drug is delivered and retained.

'he relative potency of corticosteroids depends
n the molecular structure, concentration, and
elease from the vehicle.
ndications and Usage: Chloramphenicol
hould be used only in those serious infections
or which less potentially dangerous drugs are
neffective or contraindicated. Bacteriological
tudies should be performed to determine the
ausative organisms and their sensitivity to
hloramphenicol (See Box Warning).
'or steroid-responsive inflammatory ocular
onditions for which a corticosteroid is indi-
ated and where bacterial infection or a risk of
acterial ocular infection exists.
)cular steroids are indicated in inflammatory
onditions of the palpebral and bulbar con-
unctiva, cornea, and anterior segment of the
;lobe where the inherent risk of steroid use in
ertain infective conjunctivitides is accepted to
btain a diminution in edema and inflamma-
ion. They are also indicated in chronic ante-
ior uveitis and corneal injury from chemical
adiation, thermal burns, or penetration of
oreign bodies.
'he use of a combination drug with an antiin-
ective component is indicated where the risk
f infection is high or where there is an expec-
ation that potentially dangerous numbers of
acteria will be present in the eye.
'he particular antiinfective drug in this prod-
ct is active against the following common bac-
erial eye pathogens:
taphylococcus aureus
treptococci, including *Streptococcus pneumoniae*
scherichia coli
Iaemophilus influenzae
Klebsiella/Enterobacter species
Aoraxella lacunata (Morax-Axenfeld bacillus)
Veisseria species
The product does not provide adequate cover-
ge against:
Pseudomonas aeruginosa
erratia marcescens
Contraindications: Epithelial herpes sim-
lex keratitis (dendritic keratitis), vaccinia,
aricella, and many other viral diseases of the
ornea and conjunctiva. Mycobacterial infec-
ion of the eye. Fungal diseases of ocular struc-
ures. Hypersensitivity to a component of the
nedication. (Hypersensitivity to the antibiotic
omponent occurs at a higher rate than for
ther components).
The use of these combinations is always contra-
ndicated after uncomplicated removal of a
orneal foreign body.
Warnings: SEE BOX WARNING
Prolonged use of steroids may result in glau-
oma, with damage to the optic nerve, defects
n visual acuity and fields of vision, and poste-
ior subcapsular cataract formation. Pro-
onged use may suppress the host response and
hus increase the hazard of secondary ocular
nfections. In those diseases causing thinning
f the cornea or sclera, perforations have been
nown to occur with the use of topical steroids.
n acute purulent conditions of the eye, ste-
oids may mask infection or enhance existing
nfection. If these products are used for 10 days
r longer, intraocular pressure should be rou-
inely monitored even though it may be diffi-
ult in children and uncooperative patients.
Employment of steroid medication in the treat-
nent of herpes simplex requires great caution.
Precautions: The initial prescription and
enewal of the medication order beyond 20
nilliliters should be made by a physician only
fter examination of the patient with the aid of
nagnification, such as slit lamp biomicroscopy
nd, where appropriate, fluorescein staining.
The possibility of persistent fungal infections
f the cornea should be considered after pro-
onged steroid dosing.
The prolonged use of antibiotics may occasion-
lly result in overgrowth of nonsusceptible
rganisms, including fungi. If new infections
ppear during medication, the drug should be discontinued and appropriate measures should be taken.

In all serious infections the topical use of chloramphenicol should be supplemented by appropriate systemic medication.

Adverse Reactions: Blood dyscrasias have been reported in association with the use of chloramphenicol. (See **Warnings**).

Adverse reactions have occurred with steroid/antiinfective combination drugs which can be attributed to the steroid component, the antiinfective component, or the combination. Exact incidence figures are not available since no denominator of treated patients is available.

Reactions occurring most often from the presence of the antiinfective ingredient are allergic sensitizations. The reactions due to the steroid component in decreasing order of frequency are: elevation of intraocular pressure (IOP) with possible development of glaucoma, and infrequent optic nerve damage; posterior subcapsular cataract formation; and delayed wound healing.

Secondary Infection: The development of secondary infection has occurred after use of combinations containing steroids and antimicrobials. Fungal infections of the cornea are particularly prone to develop coincidentally with long-term applications of steroid. The possibility of fungal invasion must be considered in any persistent corneal ulceration where steroid treatment has been used.

Secondary bacterial ocular infection following suppression of host responses also occurs.

Dosage and Administration: Two drops applied to the affected eye every three hours, or more frequently if deemed advisable by the prescribing physician. Administration should be continued day and night for the first 48 hours, after which the interval between applications may be increased. Treatment should be continued for at least 48 hours after the eye appears normal.

Directions for dispensing—Add 5 ml sterile distilled water to contents of vial under aseptic conditions. Shake to make uniform suspension. Place sterile dropper in vial. Each ml of suspension prepared as directed contains 2.5 mg Chloromycetin (chloramphenicol) and 5 mg Hydrocortisone Acetate.

Not more than 20 milliliters should be prescribed initially and the prescription should not be refilled without further evaluation as outlined in Precautions above.

How Supplied: N 0071-3228-36 Chloromycetin Hydrocortisone Ophthalmic (Chloramphenicol and Hydrocortisone Acetate for Suspension, USP) is supplied in a package containing dry ingredients in a 5 ml vial and also a vial containing 5 ml of Sterile Distilled Water for use as a diluent in preparation of the ophthalmic suspension. After dispensing, the product may be stored at room temperature for a period of not more than 10 days. A sterilized dropper-cap assembly for use with the vial is included in the package.

Chloromycetin, brand of chloramphenicol, Reg US Pat Off. **3228G014**

Shown in Product Identification Section, page 104

CHLOROMYCETIN® ℞

[klo "ro-mi-se "tin]

OPHTHALMIC OINTMENT, 1%

(chloramphenicol ophthalmic ointment, USP)

> **WARNING:**
> Bone marrow hypoplasia including aplastic anemia and death has been reported following local application of chloramphenicol. Chloramphenicol should not be used when less potentially dangerous agents would be expected to provide effective treatment.

Description: Each gram of Chloromycetin Ophthalmic Ointment, 1%, contains 10 mg chloramphenicol in a special base of liquid petrolatum and polyethylene. It contains no preservatives. Sterile ointment.

The chemical names for chloramphenicol are:

(1) Acetamide,2,2-dichloro-*N*-[2-hydroxy-1-(hydroxymethyl)-2-(4-nitrophenyl) ethyl]-, and

(2) D-*threo*-(–)-2,2-Dichloro-*N*-[β-hydroxy-α-(hydroxymethyl)-*p*-nitrophenethyl] acetamide

Clinical Pharmacology: Chloramphenicol is a broad-spectrum antibiotic originally isolated from *Streptomyces venezuelae.* It is primarily bacteriostatic and acts by inhibition of protein synthesis by interfering with the transfer of activated amino acids from soluble RNA to ribosomes. It has been noted that chloramphenicol is found in measurable amounts in the aqueous humor following local application to the eye. Development of resistance to chloramphenicol can be regarded as minimal for staphylococci and many other species of bacteria.

Indications and Usage: Chloramphenicol should be used only in those serious infections for which less potentially dangerous drugs are ineffective or contraindicated. Bacteriological studies should be performed to determine the causative organisms and their sensitivity to chloramphenicol (See Box Warning).

Chloromycetin (chloramphenicol) Ophthalmic Ointment, 1%, is indicated for the treatment of surface ocular infections involving the conjunctiva and/or cornea caused by chloramphenicol-susceptible organisms.

The particular antiinfective drug in this product is active against the following common bacterial eye pathogens:

Staphylococcus aureus
Streptococci, including *Streptococcus pneumoniae*
Escherichia coli
Haemophilus influenzae
Klebsiella/Enterobacter species
Moraxella lacunata (Morax-Axenfeld bacillus)
Neisseria species

The product does not provide adequate coverage against:

Pseudomonas aeruginosa
Serratia marcescens

Contraindications: This product is contraindicated in persons sensitive to any of its components.

Warnings: SEE BOX WARNING
Ophthalmic ointments may retard corneal wound healing.

Precautions: The prolonged use of antibiotics may occasionally result in overgrowth of nonsusceptible organisms, including fungi. If new infections appear during medication, the drug should be discontinued and appropriate measures should be taken.

In all serious infections the topical use of chloramphenicol should be supplemented by appropriate systemic medication.

Adverse Reactions: Allergic or inflammatory reactions due to individual hypersensitivity and occasional burning or stinging may occur with the use of Chloromycetin Ophthalmic Ointment. Blood dyscrasias have been re-

Continued on next page

The product information represents the package circular in effect July, 1991. Information on other Parke-Davis Products may be obtained by addressing PARKE-DAVIS, Division of Warner-Lambert Company, Morris Plains, New Jersey 07950

Parke-Davis—Cont.

ported in association with the use of chloramphenicol (See WARNINGS).

Dosage and Administration: A small amount of ointment placed in the lower conjunctival sac every three hours, or more frequently if deemed advisable by the prescribing physician. Administration should be continued day and night for the first 48 hours, after which the interval between applications may be increased. Treatment should be continued for at least 48 hours after the eye appears normal.

How Supplied:
N 0071-3070-07
Chloromycetin Ophthalmic Ointment, 1% (Chloramphenicol Ophthalmic Ointment, USP) is supplied, sterile, in ophthalmic ointment tubes of 3.5 grams.
Chloromycetin, brand of chloramphenicol, Reg US Pat Off
AHFS Category 52:04.04 **3070G022**

Shown in Product Identification Section, page 104

CHLOROMYCETIN® OPHTHALMIC ℞
[*klo"ro-mi-se"tin*]
(Chloramphenical for Ophthalmic Solution, USP)

> **WARNING**
> Bone marrow hypoplasia including aplastic anemia and death has been reported following local application of chloramphenicol. Chloramphenicol should not be used when less potentially dangerous agents would be expected to provide effective treatment.

Description: Each vial of Chloromycetin Ophthalmic contains 25 mg of Chloromycetin (chloramphenicol) with boric acid-sodium borate buffer. Sodium hydroxide may have been added for adjustment of pH. A 15 ml bottle of Sterile Distilled Water is included in each package for use as a diluent in the preparation of a solution of Chloromycetin suitable for ophthalmic use. By varying the quantity of diluent used solutions ranging in strength from 0.16% to 0.5% may be prepared. Both the powder for solution and the diluent contain no preservatives. Sterile powder.

The chemical names for chloramphenicol are:
(1) Acetamide,2,2-dichloro-*N*-[2-hydroxy-1-(hydroxymethyl)-2-(4-nitrophenyl) ethyl]-, and
(2) D-*threo*-(−)-2,2-Dichloro-*N*-[β-hydroxy-α-(hydroxymethyl)-*p*-nitrophenethyl] acetamide

Chloramphenicol has the following empirical and structural formulas:

$$O_2N-C_6H_4-CH(OH)-CH(NHCOCHCl_2)-CH_2OH$$

$C_{11}H_{12}Cl_2N_2O_5$ **Mol Wt 323.13**

Clinical Pharmacology: Chloramphenicol is a broad-spectrum antibiotic originally isolated from *Streptomyces venezuelae.* It is primarily bacteriostatic and acts by inhibition of protein synthesis by interfering with the transfer of activated amino acids from soluble RNA to ribosomes. It has been noted that chloramphenicol is found in measurable amounts in the aqueous humor following local application to the eye. Development of resistance to chloramphenicol can be regarded as minimal for staphylococci and many other species of bacteria.

Indications and Usage: Chloramphenicol should be used only in those serious infections for which less potentially dangerous drugs are ineffective or contraindicated. Bacteriological studies should be performed to determine the causative organisms and their sensitivity to chloramphenicol (See Box Warning).

Chloromycetin (chloramphenicol) Ophthalmic is indicated for the treatment of surface ocular infections involving the conjunctiva and/or cornea caused by chloramphenicol-susceptible organisms.

The particular antiinfective drug in this product is active against the following common bacterial eye pathogens:
Staphylococcus aureus
Streptococci, including *Streptococcus pneumoniae*
Escherichia coli
Haemophilus influenzae
Klebsiella/Enterobacter species
Moraxella lacunata (Morax-Axenfeld bacillus)
Neisseria species

The product does not provide adequate coverage against:
Pseudomonas aeruginosa
Serratia marcescens

Contraindications: This product is contraindicated in persons sensitive to any of its components.

Warnings: SEE BOX WARNING

Precautions: The prolonged use of antibiotics may occasionally result in overgrowth of nonsusceptible organisms, including fungi. If new infections appear during medication, the drug should be discontinued and appropriate measures should be taken.

In all serious infections the topical use of chloramphenicol should be supplemented by appropriate systemic medication.

Adverse Reactions: Blood dyscrasias have been reported in association with the use of chloramphenicol (See WARNINGS). Transient burning or stinging sensations may occur with use of Chloromycetin Ophthalmic Solution.

Dosage and Administration: Two drops applied to the affected eye every three hours, or more frequently if deemed advisable by the prescribing physician. Administration should be continued day and night for the first 48 hours, after which the interval between applications may be increased. Treatment should be continued for at least 48 hours after the eye appears normal.

Directions for dispensing—Prepare solution by adding sterile distilled water to the vial as follows:

Strength of solution desired	Add sterile distilled water
0.5%	5 ml
0.25%	10 ml
0.16%	15 ml

Solutions remain stable at room temperature for ten days.

How Supplied: N 0071-3213-35 Chloromycetin (chloramphenicol) Ophthalmic is supplied in a package containing dry ingredients in a 15 ml vial and also a vial containing 15 ml of Sterile Distilled Water for use as a diluent in preparing the solution for ophthalmic use. A sterilized dropper-cap assembly for use on the vial of solution is included in the package.
Store below 86°F (30°C).
Chloromycetin, brand of chloramphenicol. Reg US Pat Off
3213G012

Shown in Product Identification Section, page 104

OPHTHOCHLOR® ℞
[*ŏf'thō-klōr"*]
(chloramphenicol ophthalmic solution) 0.5%

> **Warning**
> Bone marrow hypoplasia including aplastic anemia and death has been reported following local application of chloramphenicol. Chloramphenicol should not be used when less potentially dangerous agents would be expected to provide effective treatment.

Description: Ophthochlor (Chloramphenicol Ophthalmic Solution, USP), 0.5%, is a sterile, buffered solution containing 0.5% (5 mg/ml) of chloramphenicol. It contains no preservatives.

The chemical names for chloramphenicol are
(1) Acetamide,2,2-dichloro-*N*-[2-hydroxy-1-(hydroxymethyl)-2-[4-nitrophenyl) ethyl]-and
(2) D-*threo*-(-)-2,2-Dichloro-*N*-[β-hydroxy-α-(hydroxymethyl)-*p*-nitrophenethyl] acetamide

Clinical Pharmacology: Chloramphenicol is a broad-spectrum antibiotic originally isolated from *Streptomyces venezuelae.* It is primarily bacteriostatic and acts by inhibition of protein synthesis by interfering with the transfer of activated amino acids from soluble RNA to ribosomes. It has been noted that chloramphenicol is found in measurable amounts in the aqueous humor following local application to the eye. Development of resistance to chloramphenicol can be regarded as minimal for staphylococci and many other species of bacteria.

Indications and Usage: Chloramphenicol should be used only in those serious infections for which less potentially dangerous drugs are ineffective or contraindicated. Bacteriological studies should be performed to determine the causative organisms and their sensitivity to chloramphenicol. (See Box Warning).

Ophthochlor (chloramphenicol ophthalmic solution) 0.5% is indicated for the treatment of surface ocular infections involving the conjunctiva and/or cornea caused by chloramphenicol-susceptible organisms.

The particular antiinfective drug in this product is active against the following common bacterial eye pathogens:
Staphylococcus aureus
Streptococci, including *Streptococcus pneumoniae*
Escherischia coli
Haemophilus influenzae
Klebsiella/Enterobacter species
Moraxella lacunata (Morax-Axenfeld bacillus)
Neisseria species

The product does not provide adequate coverage against:
Pseudomonas aeruginosa
Serratia marcescens

Contraindications: This product is contraindicated in persons sensitive to any of its components.

Warnings: SEE BOX WARNING

Precautions: The prolonged use of antibiotics may occasionally result in overgrowth of nonsusceptible organisms, including fungi. If new infections appear during medication, the drug should be discontinued and appropriate measures should be taken. In all serious infections the topical use of chloramphenicol should be supplemented by appropriate systemic medication.

Adverse Reactions: Blood dyscrasias have been reported in association with the use of chloramphenicol (see WARNINGS). Transient burning or stinging sensations may occur with use of Ophthochlor.

Dosage and Administration: Two drops applied to the affected eye every three hours, or more frequently if deemed advisable by the prescribing physician. Administration should be continued day and night for the first 48 hours, after which the interval between applications may be increased. Treatment should be continued for at least 48 hours after the eye appears normal.

How Supplied: N 0071-3395-11 15-ml bottle. Ophthochlor (Chloramphenicol Ophthalmic Solution, USP), 0.5%, is supplied in plastic dropper bottles and contains no preservatives. Each ml contains 5 mg chloramphenicol in a boric acid-sodium borate buffer solution. Sodium hydroxide may have been added for adjustment of pH. To protect it from light, the solution should be dispensed in the carton. This product should be stored in a refrigerator until dispensed. Discard solution within 21 days from date dispensed.

AHFS Category 52:04.04 **3395G012**

Shown in Product Identification Section, page 104

OPHTHOCORT® ℞

[*ŏf'thō-kort*]

(Chloramphenicol, Polymyxin B Sulfate, and Hydrocortisone Acetate Ophthalmic Ointment, USP)

> **WARNING**
> Bone marrow hypoplasia including aplastic anemia and death has been reported following local application of chloramphenicol. Chloramphenicol should not be used when less potentially dangerous agents would be expected to provide effective treatment.

Description: Ophthocort® (Chloramphenicol, Polymyxin B Sulfate, and Hydrocortisone Acetate Ophthalmic Ointment, USP) is a sterile antibiotic/antiinflammatory ointment for ophthalmic administration. Each gram of Ophthocort contains 10 mg chloramphenicol, 10,000 units polymyxin B (as the sulfate), and 5 mg hydrocortisone acetate in a special base of liquid petrolatum and polyethylene. It contains no preservatives.

Clinical Pharmacology: Corticoids suppress the inflammatory response to a variety of agents and they probably delay or slow healing. Since corticoids may inhibit the body's defense mechanism against infection, a concomitant antimicrobial drug may be used when this inhibition is considered to be clinically significant in a particular case.

The antiinfective components in this combination are included to provide action against specific organisms susceptible to them. Chloramphenicol is considered active against a wide spectrum of gram-negative and gram-positive organisms such as *Escherichia coli, Haemophilus influenzae, Staphylococcus aureus, Streptococcus hemolyticus,* and *Moraxella lacunata* (Morax-Axenfeld bacillus). Development of resistance to chloramphenicol can be regarded as minimal for staphylococci and many other species of bacteria. Chloramphenicol is primarily bacteriostatic and acts by inhibition of protein synthesis by interfering with the transfer of activated amino acids from soluble RNA to ribosomes. It has been noted that chloramphenicol is found in measurable amounts in the aqueous humor following local application to the eye.

Polymyxin B sulfate has a bactericidal action against almost all gram-negative bacilli except the *Proteus* group. All gram-positive bacteria, fungi, and the gram-negative cocci, *Neisseria gonorrhoeae* and *N meningitidis,* are resistant.

When a decision to administer both a corticoid and an antimicrobial is made, the administration of such drugs in combination has the advantage of greater patient compliance and convenience, with the added assurance that the appropriate dosage of both drugs is administered, plus assured compatibility of ingredients when both types of drug are in the same formulation and, particularly, that the correct volume of drug is delivered and retained.

The relative potency of corticosteroids depends on the molecular structure, concentration, and release from the vehicle.

Indications and Usage: Chloramphenicol should be used only in those serious infections for which less potentially dangerous drugs are ineffective or contraindicated. Bacteriological studies should be performed to determine the causative organisms and their sensitivity to chloramphenicol (See Boxed warning).

For steroid-responsive inflammatory ocular conditions for which a corticosteroid is indicated and where bacterial infection or a risk of bacterial ocular infection exists.

Ocular steroids are indicated in inflammatory conditions of the palpebral and bulbar conjunctiva, cornea, and anterior segment of the globe where the inherent risk of steroid use in certain infective conjunctivitides is accepted to obtain a diminution in edema and inflammation. They are also indicated in chronic anterior uveitis and corneal injury from chemical radiation, thermal burns, or penetration of foreign bodies.

The use of a combination drug with an antiinfective component is indicated where the risk of infection is high or where there is an expectation that potentially dangerous numbers of bacteria will be present in the eye.

The particular antiinfective drugs in this product are active against the following common bacterial eye pathogens:

Staphylococcus aureus
Streptococci, including *Streptococcus pneumoniae*
Escherichia coli
Hemophilus influenzae
Klebsiella/Enterobacter species
Neisseria species
Moraxella lacunata (Morax-Axenfeld bacillus)
Pseudomonas aeruginosa

The product does not provide adequate coverage against:

Serratia marcescens

Contraindications: Epithelial herpes simplex keratitis (dendritic keratitis), vaccinia, varicella, and many other viral diseases of the cornea and conjunctiva. Mycobacterial infection of the eye. Fungal diseases of ocular structures. Hypersensitivity to a component of the medication. (Hypersensitivity to the antibiotic component occurs at a higher rate than for other components.)

The use of these combinations is always contraindicated after uncomplicated removal of a corneal foreign body.

Warnings: SEE BOX WARNING

Prolonged use of steroids may result in glaucoma, with damage to the optic nerve, defects in visual acuity and fields of vision, and posterior subcapsular cataract formation. Prolonged use may suppress the host response and thus increase the hazard of secondary ocular infections. In those diseases causing thinning of the cornea or sclera, perforations have been known to occur with the use of topical steroids. In acute purulent conditions of the eye, steroids may mask infection or enhance existing infection. If these products are used for 10 days or longer, intraocular pressure should be routinely monitored even though it may be difficult in children and uncooperative patients.

Employment of steroid medication in the treatment of herpes simplex requires great caution.

Ophthalmic ointments may retard corneal wound healing.

Precautions: The initial prescription and renewal of the medication order beyond 8 grams should be made by a physician only after examination of the patient with the aid of magnification, such as slit lamp biomicroscopy and, where appropriate, fluorescein staining.

The possibility of persistent fungal infections of the cornea should be considered after prolonged steroid dosing.

The prolonged use of antibiotics may occasionally result in overgrowth of nonsusceptible organisms, including fungi. If new infections appear during medication, the drug should be discontinued and appropriate measures should be taken.

In all serious infections the topical use of chloramphenicol should be supplemented by appropriate systemic medication.

Adverse Reactions: There have been reports of punctate staining of the cornea following intensive treatment (every one to two hours during the waking day) of corneal ulcers with Ophthocort. In each reported case, the staining has disappeared after discontinuation of the medication.

Blood dyscrasias have been reported in association with the use of chloramphenicol. (See WARNINGS.)

Adverse reactions have occurred with steroid/antiinfective combination drugs which can be attributed to the steroid component, the antiinfective component, or the combination. Exact incidence figures are not available since no denominator of treated patients is available.

Reactions occurring most often from the presence of the antiinfective ingredient are allergic sensitizations. The reactions due to the steroid component in decreasing order of frequency are: elevation of intraocular pressure (IOP) with possible development of glaucoma, and infrequent optic nerve damage; posterior subcapsular cataract formation; and delayed wound healing.

Secondary Infection: The development of secondary infection has occurred after use of combinations containing steroids and antimicrobials. Fungal infections of the cornea are particularly prone to develop coincidentally with long-term applications of steroid. The possibility of fungal invasion must be considered in any persistent corneal ulceration where steroid treatment has been used.

Secondary bacterial ocular infection following suppression of host responses also occurs.

Dosage and Administration: Application of a small amount of ointment, placed in the lower conjunctival sac, is made to the affected eye every three hours, or more frequently if deemed advisable by the prescribing physician. Administration should be continued day and night for the first 48 hours, after which the interval between applications may be increased. Treatment should be continued for at least 48 hours after the eye appears normal.

Not more than 8 grams should be prescribed initially and the prescription should not be refilled without further evaluation as outlined in Precautions above.

How Supplied: N 0071-3079-07 Ophthocort (Chloramphenicol, Polymyxin B Sulfate, Hydrocortisone Acetate Ophthalmic Ointment, USP); Each gram of ointment contains 10 mg chloramphenicol, 10,000 units polymyxin B (as the sulfate), and 5 mg hydrocortisone acetate

Continued on next page

The product information represents the package circular in effect July, 1991. Information on other Parke-Davis Products may be obtained by addressing PARKE-DAVIS, Division of Warner-Lambert Company, Morris Plains, New Jersey 07950

Parke-Davis—Cont.

in a special base of liquid petrolatum and polyethylene. Supplied in 3.5 g tubes.

AHFS Category 52:04.04 **3079G012**

Shown in Product Identification Section, page 104

VIRA-A® ℞

[*vī″rā-ā′*]

(Vidarabine Ophthalmic Ointment, USP) 3%

Description: VIRA-A is the trade name for vidarabine (also known as adenine arabinoside and Ara-A), an antiviral drug for the topical treatment of epithelial keratitis caused by Herpes simplex virus. The chemical name is 9-β-D-arabinofuranosyladenine. Each gram of the ophthalmic ointment contains 30 mg of vidarabine monohydrate equivalent to 28.11 mg of vidarabine in a sterile, inert, petrolatum base.

Clinical Pharmacology: VIRA-A is a purine nucleoside obtained from fermentation cultures of *Streptomyces antibioticus.* VIRA-A possesses *in vitro* and *in vivo* antiviral activity against Herpes simplex types 1 and 2, Varicella-Zoster, and Vaccinia viruses. Except for Rhabdovirus and Oncornavirus, VIRA-A does not display *in vitro* antiviral activity against other RNA or DNA viruses, including Adenovirus.

The antiviral mechanism of action has not been established. VIRA-A appears to interfere with the early steps of viral DNA synthesis. VIRA-A is rapidly deaminated to arabinosylhypoxanthine (Ara-Hx), the principal metabolite. Ara-Hx also possesses *in vitro* antiviral activity but this activity is less than that of VIRA-A. Because of the low solubility of VIRA-A, trace amounts of both VIRA-A and Ara-Hx can be detected in the aqueous humor only if there is an epithelial defect in the cornea. If the cornea is normal, only trace amounts of Ara-Hx can be recovered from the aqueous humor.

Systemic absorption of VIRA-A should not be expected to occur following ocular administration and swallowing lacrimal secretions. In laboratory animals, VIRA-A is rapidly deaminated in the gastrointestinal tract to Ara-Hx.

In contrast to topical idoxuridine, VIRA-A demonstrated less cellular toxicity in the regenerating corneal epithelium of the rabbit.

Indications and Usage: VIRA-A Ophthalmic Ointment, 3%, is indicated for the treatment of acute keratoconjunctivitis and recurrent epithelial keratitis due to Herpes simplex virus types 1 and 2. It is also effective in superficial keratitis caused by Herpes simplex virus which has not responded to topical idoxuridine or when toxic or hypersensitivity reactions to idoxuridine have occurred. The effectiveness of VIRA-A Ophthalmic Ointment, 3%, against stromal keratitis and uveitis due to Herpes simplex virus has not been established.

The clinical diagnosis of keratitis caused by Herpes simplex virus is usually established by the presence of typical dendritic or geographic lesions on slit-lamp examination.

In controlled and uncontrolled clinical trials, an average of seven and nine days of continuous VIRA-A Ophthalmic Ointment, 3%, therapy was required to achieve corneal re-epithelialization. In the controlled trials, 70 of 81 subjects (86%) re-epithelialized at the end of three weeks of therapy. In the uncontrolled trials, 101 of 142 subjects (71%) re-epithelialized at the end of three weeks. Seventy-five percent of the subjects in these uncontrolled trials had either not healed previously or had developed hypersensitivity to topical idoxuridine therapy.

The following topical antibiotics: gentamicin, erythromycin, chloramphenicol; or topical steroids: prednisolone or dexamethasone have been administered concurrently with VIRA-A Ophthalmic Ointment, 3%, without an increase in adverse reactions.

Contraindication: VIRA-A Ophthalmic Ointment, 3%, is contraindicated in patients who develop hypersensitivity reactions to it.

Warnings: Normally, corticosteroids alone are contraindicated in Herpes simplex virus infections of the eye. If VIRA-A Ophthalmic Ointment, 3%, is administered concurrently with topical corticosteroid therapy, corticosteroid-induced ocular side effects must be considered. These include corticosteroid-induced glaucoma or cataract formation and progression of a bacterial or viral infection.

VIRA-A is not effective against RNA virus or adenoviral ocular infections. It is also not effective against bacterial, fungal, or chlamydial infections of the cornea or nonviral trophic ulcers.

Although viral resistance to VIRA-A has not been observed, this possibility may exist.

Precautions:

General—The diagnosis of keratoconjunctivitis due to Herpes simplex virus should be established clinically prior to prescribing VIRA-A Ophthalmic Ointment, 3%.

Patients should be forewarned that VIRA-A Ophthalmic Ointment, 3%, like any ophthalmic ointment, may produce a temporary visual haze.

Carcinogenesis—Chronic parenteral (IM) studies of vidarabine have been conducted in mice and rats.

In the mouse study, there was a statistically significant increase in liver tumor incidence among the vidarabine-treated females. In the same study some vidarabine-treated male mice developed kidney neoplasia. No renal tumors were found in the vehicle-treated control mice or the vidarabine-treated female mice.

In the rat study, intestinal, testicular, and thyroid neoplasia occurred with greater frequency among the vidarabine-treated animals than in the vehicle-treated controls. The increases in thyroid adenoma incidence in the high dose (50 mg/kg) males and the low dose (30 mg/kg) females were statistically significant.

Hepatic megalocytosis, associated with vidarabine treatment, has been found in short- and long-term rodent (rat and mouse) studies. It is not clear whether or not this represents a preneoplastic change.

The recommended frequency and duration of administration should not be exceeded (See Dosage and Administration).

Mutagenesis—Results of *in vitro* experiments indicate that vidarabine can be incorporated into mammalian DNA and can induce mutation in mammalian cells (mouse L5178Y cell line). Thus far, *in vivo* studies have not been as conclusive, but there is some evidence (dominant lethal assay in mice) that vidarabine may be capable of producing mutagenic effects in male germ cells.

It has also been reported that vidarabine causes chromosome breaks and gaps when added to human leukocytes *in vitro.* While the significance of these effects in terms of mutagenicity is not fully understood, there is a well-known correlation between the ability of various agents to produce such effects and their ability to produce heritable genetic damage.

Pregnancy Category C—VIRA-A parenterally is teratogenic in rats and rabbits. Ten percent VIRA-A ointment applied to 10% of the body surface during organogenesis induced fetal abnormalities in rabbits. When 10% VIRA-A ointment was applied to 2% to 3% of the body surface of rabbits, no fetal abnormalities were found. This dose greatly exceeds the total recommended ophthalmic dose in humans. The possibility of embryonic or fetal damage in pregnant women receiving VIRA-A Ophthalmic Ointment, 3%, is remote. The topical ophthalmic dose is small, and the drug relatively insoluble. Its ocular penetration is very low. However, a safe dose for a human embryo or fetus has not been established. There are no adequate and well controlled studies in pregnant women. VIRA-A should be used during pregnancy only if the potential benefit justifies the potential risk to the fetus.

Nursing Mothers—It is not known whether VIRA-A is secreted in human milk. Because many drugs are excreted in human milk and because of the potential for tumorigenicity shown for VIRA-A in animal studies, a decision should be made whether to discontinue nursing or to discontinue the drug, taking into account the importance of the drug to the mother. However, breast milk excretion is unlikely because VIRA-A is rapidly deaminated in the gastrointestinal tract.

Adverse Reactions: Lacrimation, foreign body sensation, conjunctival injection, burning, irritation, superficial punctate keratitis pain, photophobia, punctal occlusion, and sensitivity have been reported with VIRA-A Ophthalmic Ointment, 3%. The following have also been reported but appear disease-related: uveitis, stromal edema, secondary glaucoma, trophic defects, corneal vascularization, and hyphema.

Overdosage: Acute massive overdosage by oral ingestion of the ophthalmic ointment has not occurred. However, the rapid deamination to arabinosylhypoxanthine should preclude any difficulty. The oral LD_{50} for vidarabine is greater than 5020 mg/kg in mice and rats. No untoward effects should result from ingestion of the entire contents of a tube.

Overdosage by ocular instillation is unlikely because any excess should be quickly expelled from the conjunctival sac. Too frequent administration should be avoided.

Dosage and Administration: Administer approximately one half inch of VIRA-A Ophthalmic Ointment, 3%, into the lower conjunctival sac five times daily at three-hour intervals.

If there are no signs of improvement after 7 days, or complete re-epithelialization has not occurred by 21 days, other forms of therapy should be considered. Some severe cases may require longer treatment.

After re-epithelialization has occurred, treatment for an additional seven days at a reduced dosage (such as twice daily) is recommended in order to prevent recurrence.

How Supplied: N 0071-3677-07

VIRA-A Ophthalmic Ointment, 3%, is supplied sterile in ophthalmic ointment tubes of 3.5 g. The base is a 60:40 mixture of solid and liquid petrolatum.

3677G020

Shown in Product Identification Section, page 104

The product information represents the package circular in effect July, 1991. Information on other Parke-Davis Products may be obtained by addressing PARKE-DAVIS, Division of Warner-Lambert Company, Morris Plains, New Jersey 07950

Refer to contents page for information on Sutures.

Pfizer Consumer Health Care

Division of Pfizer Inc
235 EAST 42nd ST.
NEW YORK, NY 10017

VISINE® OTC
Tetrahydrozoline Hydrochloride Redness Reliever Eye Drops

Description: Visine is a sterile, isotonic, buffered ophthalmic solution containing tetrahydrozoline hydrochloride 0.05%, boric acid, sodium borate, sodium chloride and water. It is preserved with benzalkonium chloride 0.01% and edetate disodium 0.1%. Visine is a decongestant ophthalmic solution designed to provide symptomatic relief of conjunctival edema and hyperemia secondary to minor irritations, due to conditions such as smoke, dust, other airborne pollutants, swimming etc. and so-called nonspecific or catarrhal conjunctivitis. Relief is afforded by tetrahydrozoline hydrochloride, a sympathomimetic agent, which brings about decongestion by vasoconstriction. Reddened eyes are rapidly whitened by this effective vasoconstrictor, which limits the local vascular response by constricting the small blood vessels. The onset of vasoconstriction becomes apparent within minutes.
The effectiveness of Visine in relieving conjunctival hyperemia has been demonstrated by numerous clinicals, including several double-blind studies, involving more than 2,000 subjects suffering from acute or chronic hyperemia induced by a variety of conditions. Visine was found to be efficacious in providing relief from conjunctival hyperemia.
Indications: Relieves redness of the eye due to minor eye irritations.
Directions: Place 1 to 2 drops in the affected eye(s) up to four times daily.
Parents: Before using with children under 6 years of age, consult your physician. Keep this and all other medications out of the reach of children. In case of accidental ingestion, seek professional assistance or contact a poison control center immediately.
Warning: To avoid contamination, do not touch tip of container to any surface. Replace cap after using. If you experience eye pain, changes in vision, continued redness or irritation of the eye, or if the condition worsens or persists for more than 72 hours, discontinue use and consult a doctor. If you have glaucoma, do not use this product except under the advice and supervision of a doctor. Overuse of this product may produce increased redness of the eye. If solution changes color or becomes cloudy, do not use. Remove contact lenses before using.
How Supplied: In 0.5 fl. oz., 0.75 fl. oz., and 1.0 fl. oz. plastic dispenser bottle and 0.5 fl. oz. plastic bottle with dropper.

Shown in Product Identification Section, page 104

VISINE A.C.® OTC
Astringent/Redness Reliever Eye Drops

Description: Visine A.C. is a sterile, isotonic, buffered ophthalmic solution containing tetrahydrozoline hydrochloride 0.05%, zinc sulfate 0.25%, boric acid, sodium chloride, sodium citrate and purified water. It is preserved with benzalkonium chloride 0.01% and edetate disodium 0.1%. Visine A.C. is an ophthalmic solution combining the effects of the vasoconstrictor tetrahydrozoline hydrochloride with the astringent effects of zinc sulfate. The vasoconstrictor provides symtomatic relief of conjunctival edema and hyperemia secondary to minor irritation due to conditions such as dust and airborne pollutants as well as so-called nonspecific or catarrhal conjunctivitis, while zinc sulfate provides relief from hay fever, allergies, etc. Beneficial effects include amelioration of burning, irritation, pruritis, and removal of mucous from the eye. Relief is afforded by both ingredients, tetrahydrozoline hydrochloride and zinc sulfate.
Tetrahydrozoline hydrochloride is a sympathomimetic agent, which brings about decongestion by vasoconstriction. Reddened eyes are rapidly whitened by this effective vasoconstrictor, which limits the local vascular response by constricting the small blood vessels. The onset of vasoconstriction becomes apparent within minutes. Zinc sulfate is an ocular astringent which, by precipitating protein, helps to clear mucus from the outer surface of the eye.
The effectiveness of Visine A.C. in relieving conjunctival hyperemia and associated symptoms induced by allergies has been clinically demonstrated. In one double-blind study allergy sufferers experienced acute episodes of minor eye irritation. Visine A.C. produced statistically significant beneficial results versus a placebo of normal saline solution in relieving irritation of bulbar conjunctiva, irritation of palpebral conjunctiva, and mucus build-up. Treatment with Visine A.C. containing zinc sulfate also significantly improved burning and itching symptoms.
Indications: For temporary relief of discomfort and redness due to minor eye irritations.
Directions: Place 1 to 2 drops in the affected eye(s) up to 4 times daily.
Parents: Before using with children under 6 years of age, consult your physician. Keep this and all other medications out of the reach of children. In case of accidental ingestion, seek professional assistance or contact a poison control center immediately.
Warning: To avoid contamination, do not touch tip of container to any surface. Replace cap after using. If you experience eye pain, changes in vision, continued redness or irritation of the eye, or if the condition worsens or persists for more than 72 hours, discontinue use and consult a doctor. If you have glaucoma, do not use this product except under the advice and supervision of a doctor. Overuse of this product may produce increased redness of the eye. If solution changes color or becomes cloudy, do not use. Remove contact lenses before using.
How Supplied: In 0.5 fl. oz. and 1.0 fl. oz. plastic dispenser bottle.

Shown in Product Identification Section, page 104

VISINE EXTRA® OTC
Redness Reliever/Lubricant Eye Drops

Description: Visine Extra is a sterile, isotonic, buffered ophthalmic solution containing tetrahydrozoline hydrochloride 0.05%, polyethylene glycol 400 1.0%, boric acid, sodium borate, sodium chloride and water. It is preserved with benzalkonium chloride 0.013% and edetate disodium 0.1%.
Visine Extra is an ophthalmic solution combining the effects of the decongestant tetrahydrozoline hydrochloride with the demulcent effects of polyethylene glycol. It provides symptomatic relief of conjunctival edema and hyperemia secondary to ocular allergies, minor irritations and so-called nonspecific or catarrhal conjunctivitis. Tetrahydrozoline hydrochloride is a sympathomimetic agent, which brings about decongestion by vasoconstriction. Reddened eyes are rapidly whitened by this effective vasoconstrictor, which limits the local vascular response by constricting the small blood vessels. The onset of vasoconstriction becomes apparent within minutes. Additional effects include amelioration of burning, irritation, pruritus, soreness, and excessive lacrimation. Relief is afforded by polyethylene glycol.
Polyethylene glycol is an ophthalmic demulcent which has been shown to be effective for the temporary relief of discomfort of minor irritations of the eye due to exposure to wind or sun. It is effective as a protectant and lubricant against further irritation or to relieve dryness of the eye.
The effectiveness of tetrahydrozoline hydrochloride in relieving conjunctival hyperemia and associated symptoms has been demonstrated by numerous clinicals, including several double-blind studies, involving more than 2000 subjects suffering from acute or chronic hyperemia induced by a variety of conditions.
Visine Extra is a product that combines the redness relieving effects of a vasoconstrictor and the soothing moisturizing and protective effects of a demulcent.
Indications: Relieves redness of the eye due to minor eye irritations. For use as a protectant against further irritation or to relieve dryness.
Directions: Place 1 to 2 drops in the affected eye(s) up to 4 times daily.
Parents: Before using with children under 6 years of age, consult your physician. Keep this and all other medications out of the reach of children. In case of accidental ingestion, seek professional assistance or contact a poison control center immediately.
Warning: To avoid contamination, do not touch tip of container to any surface. Replace cap after using. If you experience eye pain, changes in vision, continued redness or irritation of the eye, or if the condition worsens or persists for more than 72 hours, discontinue use and consult a doctor. If you have glaucoma, do not use this product except under the advice and supervision of a doctor. Overuse of this product may produce increased redness of the eye. If solution changes color or becomes cloudy, do not use. Remove contact lenses before using.
How Supplied: In 0.5 fl. oz. and 1.0 fl. oz. plastic dispenser bottle.

Shown in Product Identification Section, page 104

VISINE L. R.™ EYE DROPS OTC
(oxymetazoline hydrochloride)

Description: Visine L. R. is a sterile, isotonic, buffered ophthalmic solution containing oxymetazoline hydrochloride 0.025%, boric acid, sodium borate, sodium chloride and water. It is preserved with benzalkonium chloride 0.01% and edetate disodium 0.1%.
Visine L. R. is produced by a process that assures sterility.
Indications: Visine L. R. is a decongestant ophthalmic solution designed for the relief of redness of the eye due to minor eye irritations. Visine L. R. is specially formulated to relieve redness of the eye in minutes with effective relief that lasts up to 6 hours.
Directions: *Adults and children 6 years of age and older*—Place 1 or 2 drops in the affected eye(s). This may be repeated as needed every 6 hours or as directed by a physician.
Parents: Before using with children under 6 years of age, consult your physician. Keep this and all other medications out of the reach of children. In case of accidental ingestion, seek professional assistance or contact a poison control center immediately.
Warning: If you experience eye pain, changes in vision, continued redness or irritation of the eye, or if the condition worsens or persists for more than 72 hours, discontinue use and consult a physician. If you have glaucoma, do not use this product except under the advice and supervision of a physician. As with any medication, if you are pregnant seek the advice of a physician before using this product.

Continued on next page

Pfizer Consumer—Cont.

Overuse of this product may produce increased redness of the eye. If solution changes color or becomes cloudy, do not use. To avoid contamination of this product, do not touch tip of container to any surface. Replace cap after using. Remove contact lenses before using this product.

Caution: Should not be used if Visine imprinted neckband on bottle is broken or missing.

Storage: Store between 2° and 30°C (36° and 86°F).

How Supplied: In 0.5 fl. oz. and 1 fl. oz. plastic dispenser bottle.

Shown in Product Identification Section, page 104

Roche Laboratories

a division of Hoffmann-La Roche Inc.
NUTLEY, NJ 07110

GANTRISIN® ℞

[gan 'trĭ-sin]

(sulfisoxazole diolamine/Roche)
OPHTHALMIC SOLUTION
OPHTHALMIC OINTMENT

The following text is complete prescribing information based on official labeling in effect May 15, 1990.

Description: Gantrisin (sulfisoxazole diolamine/Roche) Ophthalmic Solution and Ointment are antibacterial sulfonamide preparations specifically intended for topical ophthalmic use. The solution is a sterile, isotonic preparation containing 4% (40 mg/ml) sulfisoxazole in the form of the diolamine salt, and phenylmercuric nitrate 1:100,000 as a preservative. The solution has a physiologic pH, and does not cause significant stinging or burning on application. The ointment is a sterile preparation containing 4% sulfisoxazole in the form of the diolamine salt, compounded with white petrolatum, mineral oil and phenylmercuric nitrate 1:50,000 as a preservative.

Chemically, sulfisoxazole diolamine is N^1-(3,4-dimethyl-5-isoxazolyl)sulfanilamide compound with 2,2′-iminodiethanol (1:1). It is a white to off-white, odorless, crystalline powder that is freely soluble in water and soluble in alcohol. Sulfisoxazole diolamine has a molecular weight of 372.44.

Clinical Pharmacology: Sulfonamides do not appear to be appreciably absorbed from mucous membranes.

Microbiology: Sulfonamides exert a bacteriostatic effect against a wide range of gram-positive and gram-negative microorganisms. Sulfonamides inhibit bacterial synthesis of dihydrofolic acid by competing with *para*-aminobenzoic acid (PABA). Resistant strains are capable of utilizing folic acid precursors or preformed folic acid. Currently, the increasing frequency of resistant organisms is a limitation of the usefulness of antibacterial agents, including the sulfonamides.

Indications: For the treatment of conjunctivitis, corneal ulcers and other superficial ocular infections due to susceptible microorganisms, and as an adjunct in systemic sulfonamide therapy of trachoma.

Contraindications: Hypersensitivity to sulfonamides or to other ingredients in the formulation. Infants less than 2 months of age. Pregnancy at term and during the nursing period because sulfonamides pass the placenta and are excreted in the milk and may cause kernicterus.

Precautions: *General:* Ophthalmic ointments may retard corneal healing. Nonsusceptible organisms, including fungi, may proliferate with the use of these preparations. Sulfonamides are inactivated by the *para*-aminobenzoic acid present in purulent exudates. Should undesirable reactions occur, discontinue Gantrisin immediately.

Information for patients: Patients using Gantrisin Ophthalmic Solution should be instructed not to touch the dropper tip to any surface, since contamination of the solution may result.

Drug interactions: Gantrisin Ophthalmic Solution and Ointment are incompatible with preparations containing silver. *In vitro* antagonism with sulfisoxazole diolamine and gentamicin sulfate (Garamycin) has been reported.

Carcinogenesis, mutagenesis, impairment of fertility: Carcinogenesis: Carcinogenic studies have not been performed with ophthalmic preparations of sulfisoxazole. Sulfisoxazole was not carcinogenic in either sex when administered by gavage for 103 weeks at dosages up to 2000 mg/kg/day in mice or 400 mg/kg/day in rats.

Mutagenesis: Bacterial mutagenic studies have not been performed with sulfisoxazole. However, Gantrisin was not observed to be mutagenic in *E. coli* Sd-4-73 when tested in the absence of a metabolic activating system.

Impairment of fertility: Fertility studies have not been performed with ophthalmic preparations of sulfisoxazole. No effects on mating behavior, conception rate or fertility index (percent pregnant) were observed in a reproduction study in rats given oral dosages of 800 mg/kg/day sulfisoxazole

Pregnancy: Teratogenic effects: Pregnancy Category C. Teratogenic studies of ophthalmic preparations of sulfisoxazole have not been performed in laboratory animals. Sulfisoxazole was not teratogenic in either rats or rabbits at oral dosages of 800 mg/kg/day. However, in another teratogenicity study, cleft palates developed in both rats and mice after oral administration of 1000 mg/kg/day sulfisoxazole; skeletal defects were also observed in rats. This dose is 9 to 18 times the usual adult dosage for oral Gantrisin.

There are no adequate and well-controlled studies of Gantrisin in pregnant women. Gantrisin Ophthalmic Solution and Ointment should be used during pregnancy only if the potential benefit justifies the potential risk to the fetus.

Nursing mothers: See **Contraindications** section.

Pediatric use: Gantrisin Ophthalmic Solution is not recommended for use in infants younger than 2 months of age.

Adverse Reactions: Topical application of the sulfonamides may produce sensitization and preclude later systemic use of these drugs. In addition, patients who have been sensitized by systemic sulfonamide administration may exhibit hypersensitivity reactions following topical application of the drugs.

Ophthalmic: Ocular irritation, chemosis, itching.

Included in the listing that follows are adverse reactions that have not been reported with these dosage forms but have been reported for the systemically absorbed sulfonamides.

Hematologic: Agranulocytosis, aplastic anemia, thrombocytopenia, leukopenia, hemolytic anemia, purpura, hypoprothrombinemia and methemoglobinemia.

Allergic reactions: Erythema multiforme (Stevens-Johnson syndrome), generalized skin eruptions, epidermal necrolysis, urticaria, serum sickness, pruritus, exfoliative dermatitis, anaphylactoid reactions, periorbital edema, conjunctival and scleral injection, photosensitization, arthralgia and allergic myocarditis.

Gastrointestinal reactions: Nausea, emesis, abdominal pain, hepatitis, hepatocellular necrosis, diarrhea, anorexia, pancreatitis and stomatitis.

C.N.S. reactions: Headache, peripheral neuritis, mental depression, convulsions, ataxia hallucinations, tinnitus, vertigo and insomnia.

Miscellaneous reactions: Drug fever, chills, and toxic nephrosis with oliguria and anuria. Periarteritis nodosa and L.E. phenomenon have occurred.

Endocrine: The sulfonamides bear certain chemical similarities to some goitrogens, diuretics (acetazolamide and the thiazides) and oral hypoglycemic agents. Goiter production, diuresis and hypoglycemia have occurred rarely in patients receiving sulfonamides. Cross sensitivity may exist with these agents.

Dosage and Administration:

Solution: Instill two or three drops in the eye three or more times daily. Care should be taken not to touch dropper tip to any surface, since contamination of the solution may result.

Ointment: Instill small amount in the lower conjunctival sac one to three times daily and at bedtime.

How Supplied: *Gantrisin Ophthalmic Solution,* containing 4% (40 mg/ml) sulfisoxazole in the form of the diolamine salt-½ oz bottles with dropper (NDC 0004-1702-39).

Gantrisin Ophthalmic Ointment, containing 4% sulfisoxazole in the form of the diolamine salt-⅛ oz tubes (NDC 0004-1501-41).

Both dosage forms are stable at room temperature and do not require refrigeration.

Revised: August 1985

Shown in Product Identification Section, page 105

Ross Laboratories

COLUMBUS, OH 43216
Division of Abbott Laboratories, USA

CLEAR EYES® OTC

[klēr īz]

Lubricating Eye Redness Reliever

Description: Clear Eyes is a sterile, isotonic buffered solution containing the active ingredients naphazoline hydrochloride (0.012%) and glycerin (0.2%). It also contains boric acid, purified water and sodium borate. Edetate disodium (0.1%) and benzalkonium chloride (0.01%) are added as preservatives. Clear Eyes is a lubricating, decongestant ophthalmic solution specially designed for temporary relief of redness and drying due to minor eye irritation caused by dust, smoke, smog, sun glare, wearing contact lenses, colds, allergies, swimming, reading, driving, TV or close work. Clear Eyes contains laboratory tested and scientifically blended ingredients, including an effective vasoconstrictor which narrows swollen blood vessels and rapidly whitens reddened eyes in a formulation which also contains a lubricant and produces a refreshing, soothing effect. Clear Eyes is a sterile, isotonic solution compatible with the natural fluids of the eye.

Indications: For the temporary relief of redness due to minor eye irritation AND for protection against further irritation or dryness of the eye.

Warning: To avoid contamination, do not touch tip of container to any surface. Replace cap after using. If you experience eye pain, changes in vision, continued redness or irritation of the eye, or if the condition worsens or persists for more than 72 hours, discontinue use and consult a doctor. If you have glaucoma, do not use this product except under the advice and supervision of a doctor. Overuse of this product may produce increased redness of the eye. If solution changes color or becomes cloudy, do not use. Keep this and all drugs out of the reach of children. **Remove contact lenses before using.**

Dosage and Administration: Instill 1 or 2 drops in the affected eye(s) up to four times daily.
How Supplied: In 0.5-fl-oz and 1.0-fl-oz plastic dropper bottles.
(FAN 2222-03)

CLEAR EYES® ACR OTC
[*klēr īz*]
Astringent/Lubricating Eye Redness Reliever Drops

Description: Clear Eyes ACR is a sterile, isotonic, buffered solution containing the active ingredients naphazoline hydrochloride (0.012%), zinc sulfate (0.25%) and glycerin (0.2%). It also contains boric acid, purified water and sodium borate. Edetate disodium (0.1%) and benzalkonium chloride (0.01%) are added as preservatives. Clear Eyes ACR is a lubricating, decongestant, astringent ophthalmic solution specially designed for temporary relief of redness and drying due to minor eye irritation caused by dust, smoke, smog, sun glare, wearing contact lenses, colds, allergies, swimming, reading, driving, TV or close work. Clear Eyes ACR contains laboratory-tested and scientifically blended ingredients, including an effective vasoconstrictor which narrows swollen blood vessels and rapidly whitens reddened eyes in a formulation which also contains a lubricant and produces a refreshing, soothing effect. Clear Eyes ACR also contains an ocular astringent (zinc sulfate) that precipitates the sticky mucus buildup on the eye often associated with hayfever, allergies and colds and this helps clear the mucus from the outer surface of the eye. Clear Eyes ACR is a sterile, isotonic solution compatible with the natural fluids of the eye.
Indications: For the temporary relief of redness due to minor eye irritation AND for protection against further irritation or dryness of the eye.
Warnings: To avoid contamination, do not touch tip of container to any surface. Replace cap after using. If you experience eye pain, changes in vision, continued redness or irritation of the eye, or if the condition worsens or persists for more than 72 hours, discontinue use and consult a doctor. If you have glaucoma, do not use this product except under the advice and supervision of a doctor. Overuse of this product may produce increased redness of the eye. If solution changes color or becomes cloudy, do not use. Keep this and all drugs out of the reach of children.
Dosage and Administration: Instill 1 or 2 drops in the affected eye(s) up to four times daily.
How Supplied: In 0.5-fl-oz and 1.0-fl-oz plastic dropper bottles.
(FAN 2284)

Shown in Product Identification Section, page 105

MURINE® OTC
[*mur′ēn*]
Eye Lubricant

Description: Murine eye lubricant is a sterile buffered solution containing the active ingredients 1.4% polyvinyl alcohol and 0.6% povidone. Also contains benzalkonium chloride, dextrose, disodium edetate, potassium chloride, purified water, sodium bicarbonate, sodium chloride, sodium citrate and sodium phosphate (mono- and dibasic). Murine is a clear, buffered, sterile solution formulated to more closely match the natural fluid of the eye for gentle, soothing relief from minor eye irritation while moisturizing and relieving dryness. Use as desired to temporarily relieve minor eye irritation, dryness and burning due to dust, smoke, smog, sun glare, wearing contact lenses, colds, allergies, swimming, reading, driving, TV or close work.
Indications: For the temporary relief or prevention of further discomfort due to minor eye irritations and symptoms related to dry eyes.
Warning: To avoid contamination, do not touch tip of container to any surface. Replace cap after using. If you experience eye pain, changes in vision, continued redness or irritation of the eye, or if the condition worsens or persists for more than 72 hours, discontinue use and consult a doctor. If solution changes color or becomes cloudy, do not use. Keep this and all drugs out of the reach of children. **Remove contact lenses before using.**
Dosage and Administration: Instill 1 or 2 drops in the affected eye(s) as needed.
How Supplied: In 0.5-fl-oz and 1.0-fl-oz plastic dropper bottles.
(FAN 2202-04)

MURINE® PLUS OTC
[*mur′ēn*]
Lubricating Eye Redness Reliever

Description: Murine Plus is a sterile, nonstaining buffered solution containing the active ingredients 1.4% polyvinyl alcohol, 0.6% povidone and 0.05% tetrahydrozoline hydrochloride. Also contains benzalkonium chloride, dextrose, disodium edetate, potassium chloride, purified water, sodium bicarbonate, sodium chloride, sodium citrate and sodium phosphate (mono- and dibasic). Murine Plus is an isotonic, sterile, ophthalmic solution, formulated to more closely match the natural fluid of the eye. It contains demulcents for gentle, soothing relief from minor eye irritation as well as the sympathomimetic agent, tetrahydrozoline hydrochloride, which produces local vasoconstriction in the eye. Thus, the drug effectively narrows swollen blood vessels locally and provides symptomatic relief of edema and hyperemia of conjunctival tissues due to eye allergies, minor local irritations and conjunctivitis. Use up to four times daily, to remove redness due to minor eye irritation caused by dust, smoke, smog, sun glare, wearing contact lenses, colds, allergies, swimming, reading, driving, TV or close work. The effect of Murine Plus is prompt (apparent within minutes) and sustained.
Indications: For the temporary relief or prevention of further discomfort due to minor eye irritations and symptoms related to dry eyes PLUS removal of redness.
Warning: To avoid contamination, do not touch tip of container to any surface. Replace cap after using. If you experience eye pain, changes in vision, continued redness or irritation of the eye, or if the condition worsens or persists for more than 72 hours, discontinue use and consult a doctor. If you have glaucoma, do not use this product except under the advice and supervision of a doctor. Overuse of this product may produce increased redness of the eye. If solution changes color or becomes cloudy, do not use. Keep this and all drugs out of the reach of children. **Remove contact lenses before using.**
Dosage and Administration: Instill 1 or 2 drops in the affected eye(s) up to four times daily.
How Supplied: In 0.5-fl-oz and 1.0-fl-oz plastic dropper bottles.
(FAN 2202-04)

Refer to contents page for information on Instruments and Equipment

---

Schering Corporation

a wholly-owned subsidiary of Schering-Plough Corporation
GALLOPING HILL ROAD
KENILWORTH, NJ 07033

GARAMYCIN® ℞
[*gar-ah-mī′sin*]
brand of gentamicin sulfate
Ophthalmic Solution, USP—Sterile
Ophthalmic Ointment, USP—Sterile
Each ml or gram contains gentamicin sulfate, USP equivalent to 3.0 mg gentamicin

Description: Gentamicin sulfate is a water-soluble antibiotic of the aminoglycoside group active against a wide variety of pathogenic gram-negative and gram-positive bacteria.
GARAMYCIN **Ophthalmic Solution** is a sterile, aqueous solution buffered to approximately pH 7 for use in the eye. Each ml contains gentamicin sulfate, USP (equivalent to 3.0 mg gentamicin), disodium phosphate, monosodium phosphate, sodium chloride, and benzalkonium chloride as a preservative.
GARAMYCIN **Ophthalmic Ointment** is a sterile ointment, each gram containing gentamicin sulfate, USP (equivalent to 3.0 mg gentamicin) in a bland base of white petrolatum, with methylparaben and propylparaben as preservatives.
Actions: The gram-positive bacteria against which gentamicin sulfate is active include coagulase-positive and coagulase-negative staphylococci, including certain strains that are resistant to penicillin; Group A beta-hemolytic and nonhemolytic streptococci; and *Diplococcus pneumoniae.* The gram-negative bacteria against which gentamicin sulfate is active include certain strains of *Pseudomonas aeruginosa,* indole-positive and indole-negative *Proteus* species, *Escherichia coli, Klebsiella pneumoniae* (Friedlander's bacillus), *Haemophilus influenza* and *Haemophilus aegyptius* (Koch-Weeks bacillus), *Aerobacter aerogenes, Moraxella lacunata* (diplobacillus of Morax-Axenfeld), and *Neisseria* species, including *Neisseria gonorrhoeae.* Although significant resistant organisms have not been isolated from patients treated with gentamicin at the present time, this may occur in the future as resistance has been produced with difficulty *in vitro* by repeated exposures.
Indications: GARAMYCIN **Ophthalmic Solution** and **Ointment** are indicated in the topical treatment of infections of the external eye and its adnexa caused by susceptible bacteria. Such infections embrace conjunctivitis, keratitis and keratoconjunctivitis, corneal ulcers, blepharitis and blepharoconjunctivitis, acute meibomianitis, and dacryocystitis.
Contraindications: GARAMYCIN **Ophthalmic Solution** and **Ointment** are contraindicated in patients with known hypersensitivity to any of their components.
Warnings: GARAMYCIN **Ophthalmic Solution** is not for injection. It should never be injected subconjunctivally, nor should it be directly introduced into the anterior chamber of the eye.
Precautions: Prolonged use of topical antibiotics may give rise to overgrowth of nonsusceptible organisms, such as fungi. Should this occur, or if irritation or hypersensitivity to any component of the drug develops, discontinue use of the preparation and institute appropriate therapy.
Ophthalmic ointments may retard corneal healing.
Adverse Reactions: Transient irritation has been reported with the use of GARAMYCIN **Ophthalmic Solution.**

Continued on next page

Schering—Cont.

Occasional burning or stinging may occur with the use of GARAMYCIN **Ophthalmic Ointment.**

Dosage and Administration: GARAMYCIN **Ophthalmic Solution:** instill one or two drops into the affected eye every four hours. In severe infections, dosage may be increased to as much as two drops once every hour.

GARAMYCIN **Ophthalmic Ointment:** apply a small amount to the affected eye two to three times a day.

How Supplied: GARAMYCIN **Ophthalmic Solution—Sterile,** 5 ml plastic dropper bottle, box of one (NDC 0085-0899-05).

GARAMYCIN **Ophthalmic Ointment—Sterile,** 3.5 g tube, box of one (NDC 0085-0151-05).

Store GARAMYCIN Ophthalmic Ointment and Solution between 2° and 30°C (36° and 86°F).

 Rev. 4/84

METIMYD® ℞

[*met 'ĭ-mid*]

brand of prednisolone acetate, USP and sulfacetamide sodium, USP

Ophthalmic Suspension–Sterile

Ophthalmic Ointment–Sterile

Description: METIMYD **Ophthalmic Suspension** is a steroid/anti-infective sterile preparation having a pH range of 7.0 to 7.4. Each ml contains: 5 mg prednisolone acetate, USP; 100 mg sulfacetamide sodium, USP; sodium phosphate dibasic, sodium phosphate monobasic, tyloxapol, sodium thiosulfate, edetate disodium, and purified water; 5 mg phenylethyl alcohol and 0.25 mg benzalkonium chloride as preservatives.

METIMYD **Ophthalmic Ointment** is a steroid/anti-infective sterile preparation containing in each gram: 5 mg prednisolone acetate, USP and 100 mg sulfacetamide sodium, USP; 0.5 mg methylparaben and 0.1 mg propylparaben as preservatives, in a bland, unctuous base of mineral oil and white petrolatum.

The empirical formula for prednisolone acetate, a 1-unsaturated analog of hydrocortisone acetate, is $C_{23}H_{30}O_6$. The molecular weight is 402.49. Chemically it is 11β,17,21-trihydroxypregna-1,4-diene-3,20-dione 21-acetate.

Prednisolone acetate is a nearly odorless, white to practically white, crystalline powder. It is slightly soluble in acetone, alcohol, and chloroform, and practically insoluble in water.

Sulfacetamide sodium, $C_8H_9N_2NaO_3S \cdot H_2O$, is a sulfonamide antibacterial agent with a molecular weight of 254.24. Chemically it is *N*-[(4-aminophenyl) sulfonyl]-, acetamide, monosodium salt, monohydrate.

Sulfacetamide sodium is an odorless, white, crystalline powder. It is freely soluble in water, sparingly soluble in alcohol, and practically insoluble in benzene, chloroform, and ether.

Clinical Pharmacology: Corticosteroids suppress the inflammatory response to a variety of agents, and they probably delay or slow healing. Since corticosteroids may inhibit the body's defense mechanism against infection, a concomitant antimicrobial drug may be used when this inhibition is considered to be clinically significant in a particular case.

The anti-infective component in the combination is included to provide action against specific organisms susceptible to it.

When a decision is made to administer both a corticoid and an antimicrobial, the administration of such drugs in combination has the advantages of greater patient compliance and convenience and added assurance that the appropriate dosage of both drugs is administered. There is also assured compatibility of ingredients when both types of drug are in the same formulation and, particularly, that the correct volume of drug is delivered and retained.

The relative potency of corticosteroids depends on the molecular structure, concentration, and release from the vehicle.

Indications and Usage: METIMYD **Ophthalmic Suspension** or **Ointment** is indicated for steroid-responsive inflammatory ocular conditions for which a corticosteroid is indicated and where bacterial infection or a risk of bacterial ocular infection exists.

Ocular steroids are indicated in inflammatory conditions of the palpebral and bulbar conjunctivae, cornea, and anterior segment of the globe where the inherent risk of steroid use in certain infective conjunctivitides is accepted to obtain a diminution in edema and inflammation. They are also indicated in chronic anterior uveitis and corneal injury from chemical, radiation, or thermal burns, or penetration of foreign bodies.

The use of a combination drug with an anti-infective component is indicated where the risk of infection is high or where there is an expectation that potentially dangerous numbers of bacteria will be present in the eye.

The particular anti-infective drug in this product is active against the following common bacterial eye pathogens: *Pseudomonas* species, *Hemophilus influenzae, Klebsiella* species, *Staphylococcus aureus, Streptococcus pneumoniae, Streptococcus* (Viridans group), *Escherichia coli,* and *Enterobacter* species.

This product does not provide adequate coverage against: *Neisseria* species and *Serratia marcescens.*

Contraindications: METIMYD is contraindicated in: epithelial herpes simplex keratitis (dendritic keratitis), vaccinia, varicella, and many other viral diseases of the cornea or conjunctiva; mycobacterial infection of the eye; and fungal diseases of ocular structures. METIMYD is contraindicated in individuals with known or suspected hypersensitivity to any of the ingredients of the preparation, or to other sulfonamides, or other corticosteroids. (Hypersensitivity to the antibacterial component occurs at a higher rate than for other components.) The use of these combinations is always contraindicated after uncomplicated removal of a corneal foreign body.

Warnings: Prolonged use may result in glaucoma, with damage to the optic nerve, defects in visual acuity and fields of vision, and in posterior subcapsular cataract formation. Prolonged use may suppress the host response and thus increase the hazard of secondary ocular infections. In those diseases causing thinning of the cornea or sclera, perforations have been known to occur with the use of topical steroids. In acute purulent conditions of the eye, steroids may mask infection or enhance existing infection. If these products are used for 10 days or longer, intraocular pressure should be routinely monitored even though this may be difficult in children and uncooperative patients.

Employment of steroid medication in the treatment of herpes simplex requires great caution.

A significnt percentage of staphylococcal isolates are completely resistant to sulfonamides.

Precautions: The initial prescription and renewal of the medication order beyond 20 ml of METIMYD **Ophthalmic Suspension** or beyond 8 g of the **Ointment** should be made by a physician only after examination of the patient with the aid of magnification, such as slitlamp biomicroscopy and where appropriate, fluorescein staining.

The possibility of fungal infections of the cornea should be considered after prolonged steroid dosing.

Sensitization may recur when a sulfonamide is readministered irrespective of the route of administration, and cross-sensitivity among different sulfonamides may occur. (See ADVERSE REACTIONS.) Cross-allergenicity among corticosteroids has been demonstrated. If signs of hypersensitivity or other untoward reactions occur, discontinue use of the preparation.

Adverse Reactions: Adverse reactions have occurred which can be attributed to the steroid component, the anti-infective component, or the combination. Exact incidence figures are not available since no denominator of treated patients is available.

Reactions occurring most often from the presence of the anti-infective ingredient are allergic sensitizations. Instances of Stevens-Johnson syndrome and systemic lupus erythematosus (in one case producing a fatal outcome) have been reported following the use of ophthalmic sulfonamide-containing preparations.

The reactions due to the steroid component in decreasing order of frequency are: elevation of intraocular pressure (IOP) with possible development of glaucoma, and infrequent optic nerve damage; posterior subcapsular cataract formation; and delayed wound healing.

Corticosteroid-containing preparations can also cause acute anterior uveitis or perforation of the globe. Mydriasis, loss of accommodation, and ptosis have occasionally been reported following local use of corticosteroids.

Secondary Infection: The development of secondary infection has occurred after use of combinations containing steroids and antimicrobials. Fungal infections of the cornea are particularly prone to develop coincidentally with long-term applications of the steroid. The possibility of fungal invasion must be considered in any persistent corneal ulceration where steroid treatment has been used.

Secondary bacterial ocular infection following suppression of host responses also occurs.

Dosage and Administration: METIMYD **Ophthalmic Suspension:** Two or three drops should be instilled into the conjunctival sac every one to two hours during the day and at bedtime until a favorable response is obtained.

METIMYD **Ophthalmic Ointment:** A thin film should be applied three or four times daily and once at bedtime until a favorable response is obtained.

The initial prescription of METIMYD **Ophthalmic** should <u>not</u> be more than 20 ml of the **Suspension** or 8 g of the **Ointment** and the prescription should not be refilled without further evaluation as outlined in PRECAUTIONS.

Dosage should be adjusted according to the specific needs of the patient. METIMYD **Ophthalmic Suspension** or **Ointment** dosage may be reduced, but care should be taken not to discontinue therapy prematurely. In chronic conditions, withdrawal of treatment should be carried out by gradually decreasing the frequency of application.

How Supplied: METIMYD **Ophthalmic Suspension,** 5 ml dropper bottle; box of one; NDC 0085-0074-05. **Store between 2° and 30°C (36° and 86°F). Clumping may occur on long standing at high temperatures. Shake well before using. Protect from light.**

METIMYD **Ophthalmic Ointment,** 3.5 g applicator tube; box of one; NDC 0085-0695-05. **Store between 2° and 30°C (36° and 86°F).**

Revised 4/84

OCUCLEAR® EYE DROPS OTC

[*ok 'u-klēr*]

(oxymetazoline HCl) 0.025%

Description: OCUCLEAR is a sterile, isotonic buffered aqueous solution of oxymetazoline hydrochloride 0.025%; sodium chloride, edetate disodium, boric acid and benzalkonium chloride 0.01% as preservative. Sodium hydroxide is added to adjust pH to approximately 6.4.

Indication: For the relief of redness of the eye due to minor eye irritations.
Warnings: If you experience eye pain, changes in vision, continued redness or irritation of the eye, or if the condition worsens or persists for more than 72 hours, discontinue use and consult a physician. If you have glaucoma, do not use this product except under the advice and supervision of a physician. As with any drug, if you are pregnant seek the advice of a physician before using this product.
Overuse of this product may produce increased redness of the eye. If solution changes color or becomes cloudy, do not use. To avoid contamination of this product, do not touch tip of container to any surface. Replace cap after using. Remove soft contact lenses before using this product.
Directions: Adults and children 6 years of age and older: Instill 1 or 2 drops in the affected eye(s). This may be repeated as needed every 6 hours or as directed by a physician. Before using with children under 6 years of age, consult your physician.
How Supplied: In 15 ml and 30 ml plastic dispensing bottle. **Store between 2° and 30°C (36° and 86°F).**

Sodium SULAMYD® ℞
[*so 'lah-mid*]
brand of sulfacetamide sodium
Ophthalmic Solution, USP 30%—Sterile
Ophthalmic Solution, USP 10%—Sterile
Ophthalmic Ointment, USP 10%—Sterile

Description: Sodium SULAMYD is available in three ophthalmic forms:
Ophthalmic Solution 30% contains in each ml of sterile aqueous solution 300 mg sulfacetamide sodium, USP, 1.5 mg sodium thiosulfate pentahydrate, with 0.5 mg methylparaben and 0.1 mg propylparaben added as preservatives, and sodium phosphate monobasic monohydrate as buffer.
Ophthalmic Solution 10% contains in each ml of sterile aqueous solution 100 mg sulfacetamide sodium, USP, 3.1 mg sodium thiosulfate pentahydrate, and 5 mg methylcellulose, with 0.5 mg methylparaben and 0.1 mg propylparaben, added as preservatives and sodium phosphate monobasic monohydrate as buffer.
Ophthalmic Ointment 10% is a sterile ointment, each gram containing 100 mg sulfacetamide sodium, USP with 0.5 mg methylparaben, 0.1 mg propylparaben and 0.25 mg benzalkonium chloride added as preservatives, and sorbitan monolaurate and water in a bland, unctuous, petrolatum base.
Actions: Sodium SULAMYD exerts a bacteriostatic effect against a wide range of gram-positive and gram-negative microorganisms by restricting, through competition with para-aminobenzoic acid, the synthesis of folic acid which bacteria require for growth.
Indications: Sodium SULAMYD is indicated for the treatment of conjunctivitis, corneal ulcer, and other superficial ocular infections due to susceptible microorganisms, and as adjunctive treatment in systemic sulfonamide therapy of trachoma.
Contraindications: Sodium SULAMYD is contraindicated in individuals with known or suspected sensitivity to sulfonamides or to any of the ingredients of the preparations.
Precautions: Sodium SULAMYD products are incompatible with silver preparations. Ophthalmic ointments may retard corneal healing. Non-susceptible organisms, including fungi, may proliferate with the use of these preparations. Sulfonamides are inactivated by the para-aminobenzoic acid present in purulent exudates.
Sensitization may recur when a sulfonamide is re-administered irrespective of the route of administration, and cross-sensitivity between different sulfonamides may occur. If signs of sensitivity or other untoward reactions occur, discontinue use of the preparation.
Adverse Reactions: Sulfacetamide sodium may cause local irritation, stinging and burning. While the irritation may be transient, occasionally, use of the medication has to be discontinued.
Although sensitivity reactions to sulfacetamide sodium are rare, an isolated incident of Stevens-Johnson syndrome was reported in a patient who had experienced a previous bullous drug reaction to an orally administered sulfonamide, and a single instance of local hypersensitivity was reported which progressed to a fatal syndrome resembling systemic lupus erythematosus.
Dosage and Administration: Sodium SULAMYD Ophthalmic Solution 30%. *For conjunctivitis or corneal ulcer:* instill one drop into lower conjunctival sac every two hours or less frequently according to severity of infection. *For trachoma:* Two drops every two hours; concomitant systemic sulfonamide therapy is indicated.
Sodium SULAMYD Ophthalmic Solution 10%. One or two drops into the lower conjunctival sac every two or three hours during the day and less often at night.
Sodium SULAMYD Ophthalmic Ointment 10%. Apply a small amount four times daily and at bedtime. The ointment may be used adjunctively with either of the solution forms.
How Supplied: Sodium SULAMYD Ophthalmic Ointment 10%, 3.5 gram tube (NDC 0085-0066-03), box of one. **Store away from heat.**
Sodium SULAMYD Ophthalmic Solution 30%, 15 ml dropper bottle (NDC 0085-0717-06), box of one. **Store between 2° and 30°C (36° and 86°F).**
Sodium SULAMYD Ophthalmic Solution 10%, 5 ml dropper bottle (NDC 0085-0946-03), box of 25; 15 ml dropper bottle (NDC 0085-0946-06), box of one. **Store between 2° and 30°C (36° and 86°F).**
On long standing, sulfonamide solutions will darken in color and should be discarded.
 Rev. 1/86

Storz Ophthalmics, Inc.
3365 TREE COURT INDUSTRIAL BLVD.
ST. LOUIS, MO 63122-6694

Products manufactured by:

Lederle Laboratories
A Division of American Cyanamid Co.
One Cyanamid Plaza
Wayne, NJ 07470

Lederle Parenterals, Inc.
Carolina, Puerto Rico 00630

LEDERMARK® Product Identification Code
Many Lederle tablets and capsules bear an identification code. A current listing appears in the Product Information Section of the 1992 PDR for Prescription Drugs.

ACHROMYCIN® ℞
[*ak 'ro-mi "sin*]
tetracycline hydrochloride
Ophthalmic Ointment, USP,
1% Sterile

Description: ACHROMYCIN Ophthalmic Ointment, USP, 1% Sterile contains 10 mg of tetracycline hydrochloride per gram with Light Mineral Oil, White Petrolatum and Anhydrous Lanolin as inactive ingredients.
Chemically, ACHROMYCIN is: [4*S*-(4α, 4aα,5aα,6β,12aα)] -4- (dimethylamino)-1, 4, 4a, 5,5a,6,11,12a- octahydro-3, 6, 10, 12, 12a, pentahydroxy -6- methyl -1, 11- dioxo -2- naphthacenecarboxamide monohydrochloride.
Indications: For the treatment of superficial ocular infections susceptible to ACHROMYCIN.
For prophylaxis of ophthalmia neonatorum due to *Neisseria gonorrhoeae* or *Chlamydia trachomatis.* The Centers for Disease Control (USPHS) and the Committee on Drugs, the Committee on Fetus and Newborn, and the Committee on Infectious Diseases of the American Academy of Pediatrics recommend 1 percent silver nitrate solution in single-dose ampoules or single-use tubes of an ophthalmic ointment containing 0.5 percent erythromycin or 1 percent tetracycline as "effective and acceptable regimens for prophylaxis of gonococcal ophthalmia neonatorum."[1] (For infants born to mothers with clinically apparent gonorrhea, intravenous or intramuscular injections of aqueous crystalline penicillin G should be given: a single dose of 50,000 units for term infants or 20,000 units for infants of low birth weight. Topical prophylaxis alone is inadequate for these infants.[1])
The following organisms have demonstrated susceptibility to ACHROMYCIN:
Staphylococcus aureus
Streptococci including *Streptococcus pneumoniae*
Escherichia coli
Neisseria species
Chlamydia trachomatis
When treating trachoma a concomitant oral tetracycline is helpful.
Other organisms, not known to cause superficial eye infections, but with demonstrated susceptibility to ACHROMYCIN, have been omitted from the above list.
ACHROMYCIN does not provide adequate coverage against:
Haemophilus influenzae
Klebsiella/Enterobacter species
Pseudomonas aeruginosa
Serratia marcescens
Contraindications: This product is contraindicated in persons who have shown hypersensitivity to any of the tetracyclines.
Precautions: The use of antibiotics occasionally may result in overgrowth of nonsusceptible organisms. Constant observation of the patient is essential. If new infections appear during therapy, appropriate measures should be taken.
Adverse Reactions: Dermatitis and allied symptomatology have been reported.
If adverse reaction or idiosyncrasy occurs, discontinue medication and institute appropriate therapy.
Dosage and Administration: Apply directly to the affected area every 2 hours or more often, as the severity of the infection and the degree of response indicate. Severe or stubborn ocular infections may require treatment for many days, and may also require oral therapy. Mild infections may respond within 48 hours.
How Supplied: ACHROMYCIN *tetracycline HCl* Ophthalmic Ointment, USP, 1%:
NDC 0005-3501-51—⅛ oz. tube.
Store at Controlled Room Temperature 15°–30°C (59°–86°F).

Continued on next page

Information on Storz products listed on these pages is the full Prescribing Information from product literature or package inserts effective in June 1991. Information concerning all Storz products may be obtained from the Professional Services Department, Lederle Laboratories, Pearl River, New York 10965

Storz Ophthalmics, Inc.—Cont.

Reference: 1. American Academy of Pediatrics. Prophylaxis and treatment of neonatal gonococcal infections. *Pediatrics.* 1980; 65:1047.

LEDERLE LABORATORIES DIVISION
American Cyanamid Company
Pearl River, NY 10965 Rev. 8/86
12157

ACHROMYCIN® ℞

[*ak 'ro-mi "sin*]
tetracycline hydrochloride
Ophthalmic Suspension, USP,
1% Sterile

Description: ACHROMYCIN Ophthalmic Suspension, USP, 1% Sterile contains 10 mg of tetracycline hydrochloride per mL with Plastibase 50W and Light Mineral Oil as inactive ingredients.
Chemically, ACHROMYCIN is: [4S-(4α,4aα, 5aα,6β,12aα)]-4-(dimethylamino)-1, 4, 4a, 5, 5a, 6, 11, 12a-octahydro-3, 6, 10, 12, 12a-pentahydroxy -6- methyl -1, 11- dioxo -2- naphthacenecarboxamide monohydrochloride.
Indications: For the treatment of superficial ocular infections susceptible to ACHROMYCIN.
For prophylaxis of ophthalmia neonatorum due to *Neisseria gonorrhoeae* or *Chlamydia trachomatis.* The Centers for Disease Control (USPHS) and the Committee on Drugs, the Committee on Fetus and Newborn, and the Committee on Infectious Diseases of the American Academy of Pediatrics recommend 1 percent silver nitrate solution in single-dose ampoules or single-use tubes of an ophthalmic ointment containing 0.5 percent erythromycin or 1 percent tetracycline as "effective and acceptable regimens for prophylaxis of gonococcal ophthalmia neonatorum."[1] (For infants born to mothers with clinically apparent gonorrhea, intravenous or intramuscular injections of aqueous crystalline penicillin G should be given: a single dose of 50,000 units for term infants or 20,000 units for infants of low birth weight. Topical prophylaxis alone is inadequate for these infants.[1])
The following organisms have demonstrated susceptibility to ACHROMYCIN:
Staphylococcus aureus
Streptococci including *Streptococcus pneumoniae*
Escherichia coli
Neisseria species
Chlamydia trachomatis
When treating trachoma, a concomitant oral tetracycline is helpful.
Other organisms, not known to cause superficial eye infections, but with demonstrated susceptibility to ACHROMYCIN, have been omitted from the above list.
ACHROMYCIN does not provide adequate coverage against:
Haemophilus influenzae
Klebsiella/Enterobacter species
Pseudomonas aeruginosa
Serratia marcescens
Contraindications: This product is contraindicated in persons who have shown hypersensitivity to any of the tetracyclines.
Precautions: The use of antibiotics occasionally may result in overgrowth of nonsusceptible organisms. Constant observation of the patient is essential. If new infections appear during therapy, appropriate measures should be taken.
Adverse Reactions: Dermatitis and allied symptomatology have been reported.
If adverse reaction or idiosyncrasy occurs, discontinue medication and institute appropriate therapy.
Dosage and Administration: For most susceptible bacterial infections shake well, then gently squeeze the plastic dropper bottle to instill 2 drops in the affected eye, or if necessary, in both eyes, 2 or 4 times daily, or more frequently, depending upon the severity of the infection. Very severe infections may require days of treatment, whereas other cases may be cured by instillation with much less frequency for 48 hours.
In acute and chronic trachoma, instill 2 drops in each eye 2 to 4 times daily. This treatment should be continued for 1 to 2 months, except that certain individual or complicated cases may require a longer duration. A concomitant oral tetracycline is helpful.
For unit dose administration and convenience, the DISPENSER may be used. Immediately prior to use, simultaneously roll, invert and squeeze DISPENSER between thumb and fingers. Repeat several times to mix contents well. Use aseptic technique to cut the tip of the DISPENSER, thereby maintaining sterility. Discard first two drops before instilling drops in eye(s). Instill two drops in eye(s), then discard DISPENSER.
How Supplied: ACHROMYCIN *tetracycline hydrochloride* Ophthalmic Suspension, USP, 1% Sterile is supplied as follows:
NDC 0005-3505-18—4 mL plastic dropper type bottle
Store at Controlled Room Temperature 15°–30°C (59°–86° F).
Reference: 1. American Academy of Pediatrics. Prophylaxis and treatment of neonatal gonococcal infections. *Pediatrics.* 1980; 65:1047.

LEDERLE LABORATORIES DIVISION
American Cyanamid Company
Pearl River, NY 10965 Rev. 1/90
25727

Shown in Product Identification Section, page 105

AUREOMYCIN® ℞

chlortetracycline HCl
Ophthalmic Ointment 1.0%
Sterile

Description: AUREOMYCIN Ointment (Ophthalmic) contains 10 mg of Chlortetracycline HCl per gram in an anhydrous lanolin-petrolatum base.
Indications: For the treatment of superficial ocular infections susceptible to AUREOMYCIN.
The following organisms have demonstrated susceptibility to AUREOMYCIN:
Staphylococcus aureus,
Streptococcus pyogenes,
N. gonorrhoeae,
D. pneumoniae,
H. influenzae,
H. ducreyi,
Klebsiella pneumoniae,
Past. tularensis,
Past. pestis,
E. coli,
B. anthracis,
Lymphogranuloma venereum.
In the treatment of trachoma (in conjunction with oral therapy).
Contraindications: This product is contraindicated in persons who have shown hypersensitivity to any of the tetracyclines.
Precautions: The use of antibiotics occasionally may result in overgrowth of nonsusceptible organisms. Constant observation of the patient is essential. If new infections appear during therapy, appropriate measures should be taken.
Adverse Reactions: Dermatitis and allied symptomatology have been reported.
If adverse reaction or idiosyncrasy occurs, discontinue medication and institute appropriate therapy.
Dosage and Administration: Apply to the infected eye every 2 hours or oftener as the condition and response indicate. Severe or stubborn infections may require treatment for many days or oral administration in addition to local treatment. Mild infections may respond in as little as 48 hours.
How Supplied:
⅛ oz. tubes—NDC 0005-3511-51

LEDERLE LABORATORIES DIVISION
American Cyanamid Company
Pearl River, NY 10965
Rev. 11/81
03680

DIAMOX® ℞

[*di 'ah-moks*]
Acetazolamide Tablets USP and
DIAMOX Sterile Acetazolamide Sodium USP
Intravenous

Description: DIAMOX, an inhibitor of the enzyme carbonic anhydrase, is a white to faintly yellowish white crystalline, odorless powder, weakly acidic, very slightly soluble in water and slightly soluble in alcohol. The chemical name for DIAMOX is *N*-(5-Sulfamoyl-1,3,4-thiadiazol-2yl)-acetamide. Its chemical formula is $C_4H_6N_4O_3S_2$. Its molecular weight is 222.24.
DIAMOX is available as oral tablets containing 125 mg and 250 mg of acetazolamide respectively and the following inactive ingredients: Corn Starch, Dibasic Calcium Phosphate, Magnesium Stearate, Povidone, and Sodium Starch Glycolate.
DIAMOX is also available for intravenous use, and is supplied as a sterile powder requiring reconstitution. Each vial contains an amount of acetazolamide sodium equivalent to 500 mg of acetazolamide. The bulk solution is adjusted to pH 9.2 using sodium hydroxide and, if necessary, hydrochloric acid prior to lyophilization.
Clinical Pharmacology: DIAMOX is a potent carbonic anhydrase inhibitor, effective in the control of fluid secretion (eg, some types of glaucoma), in the treatment of certain convulsive disorders (eg, epilepsy), and in the promotion of diuresis in instances of abnormal fluid retention (eg, cardiac edema).
DIAMOX is not a mercurial diuretic. Rather it is a nonbacteriostatic sulfonamide possessing a chemical structure and pharmacological activity distinctly different from the bacteriostatic sulfonamides.
DIAMOX is an enzyme inhibitor which acts specifically on carbonic anhydrase, the enzyme which catalyzes the reversible reaction involving the hydration of carbon dioxide and the dehydration of carbonic acid. In the eye, this inhibitory action of acetazolamide decreases the secretion of aqueous humor and results in a drop in intraocular pressure, a reaction considered desirable in cases of glaucoma and even in certain nonglaucomatous conditions. Evidence seems to indicate that DIAMOX has utility as an adjuvant in the treatment of certain dysfunctions of the central nervous system (eg, epilepsy). Inhibition of carbonic anhydrase in this area appears to retard abnormal, paroxysmal, excessive discharge from central nervous system neurons. The diuretic effect of DIAMOX is due to its action in the kidney on the reversible reaction involving hydration of carbon dioxide and dehydration of carbonic acid. The result is renal loss of HCO_3 ion, which carries out sodium, water, and potassium. Alkalinization of the urine and promotion of diuresis are thus effected. Alteration in ammonia metabolism occurs due to increased reabsorption of ammonia by the renal tubules as a result of urinary alkalinization.
Placebo-controlled clinical trials have shown that prophylactic administration of DIAMOX at a dose of 250 mg every 8 to 12 hours (or a 500 mg controlled-release capsule once daily)

before and during rapid ascent to altitude results in fewer and/or less severe symptoms (such as headache, nausea, shortness of breath, dizziness, drowsiness, and fatigue) of acute mountain sickness (AMS). Pulmonary function (eg, minute ventilation, expired vital capacity, and peak flow) is greater in the DIAMOX treated group, both in subjects with AMS and asymptomatic subjects. The DIAMOX treated climbers also had less difficulty in sleeping.

Indications and Usage: For adjunctive treatment of: edema due to congestive heart failure; drug-induced edema; centrencephalic epilepsies (petit mal, unlocalized seizures); chronic simple (open-angle) glaucoma, secondary glaucoma, and preoperatively in acute angle-closure glaucoma where delay of surgery is desired in order to lower intraocular pressure. DIAMOX is also indicated for the prevention or amelioration of symptoms associated with acute mountain sickness in climbers attempting rapid ascent and in those who are very susceptible to acute mountain sickness despite gradual ascent.

Contraindications: DIAMOX *acetazolamide* therapy is contraindicated in situations in which sodium and/or potassium blood serum levels are depressed, in cases of marked kidney and liver disease or dysfunction, in suprarenal gland failure and in hyperchloremic acidosis. It is contraindicated in patients with cirrhosis because of the risk of development of hepatic encephalopathy.

Long-term administration of DIAMOX is contraindicated in patients with chronic noncongestive angle-closure glaucoma since it may permit organic closure of the angle to occur while the worsening glaucoma is masked by lowered intraocular pressure.

Warnings: Fatalities have occurred, although rarely, due to severe reactions to sulfonamides including Stevens-Johnson syndrome, toxic epidermal necrolysis, fulminant hepatic necrosis, agranulocytosis, aplastic anemia, and other blood dyscrasias. Sensitizations may recur when a sulfonamide is readministered irrespective of the route of administration. If signs of hypersensitivity or other serious reactions occur, discontinue use of this drug.

Caution is advised for patients receiving concomitant high-dose aspirin and DIAMOX, as anorexia, tachypnea, lethargy, coma and death have been reported.

Precautions: *General:* Increasing the dose does not increase the diuresis and may increase the incidence of drowsiness and/or paresthesia. Increasing the dose often results in a decrease in diuresis. Under certain circumstances, however, very large doses have been given in conjunction with other diuretics in order to secure diuresis in complete refractory failure.

Information for Patients: Adverse reactions common to all sulfonamide derivatives may occur: anaphylaxis, fever, rash (including erythema multiforme, Stevens-Johnson syndrome, toxic epidermal necrolysis), crystalluria, renal calculus, bone marrow depression, thrombocytopenic purpura, hemolytic anemia, leukopenia, pancytopenia, and agranulocytosis. Precaution is advised for early detection of such reactions, and the drug should be discontinued and appropriate therapy instituted.

In patients with pulmonary obstruction or emphysema where alveolar ventilation may be impaired, DIAMOX, which may precipitate or aggravate acidosis, should be used with caution.

Gradual ascent is desirable to try to avoid acute mountain sickness. If rapid ascent is undertaken and DIAMOX *acetazolamide* is used, it should be noted that such use does not obviate the need for prompt descent if severe forms of high altitude sickness occur, ie, high altitude pulmonary edema (HAPE) or high altitude cerebral edema.

Caution is advised for patients receiving concomitant high-dose aspirin and DIAMOX, as anorexia, tachypnea, lethargy, coma and death have been reported (see **Warnings**).

Laboratory Tests: To monitor for hematologic reactions common to all sulfonamides, it is recommended that a baseline CBC and platelet count be obtained on patients prior to initiating DIAMOX therapy and at regular intervals during therapy. If significant changes occur, early discontinuance and institution of appropriate therapy are important. Periodic monitoring of serum electrolytes is recommended.

Carcinogenesis, Mutagenesis, Impairment of Fertility: Long-term studies in animals to evaluate the carcinogenic potential of DIAMOX have not been conducted. In a bacterial mutagenicity assay, DIAMOX was not mutagenic when evaluated with and without metabolic activation.

The drug had no effect on fertility when administered in the diet to male and female rats at a daily intake of up to four times the recommended human dose of 1000 mg in a 50 kg individual.

Pregnancy: Pregnancy Category C: Acetazolamide, administered orally or parenterally, has been shown to be teratogenic (defects of the limbs) in mice, rats, hamsters and rabbits. There are no adequate and well-controlled studies in pregnant women. Acetazolamide should be used in pregnancy only if the potential benefit justifies the potential risk to the fetus.

Nursing Mothers: Because of the potential for serious adverse reaction in nursing infants from DIAMOX, a decision should be made whether to discontinue nursing or to discontinue the drug taking into account the importance of the drug to the mother.

Pediatric Use: The safety and effectiveness of DIAMOX *acetazolamide* in children have not been established.

Adverse Reactions: Adverse reactions, occurring most often early in therapy, include paresthesias, particularly a "tingling" feeling in the extremities, hearing dysfunction or tinnitus, loss of appetite, taste alteration and gastrointestinal disturbances such as nausea, vomiting and diarrhea; polyuria, and occasional instances of drowsiness and confusion. Metabolic acidosis and electrolyte imbalance may occur.

Transient myopia has been reported. This condition invariably subsides upon diminution or discontinuance of the medication.

Other occasional adverse reactions include urticaria, melena, hematuria, glycosuria, hepatic insufficiency, flaccid paralysis, photosensitivity and convulsions. Also see **Precautions:** *Information for Patients* for possible reactions common to sulfonamide derivatives. Fatalities have occurred although rarely, due to severe reactions to sulfonamides including Stevens-Johnson syndrome, toxic epidermal necrolysis, fulminant hepatic necrosis, agranulocytosis, aplastic anemia and other blood dyscrasias (see **Warnings**).

Overdosage: No data are available regarding DIAMOX overdosage in humans as no cases of acute poisoning with this drug have been reported. Animal data suggest that DIAMOX is remarkably nontoxic. No specific antidote is known. Treatment should be symptomatic and supportive.

Electrolyte imbalance, development of an acidotic state, and central nervous effects might be expected to occur. Serum electrolyte levels (particularly potassium) and blood pH levels should be monitored.

Supportive measures are required to restore electrolyte and pH balance. The acidotic state can usually be corrected by the administration of bicarbonate.

Despite its high intraerythrocytic distribution and plasma protein binding properties, DIAMOX may be dialyzable. This may be particularly important in the management of DIAMOX overdosage when complicated by the presence of renal failure.

Dosage and Administration: *Preparation and Storage of Parenteral Solution:* Each 500 mg vial containing DIAMOX parenteral should be reconstituted with at least 5 mL of Sterile Water for Injection prior to use. Reconstituted solutions retain potency for 1 week if refrigerated. Since this product contains no preservative, use within 24 hours of reconstitution is strongly recommended. The direct intravenous route of administration is preferred. Intramuscular administration is not recommended.

Glaucoma: DIAMOX *acetazolamide* should be used as an adjunct to the usual therapy. The dosage employed in the treatment of *chronic simple (open-angle) glaucoma* ranges from 250 mg to 1 g of DIAMOX per 24 hours, usually in divided doses for amounts over 250 mg. It has usually been found that a dosage in excess of 1 g per 24 hours does not produce an increased effect. In all cases, the dosage should be adjusted with careful individual attention both to symptomatology and ocular tension. Continuous supervision by a physician is advisable.

In treatment of secondary glaucoma and in the preoperative treatment of some cases of *acute congestive (closed-angle) glaucoma,* the preferred dosage is 250 mg every 4 hours, although some cases have responded to 250 mg twice daily on short-term therapy. In some acute cases, it may be more satisfactory to administer an initial dose of 500 mg followed by 125 or 250 mg every 4 hours depending on the individual case. Intravenous therapy may be used for rapid relief of ocular tension in acute cases. A complementary effect has been noted when DIAMOX has been used in conjunction with miotics or mydriatics as the case demanded.

Epilepsy: It is not clearly known whether the beneficial effects observed in epilepsy are due to direct inhibition of carbonic anhydrase in the central nervous system or whether they are due to the slight degree of acidosis produced by the divided dosage. The best results to date have been seen in petit mal in children. Good results, however, have been seen in patients, both children and adult, in other types of seizures such as grand mal, mixed seizure patterns, myoclonic jerk patterns, etc. The suggested total daily dose is 8 to 30 mg per kg in divided doses. Although some patients respond to a low dose, the optimum range appears to be from 375 to 1000 mg daily. However, some investigators feel that daily doses in excess of 1 g do not produce any better results than a 1 g dose. When DIAMOX is given in combination with other anticonvulsants it is suggested that the starting dose should be 250 mg once daily in addition to the existing medications. This can be increased to levels as indicated above.

The change from other medication to DIAMOX should be gradual and in accordance with usual practice in epilepsy therapy.

Continued on next page

Information on Storz products listed on these pages is the full Prescribing Information from product literature or package inserts effective in June 1991. Information concerning all Storz products may be obtained from the Professional Services Department, Lederle Laboratories, Pearl River, New York 10965

Storz Ophthalmics, Inc.—Cont.

Congestive Heart Failure: For diuresis in congestive heart failure, the starting dose is usually 250 to 375 mg once daily in the morning (5 mg/kg). If after an initial response, the patient fails to continue to lose edema fluid, do not increase the dose but allow for kidney recovery by skipping medication for a day. DIAMOX *acetazolamide* yields best diuretic results when given on alternate days, or for 2 days alternating with a day of rest.
Failures in therapy may be due to overdosage or too frequent dosage. The use of DIAMOX does not eliminate the need for other therapy such as digitalis, bed rest, and salt restriction.
Drug-Induced Edema: Recommended dosage is 250 to 375 mg of DIAMOX once a day for 1 or 2 days, alternating with a day of rest.
Acute Mountain Sickness: Dosage is 500 mg to 1000 mg daily, in divided doses using tablets or sustained-release capsules as appropriate. In circumstances of rapid ascent, such as in rescue or military operations, the higher dose level of 1000 mg is recommended. It is preferable to initiate dosing 24 to 48 hours before ascent and to continue for 48 hours while at high altitude, or longer as necessary to control symptoms.
Note: The dosage recommendations for glaucoma and epilepsy differ considerably from those for congestive heart failure, since the first two conditions are not dependent upon carbonic anhydrase inhibition in the kidney which requires intermittent dosage if it is to recover from the inhibitory effect of the therapeutic agent.
Parenteral drug products should be inspected visually for particulate matter and discoloration prior to administration, whenever solution and container permit.
How Supplied: *Tablets* 125 mg–Round, flat-faced, beveled, white tablets engraved with DIAMOX and 125 on one side and scored in half on the other side. Engraved with LL on the right of the score and D1 on the left, are supplied as follows:
NDC 57706-754-23—Bottle of 100
250 mg—Round, convex, white tablets engraved with DIAMOX *acetazolamide* and 250 on one side and scored in quarters on the other side. Engraved with LL in the upper right quadrant and D2 in the lower left quadrant, are supplied as follows:
NDC 57706-755-23—Bottle of 100
NDC 57706-755-34—Bottle of 1000
NDC 57706-755-60—Unit Dose 10 × 10
Store at Controlled Room Temperature 15°–30°C (59°–86°F).
Manufactured for
STORZ OPHTHALMICS, INC.
St. Louis, MO 63122
by
LEDERLE LABORATORIES DIVISION
American Cyanamid Company
Pearl River, NY 10965
Intravenous –Sterile intravenous (lyophilized) powder.
NDC 57706-762-96–500 mg vial
Store at Controlled Room Temperature 15°–30°C (59°–86° F).
MILITARY DEPOT:
NSN 6505-00-064-8724 —Parenteral, 500 mg vial
Manufactured for
STORZ OPHTHALMICS, INC.
St. Louis, MO 63122
by
LEDERLE PARENTERALS, INC.
Carolina, Puerto Rico 00630 Rev. 3/91
10248-91

Shown in Product Identification Section, page 105

DIAMOX® Acetazolamide SEQUELS® Sustained-Release Capsules ℞

Description: DIAMOX is an inhibitor of the enzyme carbonic anhydrase.
DIAMOX is a white to faintly yellowish white crystalline, odorless powder, weakly acidic, very slightly soluble in water and slightly soluble in alcohol. The chemical name for DIAMOX is N-(5-Sulfamoyl-1,3,4-thiadiazol-2yl)-acetamide.
DIAMOX SEQUELS are sustained-release capsules, for oral administration, each containing 500 mg of acetazolamide and the following inactive ingredients: Beeswax, Benzoin Gum, Corn Starch, Ethylcellulose, FD&C Blue No. 1, FD&C Yellow No. 6, Gelatin, Glycerin, Magnesium Stearate, Methylparaben, Mineral Oil, Mono- and Diglycerides, Propylene Glycol, Propylparaben, Silica, Sucrose, Talc, Terpene Resin, and Vanillin.
Clinical Pharmacology: DIAMOX is a potent carbonic anhydrase inhibitor, effective in the control of fluid secretion (eg, some types of glaucoma), in the treatment of certain convulsive disorders (eg, epilepsy), and in the promotion of diuresis in instances of abnormal fluid retention (eg, cardiac edema).
DIAMOX is not a mercurial diuretic. Rather it is a nonbacteriostatic sulfonamide possessing a chemical structure and pharmacological activity distinctly different from the bacteriostatic sulfonamides.
DIAMOX is an enzyme inhibitor that acts specifically on carbonic anhydrase, the enzyme which catalyzes the reversible reaction involving the hydration of carbon dioxide and the dehydration of carbonic acid. In the eye, this inhibitory action of acetazolamide decreases the secretion of aqueous humor and results in a drop in intraocular pressure, a reaction considered desirable in cases of glaucoma and even in certain nonglaucomatous conditions. Evidence seems to indicate that DIAMOX has utility as an adjuvant in the treatment of certain dysfunctions of the central nervous system (eg, epilepsy). Inhibition of carbonic anhydrase in this area appears to retard abnormal, paroxysmal, excessive discharge from central nervous system neurons. The diuretic effect of DIAMOX is due to its action in the kidney on the reversible reaction involving hydration of carbon dioxide and dehydration of carbonic acid. The result is renal loss of HCO_3 ion, which carries out sodium, water, and potassium. Alkalinization of the urine and promotion of diuresis are thus effected. Alteration in ammonia metabolism occurs due to increased reabsorption of ammonia by the renal tubules as a result of urinary alkalinization.
DIAMOX SEQUELS sustained-release capsules provide prolonged action to inhibit aqueous humor secretion for 18 to 24 hours after each dose, whereas tablets act for only 8 to 12 hours. The prolonged continuous effect of SEQUELS permits a reduction in dosage frequency.
Plasma concentrations of acetazolamide peak between 3 to 6 hours after administration of DIAMOX SEQUELS, compared to 1 to 4 hours with tablets.
Placebo-controlled clinical trials have shown that prophylactic administration of DIAMOX at a dose of 250 mg every 8 to 12 hours (or a 500 mg controlled-release capsule once daily) before and during rapid ascent to altitude results in fewer and/or less severe symptoms (such as headache, nausea, shortness of breath, dizziness, drowsiness, and fatigue) of acute mountain sickness (AMS). Pulmonary function (eg, minute ventilation, expired vital capacity, and peak flow) is greater in the DIAMOX treated group, both in subjects with AMS and asymptomatic subjects. The DIAMOX treated climbers also had less difficulty in sleeping.
Indications and Usage: For adjunctive treatment of: chronic simple (open-angle) glaucoma, secondary glaucoma, and preoperatively in acute angle-closure glaucoma where delay of surgery is desired in order to lower intraocular pressure. DIAMOX is also indicated for the prevention or amelioration of symptoms associated with acute mountain sickness in climbers attempting rapid ascent and in those who are very susceptible to acute mountain sickness despite gradual ascent.
Contraindications: Acetazolamide therapy is contraindicated in situations in which sodium and/or potassium blood serum levels are depressed, in cases of marked kidney and liver disease or dysfunction, in suprarenal gland failure, and in hyperchloremic acidosis. It is contraindicated in patients with cirrhosis because of the risk of development of hepatic encephalopathy.
Long-term administration of DIAMOX *acetazolamide* is contraindicated in patients with chronic noncongestive angle-closure glaucoma since it may permit organic closure of the angle to occur while the worsening glaucoma is masked by lowered intraocular pressure.
Warnings: Fatalities have occurred, although rarely, due to severe reactions to sulfonamides including Stevens-Johnson syndrome, toxic epidermal necrolysis, fulminant hepatic necrosis, agranulocytosis, aplastic anemia, and other blood dyscrasias. Sensitizations may recur when a sulfonamide is readministered irrespective of the route of administration. If signs of hypersensitivity or other serious reactions occur, discontinue use of this drug.
Caution is advised for patients receiving concomitant high-dose aspirin and DIAMOX, as anorexia, tachypnea, lethargy, coma, and death have been reported.
Precautions: General: Increasing the dose does not increase the diuresis and may increase the incidence of drowsiness and/or paresthesia. Increasing the dose often results in a decrease in diuresis. Under certain circumstances, however, very large doses have been given in conjunction with other diuretics in order to secure diuresis in complete refractory failure.
Information for Patients: Adverse reactions common to all sulfonamide derivatives may occur: anaphylaxis, fever, rash (including erythema multiforme, Stevens-Johnson syndrome, toxic epidermal necrolysis), crystalluria, renal calculus, bone marrow depression, thrombocytopenic purpura, hemolytic anemia, leukopenia, pancytopenia, and agranulocytosis. Precaution is advised for early detection of such reactions, and the drug should be discontinued and appropriate therapy instituted.
In patients with pulmonary obstruction or emphysema where alveolar ventilation may be impaired, DIAMOX *acetazolamide,* which may aggravate acidosis, should be used with caution.
Gradual ascent is desirable to try to avoid acute mountain sickness. If rapid ascent is undertaken and DIAMOX is used, it should be noted that such use does not obviate the need for prompt descent if severe forms of high altitude sickness occur, ie, high altitude pulmonary edema (HAPE) or high altitude cerebral edema.
Caution is advised for patients receiving concomitant high-dose aspirin and DIAMOX, as anorexia, tachypnea, lethargy, coma, and death have been reported (see **Warnings**).
Laboratory Tests: To monitor for hematologic reactions common to all sulfonamides, it is recommended that a baseline CBC and platelet count be obtained on patients prior to initiating DIAMOX therapy and at regular intervals during therapy. If significant changes occur, early discontinuance and institution of appropriate therapy are important.

Periodic monitoring of serum electrolytes is recommended.

Carcinogenesis, Mutagenesis, Impairment of Fertility: Long-term studies in animals to evaluate the carcinogenic potential of DIAMOX have not been conducted. In a bacterial mutagenicity assay, DIAMOX was not mutagenic when evaluated with and without metabolic activation. The drug had no effect on fertility when administered in the diet to male and female rats at a daily intake of up to four times the maximum recommended human dose of 1000 mg in a 50 kg individual.

Pregnancy Category C. Acetazolamide, administered orally or parenterally, has been shown to be teratogenic (defects of the limbs) in mice, rats, hamsters and rabbits. There are no adequate and well-controlled studies in pregnant women. Acetazolamide should be used in pregnancy only if the potential benefit justifies the potential risk to the fetus.

Nursing Mothers: Because of the potential for serious adverse reactions in nursing infants from DIAMOX, a decision should be made whether to discontinue nursing or to discontinue the drug taking into account the importance of the drug to the mother.

Pediatric Use: The safety and effectiveness of DIAMOX in children have not been established.

Adverse Reactions: Adverse reactions, occurring most often early in therapy, include paresthesia, particularly a "tingling" feeling in the extremities, hearing dysfunction or tinnitus, loss of appetite, taste alteration and gastrointestinal disturbances such as nausea, vomiting and diarrhea; polyuria, and occasional instances of drowsiness and confusion. Metabolic acidosis and electrolyte imbalance may occur.

Transient myopia has been reported. This condition invariably subsides upon diminution or discontinuance of the medication.

Other occasional adverse reactions include urticaria, melena, hematuria, glycosuria, hepatic insufficiency, flaccid paralysis, photosensitivity and convulsions. Also see **Precautions: Information for Patients** for possible reactions common to sulfonamide derivatives. Fatalities have occurred although rarely, due to severe reactions to sulfonamides including Stevens-Johnson syndrome, toxic epidermal necrolysis, fulminant hepatic necrosis, agranulocytosis, aplastic anemia and other blood dyscrasia (see **Warnings**).

Overdosage: No data are available regarding DIAMOX *acetazolamide* overdosage in humans as no cases of acute poisoning with this drug have been reported. Animal data suggest that DIAMOX is remarkably nontoxic. No specific antidote is known. Treatment should be symptomatic and supportive.

Electrolyte imbalance, development of an acidotic state, and central nervous effects might be expected to occur. Serum electrolyte levels (particularly potassium) and blood pH levels should be monitored.

Supportive measures are required to restore electrolyte and pH balance. The acidotic state can usually be corrected by the administration of bicarbonate.

Despite its high intraerythrocytic distribution and plasma protein binding properties, DIAMOX may be dialyzable. This may be particularly important in the management of DIAMOX overdosage when complicated by the presence of renal failure.

Dosage and Administration: Glaucoma: The recommended dose is one capsule (500 mg) two times a day. Usually one capsule is administered in the morning and one capsule in the evening. It may be necessary to adjust the dose but it has usually been found that dosage in excess of two capsules (1 g) does not produce an increased effect. The dosage should be adjusted with careful individual attention both to symptomatology and intraocular tension. In all cases, continuous supervision by a physician is advisable.

In those unusual instances where adequate control is not obtained by the twice-a-day administration of DIAMOX *acetazolamide* SEQUELS sustained-release capsules, the desired control may be established by means of DIAMOX (tablets or parenteral). Use tablets or parenteral in accordance with the more frequent dosage schedules recommended for these dosage forms, such as 250 mg every 4 hours, or an initial dose of 500 mg followed by 250 mg or 125 mg every 4 hours, depending on the case in question.

Acute Mountain Sickness: Dosage is 500 mg to 1000 mg daily, in divided doses using tablets or sustained-release capsules as appropriate. In circumstances of rapid ascent, such as in rescue or military operations, the higher dose level of 1000 mg is recommended. It is preferable to initiate dosing 24 to 48 hours before ascent and to continue for 48 hours while at high altitude, or longer, as necessary to control symptoms.

How Supplied:

DIAMOX SEQUELS, 500 mg orange capsules printed with DIAMOX over D3, are supplied as follows:

NDC 57706-753-13—Bottle of 30

NDC 57706-753-23—Bottle of 100

Store at Controlled Room Temperature 15°–30°C (59°–86°F).

Military and VA Depots: NSN 6505-00-880-4949—(100s)

Manufactured for
STORZ OPHTHALMICS
St. Louis, MO 63122
by
LEDERLE LABORATORIES DIVISION
American Cyanamid Company
Pearl River, NY 10965

Rev. 11/90
28463

Shown in Product Identification Section, page 105

NEPTAZANE® ℞

[*nĕp-ta 'zāne*]

methazolamide

Tablets

Description: NEPTAZANE, a sulfonamide derivative, is a white crystalline powder, weakly acid, and slightly soluble in water. It is available as 25 mg and 50 mg tablets. The chemical name for methazolamide is: *N*-[5-(aminosulfonyl) -3- methyl-1, 3, 4- thiadiazol-2(3*H*)-ylidene]-acetamide.

NEPTAZANE tablets contain the following inactive ingredients: Acacia, Alginic Acid, Corn Starch, Dibasic Calcium Phosphate, Gelatin, and Magnesium Stearate.

Clinical Pharmacology: NEPTAZANE is a potent inhibitor of the enzyme carbonic anhydrase. It is absorbed somewhat slowly from the gastrointestinal tract and disappears more slowly from the plasma than does acetazolamide, which may account for the delay in onset and duration of its activity. It is distributed throughout the body, and can be assayed in the blood plasma, the cerebrospinal fluid, the aqueous humor of the eye, the red blood cell, in the bile, and the extracellular fluid. Urinary excretion accounts for only 15% of NEPTAZANE in man. It is not cumulative in its concentration. The drug is considered non-bactericidal. Although concentration in the cerebrospinal fluid is high, it is not considered an effective anticonvulsant.

NEPTAZANE does have a diuretic effect, resulting in increase in urinary volume, with excretion of sodium and potassium and chloride, but it is less active than acetazolamide. This effect is transient and of low degree, and the drug is not used as a diuretic. Serum electrolyte changes in sodium, potassium, and chloride are minimal and return to pretreatment levels after daily administration for 3 to 4 days. Inhibition of renal bicarbonate reabsorption produces an alkaline urine. Plasma bicarbonate decreases temporarily, and a relative and transient metabolic acidosis may occur due to a disequilibrium in CO_2 transport in the red cell. This is quickly restored to balance by the initiation of compensatory mechanisms. Urinary citrate excretion is decreased by 40% on doses of 100 mg every 8 hours with variations in urinary volume output. Uric acid output was decreased 36% in the first 24-hour period and varied thereafter. The oral administration of the drug by inhibition of carbonic anhydrase in the various tissues of the eye causes a decrease in the rate of aqueous humor formation. Various authors differ somewhat as to the time of onset of intraocular pressure fall, of the peak of activity, and the duration of the effect on the pressure, of a 24-hour period of ingestion, but on the average, the onset of fall in intraocular pressure occurs within 2 to 4 hours, with a peak of fall in 6 to 8 hours, the effect lasting from 10 to 18 hours.

Indications and Usage: For adjunctive treatment of: chronic simple (open-angle) glaucoma, secondary glaucoma, and preoperatively in acute angle-closure glaucoma where delay of surgery is desired in order to lower intraocular pressure.

Contraindications: Severe or absolute glaucoma and chronic noncongestive angle-closure glaucoma. It is of doubtful use in glaucoma due to severe peripheral anterior synechiae or hemorrhagic glaucoma.

NEPTAZANE is contraindicated in patients with adrenocortical insufficiency, hepatic insufficiency, renal insufficiency, or an electrolyte imbalance state such as hyperchloremic acidosis, and sodium and potassium depletion states.

Warnings: Studies in rats have demonstrated teratogenic effects (skeletal anomalies) at high doses. There is no evidence of these effects in human beings and no fetal defects have been reported. However, NEPTAZANE should not be used in women of childbearing potential or in pregnancy, especially in the first trimester, unless the benefits to be gained in the control of glaucoma outweigh potential adverse effects.

Precautions: Potassium excretion is increased initially, upon administration of NEPTAZANE, and in patients with cirrhosis or hepatic insufficiency could precipitate a hepatic coma. It should be used with caution in patients on steroid therapy because of the potentiality of a hypokalemic state.

Adequate and balanced electrolyte intake is essential in all patients whose concomitant clinical condition may occasion electrolyte imbalance.

In patients with pulmonary obstruction or emphysema where alveolar ventilation may be impaired, NEPTAZANE *methazolamide*, which may precipitate or aggravate acidosis, should be used with caution.

Adverse reactions common to all sulfonamide derivatives may occur: anaphylaxis, fever, rash (including erythema multiforme, Stevens-Johnson syndrome, toxic epidermal necrolysis), crystalluria, renal calculus, bone marrow depression, thrombocytopenic purpura, hemolytic anemia, leukopenia, pancytopenia, and

Continued on next page

Information on Storz products listed on these pages is the full Prescribing Information from product literature or package inserts effective in June 1991. Information concerning all Storz products may be obtained from the Professional Services Department, Lederle Laboratories, Pearl River, New York 10965

Storz Ophthalmics, Inc.—Cont.

agranulocytosis. Precaution is advised for early detection of such reactions, and the drug should be discontinued and appropriate therapy instituted.

Adverse Reactions: Most adverse reactions to NEPTAZANE have been relatively mild in character and disappear upon withdrawal of the drug or adjustment of dosage. They are as follows: anorexia, nausea, vomiting, malaise, fatigue or drowsiness, headache, vertigo, mental confusion, depression, and paresthesia of fingers, toes, hands or feet and occasionally at the mucocutaneous junction of the lips, mouth, and anus. Rarely, photosensitivity has been reported.
Urinary citrate excretion is decreased during the administration of NEPTAZANE as is uric acid output, but urinary calculi have been reported only rarely. The effect on citrate excretion is less than that reported from the administration of acetazolamide.
In order to monitor for hematologic reactions common to all sulfonamides, it is recommended that a baseline CBC and platelet count be obtained on all patients prior to initiating NEPTAZANE therapy and at regular intervals during therapy. Early detection of such reactions is important, and the drug should be discontinued, and appropriate therapy instituted if significant changes occur in these laboratory parameters.

Dosage and Administration: The effective therapeutic dose administered in tablet form varies from 50 mg to 100 mg two to three times daily. The drug may be used concomitantly with miotic and osmotic agents. It is not available for parenteral use.

How Supplied: NEPTAZANE *methazolamide* Tablets, 25 mg, are square, white tablets with engraved N2 on one side and embossed large N on the other side, supplied as follows:
NDC 0005-4565-23—Bottle of 100
NEPTAZANE Tablets, 50 mg, are round, scored, white tablets engraved with LL on one side and N above and 1 below the score on the other side, supplied as follows:
NDC 0005-4570-23—Bottle of 100
Store at Controlled Room Temperature 15°–30°C (59°–86°F).

Military Depot:
NSN 6505-00-065-4205—50 mg (100s)
LEDERLE LABORATORIES DIVISION
American Cyanamid Company
Pearl River, NY 10965 Rev. 2/88
22290

Shown in Product Identification Section, page 105

OCCUCOAT®
2% Hydroxypropylmethylcellulose

Description: OCCUCOAT is a sterile, isotonic, nonpyrogenic viscoelastic solution of highly purified, noninflammatory, 2% hydroxypropylmethylcellulose with a high molecular weight greater than 80,000 daltons. OCCUCOAT is supplied in 1 mL syringes. Each mL provides 20 mg/mL of hydroxypropylmethylcellulose dissolved in a physiological balanced salt solution containing 0.49% sodium chloride, 0.075% potassium chloride, 0.048% calcium chloride, 0.03% magnesium chloride, 0.39% sodium acetate, 0.17% sodium citrate and water for injection. The osmolarity of OCCUCOAT is 285±32 mOsM; the viscosity is 4000±1500 cst; and the pH is 7.2±0.4.

Characteristics: OCCUCOAT is an ophthalmic surgical aid for use in anterior segment surgery.
OCCUCOAT:
1. Is a space occupying, tissue protective substance
2. Exhibits excellent flow properties
3. Is completely transparent
4. Is nonantigenic
5. Is easily removed from the anterior chamber
6. Contains no proteins which may cause inflammation or foreign body reactions
7. Requires no refrigeration or restrictive storage conditions
8. Does not interfere with normal wound healing process
9. Clears the trabecular meshwork in 24 hours (98% clearance rate)

Indications: OCCUCOAT is indicated for use as an ophthalmic surgical aid in anterior segment surgical procedures including cataract extraction and intraocular lens implantation. OCCUCOAT maintains a deep chamber during anterior segment surgery and thereby allows for more efficient manipulation with less trauma to the corneal endothelium and other ocular tissues. The viscoelasticity of OCCUCOAT helps the vitreous face to be pushed back, thus preventing formation of a postoperative flat chamber.

Contraindications: At present, there are no known contraindications to the use of OCCUCOAT when used as recommended.

Precautions: Precautions are limited to those normally associated with the ophthalmic surgical procedure being performed. There may be transient increased intraocular pressure following surgery because of pre-existing glaucoma or due to the surgery itself. For these reasons, the following precautions should be considered:
- OCCUCOAT should be removed from the anterior chamber at the end of surgery.
- If the postoperative intraocular pressure increases above expected values, appropriate therapy should be administered.

Adverse Reactions: Clinical testing of OCCUCOAT showed it to be extremely well tolerated after injection into the human eye. A transient rise in intraocular pressure postoperatively has been reported in some cases.

Clinical Applications: In anterior segment surgery, OCCUCOAT should be carefully introduced into the anterior chamber using a 20 gauge or larger cannula. OCCUCOAT may be injected into the chamber prior to or following delivery of the crystalline lens. Injection of OCCUCOAT prior to lens delivery will provide additional protection to the corneal endothelium and other ocular tissues. Injection of the material at this point is significant in that a coating of OCCUCOAT may protect the corneal endothelium from possible damage arising from surgical instrumentation during the cataract extraction surgery.
OCCUCOAT 2% *hydroxypropylmethylcellulose* may also be used to coat an intraocular lens as well as tips of surgical instruments prior to implantation surgery. Additional OCCUCOAT may be injected during anterior segment surgery to fully maintain the chamber, or to replace fluid lost during the surgical procedure. OCCUCOAT should be removed from the anterior chamber at the end of surgery.

How Supplied: OCCUCOAT is a sterile, nonpyrogenic viscoelastic preparation supplied in a 1 mL single use glass syringe with a Luer tip and a cannula.
OCCUCOAT syringes are aseptically packaged and terminally sterilized.
Store at room temperature; avoid excessive heat (60°C). Protect from light. For intraocular use.

Directions for Use—Syringe Assembly: Use sterile opening technique.
Open pouch and drop sterile contents onto sterile field.
- Assembly

Insert glass cartridge into plastic holder.

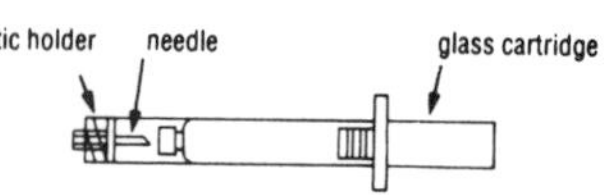

Screw in plunger rod clockwise, and squeeze plunger so that needle perforates glass cartridge membrane.

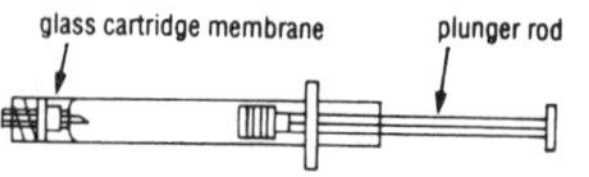

Connect cannula to syringe tip, twist firmly in place, and check for proper function. Allow air bubbles, if any, to rise to the surface, and push plunger rod slightly to release any air bubbles from syringe tip and cannula.

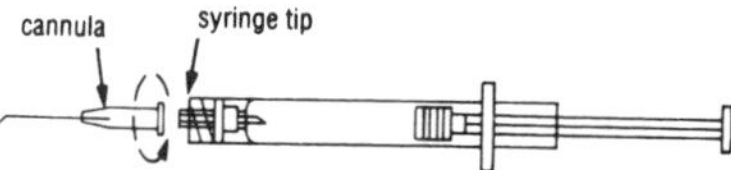

Caution: Federal (USA) law restricts this device to sale by or on the order of a physician. For intraocular use only. Discard unused contents of OCCUCOAT 2% *hydroxypropylmethylcellulose* syringe after each use. Do not re-sterilize.
Storz Ophthalmics, Inc.
A Division of American Cyanamid Company
3365 Tree Court Industrial Blvd.
St. Louis, MO 63122-6694

Shown in Product Identification Section, page 105

OCUVITE® Vitamin and Mineral Supplement

Description: Each OCUVITE tablet provides:
[See table on next page.]
Indications: OCUVITE is specifically formulated to supplement the diets of people who may have or be at risk of deficiencies of the vitamins and minerals found in the OCUVITE formulation.
Recommended Intake: Adults should take one tablet one or two times per day, or as directed by their physicians.
How Supplied: Two-tone peach, eye shaped, film coated tablet engraved LL on one side, O4 on the other side.
NDC 0005-4550-19—Bottle of 60
Store at Controlled Room Temperature 15°–30°C (59°–86°F).
LEDERLE LABORATORIES DIVISION
American Cyanamid Company
Pearl River, NY 10965

RĒV-EYES™ ℞
[*reev-eyes*]
dapiprazole hydrochloride
Ophthalmic Eyedrops, 0.5%—Sterile

Description: For ophthalmic use only.
RĒV-EYES is an alpha-adrenergic blocking agent.
Dapiprazole hydrochloride is 5,6,7,8-tetrahydro -3- [2-(4-o.tolyl -1- piperazinyl) ethyl]-s-triazolo[4,3-a] pyridine hydrochloride.
Dapiprazole hydrochloride has the empirical formula $C_{19}H_{27}N_5$ HCl and a molecular weight of 361.93.
Dapiprazole hydrochloride is a sterile, white, lyophilized powder soluble in water.

Vitamin or Mineral	Source	Amount	Adult— US RDA
Zinc	Zinc Oxide*	40 mg (elemental)	267%
Copper	Cupric Oxide	2 mg (elemental)	100%
Vitamin C	Ascorbic Acid	60 mg	100%
Vitamin E	dl-Alpha Tocopheryl Acetate	30 IU	100%
Vitamin A	Beta Carotene	5000 IU	100%
Selenium	Sodium Selenate	40 mcg (elemental)	**

*Zinc Oxide is the most concentrated form of zinc and contains more elemental zinc than any other zinc salt (ie, zinc sulfate or zinc gluconate).
**No US RDA established.

RĒV-EYES Eyedrops is a clear, colorless, slightly viscous solution for topical application. Each mL (when reconstituted as directed) contains 5 mg of dapiprazole hydrochloride as the active ingredient.
The reconstituted solution has a pH of approximately 6.6 and an osmolarity of approximately 415 mOsm.
The inactive ingredients include: Mannitol (2%), Sodium Chloride, Hydroxypropyl Methylcellulose (0.4%), Edetate Sodium (0.01%), Sodium Phosphate Dibasic, Sodium Phosphate Monobasic, Water for Injection, and Benzalkonium Chloride (0.01%) as a preservative.
RĒV-EYES Eyedrops, 0.5% is supplied in a kit consisting of one vial of dapiprazole hydrochloride (25 mg), one vial of diluent (5 mL) and one dropper for dispensing.

Clinical Pharmacology: Dapiprazole acts through blocking the alpha-adrenergic receptors in smooth muscle. Dapiprazole produces miosis through an effect on the dilator muscle of the iris.
Dapiprazole does not have any significant activity on ciliary muscle contraction and therefore does not induce a significant change in the anterior chamber depth or the thickness of the lens.
Dapiprazole has demonstrated safe and rapid reversal of mydriasis produced by phenylephrine and to a lesser degree tropicamide. In patients with decreased accommodative amplitude due to treatment with tropicamide the miotic effect of dapiprazole may partially increase the accommodative amplitude.
Eye color affects the rate of pupillary constriction. In individuals with brown irides, the rate of pupillary constriction may be slightly slower than in individuals with blue or green irides. Eye color does not appear to affect the final pupil size.
Dapiprazole does not significantly alter intraocular pressure in normotensive or in eyes with elevated intraocular pressure.

Indications and Usage: Dapiprazole is indicated in the treatment of iatrogenically induced mydriasis produced by adrenergic (phenylephrine) or parasympatholytic (tropicamide) agents. Dapiprazole is not indicated for the reduction of intraocular pressure or in the treatment of open angle glaucoma.

Contraindications: Miotics are contraindicated where constriction is undesirable; such as acute iritis, and in those subjects showing hypersensitivity to any component of this preparation.

Warning: For Topical Ophthalmic Use Only. NOT FOR INJECTION. Do not touch the dropper up to lids or any surface, as this may contaminate the solution. Dapiprazole should not be used in the same patient more frequently than once a week.

Precautions:

Information to Patients: Miosis may cause difficulty in dark adaptation and may reduce the field of vision. Patients should exercise caution when involved in night driving or other activities in poor illumination.

Carcinogenesis, Mutagenesis, Impairment of Fertility: Dapiprazole has been shown to significantly increase the incidence of liver tumors in rats after continuous dietary administration for 104 weeks. This effect was found only in male rats treated with the highest dose administered in the study, i.e., 300 mg/kg/day, (80,000 times the human dose) and was not observed in male and female rats at doses of 30 and 100 mg/kg/day and female rats at doses of 300 mg/kg/day.
Negative results have been reported on the mutagenicity and impairment of fertility studies with dapiprazole.

Pregnancy: *Pregnancy Category B:* Reproduction studies have been performed in rats and rabbits at doses up to 128,000 (rat) and 27,000 (rabbit) times the human ophthalmic dose and revealed no evidence of impaired fertility or harm to the fetus due to dapiprazole. There are, however, no adequate and well-controlled studies in pregnant women. Because animal reproduction studies are not always predictive of human response, this drug should be used during pregnancy only if clearly needed.

Nursing Mothers: It is not known whether this drug is excreted in human milk. Because many drugs are excreted in human milk, caution should be exercised when dapiprazole is administered to a nursing woman.

Pediatric Use: Safety and effectiveness in children has not been established.

Adverse Reactions: In controlled studies the most frequent reaction to dapiprazole was conjunctival injection lasting 20 minutes in over 80% of patients. Burning on instillation of dapiprazole was reported in approximately half of all patients. Reactions occurring in 10% to 40% of patients included ptosis, lid erythema, lid edema, chemosis, itching, punctate keratitis, corneal edema, browache, photophobia and headaches. Other reactions reported less frequently included dryness of eyes, tearing and blurring of vision.

Dosage and Administration: Two drops followed 5 minutes later by an additional two drops applied topically to the conjunctiva of each eye should be administered after the ophthalmic examination to reverse the diagnostic mydriasis. Dapiprazole should not be used in the same patient more frequently than once per week.

Directions for Preparing Eyedrops:

1. Use aseptic technique.
2. Tear off aluminum seals, remove and discard rubber plugs from both drug and diluent vials.
3. Pour diluent into drug vial.
4. Remove dropper assembly from its sterile wrapping and attach to the drug vial.
5. Shake container for several minutes to ensure mixing.

Storage and Stability of Eyedrops: Once the eyedrops have been reconstituted they may be stored at room temperature 15°–30°C (59°–86°F) for 21 days. Discard any solution that is not clear and colorless.

How Supplied: RĒV-EYES *dapiprazole hydrochloride* Eyedrops, 0.5%
NDC 57706-761-62
Each package contains RĒV-EYES (25 mg), diluent (5 mL) and dropper for dispensing.
Patented U.S. Patent No. 4,252,721
Caution: Federal (USA) law prohibits dispensing without prescription.

Manufactured by
Abbott Laboratories
North Chicago, IL 60064
For
Angelini Pharmaceuticals Inc.
River Edge, NJ 07661
Marketed by
Storz Ophthalmics, Inc./Lederle Laboratories Division
American Cyanamid Company
Pearl River, NY 10965

Rev. 1/91
01-2508-R1

Information on Storz products listed on these pages is the full Prescribing Information from product literature or package inserts effective in June 1991. Information concerning all Storz products may be obtained from the Professional Services Department, Lederle Laboratories, Pearl River, New York 10965.

Walker Pharmacal Company
4200 LACLEDE AVENUE
ST. LOUIS, MO 63108

SUCCUS CINERARIA MARITIMA ℞
[*suk 'us si-ne 'ra "ria mar "i-te 'ma*]
(Senecio Cineraria Compound Solution)
SCM—WALKER™
Sterile—Ophthalmic

Description: Succus Cineraria Maritima is an aqueous and glycerin solution of the total extractives of the fresh Senecio Cineraria USPH 8th (Senecio Compositae) with extract of Hamamelis V. (Witch Hazel) and boric acid USP. The Alkaloids included in the total extract include Senecine and Senecionine. Total nonvolatiles are approximately 20%. The pH is adjusted to 4.1 pH; osmotic pressure is 5.5 osmols.

Actions and Uses: Succus Cineraria Maritima applied locally to the eyes acts as a safe lymphagogue, increasing circulation in the intraocular tissues, also stimulating collateral circulation and normal metabolism, functions so necessary from the standpoint of the physiology of the eye. Clinical observation indicates the definite value of local applications of Succus Cineraria Maritima in checking, or even aborting existing opacities. The benefits attained are obviously more satisfactory when treatment is instituted in the early stage of cataract. In cases of well advanced opacity, and where pathological changes caused by the deterioration of the metabolic functions have occurred, as is characteristic in senility, less favorable results can be expected.
The use of Succus Cineraria Maritima, however, is justified in certain cases well past the incipient stage, particularly when an operation is not contemplated or is contraindicated. It gives comfort to the patient to know that something potentially beneficial is being done. Clinical studies of advanced stages of cataract treated with Succus Cineraria Maritima indicated that in 22.5% of these cases beneficial results were obtained. In many of the cases which did not show improvement the process of the opacity was retarded or checked. In certain

Continued on next page

Walker—Cont.

cases Succus Cineraria Maritima only gives temporary relief or serves to postpone the surgical removal.
Indications: Succus Cineraria Maritima is indicated in the treatment of various cases of optic opacity caused by cataract.
Contraindications: A history of a previous hypersensitivity reaction to any of the Senecio Alkaloids or to Hamamelis V. is a contraindication.
Warning: The possibility of sensitivity reactions should be considered in patients with a history of allergy. If excessive irritation occurs it may be advisable to dilute the dosage, or discontinue treatment. (pH of 4.1 may cause minor irritation.) For topical ophthalmic use only. If excessive irritation should develop, patient should consult the prescribing physician.
Caution: Federal Law prohibits dispensing without prescription.
Caution: Not intended for use in glaucoma.
Dosage and Administration: Succus Cineraria Maritima should be instilled in the affected eye, two drops morning and evening, or as directed by physician. Do not touch dropper tip to any surface, since this may contaminate the solution.
Supplied: In sterile ¼ oz. dropper vial (7cc). NDC 619-4021-38.

Wyeth-Ayerst Laboratories

Division of American Home Products Corporation
P.O. BOX 8299
PHILADELPHIA, PA 19101

As a result of a merger of Wyeth Laboratories and Ayerst Laboratories, all prescription products of both companies and all nonprescription products formerly of Wyeth are products of Wyeth-Ayerst Laboratories. All nonprescription products formerly of Ayerst Laboratories are products of Whitehall Laboratories.

COLLYRIUM for FRESH EYES — OTC

[*ko-lir 'e-um*]
EYE WASH
A neutral borate solution

Description: Soothing Collyrium Eye Wash for Fresh Eyes is specially formulated to soothe, refresh, and cleanse irritated eyes. Collyrium Eye Wash is a neutral borate solution that contains boric acid, sodium borate, thimerosal (not more than 0.002% as a preservative) and water.
Indications: Patients are advised of the following. Use Collyrium Eye Wash to cleanse the eye, loosen foreign material, air pollutants or chlorinated water.
Recommended Uses:
Home—For emergency flushing of foreign bodies or whenever a soothing eye rinse is necessary.
Hospitals, dispensaries and clinics—For emergency flushing of chemicals or foreign bodies from the eye.
Directions: Patients are advised of the following. Puncture bottle by twisting clear cap down onto bottle; then remove clear cap from bottle and discard. Remove the eyecup from plastic bag. Rinse blue eyecup with clear water immediately before and after each use. Avoid contamination of rim and interior surfaces of cup. Fill blue eyecup one-half full with Collyrium Eye Wash. Apply cup tightly to the affected eye to prevent escape of the liquid and tilt head backward. Open eyelid wide and rotate eyeball to thoroughly wash eye.
Warnings: Patients are advised of the following. Do not use if solution changes color or becomes cloudy, or with a wetting solution for contact lenses or other eye care products containing polyvinyl alcohol. This product contains thimerosal (not more than 0.002% as a preservative). Do not use this product if you are sensitive to mercury.
To avoid contamination do not touch tip of container to any surface. Replace cap after using. If you experience eye pain, changes in vision, continued redness, irritation of the eye, or if the condition worsens or persists, consult a doctor. Obtain immediate medical treatment for all open wounds in or near the eyes.
The Collyrium for Fresh Eyes bottle is sealed for your protection. Prior to first use, remove cap and squeeze bottle. If bottle leaks, do not use.
Keep this and all medication out of the reach of children. Keep bottle tightly closed at Room Temperature, Approx. 77° F (25° C).
How Supplied: Bottles of 4 FL. OZ. (118 mL) with eyecup.

Shown in Product Identification Section, page 105

COLLYRIUM FRESH™ — OTC

[*ko-lir 'e-um*]
Sterile Eye Drops
Lubricant • Redness Reliever

Description: Collyrium Fresh is a specially formulated sterile eye drop which can be used up to 4 times daily, to relieve redness and discomfort due to minor eye irritations caused by dust, smoke, smog, swimming, or sun glare. The active ingredients are tetrahydrozoline HCl (0.05%) and glycerin (1.0%). Other ingredients include benzalkonium chloride (0.01%) and edetate disodium (0.1%) as preservatives, boric acid, hydrochloric acid and sodium borate.
Indications: Patients are advised of the following. For the temporary relief of redness due to minor eye irritations or discomfort due to burning or exposure to wind or sun.
Directions: Patients are advised of the following. Tilt head back and squeeze 1 to 2 drops into each eye up to 4 times daily, or as directed by a physician.
Warnings: Patients are advised of the following. Do not use if solution changes color or becomes cloudy. Remove contact lenses before using. If you have glaucoma, do not use this product except under the advice and supervision of a physician. Overuse of this product may produce increased redness of the eye. To avoid contamination, do not touch tip of container to any surface. Replace cap after using. If you experience eye pain, changes in vision, continued redness or irritation of the eye, or if the condition worsens or persists for more than 72 hours, discontinue use and consult a physician.
Keep this and all medication out of the reach of children. The product's carton should be retained for complete product information.
Keep bottle tightly closed at Room Temperature, Approx. 77° F (25° C).
How Supplied: Bottles of 0.5 FL. OZ. (15 mL) with built-in eye dropper.

Shown in Product Identification Section, page 105

FLUOR-I-STRIP® — ℞

[*floo-or 'a "strip*]
(Fluorescein Sodium Ophthalmic Strips)

Composition (per strip):

Fluorescein Sodium 9 mg	diagnostic dye
Chlorobutanol (chloral derivative) 0.5%	preservative
Polysorbate 80	surface active agent
Potassium Chloride / Boric Acid / Sodium Carbonate	buffering agents

Description: FLUOR-I-STRIP is a specially prepared sterile ophthalmic strip for diagnostic use.
Indications: For staining the anterior segment of the eye when:
a) delineating a corneal injury, herpetic lesion or foreign body,
b) determining the site of an intraocular injury,
c) fitting contact lenses,
d) making the fluorescein test to ascertain postoperative closure of the sclerocorneal (also referred to as corneoscleral) wound in delayed anterior chamber reformation,
e) making the lacrimal drainage test.

Directions for Use: To open envelope, grasp pull-tabs firmly and separate slowly. Separate the two strips by tearing off white tab end. Moisten end of strip with a drop of sterile water. Place moistened strip at the fornix in the lower cul-de-sac close to the punctum. For best results, patient should close lid tightly over strip until desired amount of staining is obtained. Another method is to retract upper lid and touch tip of strip to the bulbar conjunctiva on the temporal side until an adequate amount of stain is available for a clearly defined end point reading.
Warning: Never use fluorescein while the patient is wearing *soft contact lenses* because the lenses may become stained. Whenever fluorescein is used, flush the eyes with sterile, normal saline solution, and wait at least one hour before replacing the lenses.
Storage: Store at room temperature (approximately 25°C).
How Supplied: Boxes of 300 strips in individual envelopes (NDC 0046-1028-83).

Shown in Product Identification Section, page 105

FLUOR-I-STRIP® -A.T. — ℞

[*floo-or 'a "strip*]
(Fluorescein Sodium Ophthalmic Strips)
For Applanation Tonometry

Composition (Per Strip):

Fluorescein Sodium 1 mg	diagnostic dye
Chlorobutanol (chloral derivative) 0.5%	preservative
Polysorbate 80	surface active agent
Boric Acid / Potassium Chloride / Sodium Carbonate	buffering agents

Description: FLUOR-I-STRIP-A.T. consists of sterile ophthalmic strips, specially prepared for diagnostic use in applanation tonometry.
Indications: For staining the anterior segment of the eye when:
a) delineating a corneal injury, herpetic lesion or foreign body,
b) determining the site of an intraocular injury,
c) fitting contact lenses,
d) making the fluorescein test to ascertain postoperative closure of the sclerocorneal (also referred to as corneoscleral) wound in delayed anterior chamber reformation,
e) making the lacrimal drainage test.

Directions for Use: To open envelope, grasp pull-tabs firmly and separate slowly. Separate the two strips by tearing off white tab end. Anesthetize the eyes. Retract upper lid and touch tip of strip to the bulbar conjunctiva on the temporal side until an adequate amount of stain is available for a clearly defined end-point reading.
Warning: Never use fluorescein while the patient is wearing *soft contact lenses* because the lenses may become stained. Whenever fluorescein is used, flush the eyes with sterile, normal saline solution, and wait at least one hour before replacing the lenses.

Storage: Store at room temperature (approximately 25°C).
How Supplied: Boxes of 300 strips, 2 in each envelope (NDC 0046-1048-83).

Shown in Product Identification Section, page 105

OPHTHALGAN® ℞
[*of″thal′găn*]
(glycerin ophthalmic solution)*
STERILE

Caution: Federal law prohibits dispensing without prescription.

Description: Glycerin is 1,2,3-propanetriol:

$CH_2OH—CHOH—CH_2OH$

It is a clear, colorless, viscous liquid.
OPHTHALGAN is a sterile glycerin ophthalmic solution.

Clinical Pharmacology: OPHTHALGAN (glycerin ophthalmic solution) is used only for topical application to the cornea. By virtue of its osmotic action, it promptly reduces edema and causes clearing of corneal haze. The action of OPHTHALGAN is transient, and it is, therefore, used primarily for diagnostic purposes.

Indications and Usage: OPHTHALGAN is indicated to clear an edematous cornea in order to facilitate ophthalmoscopic and gonioscopic examination especially in acute glaucoma, bullous keratitis, Fuchs's endothelial dystrophy, and so forth. In gonioscopy of an edematous cornea, additional OPHTHALGAN may be used as the lubricant. A local anesthetic should be instilled shortly before use of OPHTHALGAN.

Contraindications: Hypersensitivity to the active or inactive ingredients.

Precautions: Because OPHTHALGAN (glycerin ophthalmic solution) is an irritant and may cause pain, a local anesthetic should be instilled shortly before its use.
Carcinogenesis, Mutagenesis, Impairment of Fertility: No long-term studies in animals or humans have been conducted.
Pregnancy Category C: Animal reproduction studies have not been conducted with OPHTHALGAN. It is also not known whether OPHTHALGAN can cause fetal harm when administered to a pregnant woman or can affect reproduction capacity. OPHTHALGAN should be given to a pregnant woman only if clearly needed.
Nursing Mothers: It is not known whether this drug is excreted in human milk. Because many drugs are excreted in human milk, caution should be exercised when OPHTHALGAN is administered to a nursing woman.
Pediatric Use: Safety and effectiveness in children have not been established.

Adverse Reactions: Some pain and/or irritation may occur upon instillation.

Dosage and Administration: One or two drops prior to examination. In gonioscopy of an edematous cornea, additional OPHTHALGAN (glycerin ophthalmic solution) may be used as the lubricant.
DISCARD THIS PRODUCT SIX MONTHS AFTER DROPPER IS FIRST PLACED IN THE DRUG SOLUTION.

How Supplied: OPHTHALGAN is available in dropper-screw cap bottles of 7.5 mL (NDC 0046-1013-07).
Note: Keep bottle tightly closed.

Shown in Product Identification Section, page 105

---

*OPHTHALGAN contains not more than 1.0% water. Chlorobutanol (chloral derivative) 0.55% is incorporated as preservative. The pH of this solution may differ from that specified in the U.S.P.

PHOSPHOLINE IODIDE® ℞
[*fos″fo′lĭn i″o-dīd*]
(echothiophate iodide for ophthalmic solution)

Caution: Federal law prohibits dispensing without prescription.

Description: Chemical name: (2-mercaptoethyl) trimethylammonium iodide O,O-diethyl phosphorothioate.
PHOSPHOLINE IODIDE occurs as a white, crystalline, water-soluble, hygroscopic solid having a slight mercaptan-like odor. When freeze-dried in the presence of potassium acetate, the mixture appears as a white amorphous deposit on the walls of the bottle.
Each package contains materials for dispensing 5 mL of eyedrops: (1) bottle containing sterile PHOSPHOLINE IODIDE in one of four potencies [1.5 mg (0.03%), 3 mg (0.06%), 6.25 mg (0.125%), or 12.5 mg (0.25%)] as indicated on the label, with 40 mg potassium acetate in each case. Sodium hydroxide or acetic acid may have been incorporated to adjust pH during manufacturing; (2) a 5 mL bottle of sterile diluent containing chlorobutanol (chloral derivative), 0.55%; mannitol, 1.2%; boric acid, 0.06%; and exsiccated sodium phosphate, 0.026%; (3) sterilized dropper.

Clinical Pharmacology: PHOSPHOLINE IODIDE is a long-acting cholinesterase inhibitor for topical use which enhances the effect of endogenously liberated acetylcholine in iris, ciliary muscle, and other parasympathetically innervated structures of the eye. It thereby causes miosis, increase in facility of outflow of aqueous humor, fall in intraocular pressure, and potentiation of accommodation.
PHOSPHOLINE IODIDE (echothiophate iodide) will depress both plasma and erythrocyte cholinesterase levels in most patients after a few weeks of eyedrop therapy.

Indications and Usage: GLAUCOMA—Chronic open-angle glaucoma. Subacute or chronic angle-closure glaucoma after iridectomy or where surgery is refused or contraindicated. Certain non-uveitic secondary types of glaucoma, especially glaucoma following cataract surgery.
ACCOMMODATIVE ESOTROPIA—Concomitant esotropias with a significant accommodative component.

Contraindications:
1. Active uveal inflammation.
2. Most cases of angle-closure glaucoma, due to the possibility of increasing angle block.
3. Hypersensitivity to the active or inactive ingredients.

Warnings:
1. Succinylcholine should be administered only with great caution, if at all, prior to or during general anesthesia to patients receiving anticholinesterase medication because of possible respiratory or cardiovascular collapse.
2. Caution should be observed in treating glaucoma with PHOSPHOLINE IODIDE (echothiophate iodide) in patients who are at the same time undergoing treatment with systemic anticholinesterase medications for myasthenia gravis, because of possible adverse additive effects.

(See Precautions—Drug interactions for further information.)

Precautions:
General
1. Gonioscopy is recommended prior to initiation of therapy. Routine examination to detect lens opacity should accompany clinical use of PHOSPHOLINE IODIDE.
2. Where there is a quiescent uveitis or a history of this condition, anticholinesterase therapy should be avoided or used cautiously because of the intense and persistent miosis and ciliary muscle contraction that may occur.
3. While systemic effects are infrequent, proper use of the drug requires digital compression of the nasolacrimal ducts for a minute or two following instillation to minimize drainage into the nasal chamber with its extensive absorption area. To prevent possible skin absorption, hands should be washed following instillation.
4. Temporary discontinuance of medication is necessary if cardiac irregularities occur.
5. Anticholinesterase drugs should be used with extreme caution, if at all, in patients with marked vagotonia, bronchial asthma, spastic gastrointestinal disturbances, peptic ulcer, pronounced bradycardia and hypotension, recent myocardial infarction, epilepsy, parkinsonism, and other disorders that may respond adversely to vagotonic effects.
6. Anticholinesterase drugs should be employed prior to ophthalmic surgery only as a considered risk because of the possible occurrence of hyphema.
7. PHOSPHOLINE IODIDE (echothiophate iodide) should be used with great caution, if at all, where there is a prior history of retinal detachment.
8. Temporary discontinuance of medication is necessary if salivation, urinary incontinence, diarrhea, profuse sweating, muscle weakness, or respiratory difficulties occur.
9. Patients receiving PHOSPHOLINE IODIDE who are exposed to carbamate- or organophosphate-type insecticides and pesticides (professional gardeners, farmers, workers in plants manufacturing or formulating such products, etc.) should be warned of the additive systemic effects possible from absorption of the pesticide through the respiratory tract or skin. During periods of exposure to such pesticides, the wearing of respiratory masks, and frequent washing and clothing changes may be advisable.

Drug Interactions: PHOSPHOLINE IODIDE potentiates other cholinesterase inhibitors such as succinylcholine or organophosphate and carbamate insecticides. Patients undergoing systemic anticholinesterase treatment should be warned of the possible additive effects of PHOSPHOLINE IODIDE.

Carcinogenesis, Mutagenesis, Impairment of Fertility: No data is available regarding carcinogenesis, mutagenesis, and impairment of fertility.

Pregnancy:
Teratogenic Effects:
Pregnancy Category C: Animal reproduction studies have not been conducted with PHOSPHOLINE IODIDE. It is also not known whether PHOSPHOLINE IODIDE can cause fetal harm when administered to a pregnant woman or can affect reproduction capacity. PHOSPHOLINE IODIDE (echothiophate iodide) should be given to a pregnant woman only if clearly needed.

Nursing Mothers:
Because of the potential for serious adverse reactions in nursing infants from PHOSPHOLINE IODIDE, a decision should be made whether to discontinue nursing or to discontinue the drug, taking into account the importance of the drug to the mother.

Adverse Reactions:
1. Although the relationship, if any, of retinal detachment to the administration of PHOSPHOLINE IODIDE has not been established, retinal detachment has been reported in a few cases during the use of PHOSPHOLINE IODIDE in adult patients without a previous history of this disorder.
2. Stinging, burning, lacrimation, lid muscle twitching, conjunctival and ciliary redness, browache, induced myopia with visual blurring may occur.

Continued on next page

Wyeth-Ayerst—Cont.

3. Activation of latent iritis or uveitis may occur.
4. Iris cysts may form, and if treatment is continued, may enlarge and obscure vision. This occurrence is more frequent in children. The cysts usually shrink upon discontinuance of the medication, reduction in strength of the drops or frequency of instillation. Rarely, they may rupture or break free into the aqueous. Regular examinations are advisable when the drug is being prescribed for the treatment of accommodative esotropia.
5. Prolonged use may cause conjunctival thickening, obstruction of nasolacrimal canals.
6. Lens opacities occurring in patients under treatment for glaucoma with PHOSPHOLINE IODIDE have been reported and similar changes have been produced experimentally in normal monkeys. Routine examinations should accompany clinical use of the drug.
7. Paradoxical increase in intraocular pressure may follow anticholinesterase instillation. This may be alleviated by prescribing a sympathomimetic mydriatic such as phenylephrine.
8. Cardiac irregularities.

Dosage and Administration:

Directions for Preparing Eyedrops

1. Use aseptic technique.
2. Tear off aluminum seals, and remove and discard rubber plugs from both drug and diluent containers.
3. Pour diluent into drug container.
4. Remove dropper assembly from its sterile wrapping. Holding dropper assembly by the screw cap and, WITHOUT COMPRESSING RUBBER BULB, insert into drug container and screw down tightly.
5. Shake for several seconds to ensure mixing.
6. Do not cover or obliterate instructions to patient regarding storage of eyedrops.

GLAUCOMA—

Selection of Therapy: The *medication prescribed* should be that which will control the intraocular pressure around-the-clock with the least risk of side effects or adverse reactions. "Tonometric glaucoma" (ocular hypertension without other evidence of the disease) is frequently not treated with any medication, and PHOSPHOLINE IODIDE (echothiophate iodide) is certainly not recommended for this condition. In early chronic simple glaucoma with field loss or disc changes, pilocarpine is generally used for initial therapy and can be recommended so long as control is thereby maintained over the 24 hours of the day.

When this is not the case, PHOSPHOLINE IODIDE 0.03% may be effective and probably has no greater potential for side effects. If this dosage is inadequate, epinephrine and a carbonic anhydrase inhibitor may be added to the regimen. When still more effective medication is required, the higher strengths of PHOSPHOLINE IODIDE may be prescribed with the recognition that the control of the intraocular pressure should have priority regardless of potential side effects. In secondary glaucoma following cataract surgery, the higher strengths of the drug are frequently needed and are ordinarily very well tolerated. The *dosage regimen* prescribed should call for the lowest concentration that will control the intraocular pressure around-the-clock. Where tonometry around-the-clock is not feasible, it is suggested that appointments for tension-taking be made at different times of the day so that inadequate control may be more readily detected. Two doses a day are preferred to one in order to maintain as smooth a diurnal tension curve as possible, although a single dose per day or every other day has been used with satisfactory results. Because of the long duration of action of the drug, it is never necessary or desirable to exceed a schedule of twice a day. The daily dose or one of the two daily doses should always be instilled just before retiring to avoid inconvenience due to the miosis.

Early Chronic Simple Glaucoma:
PHOSPHOLINE IODIDE (echothiophate iodide) 0.03% instilled twice a day, just before retiring and in the morning, may be prescribed advantageously for cases of early chronic simple glaucoma that are not controlled around-the-clock with other less potent agents. Because of prolonged action, control during the night and early morning hours may then sometimes be obtained. A change in therapy is indicated if, at any time, the tension fails to remain at an acceptable level on this regimen.

Advanced Chronic Simple Glaucoma and Glaucoma Secondary to Cataract Surgery: These cases may respond satisfactorily to PHOSPHOLINE IODIDE 0.03% twice a day as above. When the patient is being transferred to PHOSPHOLINE IODIDE (echothiophate iodide) because of unsatisfactory control with pilocarpine, carbachol, epinephrine, etc., one of the higher strengths, 0.06%, 0.125%, or 0.25% will usually be needed. In this case, a brief trial with the 0.03% eyedrops will be advantageous in that the higher strengths will then be more easily tolerated.

Concomitant Therapy: PHOSPHOLINE IODIDE may be used concomitantly with epinephrine, a carbonic anhydrase inhibitor, or both.

Technique: Good technique in the administration of PHOSPHOLINE IODIDE requires that finger pressure at the inner canthus should be exerted for a minute or two following instillation of the eyedrops, to minimize drainage into the nose and throat. Excess solution around the eye should be removed with tissue and any medication on the hands should be rinsed off.

ACCOMMODATIVE ESOTROPIA (PEDIATRIC USE)

In Diagnosis: One drop of 0.125% may be instilled once a day in both eyes on retiring, for a period of two or three weeks. If the esotropia is accommodative, a favorable response will usually be noted which may begin within a few hours.

In Treatment: PHOSPHOLINE IODIDE (echothiophate iodide) is prescribed at the lowest concentration and frequency which gives satisfactory results. After the initial period of treatment for diagnostic purposes, the schedule may be reduced to 0.125% every other day or 0.06% every day. These dosages can often be gradually lowered as treatment progresses. The 0.03% strength has proven to be effective in some cases. The maximum usually recommended dosage is 0.125% once a day, although more intensive therapy has been used for short periods.

Technique: (See Dosage and Administration—Glaucoma.)

Duration of Treatment:
In diagnosis, only a short period is required and little time will be lost in instituting other procedures if the esotropia proves to be unresponsive. In therapy, there is no definite limit so long as the drug is well tolerated. However, if the eyedrops, with or without eyeglasses, are gradually withdrawn after about a year or two and deviation recurs, surgery should be considered. As with other miotics, tolerance may occasionally develop after prolonged use. In such cases, a rest period will restore the original activity of the drug.

How Supplied: Each package contains sterile PHOSPHOLINE IODIDE (echothiophate iodide), sterile diluent, and dropper for dispensing 5 mL eyedrops of the strength indicated on the label. Four potencies are available:

NDC 0046-1062-05...............1.5 mg package for 0.03%
White amorphous deposit on bottle walls. Aluminum crimp seal is blue.
NDC 0046-1064-05.....3 mg package for 0.06%
White amorphous deposit on bottle walls. Aluminum crimp seal is red.
NDC 0046-1065-05............6.25 mg package for 0.125%
White amorphous deposit on bottle walls. Aluminum crimp seal is green.
NDC 0046-1066-05............12.5 mg package for 0.25%
White amorphous deposit on bottle walls. Aluminum crimp seal is yellow.

Handling and Storage:
Store at room temperature (approximately 25°C).

After reconstitution, keep eyedrops in refrigerator to obtain maximum useful life of 6 months. Room temperature is acceptable if drops will be used within a month.

Shown in Product Identification Section, page 105

SECTION 9

Lenses and Lens Care

In an attempt to make this publication more useful we have organized the Lens Section in four parts:

Part 1—Contact Lenses (Hard and Soft)

Part 2—Intraocular Lenses

Part 3—Lens Care Products

Part 4—Spectacle Lenses and Products

Part 1 - Contact Lenses (Hard and Soft)

Bausch & Lomb Inc.
Contact Lens Division
1400 NORTH GOODMAN STREET
ROCHESTER, NY 14692

POLYMACON HYDROPHILIC CONTACT LENSES

For all Bausch & Lomb polymacon hydrophilic contact lenses, which include the following types:

MEDALIST™ (polymacon) Visibility Tinted Contact Lenses, SOFLENS® (polymacon) Daily Wear, OPTIMA 38™ Daily Wear, SOFSPIN® Daily Wear, P.A. 1™ Bifocal Daily Wear, BI-TECH™ Bifocal Daily Wear, 03/04® Extended Wear, OPTIMA® FW* Extended Wear Contact Lenses (Clear and Tinted); and SOFLENS® Therapeutic Daily Wear and Extended Wear Contact Lenses. NaturalTint® (polymacon) Daily Wear, P.A. 1™ Bifocal Daily Wear, 03/04® Extended Wear and OPTIMA® FW Extended Wear Contact LENSES.

IMPORTANT: This package insert is effective as of November, 1990 and supersedes all prior inserts for the products described below. Please read carefully and keep this information for future use.

CAUTION: Federal Law Prohibits Dispensing Without Prescription.

Vision Correction Use: For all Bausch & Lomb polymacon hydrophilic contact lenses, which include the following types: SOFLENS® (polymacon) Daily Wear, OPTIMA 38™ Daily Wear, SOFSPIN® Daily Wear, P.A. 1™ Bifocal Daily Wear, BI-TECH™ Bifocal Daily Wear, 03/04® Extended Wear, OPTIMA® FW* Extended Wear Contact Lenses (Clear and Tinted); and SOFLENS® Therapeutic Daily Wear and Extended Wear Contact Lenses. NaturalTint® (polymacon) Daily Wear, P.A. 1™ Bifocal Daily Wear, 03/04® Extended Wear OPTIMA® FW Extended Wear Contact Lenses and MEDALIST™ (polymacon) Visibility Tinted Contact Lenses.

*Formerly named OPTIMA® EW. All literature referring to OPTIMA® FW is applicable to OPTIMA® EW.

Description: All Bausch & Lomb SOFLENS® (clear and tinted), NaturalTint® and MEDALIST ™ Visibility Tinted Contact Lenses are available as spherical lenses. These lenses are hemispherical flexible shells of the following dimensions:

- Chord diameter: 12.0mm to 18.0mm
- Center thickness: 0.02mm to 1.0mm
- Posterior Apical Radius: 5.00mm to 12.0mm
- Powers: See "Indications" for each lens.

The lens material, polymacon, is a hydrophilic polymer of poly (2-hydroxyethylmethacrylate) 61.4%, and 38.6% water.

The physical properties of the lens are:

Refractive Index: 1.43

Surface Character: Hydrophilic

Water Content: 38.6%

Oxygen Permeability (DK): Method for determination is the polarographic method. The numbers are expressed in units X • 10^{-11}. (cm^3O_2 • cm/sec • cm^2 • mmHg) at 34°C

SOFLENS® Contact Lens
—8.4

SOFLENS® Tinted Contact Lens
—8.5
(includes BI-TECH, PA1, SOFSPIN, 03/04, OPTIMA 38 & OPTIMA FW)

MEDALIST™ Visibility Tinted Contact Lens
—8.5

NaturalTint® Contact Lens
—Blue —9.6
—Aqua—9.2
—Green—9.0
—Brown—9.3

Light Transmittance: C.I.E. Y value:

SOFLENS® Contact Lenses—approximately 98%

SOFLENS® Tinted Contact Lens—approximately 96% (includes BI-TECH, P.A.1., Sofspin, 03/04, OPTIMA 38 & OPTIMA FW)

MEDALIST™ Visibility Tinted Contact Lens—approximately 86% to 98%*

* CIE light transmittance will differ by average thickness across the optical zone for lenses tinted with Reactive Blue 246. For example, for lenses tinted with Reactive Blue 246, a lens with a center thickness of 0.6mm has a visible light transmittance of 86%, while a lens with a center thickness of 0.026mm has a visible light transmittance of 98%. A typical lens tinted with Reactive Blue No. 4 yields a light transmittance of approximately 96%.

NaturalTint® Contact Lenses
Blue—approximately 82%
Aqua—approximately 84%
Green—approximately 76%
Brown—approximately 62%

SOFLENS® Tinted Contact Lenses (includes BI-TECH™, P.A.1™, SOFSPIN®, 03®/04®, OPTIMA® 38 & OPTIMA® FW) and MEDALIST™ Visibility Tinted Contact Lenses are tinted blue using Reactive Blue No. 4 or 1,4-bis[4-(2-methacryloxyethyl) phenylamino] anthraquinone (Reactive Blue 246) to make the lens more visible for handling purposes. The apparent color of the SOFLENS® Tinted Contact Lens or MEDALIST™ Visibility Tinted Contact Lens may decrease slightly following repeated disinfection. This will not affect the safety or performance of the lens.

Continued on next page

Bausch & Lomb—Cont.

NaturalTint® Contact Lenses are tinted with any of, or with combinations of, the following lens colors: blue, green, aqua, brown and yellow. These lenses are tinted with synthetic dyes
(blue—7,16-Dichloro-6,15-dihydro-5, 9, 14, 18-anthrazietetrone,
green—16,17-Dimethoxydinaphtho (1,2,3-cd: 3′,2′,1′-lm) perylene-5,10-dione,
brown—16,23-Dihydrodinaphtho (2,3-a:2′,3′-i[, napth]2′,3′:6,7) indolo(2,3-c) carbazole-5,10, 15,17,22,24-hexone or
yellow—N,N′-(9, 10-Dihydro-9, 10-dioxo-1,5-anthracenediyl) bisbenzamide) that impart colors to the lens which combine with eye color to produce a natural appearance. See WARNINGS for Cosmetically Tinted Contact Lenses.
Therapeutic: When placed on the human cornea for therapeutic use, a SOFLENS® (polymacon) Contact Lens acts as a bandage to protect the cornea. When the patient needs improved visual acuity while the eye is healing, the lens with power acts as a refracting medium to focus light rays on the retina.

Indications:

Daily Wear: SOFLENS® Contact Lenses (Clear and Tinted), including OPTIMA® 38 and SOFSPIN®, are indicated for vision correction use in myopic and hyperopic patients with non-diseased eyes and in aphakic patients, who exhibit astigmatism of 2.00 diopters or less and can obtain satisfactory visual acuity, in a power range of −20.00 to +20.00 diopters.

SOFLENS® P.A. 1 Bifocal Contact Lenses (Clear and Tinted) are indicated for hyperopic and myopic, phakic, presbyopic patients with non-diseased eyes, who exhibit astigmatism of 2.00 diopters or less and can obtain satisfactory visual acuity. The bifocal lens is indicated for patients requiring up to 2.00 diopters of refractive add. The design of the bifocal lens is a progressive add which continuously increases up to 2.50 diopters at 3 mm from the optical center of the lens, depending upon the lens power. As a patient's add requirement increases, the probability of the patient achieving good visual acuity decreases. The lens provides a nominal functional add of 1.50 diopters in a power range of −6.00 to +6.00 diopters.

NaturalTint® Contact Lenses are indicated for emmetropic daily wear and daily wear correction of myopia and hyperopia in aphakic and phakic patients with non-diseased eyes, who exhibit astigmatism of 1.50 diopters or less and can obtain satisfactory visual acuity, in a power range of −9.00 to +15.00 diopters. These may also be used for color enhancement of the eye and for ocular masking.

SOFLENS® TINTED BI-TECH® Contact Lens is indicated for hyperopic, myopic and emmetropic phakic presbyopic patients with non-diseased eyes, who may exhibit astigmatism of 1.50 diopters or less and can obtain satisfactory visual acuity. The bifocal lens is indicated for patients requiring up to + 3.50 diopters of refractive add in a power range of +6.00 to −6.00 diopters. The design of the TINTED BI-TECH Contact Lens, is an alternating vision lens. There are two discrete optical zones. The upper zone is before the the pupil in primary (straight-ahead) gaze. The bifocal add is before the pupil in the downgaze. These zones have coaxial optical centers, thus eliminating image "jump" and double images as the gaze transmits from one zone to the other. The lens is ballasted and truncated to achieve proper orientation for distance viewing and translation into the add zone for near vision.

Extended Wear: SOFLENS® 03/04 Extended Wear Contact Lenses (Clear and Tinted), NaturalTint 03/04 Extended Wear Contact Lenses, SOFLENS® OPTIMA® FW Extended Wear Contact Lenses (Clear and Tinted) and MEDALIST™ Visibility Tinted Contact Lenses are indicated for extended wear from 1 to 7 days between removals for cleaning and disinfection, as recommended by the eye care practitioner. (However, see the "WARNINGS" reference to the relationship between the lens wearing schedule and corneal complications.) The lenses are indicated for the correction of visual acuity of myopic and hyperopic, phakic patients with non-diseased eyes who exhibit astigmatism of 2.00 diopters or less and can obtain satisfactory visual acuity, in a power range of +4.00 to −9.00 diopters.

Therapeutic: SOFLENS® (polymacon) Contact Lens is indicated in the treatment and management of the following categories of disorders of the corneal epithelium:

- bullous keratopathy
- recurrent indolent ulcers
- erosions secondary to trichiasis and epithelial defects including:
  —postoperative keratoplasties
  —recurrent erosions
  —abrasions
  —chemical and thermal burns.

The SOFLENS® (polymacon) Contact Lens for therapeutic use is available in a power range of −20.00 to +20.00 diopters.

NOTE: SOFLENS® (polymacon) Contact Lens for therapeutic use is not to be fitted solely for vision correction.

Contraindications: Bausch & Lomb SOFLENS, NaturalTint and MEDALIST Contact Lenses are contraindicated when any of the following conditions exist:

- Inflammation in the anterior chamber of the eye.
- Active disease, injury or abnormality affecting the cornea, conjunctiva, or eyelids.
- Microbial infection of the eye
- Insufficiency of lacrimal secretion
- Corneal hypoesthesia
- Use of a medication that is contraindicated, including eye medications.
- Patient history of reoccurring eye or eyelid infections including sties, or of adverse effects associated with contact lens wear, or of intolerance or abnormal ocular response to contact lens wear.
- History of patient non-compliance with contact lens care and disinfection regimens, wearing restrictions, wearing schedule, or follow-up visit schedule.
- Patient inability or unwillingness, because of age, infirmity, or other mental or physical conditions, or an adverse working or living environment, to understand or comply with any warnings, precautions, restrictions, or directions.

Warnings: Serious eye injury and loss of vision may result from problems associated with wearing contact lenses and using contact lens care products. Therefore, after a thorough eye examination, including appropriate medical background, patients must be fully apprised by the prescribing practitioner of all the risks associated with contact lens wear. To minimize these risks, the need for strict compliance with the care and disinfection regimen including cleaning of the lens case, wearing restrictions, wearing schedules, and follow-up visit schedule must be emphasized to the patient. (See the considerations listed under Contraindications and Precautions.) Since eye injury can develop rapidly, it is most important that patients be instructed in the possible signs or symptoms of problems and the need to remove the lenses and be examined by the prescribing eye care practitioner or a corneal specialist immediately if they experience any symptoms such as those listed below under Adverse Effects. (Practitioners examining patients presenting such symptoms should see below Important Treatment Information for Adverse Effects.)

Daily Wear: Daily wear lenses are not indicated for overnight wear and should not be worn while sleeping. Clinical studies have shown that the risk of serious adverse reactions is significantly increased when these lenses are worn overnight.

Extended Wear: The risk of ulcerative keratitis has been shown to be greater among users of extended wear lenses than among users of daily wear lenses. The risk among extended wear lens users increases with the number of consecutive days that lenses are worn between removals, beginning with the first overnight use. Some researchers believe that these complications are caused by one or more of the following: a weakening of the cornea's resistance to infections, particularly during a closed-eye condition, as a result of hypoxia; an eye environment which is somewhat more conducive to the growth of bacteria and other microorganisms, particularly when a regular periodic lens removal and disinfection schedule has not been adhered to by the patient; improper lens disinfection or cleaning by the patient; contamination of lens care products; poor personal hygiene by the patient; patient unsuitability to the particular lens or wearing schedule; accumulation of lens deposits; damage to the lens; improper fitting; length of wearing time; and the presence of ocular debris or environmental contaminants.

Additionally, smoking increases the risk of ulcerative keratitis for contact lens users.

While the great majority of patients successfully wear contact lenses, extended wear of lenses also is reported to be associated with a higher incidence and degree of epithelial microcysts and infiltrates, and endothelial polymegathism, which require consideration of discontinuation or restriction of extended wear. The epithelial conditions are reversible upon discontinuation of lens wear.

The reversibility of endothelial effects of contact lens wear has not yet been established. As a result, practitioner's views of extended wearing times vary from not prescribing extended wear at all to prescribing flexible wearing times from occasional overnight wear to prescribing extended wearing periods from 1 to 7 days with specified intervals of no lens wear for certain patients, with follow-up visits and a proper care regimen. Some practitioners also recommend frequent replacement of lenses at intervals such as every one or two weeks. Other practitioners may prescribe disposable contact lens wear, where lenses are disposed of at each removal.

Cosmetically Tinted Contact Lenses: NaturalTint® Contact Lenses reduce the amount of light entering the eye and should not be used under reduced illumination conditions such as night driving.

Bifocal Contact Lenses: Bifocal contact lens patients frequently require a longer adaptation than patients wearing conventional soft contact lenses. Patients wearing the SOFLENS® TINTED BI-TECH, SOFLENS® P.A. 1 Bifocal or NaturalTint® P.A. 1 Bifocal Contact Lens during the adaptation period should use caution while driving a car or while performing other critical visual fuctions until the adaptive symptoms disappear. Adaptive symptoms may include flare or reduced contrast around objects during distance gaze, especially in dim light.

Precautions: In prescribing contact lenses, the Precautions should be carefully observed. It is also strongly recommended that the practitioner review with the patient the Patient Information Booklet available from Bausch & Lomb prior to dispensing the lenses and assure that the patient understands its contents. If the practitioner prescribes a SOFLENS® Therapeutic Contact Lens, the practitioner must thoroughly explain any instructions which are different from those described in the Patient Information Booklet.

- Contact lens wear may not be suitable for certain occupations, or, in other instances, may require eye protection equipment.
- Environmental fumes, smoke, dust, and vapors, and windy conditions, must be avoided, in order to minimize the chances of lens contamination or physical trauma to the cornea.
- Hard contact lens solutions not indicated for use with soft lenses may not be used in the soft lens care system. If a soft hydrophilic contact lens is worn after soaking in a hard contact lens solution, serious corneal injury may result.
- Chemical disinfection solution may not be used with heat unless specifically indicated in the labeling for heat and chemical disinfection.
- Bausch & Lomb recommends that sterile solutions be used in the soft lens care system. Sterile non-preserved solutions should be used if the patient is allergic to preservatives. When used, sterile non-preserved solutions must be discarded after the time specified in their label directions.
- Eye injury from irritation or infection and damage to lenses may result if cosmetics, lotion, soaps, creams, hair sprays or deodorants come in contact with lenses.
- Eye injury from irritation or infection may result from lens contamination.
- Tweezers or other tools should not be used by patients to remove a lens from the lens container. The lens should be poured into the hand.
- Patients must be instructed on and demonstrate the ability of prompt removal of the lenses. For patients wearing SOFLENS® Therapeutic Contact Lenses, patients may need to have access to someone who can promptly remove their lenses.
- Fluorescein should not be used while the lenses are on the patient's eye. The lenses absorb this dye and become discolored. Fluorescein in the eye should be thoroughly flushed with a sterile saline solution; and the lens should be reinserted only after at least one hour.
- Aphakic patients should not be fitted with contact lenses during the post operative period until, in the opinion of the surgeon, the eye has healed completely.
- A lens must move freely on the eye for a proper fit. For further information, see the Bausch & Lomb Fitting Guides.
- Some patients will not be able to tolerate extended wear even if able to tolerate the same or another lens on a daily wear basis. Patients should be carefully evaluated for extended wear prior to prescription and dispensing, and practitioners should conduct early and frequent follow-up examination to determine ocular response to extended wear.
- After removal of lenses from the lens case, to prevent contamination and to help avoid serious eye injury, always empty and rinse lens case with fresh rinsing solution and allow to air dry between each lens disinfection cycle.

Adverse Effects: The following symptoms may occur:

- eye pain
- eyes sting, burn, or itch (irritation)
- comfort is less than when lens was first placed on eye
- feeling of something in the eye (foreign body, scratched area)
- excessive watering (tearing) of the eyes
- unusual eye secretions
- redness of the eyes
- reduced sharpness of vision (poor visual acuity)
- blurred vision, rainbows, or halos around objects
- change in sensitivity to light (photophobia)
- feeling of dryness

The patient should be instructed that if any of the above symptoms occur:

- Immediately remove the lenses.
- If the discomfort or problems stops, then look closely at the lens.
- If the lens is in any way damaged, do not put the lens back on the eye. Place the lens in the storage case and contact the eye care practitioner.
- If the lens has dirt, an eyelash, or foreign body on it, or the problem stops and the lens appears undamaged, thoroughly clean, rinse and disinfect the lenses; then reinsert them.
- If the above symptoms continue after removal or upon reinsertion of the lens, the lenses should be removed immediately and the patient should immediately contact their eye care practitioner or a physician, who must determine the need for examination, treatment or referral without delay. (See Important Treatment Information for Adverse Effect, below). A serious condition such as infection, corneal ulcer, corneal vascularization, or iritis may be present, and may progress rapidly. Less serious reactions such as abrasions, epithelial staining and bacterial conjunctivitis must be managed and treated carefully to avoid complications.

If the patient is wearing a SOFLENS® Therapeutic Contact Lens, the practitioner should provide instructions for the patient to follow.

Important Treatment Information For Adverse Effects: Sight-threatening ocular complications associated with contact lens wear can develop rapidly, and therefore early recognition and treatment of problems are critical. Infectious corneal ulceration is one of the most serious potential complications, and may be ambiguous in its early stage. Signs and symptoms of infectious corneal ulceration include discomfort, pain, inflammation, purulent discharge, sensitivity to light, cells and flare and corneal infiltrates.

Initial symptoms of a minor abrasion and an early infected ulcer are sometimes similar. Accordingly, such epithelial defects if not treated properly, may develop into an infected ulcer. In order to prevent serious progression of these conditions, a patient presenting symptoms of abrasions or early ulcers should be evaluated as a potential medical emergency, treated accordingly, and be referred to a corneal specialist when appropriate. Standard therapy for corneal abrasions such as eye patching, or the use of steroids or steroid/antibiotic combinations may exacerbate the condition. If the patient is wearing a contact lens on the affected eye when examined, the lens should be removed immediately and the lens and lens care products retained for analysis and culturing.

Fitting Guides And Patient Information Booklets: Bausch & Lomb Fitting Guides provide detailed fitting information for all Bausch & Lomb Contact Lenses. When lenses are dispensed for vision correction, the patient must be supplied with an appropriate cleaning and disinfection regimen, with appropriate written instructions for the care products prescribed. The patient must fully understand all lens care and handling instructions. In addition, it is very important for the eye care practitioner to give the patient a Patient Information Booklet and review it with the patient. Copies of Fitting Guides and Patient Information Booklets for Bausch & Lomb Contact Lenses are available without charge from: Contact Lens Division, Bausch & Lomb Incorporated, Rochester, New York 14692. Toll free number: In the U.S. 1-800-828-9030; In New York State 1-800-462-1720.

Wearing Schedules: It is recommended that contact lens wearers see their eye care practitioner twice each year or if directed, more frequently.

Daily Wear: There may be a tendency for the daily wear patient to overwear the lenses initially. Therefore, the importance of adhering to a proper, initial daily wearing schedule should be stressed to these patients.

The wearing schedule should be determined by the eye care practitioner. The wearing schedule chosen by the eye care practitioner should be provided to the patient.

Extended Wear (greater than 24 hours, or while asleep): Wearing schedule should be determined by the prescribing eye care practitioner for each individual patient, based upon a full examination and patient history as well as the practitioner's experience and professional judgment. Bausch & Lomb recommends beginning extended wear patients with the initial daily wear schedule recommended by the eye care practitioner, followed by a period of daily wear, and then the gradual introduction of extended wear one night at a time, unless individual considerations indicate otherwise. The practitioner should examine the patient in the early stages of extended wear in order to determine corneal response. The lens must be removed for cleaning and disinfecting at least once every 7 days or more frequently, as determined by the prescribing eye care practitioner. (See the factors discussed in the WARNINGS section.) Once removed the lens should remain out of the eye for a period of rest overnight or longer, as determined by the prescribing eye care practitioner.

Therapeutic: For therapeutic use, a SOFLENS® (polymacon) Contact Lens may be worn either intermittently or for extended periods of time. The lens should be put on and taken off only as the eye care practitioner has instructed. Close practitioner supervision is necessary for therapeutic use of the SOFLENS® (polymacon) Contact Lens. The frequency of removal of the lens depends on the eye care practitioner's recommendation. The eye care practitioner should specify to the patient both the frequency of removal according to the patient's needs and the frequency of removal to clean and disinfect or replace the therapeutic lens.

Removal of the lens from the wearer's eye is not always necessary at follow-up visits. The lens can be examined on the eye when a slit lamp is used.

Although instructions for wear will vary depending upon treatment purposes, all wearers should be able to remove their lenses or have access to someone who can promptly remove their lenses should adverse effects occur and prompt removal be necessary.

Lens Care Directions: The products and procedures in this insert are recommended by Bausch & Lomb for the care of Bausch & Lomb SOFLENS, NaturalTint and MEDALIST Contact Lenses. Each Bausch & Lomb lens solution and other care products referred to in this insert has an individually packaged insert or brochure containing instructions and warnings for its use, which must be read and followed. An eye care practitioner may recommend alternative products and procedures for lens care. If other products and procedures are recommended, specific information on those products should be provided to the patient.

Patients must adhere to the recommended care regimen. Failure to follow the regimen may result in development of serious ocular complications as discussed in the WARNINGS. Patients who require only vision correction and who would not, or could not, adhere to a recommended care regimen for the lenses, or who are unable to place and remove lenses, should not be provided with them.

Continued on next page

Bausch & Lomb—Cont.

When lenses are dispensed, the patient must be provided with an appropriate cleaning and disinfection regimen and appropriate and adequate instructions and warnings for lens care, handling, cleaning, and disinfection. The eye care practitioner should recommend appropriate and adequate procedures and products for each individual patient in accordance with the particular lens, wearing schedule, and disinfection system selected by the practitioners, the specific instructions for such products, and the particular characteristics of the patient.

Basic Instructions for Patient Cleaning and Disinfecting: The eye care practitioner's instructions to the patient concerning cleaning and disinfecting contact lenses should include the following:

- Bausch & Lomb recommends that the patient use one system of lens care, either thermal (heat) or chemical. Unless specifically indicated in the labeling, do not alternate, change, or mix lens care systems for any one pair of lenses.
- Do not reuse solutions. Use fresh solutions for each step.
- Do not use saliva, tap water, distilled water, or anything other than the recommended sterile solutions labeled for the care of soft lenses.
- Carefully read and follow the Patient Information Booklet.
- Lenses must be both cleaned and disinfected each time they are removed, for any reason. If removed while the patient is away from the lens care products, the lenses may not be re-inserted, but should be stored until they can be cleaned and disinfected. Cleaning is necessary to remove mucus and film from the lens surface. Disinfecting is necessary to destroy harmful microorganisms.
- Clean one lens first (always the same lens first to avoid mixups), rinse the lens thoroughly with sterile saline or disinfecting solution to remove the cleaning solution, mucus, and film from the lens surface, and put that lens into the correct chamber of the lens storage case. Then repeat the procedure for the second lens.
- Stored lenses must be disinfected and left in the closed case until ready to wear.
- If the lenses have been stored for more than 24 hours, disinfect immediately before wearing and at least once a week. Put fresh solution inside the lens chambers, completely covering the lenses, before each disinfection.
- After removal of lenses from the lens case, the case should be emptied, rinsed with sterile saline or disinfecting solution, and allowed to air dry. At the next use of the case, fill it with fresh solution. (See precautions for care of lens case.)

Lens Deposits and Use of the Enzymatic Cleaning Procedure: Some wearers, who tend to secrete unusually large amounts of mucus in the lacrimal fluid, may experience a buildup of lens deposits within a few weeks, despite adequate cleaning measures. If medium to heavy surface accumulations of non-removable materials are observed, the affected lenses must be replaced to prevent an increased risk of adverse effects. To minimize deposit accumulation, the practitioner may prescribe an enzymatic cleaning regimen in addition to the regular cleaning regimen.

Deposits characterized as medium, or heavy, have been reported to occur on lenses worn for approximately one year. The occurrence of these deposits appears to increase with duration of lens use. These medium or heavy deposits, when they do exist, can be detected by means of slit lamp biomicroscope examination. In order to remove protein deposits which may form on the lenses, wearers should use enzymatic contact lens cleaning tablets according to the directions for use which accompany the tablets. To help remove tear residues, mucus and other deposits that tend to accumulate on the lens surface, patients should use the recommended cleaning solution according to the directions for use which accompany the product. The practitioner's instructions should emphasize that the lenses must be disinfected after completing all cleaning procedures, including enzymatic cleaning.

Thermal (Heat) Lens Disinfection:

- Prepare the empty lens storage case by filling the lens chambers with sterile saline solution.
- Clean the contact lenses with a recommended cleaning solution and thoroughly rinse the contact lenses with sterile saline solution.
- Put each lens into its correct chamber.
- Fill the chamber of the case ⅔ full with the fresh sterile saline solution. Completely cover the lenses.
- Tightly close the top on each chamber of the lens storage case.
- To disinfect, follow the directions accompanying the disinfection unit and the care regimen recommended by the eye care practitioner. (Discoloration and cracking of lens carrying cases have been reported after varying periods of use. If such occurs, replacement is indicated to avoid interference with the disinfection procedure. The patient should also check the unit as directed in the unit instructions to assure that it is operating at each cycle. Malfunctioning units may not be used, and must be replaced.)
- Leave the lenses in the unopened storage case unitl cool and the patient is ready to place the lenses on the eyes.

Emergency Method for Heat Disinfection: If a heat disinfection unit is not available, tightly close the lens case and place in a pan of already boiling water. Leave the closed lens case in the pan of boiling water for at least 10 minutes. (Above an altitude of 7,000 feet, boil for at least 15 minutes.) Care must be exercised to not allow the water in the pan to boil away. Remove the pan from the heat and allow it to cool for 30 minutes to complete the disinfection of the lenses. USE OF HEAT DISINFECTION UNIT SHOULD BE RESUMED AS SOON AS POSSIBLE.

Chemical Lens Disinfection (Including Hydrogen Peroxide):

- Clean the contact lenses with the recommended cleaning solution and thoroughly rinse the contact lenses with the recommended rinsing solution.
- To disinfect, carefully follow the instructions accompanying the disinfection solution in the care regimen recommended by the eye care practitioner.
- Thoroughly rinse lenses with a fresh solution recommended for rinsing before inserting and wearing.
- **Do not** heat the disinfection solution and lenses.
- Leave the lenses in the unopened storage case until ready to put on eyes.

Lenses that are chemically disinfected may absorb ingredients from the disinfecting solution which may be irritating to the eyes. A 20-second rinse in fresh sterile saline solution should reduce the potential for irritation.

Care For a Dehydrated Lens: If a soft, hydrophilic contact lens is exposed to air while off the eye, it may become dry and brittle and need to be rehydrated. If the lens is adhering to a surface, such as a counter top, apply saline before handling.

To rehydrate the lens:

- Handle the lens carefully.
- Place the lens in its storage case and soak the lens in a recommended rinsing and storage solution for at least one hour until it returns to a soft state.
- Clean and disinfect the rehydrated lens using the recommended lens care system.
- If after soaking, the lens does not become soft, the lens should not be used until examined by the eye care practitioner.

Lens Care Products Chart: Bausch & Lomb offers a complete line of quality care products that make soft lens maintenance quick and easy. The following solutions are recommended by Bausch & Lomb for use with all Bausch & Lomb SOFLENS, NaturalTint and MEDALIST Contact Lenses; however, eye care practitioners may recommend alternative products and procedures for their patients. All components necessary for lens disinfection cleaning and storage are available in BAUSCH & LOMB® Care Kits.

Thermal Lens Care System

Action	Care Product
Disinfection Unit	BAUSCH & LOMB® Compact Disinfecting Unit BAUSCH & LOMB Disinfecting Unit
Cleaning	BAUSCH & LOMB® SENSITIVE EYES® Daily Cleaner
Rinsing, Disinfecting & Storing*	BAUSCH & LOMB® Compact Disinfecting Unit or Disinfecting Unit used with: BAUSCH & LOMB® ReNu® Saline Solution BAUSCH & LOMB® SENSITIVE EYES Sterile Saline Spray BAUSCH & LOMB® SENSITIVE EYES® Saline Solution
Enzymatic Protein Removal	BAUSCH & LOMB® ReNu® Thermal Enzymatic Contact Lens Cleaner BAUSH & LOMB® ReNu® Effervescent Enzymatic Contact Lens Cleaner

* See Lens Storage section.

Chemical (Not Heat) Lens Care System

Action	Care Product
Cleaning	BAUSCH & LOMB® ReNu® Multi-Purpose Solution BAUSCH & LOMB® SENSITIVE EYES® Daily Cleaner
Disinfecting & Storing	BAUSCH & LOMB® ReNu® Multi-Purpose Solution
Rinsing	BAUSCH & LOMB® ReNu® Multi-Purpose Solution BAUSCH & LOMB® SENSITIVE EYES® Saline Solution BAUSCH & LOMB® ReNu® Saline Solution BAUSCH & LOMB® SENSITIVE EYES® Sterile Saline Spray
Enzymatic Protein Removal	BAUSCH & LOMB® ReNu® Effervescent Enzymatic Contact Lens Cleaner

All Lens Care Systems

Action	Care Product
Rewetting	BAUSCH & LOMB® ReNU® Rewetting Drops BAUSCH & LOMB® SENSITIVE EYES® Drops

Practitioner Disinfection of Open Lenses: All lenses that have been opened must be heat disinfected after each fitting and at least once each week. Unopened lenses are sterile and need not be disinfected until the vial seal has been broken.

How Supplied:

1. Each Bausch & Lomb SOFLENS® and MEDALIST™ Contact Lens is supplied in sterile normal saline solution or 0.85% sodium chloride and 0.1% polyvinyl alcohol. The package is marked with the manufacturing lot number of the lens, the dioptric power, the lens series and expiration date. Add power and sagittal depth designations are included for BI-TECH™ Contact Lenses. A sagittal depth designation is included for OPTIMA® 38.
2. Each Bausch & Lomb NaturalTint® (polymacon) Contact Lens is supplied in a glass vial containing sterile normal buffered saline solution. The glass vial is marked with the manufacturing lot number of the lens, dioptric power, lens series, lens color, and expiration date. A sagittal depth designation is included for OPTIMA® 38 Contact Lenses.

Vistakon

Johnson & Johnson Vision Products, Inc.
4500 SALISBURY ROAD
JACKSONVILLE, FL 32216

ACUVUE®
(etafilcon A)
Soft Hydrophilic Contact Lens

Description: The **ACUVUE®** (etafilcon A) Soft Hydrophilic Contact Lens is available as a spherical lens. The lens is intended to be used within the Vistakon system for planned lens replacement. This sytem allows flexiblity to prescribe the lens replacement and wearing schedule that best meets the needs of the patient. The lens may be prescribed for either Disposable Wear (up to 7 days/6 nights) or Scheduled Replacement Wear (recommended Two Week Replacement).

The **ACUVUE** (etafilcon A) Contact Lens has the following properties and parameters:

- **Lens Material:** 58% water and 42% etafilcon A polymer (2-hydroxyethyl methacrylate and methacrylic acid crosslinked with 1, 1, 1 -trimethylol propane trimethacrylate and ethylene glycol dimethacrylate).
- **Lens Properties:**

• wet refractive index	1.40 ± .01
• visible light transmittance	95% minimum
• oxygen permeability (Dk)	28.0 ± 2.0 × 10 (cm_2/sec) $(ml\ O_2{}^{-11}/ml \times mm\ Hg)$ at 35°C

- **Lens Parameters:**

[See table above.]

- **How Supplied:**

Each sterile lens is supplied in a foil-sealed plastic package containing buffered saline solution. The plastic package is marked with the lens power, manufacturing expiration date, base curve/diameter series identification and manufacturing lot number.

Parameters	Minus Lens	Plus Lens
• power range (increments)	−0.50 D to −6.00 D (in 0.25 D increments) −6.50 D to −9.00 D (in 0.50 D increments)	+.50 D to +6.00 D (in 0.25 D increments)
• series	II	III
base curve	8.8 mm	9.1 mm
diameter	14.0 mm	14.4 mm
• center thickness range (varies with power)	.07 to .11 mm	.12 to .23 mm

Indications: The **ACUVUE** (etafilcon A) Contact Lens for Daily Wear is indicated for the correction of visual acuity in not-aphakic persons with nondiseased eyes who are myopic or hyperopic and may have 1.00 diopter or less of astigmatism that does not interfere with visual acuity. The lens ranges in power from −0.50 to −9.00 and +0.50 to +6.00 diopters.

The **ACUVUE** (etafilcon A) Contact Lens for Extended Wear is indicated for the correction of visual acuity in not-aphakic persons with nondiseased eyes who are myopic or hyperopic and have 1.00 diopter or less of astigmatism that does not intefere with visual acuity. The **ACUVUE** (etafilcon A) Contact Lens is indicated for Extended Wear from 1 to 7 days between removals for disposal (Disposal Wear) or cleaning, disinfection and disposal (Scheduled Replacement Wear), as recommended by the eye care practitioner (See LENS REPLACEMENT section for an additional description of these wear schedules). The lens ranges in power from −0.50 to −9.00 and +0.50 to +6.00 diopters.

Contraindications: The **ACUVUE** (etafilcon A) Contact Lens is contraindicated by the presence of any of the following conditions:

1. Acute and subacute inflammation of the anterior segment of the eye.
2. Any eye disease which affects the cornea or conjunctiva.
3. Insufficiency of lacrimal secretion (dry eye).
4. Corneal hypoesthesia (reduced corneal sensitivity).
5. Any systemic disease or allergy which may affect the eye or be exaggerated by wearing contact lenses.
6. Ocular irritation due to allergic reactions which may be caused by or exaggerated by the wearing of contact lenses and/or the use of contact lens solutions that may contain chemicals or preservatives such as thimerosal or other mercury compounds to which some people may be allergic.
7. Any medication that contraindicates contact lens wear.

Warnings: Problems with contact lenses or lens care products could result in serious injury to the eye. Patients should be cautioned that proper use and care of contact lenses and lens care products, including lens cases, are essential for the safe use of these products.

Eye problems, including corneal ulcers, can develop rapidly and lead to loss of vision. The results of a study[1] indicate the following:

- The overall annual incidence of ulcerative keratitis in daily wear contact lens users is estimated to be about 4.1 per 10,000 persons and about 20.9 per 10,000 persons in extended wear contact lens users.
- The risk of ulcerative keratitis is 4 to 5 times greater for extended wear contact lens users than for daily wear users. When daily wear users who wear their lenses overnight and extended wear users who wear their lenses on a daily basis are excluded from the comparison, the risk among extended wear users is 10 to 15 times greater than among daily wear users.
- The risk among extended wear lens users increases with the number of consecutive days that lenses are worn between removals, beginning with the first overnight use.
- The overall risk of ulcerative keratitis may be reduced by carefully following directions for emergency lens care, including cleaning of the lens case (for Disposable Wear) and for routine lens care, including cleaning of the lens case (for Scheduled Replacement Wear).
- The risk of ulcerative keratitis among contact lens users who smoke is estimated to be 3 to 8 times greater than among nonsmokers.

If patients experience eye discomfort, excessive tearing, vision changes, redness of the eye or other problems, they should be instructed to immediately remove their lenses and promptly contact their eye care practitioner. It is recommended that contact lens wearers see their eye care practitioners routinely as directed.

Precautions: These precautions should be carefully observed when prescribing contact lenses.

- The lens must move sufficiently on the eye to help assure proper fit.
- Before leaving the eye care practitioner's office, the patient should demonstrate the ability to properly insert and remove the lens.
- The patient should be instructed against the use of tweezers or other tools to remove the lens from the lens container to avoid damaging the lens.
- The patient should be instructed to promptly remove the lens in the event that dust, a foreign body or other contaminant gets between the lens and the eye to avoid any serious injury.
- The patient should be instructed to replace any lens which becomes dehydrated or damaged.
- The patient should be informed that eye irritation may result if cosmetics, lotions, soaps, creams and deodorants come in contact with the lens or the lens is contaminated through some other means.
- The patient should be instructed to avoid using aerosol products such as hair spray while wearing lenses. If sprays are used, eyes should be kept closed until the spray has settled.
- The patient who is prescribed **ACUVUE** (etafilcon A) Contact Lenses on a Daily Wear schedule should be cautioned to remove the lenses before sleeping.
- Not every patient is able to wear a lens on an extended wear basis, even if he or she is able to wear the same lens on a daily wear basis.

[1] Data on file.

- Periodic eye examinations are extremely important, especially for a patient on an extended wear schedule.
- The patient should be instructed to remove the lenses before getting into a hot tub, going swimming or in the presence of noxious or irritating vapors. The patient who swims frequently may be placed on recommended Two Week Replacement Wear.
- The patient should be instructed to inform his or her employer that contact lenses are worn, as some jobs may require the use of eye protection equipment or that contact lenses not be worn.
- The patient should be instructed to inform his or her physician that contact lenses are worn and to consult his or her eye care practitioner before using any medication in the eye.
- Certain medications such as antihistamines, decongestants, diuretics, muscle relaxants, transquilizers, and those for motion sickness may cause dryness of the eye, increased lens awareness or blurred vision. Should such conditions exist proper remedial measures should be prescribed. Depending on the severity, this could include the use of lubricat-

Continued on next page

Vistakon—Cont.

ing drops that are indicated for use with soft contact lenses or the temporary discontinuance of contact lens wear while such medication is being used.
- Oral contraceptive users could develop visual changes or changes in lens tolerance when using contact lenses. Patients should be cautioned accordingly.
- Regular fluorescein should not be used while the lenses are on the patient's eyes. When fluorescein is used, the patient's eyes should be flushed with a sterile normal saline solution following such use.

Adverse Reactions: The following problems may occur when wearing contact lenses:
- The eye may burn, sting or itch.
- There may be less comfort than when the lens was first placed on the eye.
- There may also be excessive watering, unusual eye secretions, or redness of the eye.
- Poor visual acuity, blurred vision, rainbows or halos around objects, photophobia, or dry eyes may also occur if the lenses are worn continuously for too long a time.

Removal of the lens and a rest period of at least one hour generally relieves these symptoms. If, upon re-insertion of the lens the problem continues, the patient should be instructed to promptly remove the lens and contact the eye care practitioner.

Fitting: Conventional methods of fitting soft contact lenses to the **ACUVUE** (etafilcon A) Contact Lens. For a detailed description of the fitting technique, refer to the **ACUVUE** Lens Fitting and Patient Management Guide for the Professional, copies of which are available from:

Vistakon
P.O. Box 10157
Jacksonville, Florida 32247-0157

CAUTION: FEDERAL LAW PROHIBITS DISPENSING WITHOUT A PRESCRIPTION FROM AN EYE CARE PRACTITIONER.

Lens Replacement: The **ACUVUE** (etafilcon A) Contact Lens may be prescribed for either Disposable Wear (up to 7 days/6 nights) or Scheduled Replacement Wear (recommended Two Week Replacement) within the Vistakon system for planned lens replacement.
- **Disposable Wear**—This includes only single-use wear of the product. The lens is not recommended for routine cleaning and disinfection. It is recommended that the lens be worn for up to 7 days/6 nights before removal for disposal and replacement (see wear schedule below).
- **Scheduled Replacement Wear**—This includes reuse of the product and planned replacement wear. It is recommended that lenses be replaced at least every 2 weeks (see wear schedule below). The lens is to be cleaned and disinfected each time it is removed from the patient's eye and discarded after the wearing period prescribed by the eye care practitioner. The lens may be worn for Daily Wear or Extended Wear (1 to 7 days/6 nights).

Wear Schedule: DAILY WEAR (periods less than 24 hours while awake)—The maximum suggested wearing time each day for the **ACUVUE** (etafilcon A) Contact Lens when worn on a daily wear basis should be determined by the eye care practitioner based upon the patient's physiological eye condition, because individual response to contact lenses vary.

EXTENDED WEAR (periods greater than 24 hours, including while asleep)—The **ACUVUE** (etafilcon A) Contact Lens for extended wear is recommended for 1 to 7 days/6 nights of continuous wear. Once the lens is removed, it is recommended that the patient's eye should have a rest period of overnight or longer. It is recommended that the new contact lens wearer first be evaluated on a daily wear schedule. If, in the opinion of the eye care practitioner, the patient is determined to be an acceptable extended wear candidate, the eye care practitioner is encouraged to determine a wearing schedule based upon the response of the patient.

LENS CARE DIRECTIONS (FOR RECOMMENDED TWO WEEK REPLACEMENT WEAR AND ON AN EMERGENCY BASIS FOR DISPOSABLE WEAR)

For Scheduled Replacement Wear (recommended Two Week Replacement), lenses must be both cleaned and disinfected according to the labeling instructions specified with the solutions recommended by the eye care practitioner. The chemical method of disinfection, including hydrogen peroxide, is recommended. The heat method of disinfection is generally not advised. For Disposable Wear the lenses should only be cleaned and disinfected on an emergency basis when replacement lenses are not available.

The eye care practitioner should review the following instructions with the patients:
- Always wash and rinse hands before handling lenses.
- Only use fresh sterile cleaning, disinfecting and rinsing solutions which are indicated for use with soft contact lenses according to the labeling instructions provided.
- Never use conventional hard contact lens solutions unless also indicated for use with soft contact lenses.
- Do not use saliva, tap water, homemade saline solution, or anything other than the recommended solutions to wet lenses.
- To help avoid serious eye injury from contamination, always empty and rinse the lens case with fresh sterile rinsing solution and allow to air dry.

FOR ADDITIONAL INFORMATION

For additional information concerning the **ACUVUE** (etafilcon A) Contact Lens, call us toll free at 1-800-843-2020.

ACUVUE and VISTAKON are trademarks of Johnson & Johnson Vision Products, Inc.

A-05-91-00 May, 1991

SUREVUE™
(etafilcon A)
Soft Hydrophilic Contact Lens

Description: The **SUREVUE®** (etafilcon A) Soft Hydrophilic Contact Lens is available as a spherical lens. The lens is intended to be used on a Daily Wear Two Week Replacement schedule.

The **SUREVUE** (etafilcon A) Contact Lens has the following properties and parameters:
- **Lens Material:** 58% water and 42% etafilcon A polymer (2-hydroxyethyl methacrylate and methacrylic acid crosslinked with 1, 1, 1 -trimethylol propane trimethacrylate and ethylene glycol dimethacrylate).
- **Lens Properties:**

• wet refractive index	$1.40 \pm .01$
• visible light transmittance	95% minimum
• oxygen permeability (Dk)	$28.0 \pm 2.0 \times 10^{-11}$ (cm_2/sec) (ml O_2/ml $\times$ mm Hg) at 35°C

- **Lens Parameters:**

Parameters	Minus Lens
• power range (increments)	−0.50 D to −6.00 D (in 0.25 D increments) −6.50 D to −9.00 D (in 0.50 D increments)
• base curve	8.8 mm
• diameter	14.0 mm
• center thickness range (varies with power)	.10 to .16 mm

• How Supplied:
Each sterile lens is supplied in a foil-sealed plastic package containing buffered saline solution. The plastic package is marked with the lens power, manufacturing expiration date base curve, diameter and manufacturing lot number.

Indications:
DAILY WEAR
The **SUREVUE** (etafilcon A) Contact Lens is indicated for Daily Wear (less than 1 day while awake) for the correction of visual acuity in non-aphakic persons with nondiseased eyes who are myopic and may have 1.00 diopter or less of astigmatism that does not interfere with visual acuity. The **SUREVUE** Contact Lens is indicated for scheduled replacement as recommended by the eye care practitioner. The lens ranges in power from −0.50 to −9.00 diopters.

Contraindications: The **SUREVUE** (etafilcon A) Contact Lens is contraindicated by the presence of any of the following conditions:
1. Acute and subacute inflammation of the anterior segment of the eye.
2. Any eye disease which affects the cornea or conjunctiva.
3. Insufficiency of lacrimal secretion (dry eye).
4. Corneal hypoesthesia (reduced corneal sensitivity).
5. Any systemic disease or allergy which may affect the eye or be exaggerated by wearing contact lenses.
6. Ocular irritation due to allergic reactions which may be caused by or exaggerated by the wearing of contact lenses and/or the use of contact lens solutions that may contain chemicals or preservatives such as thimerosal or other mercury compounds to which some people may be allergic.
7. Any medication that contraindicates contact lens wear.

Warnings: Problems with contact lenses or lens care products could result in serious injury to the eye. Patients should be cautioned that proper use and care of contact lenses and lens care products, including lens cases, are essential for the safe use of these products.

Eye problems, including corneal ulcers, can develop rapidly and lead to loss of vision. The results of a study[1] indicate the following:
- The overall annual incidence of ulcerative keratitis in daily wear contact lens users is estimated to be about 4.1 per 10,000 persons and about 20.9 per 10,000 persons in extended wear contact lens users.
- The risk of ulcerative keratitis is 4 to 5 times greater for extended wear contact lens users than for daily wear users. When daily wear users who wear their lenses overnight and extended wear users who wear their lenses on a daily basis are excluded from the comparison, the risk among extended wear users is 9 to 15 times greater than among daily wear users.
- When daily wear users wear their lenses overnight (outside the approved indication), the risk of ulcerative keratitis is nine times greater than among those who do not wear them overnight.
- The overall risk of ulcerative keratitis may be reduced by carefully following directions for lens care, including cleaning of the lens case.
- The risk of ulcerative keratitis among contact lens users who smoke is estimated to be 3 to 8 times greater than among nonsmokers.

If patients experience eye discomfort, excessive tearing, vision changes, redness of the eye or other problems, they should be instructed to immediately remove their lenses and promptly contact their eye care practitioner. It is recommended that contact lens wearers see their eye care practitioners routinely as directed.

Precautions: These precautions should be carefully observed when prescribing contact lenses.

- The lens must move sufficiently on the eye to help assure proper fit.
- Before leaving the eye care practitioner's office, the patient should demonstrate the ability to properly insert and remove the lenses.
- The patient should be instructed against the use of tweezers or other tools to remove the lens from the lens container to avoid damaging the lens.
- The patient should be instructed to promptly remove the lens in the event that dust, a foreign body or other contaminant gets between the lens and the eye to avoid any serious injury.
- The patient should be instructed to replace any lens which becomes dehydrated or damaged.
- The patient should be informed that eye irritation may result if cosmetics, lotions, soaps, creams and deodorants come in contact with the lens or the lens is contaminated through some other means.
- The patient should be instructed to avoid using aerosol products such as hair spray while wearing lenses. If sprays are used, eyes should be kept closed until the spray has settled.
- The patient who is prescribed **SUREVUE** (etafilcon A) Contact Lenses should be cautioned to remove the lenses before sleeping.
- Periodic eye examinations are extremely important.
- The patient should be instructed to remove the lenses before getting into a hot tub, going swimming or in the presence of noxious or irritating vapors.
- The patient should be instructed to inform his or her employer that contact lenses are worn, as some jobs may require the use of eye protection equipment or that contact lenses not be worn.
- The patient should be instructed to inform his or her physician that contact lenses are worn and to consult his or her eye care practitioner before using any medication in the eye.
- Certain medications such as antihistamines, decongestants, diuretics, muscle relaxants, tranquilizers, and those for motion sickness may cause dryness of the eye, increased lens awareness or blurred vision. Should such conditions exist proper remedial measures should be prescribed. Depending on the severity, this could include the use of lubricating drops that are indicated for use with soft contact lenses or the temporary discontinuance of contact lens wear while such medication is being used.
- Oral contraceptive users could develop visual changes or changes in lens tolerance when using contact lenses. Patients should be cautioned accordingly.
- Regular fluorescein should not be used while the lenses are on the patient's eyes. When fluorescein is used, the patient's eyes should be flushed with a sterile normal saline solution following such use.

Adverse Reactions: The following problems may occur when wearing contact lenses:

- The eye may burn, sting or itch.
- There may be less comfort than when the lens was first placed on the eye.
- There may also be excessive watering, unusual eye secretions, or redness of the eye.
- Poor visual acuity, blurred vision, rainbows or halos around objects, photophobia, or dry eyes may also occur if the lenses are worn continuously for too long a time.

Removal of the lens and a rest period of at least one hour generally relieves these symptoms. If, upon re-insertion of the lens the problem continues, the patient should be instructed to promptly remove the lens and contact the eye care practitioner.

Fitting: Conventional methods of fitting soft contact lenses apply to the **SUREVUE** (etafilcon A) Contact Lens. For a detailed description of the fitting technique, refer to the **SUREVUE** Fitting and Patient Management Guide for the Professional, copies of which are available from:

VISTAKON
Johnson & Johnson Vision Products, Inc.
P.O. Box 10157
Jacksonville, Florida 32247-0157

CAUTION: FEDERAL LAW PROHIBITS DISPENSING WITHOUT A PRESCRIPTION FROM AN EYE CARE PRACTITIONER.

Lens Replacement: The **SUREVUE** (etafilcon A) Contact Lens is to be prescribed within the Vistakon system for planned lens replacement. The lens is to be cleaned and disinfected each time it is removed from the patient's eye, and discarded after the wearing period prescribed by the eye care practitioner. It is recommended that lenses be replaced at least every two weeks (see wear schedule below).

Wear Schedule: DAILY WEAR (periods less than 1 day while awake)—The maximum suggested wearing time each day for the **SUREVUE** (etafilcon A) Contact Lens worn on a daily wear basis should be determined by the eye care practitioner based upon the patient's physiological eye condition, because individual response to contact lenses vary.

Lens Care Directions: Lenses must be both cleaned and disinfected according to the labeling instructions specified with the solutions recommended by the eye care practitioner. The chemical method of disinfection is recommended. The heat method of disinfection is generally not advised.

The eye care practitioner should review the following instructions with the patients:

- Always wash and rinse hands before handling lenses.
- Only use fresh sterile lens care solutions which are indicated for use with soft contact lenses according to the labeling instructions provided.
- Never use conventional hard contact lens solutions unless also indicated for use with soft contact lenses.
- Do not use saliva, tap water, homemade saline solution, or anything other than the recommended solutions to wet lenses.
- To help avoid serious eye injury from contamination, always empty and rinse the lens case with fresh sterile rinsing solution and allow to air dry.

For Additional Information: For additional information concerning the **SUREVUE** (etafilcon A) Contact Lens, call us toll free at 1-800-843-2020.

SUREVUE and VISTAKON are trademarks of Johnson & Johnson Vision Products, Inc.

Printed in U.S.A. February, 1991

[1] Data on file.

Part 2 - Intraocular Lenses

Alcon Surgical, Inc.

6201 SOUTH FREEWAY
FT. WORTH, TX 76134

Address Inquiries to:
Marketing Department (817) 293-0450
1-800-TO-ALCON
(1-800-862-5266)

ALCON® INTRAOCULAR LENSES

Alcon Surgical manufactures single-piece all PMMA anterior and posterior chamber lenses and multi-piece posterior chamber lenses with either polypropylene or MonoFlex™ PMMA haptics. All optics are lathe cut from high molecular weight clear and UV-absorbing PMMA and come in a wide range of diameters and styles (convexoplano, meniscus, ridged or biconvex). For additional information please contact Alcon Surgical, Marketing Department at 1-800-TO-ALCON.

IOLAB Corporation

a Johnson & Johnson Company
500 IOLAB DRIVE
CLAREMONT, CA 91711

Address inquiries to:
Marketing Services (800) 423-1871
CA only (800) 352-1891

IOLAB, a Johnson & Johnson company, manufactures a complete line of ophthalmic products including Intraocular Lenses, Microsurgical Equipment, Viscoelastics and Pharmaceuticals.

IOLAB intraocular lens products include the new SLIMFIT™ Ovoid Optic Lenses and EZ-VUE™ Violet Haptic Lenses. IOLAB also distributes AMVISC® and AMVISC® Plus Sodium Hyaluronate.

IOLAB provides the widest selection of Pre-Market Approved lenses available for the posterior and anterior chamber. IOLs are available in many styles including one-piece designs and special high and low diopter powers. All models are available with the preferred class I UV filtration. Many models are available with or without positioning holes as well as a variety of optic sizes. These range from 5.5mm round, 5 × 6 mm to 7mm round.

For current information on intraocular lenses or any other product please contact your IOLAB Sales Representative or IOLAB directly.

AMVISC® PLUS ℞
(sodium hyaluronate)

Description: AMVISC® PLUS is a sterile nonpyrogenic solution of sodium hyaluronate. AMVISC® PLUS contains 16 mg/mL of sodium hyaluronate adjusted to yield approximately 55,000 centistokes dissolved in physiological saline and exhibits an osmolality of approximately 340 milliosmoles.

Continued on next page

IOLAB Corporation—Cont.

Characteristics: Sodium hyaluronate is a high molecular weight polysaccharide composed of sodium glucuronate and N-acetylglucosamine. Sodium hyaluronate is ubiquitously distributed throughout the tissues of the body and is present in high concentrations in such tissues as vitreous humor, synovial fluid, umbilical cord and the dermis of rooster combs. Sodium hyaluronate functions as a tissue lubricant (1,2) and it is thought to play an important role in modulating the interactions between adjacent tissues. It can also act as a viscoelastic support maintaining a separation between tissues. Sodium hyaluronates prepared from different tissues may have different molecular weights but are thought to have the same chemical structure. The sodium hyaluronate in AMVISC® PLUS is prepared from the dermis of rooster combs (3). It has a molecular weight greater than 1,000,000, is reported to be nonantigenic (4,5), does not cause foreign body reactions, is nonpyrogenic and is well tolerated in human eyes (6). AMVISC® PLUS does not interfere with normal wound healing processes.

Indications: AMVISC® PLUS is indicated for use as a surgical aid in ophthalmic anterior (7) and posterior (6) segment procedures including • glaucoma filtering surgery • surgical procedures to reattach the retina • implantation of an intraocular lens (IOL) • extraction of a cataract • corneal transplantation surgery. Due to its lubricating and viscoelastic properties, transparency and ability to protect corneal endothelial cells (8), AMVISC® PLUS helps maintain anterior chamber depth and visibility, minimizes interaction between tissues, and acts as a tamponade and vitreous substitute during retina reattachment surgery. AMVISC® PLUS also preserves tissue integrity and good visibility when used to fill the anterior and posterior segments of the eye following open sky procedures.

Contraindications: At the present time there are no contraindications to the use of AMVISC® PLUS when used as recommended as an intraocular implant.

Applications:

1. Cataract surgery and IOL implantation—The required amount of AMVISC® PLUS is slowly infused through a needle or cannula into the anterior chamber. The protective effect of AMVISC® PLUS as an aid is optimized when the injection is performed prior to cataract extraction and insertion of the IOL and is effective for both intra- and extracapsular cataract procedures. AMVISC® PLUS may be applied to the IOL prior to insertion. Additional AMVISC® PLUS can be injected as required to facilitate surgical procedures (see precautions).
2. Corneal transplant surgery—The corneal button is removed and the anterior chamber filled with AMVISC® PLUS until it is level with the surface of the cornea. The donor graft is then placed on top of the AMVISC® PLUS and sutured into place. Additional AMVISC® PLUS can be used as required to aid in surgical procedures (see precautions).
3. Glaucoma filtration surgery—AMVISC® PLUS is injected through a corneal paracentesis to restore and maintain anterior chamber volume during the performance of the trabeculectomy. Additional AMVISC® PLUS can be used as required to aid in the surgical procedures (see precautions).
4. Intraocular injection in conjunction with scleral buckling procedures for retina reattachment—After release of subretinal fluid and development of buckling by tying the mattress sutures, air is injected into the vitreous cavity and then exchanged with AMVISC® PLUS injected through a needle (22 to 30 gauge) passed via the pars plana epithelium. The volume of AMVISC® PLUS injected (2–4 ml) will vary with the volume of the subretinal fluid released and the space occupied by the buckle.

Precautions: Those precautions normally considered during anterior segment and retina reattachment procedures are recommended. There may be increased intraocular pressure following surgery (9) caused by preexisting glaucoma or by the surgery itself. For these reasons the following precautions should be considered.

- An excess quantity of AMVISC® PLUS should not be used. • AMVISC® PLUS should be removed from the anterior chamber at the end of surgery. • If the postoperative intraocular pressure increases above expected values, correcting therapy should be administered. • AMVISC® PLUS is prepared from a biological source and the physician should be aware of the possible effects of using any biological materials. • Reuse of cannula should be avoided. Even after cleaning and rinsing, resterilized cannula could release particulate matter as AMVISC® PLUS is injected. It is recommended that disposable cannula be used when administering AMVISC® PLUS. • There have been isolated reports of diffuse particulates or haziness appearing after injection of AMVISC® PLUS into the eye. While such reports are infrequent and seldom associated with any effects on ocular tissues, the physician should be aware of this occurrence. If observed, the particulate matter should be removed by irrigation and/or aspiration.

Adverse Reactions: Sodium hyaluronate is a natural component of the tissues of the body and is extremely well tolerated in human eyes. Transient postoperative inflammatory reactions were reported in clinical trials (6) and oral and topical steroid preparations were administered. AMVISC® PLUS is tested in animals to determine that each batch is essentially noninflammatory. Since sodium hyaluronate molecules are noninflammatory, and phlogistic response is considered to be caused by the surgical procedures. The best index of the degree of phlogistic response is the postoperative clarity of the vitreous cavity. As outlined above a transient postoperative increase in intraocular pressure has been observed following the use of sodium hyaluronate in anterior segment surgery. On rare occasions postoperative reactions including inflammation, corneal edema and corneal decompensation have been reported. The relationship to the use of AMVISC® PLUS has not been established.

How Supplied: AMVISC® PLUS is a sterile viscoelastic preparation supplied in a disposable glass syringe delivering either 0.25 ml, 0.5 ml or 0.8 ml of sodium hyaluronate dissolved in physiological saline. Each ml of AMVISC® PLUS contains 16 mg of sodium hyaluronate adjusted to yield approximately 55,000 centistokes, 9 mg of Sodium Chloride and q.s. Sterile Water for Injection USP. AMVISC® PLUS exhibits an osmolality of approximately 340 milliosmoles. Sodium hydroxide and/or hydrochloric acid are added to adjust pH (if necessary). AMVISC® PLUS syringes are terminally sterilized and aseptically packaged. Contents of unopened and undamaged pouches are sterile. Refrigerated AMVISC® PLUS should be allowed to reach room temperature (approximately 20 to 45 minutes, depending on volume) prior to use.

For Intraocular Use: Store at 2–8°C. Protect from freezing.

Caution: Federal law restricts this device to sale by or on the order of a physician.

References:

1. Swann DA, Radin El, Nazimiec, Weisser PA, Curran N, Lewinneck G. Role of hyaluronic acid in joint lubrication. Ann Rheum Dis 1974; 33:318.
2. Radin EL, Paul IL, Swann DA, Schottstaedt ES. Lubrication of synovial membrane. Ann Rheum Dis 1971; 30:322.
3. Swann DA, Studies of Hyaluronic Acid. I. The preparation and properties of rooster comb hyaluronic acid. Biochim Biophys Acta 1968; 156:17.
4. Richter W. Non-immunogenicity of purified hyaluronic acid preparations tested by passive cutaneous anaphylaxis. Int Arch Allergy 1974; 47:211.
5. Richter, W, Ryde EM, Zetterstrom EO. Non-immunogenicity of a purified sodium hyaluronate preparation in man. Int Arch Appl Immunol 1979; 59:45.
6. Pruett RC, Schepens CL, Swann DA, Hyaluronic acid vitreous substitute. A six-year clinical evaluation. Arch Ophthalmol 1979; 97:2325.
7. Pape LG, Balazs EA. The use of sodium hyaluronate (Healon®) in human anterior segment surgery. Ophthalmol 1980; 87:699.
8. Miller D, Stegmann R. Use of Na-hyaluronate in anterior segment eye surgery. Am Intra-Ocular Implant Soc J 1980; 6:13.
9. Miller D, Stegmann R. The use of Healon® in intraocular lens implantation. Int Ophthalmol Clinics 1982; 22:177.

Manufactured by:
MedChem Products, Inc.
232 West Cummings Park
Woburn, MA 01801

Size	Reorder #
0.5 ml	60051
0.8 ml	60081

Distributed by:
IOLAB
a Johnson & Johnson company
500 Iolab Drive
Claremont, CA 91711
Toll-free: 800/423-1871 • In CA: 800/352-1891
Revised July 1988

For more information regarding AMVISC Plus or AMVISC viscoelastics contact: IOLAB, 500 IOLAB Drive, Claremont, California 91711. Toll free: 800-423-1871 ext. 1250. • In California: 800-352-1891 ext. 1250.

AMVISC® ℞

Information listed for AMVISC Plus also applies to AMVISC with the following exceptions.

- AMVISC contains 12 mg/ml sodium hyaluronate adjusted to yield approximately 40,000cs dissolved in physiological saline.
- AMVISC is a sterile viscoelastic preparation supplied in a disposable glass syringe delivering either 0.50ml or 0.80ml sodium hyaluronate dissolved in physiological saline. Each ml of AMVISC contains 12mg sodium hyaluronate adjusted to yield approximately 40,000cs, 9.0mg of sodium chloride and sterile water for injection. U.S.P.q.s.

For more information regarding AMVISC Plus or AMVISC viscoelastics contact: IOLAB, 500 IOLAB Drive, Claremont, California 91711. Toll free: 800-423-1871 ext. 1250. • In California: 800-352-1891 ext. 1250.

Refer to contents page for information on Pharmaceutical Products.

Optical Radiation Corporation

1300 OPTICAL DRIVE
AZUSA, CA 91702

ORCOLON®
(polyacrylamide)
For Anterior Segment Use Only

Description: ORCOLON (polyacrylamide) is a sterile, nonpyrogenic, viscoelastic preparation of highly purified, noninflammatory, high molecular weight polymer of polyacrylamide. ORCOLON contains 4.5% polyacrylamide dissolved in a physiologic balanced salt solution. Polyacrylamide is a linear homopolymer of acrylamide, made of carbon atoms which are commonly found in fatty acids, carotinoids and natural rubber. ORCOLON is essentially nonionic with a pH 7.2 ± 0.3 and a molecular weight of approximately one million. It is completely transparent and has a viscosity of 40,000 ± 10,000 centipoise and osmolarity of 340 (+40, −25) mOsm.
Indications: ORCOLON is indicated for use as a surgical aid in anterior segment procedures including cataract extractions and intraocular lens (IOL) implantation.
Actions: In cataract extractions, the instillation of ORCOLON may protect the corneal endothelium. When applied to the intraocular lens during primary or secondary lens implantation, ORCOLON may facilitate insertion. In all of these surgical procedures ORCOLON serves to maintain a deep anterior chamber during surgery, allowing for efficient manipulation with less trauma to the corneal endothelium and surrounding ocular structures.

Contraindications: Presently there are no known contrainindications to the use of ORCOLON when used as recommended.

Precautions: Precautions normally associated with the ophthalmic surgical procedure being performed are recommended.
There may be transient increased postoperative intraocular pressure as a result of preexisting glaucoma or due to the operative procedure itself. For these reasons, the following precautions should be considered:
- ORCOLON should be removed from the anterior chamber at the end of surgery by irrigation and aspiration.
- The intraocular pressure of postoperative patients should be carefully monitored.
- If the postoperative intraocular pressure increases above expected values, appropriate therapy should be administered.

Testing has not been done on the safety of ORCOLON with soft lens material.

Adverse Reactions: ORCOLON has been well tolerated after injection into human eyes. A transient rise in intraocular pressure postoperatively has been reported in some cases. Any adverse reactions observed, including but not limited to uncontrolled intraocular pressure, should be reported to Optical Radiation Corporation, 800 423-1887 (National) or 818 969-3355.

Clinical Application: ORCOLON may be injected into the anterior chamber prior to or following delivery of the crystalline lens. ORCOLON should be introduced slowly through a needle or cannula into the anterior chamber. In addition to maintaining a deep anterior chamber, the instillation of ORCOLON *prior* to delivery of the cataractous lens may provide additional protection to the corneal endothelium and other ocular tissues. ORCOLON may also be used to coat surgical instruments and intraocular lenses prior to insertion. ORCOLON may be injected at any time during intraocular surgery to maintain the anterior chamber or to replace fluids lost during the surgical procedure.
How Supplied: ORCOLON is a sterile, nonpyrogenic viscoelastic preparation of polyacrylamide supplied in disposable glass syringes, delivering 0.5 ml or 0.75 ml ployacrylamide dissolved in physiologic balanced salt solution). Each milliliter of ORCOLON contains 0.39% sodium chloride, 0.06% potassium chloride, 0.04% calcium chloride dihydrate, 0.02% magnesium chloride hexahydrate, 0.17% sodium citrate dihydrate, 0.39% sodium acetate trihydrate, 4.5% purified polyacrylamide polymer and sterile water. The containers are marked with lot number and expiration date. A sterile single-use cannula is also provided for instilling ORCOLON. ORCOLON is terminally sterilized.
Caution: Federal law (USA) restricts this device to sale by or on the order of a licensed physician.
For intraocular use.
Single use only.
Do not autoclave.
Store at room temperature (20°–35°C).
No refrigeration required.

Part 3 - Lens Care Products

Allergan Optical

A Division of Allergan, Inc.
2525 DUPONT DRIVE
P.O. BOX 19534
IRVINE, CA 92713-9534

ALLERGAN® HYDROCARE®
CLEANING AND DISINFECTING SOLUTION
For use with clear and tinted soft (hydrophilic) contact lenses in a chemical (not heat) lens care system.

Description: (Ingredients): Allergan HYDROCARE Cleaning and Disinfecting Solution is a sterile, isotonic, buffered solution that contains sodium bicarbonate; sodium phosphate, dibasic, anhydrous; sodium phosphate, monobasic; propylene glycol; polysorbate 80; special soluble polyhema; and hydrochloric acid with tris (2-hydroxyethyl) tallow ammonium chloride (0.013%); thimerosal (0.002%); and bis (2-hydroxyethyl) tallow ammonium chloride as preservatives.
Actions: Allergan HYDROCARE Cleaning and Disinfecting Solution loosens and removes accumulations of film, deposits and debris from your lenses and destroys harmful microorganisms on the surface of your lenses.
Indications (Uses): Use Allergan HYDROCARE Cleaning and Disinfecting Solution to clean, disinfect and store your soft (hydrophilic) contact lenses.
Contraindications (Reasons Not to Use): If you are allergic to mercury, which is in thimerosal, quaternary ammonium compounds, or to any other ingredient in Allergan HYDROCARE Cleaning and Disinfecting Solution, do not use this product.
Warnings: Problems with contact lenses and lens care products could result in serious injury to the eye. It is essential that you follow your eye care practitioner's directions and all labeling instructions for proper use and care of your lenses and lens care products, including the lens case. Eye problems, including corneal ulcers, can develop rapidly and lead to loss of vision.
Daily wear lenses are not indicated for overnight wear and should not be worn while sleeping. Clinical studies have shown the risk of serious adverse reactions is increased when these lenses are worn overnight.
Extended wear lenses should be regularly removed for cleaning and disinfection or for disposal and replacement on the schedule prescribed by your eye care practitioner. Clinical studies have shown that there is an increased incidence of serious adverse reactions in extended wear contact lens users as compared to daily wear contact lens users. Studies have also shown that the risk of serious adverse reactions increases the longer extended wear lenses are worn before removal for cleaning and disinfection or for disposal and replacement.
Studies have also shown that smokers had a higher incidence of adverse reactions.
If you experience eye discomfort, excessive tearing, vision changes, or redness of the eye, immediately remove your lenses and promptly contact your eye care practitioner.
It is recommended that contact lens wearers see their eye care practitioner twice each year or if directed, more frequently.
To avoid contamination, do not touch tip of container to any surface. Replace cap after using.
Precautions:
- Do not put this product in the eye. The red tip is to remind you not to put this product in your eye.
- Never reuse this solution.
- Keep out of the reach of children.
- Always wash, rinse and dry hands before handling lenses.
- After reapplying your lenses, always empty your lens storage case, rinse with sterile rinsing solution and allow to air dry.
- After using ALLERGAN® ENZYMATIC Contact Lens Cleaner for soft (hydrophilic) lenses each week to remove accumulated protein deposits, thoroughly rinse your lenses with LENS PLUS® Sterile Saline Solution, Allergan® HYDROCARE® Preserved Saline Solution, or other appropriate sterile saline solution before disinfecting.
- Do not let Allergan® HYDROCARE® Cleaning and Disinfecting Solution dry on the lenses.
- Store at room temperature.
- Use before the expiration date marked on the bottle and carton.

Note: This product is not recommended for use with crofilcon A (CSI® and AZTECH™)* lenses.
Adverse Reactions (Possible Problems) and What to Do:
The following problems may occur:
- Eyes stinging, burning, or itching (irritation).
- Excessive watering (tearing) of the eyes.
- Unusual eye secretions.
- Redness of the eyes.
- Reduced sharpness of vision (visual acuity).
- Blurred vision.
- Sensitivity to light (photophobia).
- Dry eyes.

If you notice any of the above problems, immediately remove and examine your lenses. If a lens appears to be damaged, do not reapply; consult your eye care practitioner. If the problem stops and the lenses appear to be undamaged, thoroughly clean, rinse and disinfect the lenses and reapply them. If the problem continues, immediately remove your lenses and consult your eye care practitioner.
If any of the above symptoms occur, a serious condition such as infection, corneal ulcer, neovascularization, or iritis may be present. Immediately remove your lenses and seek imme-

Continued on next page

Allergan Optical—Cont.

diate professional identification of the problem and begin treatment, if necessary, to avoid serious eye damage. For more information, see your **Instructions for Wearers** booklet for your specific contact lens type.

Directions For Use:

- Clean, rinse and disinfect your lenses each time you remove them.
- Always wash, rinse and dry hands before handling contact lenses.
- Always remove and clean the same lens first to avoid any mix-ups.

Prepare The Storage Case For Lens Disinfection:

- Fill each chamber of your lens storage case with Allergan® HYDROCARE® Cleaning and Disinfecting Solution.

Clean and Rinse Your Lenses:

- After you remove one lens, place it in the palm of your hand. Place 3 drops of LENS PLUS® Daily Cleaner or Allergan® HYDROCARE® Cleaning and Disinfecting Solution on each lens surface and rub for 20 seconds in the palm with your forefinger or between your thumb and forefinger. Then rinse the lens with LENS PLUS® Sterile Saline Solution. Place the lens in the appropriate chamber of your lens storage case. Repeat the cleaning and rinsing procedure with your other lens and place it in the proper chamber.

Disinfect and Store Your Lenses:

- Allow your lenses to soak a minimum of 4 hours in the cleaning and disinfecting solution for proper disinfection.
- Your lenses should always be stored in Allergan HYDROCARE Cleaning and Disinfecting Solution when you are not wearing them. If you do not intend to wear your lenses immediately following disinfection, you may store them in the unopened storage case until ready to wear later in the day.
  If the lenses have been stored in the unopened case for more than 24 hours, disinfect before wearing. Put fresh solution inside the lens storage case, completely covering the lenses, before disinfecting.
  If lenses will be stored for longer periods of time, disinfect once a week and before wearing.

Rinse and Wear:

- Since Allergan HYDROCARE Cleaning and Disinfecting Solution is not intended for use directly in the eye, lenses should be rinsed thoroughly with LENS PLUS® Sterile Saline Solution, Allergan® HYDROCARE® Preserved Saline solution or other appropriate saline solution before wearing.
  To prevent contamination and to help avoid serious eye injury, always empty and rinse lens case with sterile rinsing solution and allow to air dry.

How Supplied: Allergan HYDROCARE Cleaning and Disinfecting Solution is supplied in sterile 8 fl oz and 12 fl oz plastic bottles. The bottles and cartons are marked with lot number and expiration date.

Lenses: Allergan HYDROCARE Cleaning and Disinfecting Solution is for use with clear and tinted soft (hydrophilic) contact lenses.

* Trademarks of Sola/Barnes-Hind.

ALLERGAN® HYDROCARE® PRESERVED SALINE SOLUTION

For rinsing in conjunction with chemical disinfection and for rinsing, heat disinfection and storage of soft (hydrophilic) contact lenses. Regular use in your heat disinfection unit prevents calcium deposits from forming on soft contact lenses.

Description: Allergan HYDROCARE Preserved Saline Solution is a sterile, buffered, isotonic solution containing sodium chloride, sodium hexametaphosphate, boric acid and sodium borate with edetate disodium (0.01%) and thimerosal (0.001%) as preservatives and sodium hydroxide to adjust the pH.

Actions: Rinsing lenses with Allergan HYDROCARE Preserved Saline Solution after cleaning will remove loosened debris and traces of daily cleaning products. Disinfection of lenses is accomplished by immersing your lenses in Allergan HYDROCARE Preserved Saline Solution in an appropriate carrying case and heating them in your heat disinfection (heating) unit.

When used with your heat disinfection unit, the special sequestering agent in Allergan HYDROCARE Preserved Saline Solution prevents inorganic deposits such as calcium and rust from attaching to your soft contact lenses.

Indications (Uses): Allergan HYDROCARE Preserved Saline Solution is for use with soft (hydrophilic) contact lenses. It can be used for rinsing, heat disinfection, and storage. It may also serve as a rinsing solution in conjunction with chemical disinfection.

Regular use in your heat disinfection unit prevents calcium deposits from forming on soft contact lenses.

Contraindications (Reasons Not to Use):
If you are allergic to mercury, which is in thimerosal, or to any other ingredient in Allergan HYDROCARE Preserved Saline Solution, do not use this product.

Warnings: PROBLEMS WITH CONTACT LENSES AND LENS CARE PRODUCTS COULD RESULT IN SERIOUS INJURY TO THE EYE. It is essential that you follow your eye care practitioner's directions and all labeling instructions for proper use of your lenses and lens care products. **EYE PROBLEMS, INCLUDING CORNEAL ULCERS, CAN DEVELOP RAPIDLY AND LEAD TO LOSS OF VISION; THEREFORE, IF YOU EXPERIENCE EYE DISCOMFORT, EXCESSIVE TEARING, VISION CHANGES, OR REDNESS OF THE EYE, IMMEDIATELY REMOVE YOUR LENSES AND PROMPTLY CONTACT YOUR EYE CARE PRACTITIONER.**

All contact lens wearers must see their eye care practitioner as directed. If your lenses are for extended wear, your eye care practitioner may prescribe more frequent visits.

To avoid contamination, do not touch tip of container to any surface. Replace cap after using.

Precautions:

- Always wash, rinse and dry hands before handling lenses.
- Fresh Allergan HYDROCARE Preserved Saline Solution should be used daily. **Never reuse the solution.**
- To prevent buildup of calcium deposits which can damage lenses, this solution should be used daily. Do not wait until buildup occurs, since removal of established calcium deposits may reveal that permanent damage to your lenses has already occurred.
- After reapplying your lenses, always empty your lens storage case, rinse with sterile rinsing solution, and allow to air dry.
- Store at room temperature.
- Use before the expiration date marked on bottle and carton.

Adverse Reactions (Possible Problems) and What to Do:
The following problems may occur:

- Eyes stinging, burning, or itching (irritation)
- Excessive watering (tearing) of the eye
- Unusual eye secretions
- Redness of the eyes
- Reduced sharpness of vision (visual acuity)
- Blurred vision
- Sensitivity to light (photophobia)
- Dry eyes

If you notice any of the above problems, immediately remove and examine your lenses. If a lens appears to be damaged, do not reapply; consult your eye care practitioner. If the problem stops and the lenses appear to be undamaged, thoroughly clean, rinse and disinfect the lenses and reapply them. If the problem continues, immediately remove your lenses and consult your eye care practitioner.

If any of the above symptoms occur, a serious condition such as infection, corneal ulcer, neovascularization, or iritis may be present. Seek immediate professional identification of the problem and begin treatment, if necessary, to avoid serious eye damage. For more information, see your **Instructions for Wearers** booklet for your specific contact lens type.

Directions For Use:

- Always wash, rinse and dry hands before you handle your lenses.
- Clean, rinse, and disinfect your lenses each time you remove them.
- Clean and rinse one lens first (always the same lens first to avoid mix-ups) and put that lens into the correct chamber (section) of the lens storage case. Then repeat the procedure for the second lens.
- After you clean your lens, rinse it thoroughly with Allergan® HYDROCARE® Preserved Saline Solution by holding the lens between the forefinger and thumb of one hand and directing a steady stream onto the lens or placing the lens in the palm of one hand and directing a steady stream of Allergan HYDROCARE Preserved Saline Solution onto the lens.

Chemical Disinfection (Not Heat)

- Disinfect and store your lenses as directed by your eye care practitioner.
- Before reapplying your lenses, rinse the lenses thoroughly with Allergan® HYDROCARE® Preserved Saline Solution.
- After you remove your lenses from the lens case, empty and rinse your lens storage case with sterile saline solution and allow it to air dry. When you next use the case, refill it with fresh disinfecting solution.

Heat (Thermal) Disinfection

- Prepare the empty lens storage case. Wet the chambers of the case with Allergan HYDROCARE Preserved Saline Solution.
- Place each lens in its correct chamber of the storage case.
- Fill the chamber using enough Allergan HYDROCARE Preserved Saline Solution to completely cover the lens.
- Tightly close the top on the chamber.
- Repeat the above procedure for the second lens.
- Put the lens storage case into the disinfection unit and follow the directions for operating your unit.

Emergency (Alternate) Method for Heat (Thermal) Disinfection
If your heat disinfection unit is not available, place the tightly closed lens storage case which contains the lenses into a pan of already boiling water. Leave the closed lens case in the pan of boiling water for at least 10 minutes. (Above an altitude of 7,000 feet, boil for at least 15 minutes.) Be careful not to allow the water to boil away. Remove the pan from the heat and allow it to cool for 30 minutes to complete the disinfection of the lenses.

NOTE: USE OF THE HEAT DISINFECTION UNIT SHOULD BE RESUMED AS SOON AS POSSIBLE.

- Leave the lenses in the unopened storage case until ready to put on your eyes. Before reapplying the lenses, rinsing is not necessary unless your eye care practitioner recommends rinsing.
  Clean soft contact lenses weekly with ALLERGAN® ENZYMATIC Contact Lens

Cleaner to remove tear protein deposits which can damage your lenses, impair your vision and reduce comfort.

How Supplied: Allergan HYDROCARE Preserved Saline Solution is supplied in 8 fl oz and 12 fl oz plastic bottles. Bottles and cartons are marked with lot number and expiration date.

Lenses: Allergan HYDROCARE Preserved Saline Solution is for use with soft (hydrophilic) contact lenses.

U.S. Patent No. 4,395,346

ALLERGAN® ENZYMATIC

Contact Lens Cleaner

For use with soft (hydrophilic) contact lenses.

Description: ALLERGAN® ENZYMATIC Contact Lens Cleaner is a round tablet containing the enzyme papain, sodium chloride, sodium carbonate, sodium borate, and edetate disodium.

Action: ALLERGAN® ENZYMATIC Contact Lens Cleaner removes protein deposits from the surface of daily wear and extended wear soft (hydrophilic) contact lenses. It safely and effectively removes protein and reduces its buildup on your lenses when used as directed.

Indications: Use ALLERGAN® ENZYMATIC Contact Lens Cleaner prepared with **sterile saline solution** once a week to reduce protein buildup for clear vision and comfortable lens wear.

Contraindications: Do not use this product if you are allergic to any of its ingredients. If you are allergic to any ingredient in one sterile saline solution, use another appropriate sterile saline solution for soft contact lenses to prepare the enzymatic cleaning solution.

Warnings: This product contains the enzyme papain. Do not use this product if you are allergic to papain.

LENSES MUST BE RINSED AND DISINFECTED FOLLOWING EACH ENZYMATIC CLEANING CYCLE. FAILURE TO DISINFECT MAY CAUSE IRRITATION AND DISCOMFORT. DO NOT INSTILL THE ENZYMATIC CLEANING SOLUTION DIRECTLY INTO THE EYE.

NEVER USE DISTILLED WATER TO DISSOLVE THE TABLETS. DISTILLED WATER IS NOT STERILE. USE OF A NON-STERILE PRODUCT IN THE PREPARATION OF SOFT CONTACT LENS SOLUTIONS MAY LEAD TO MICROBIAL CONTAMINATION OF LENSES WHICH CAN CAUSE SERIOUS EYE INFECTIONS.

PROBLEMS WITH CONTACT LENSES AND LENS CARE PRODUCTS COULD RESULT IN SERIOUS INJURY TO THE EYE. It is essential that you follow your eye care practitioner's directions and all labeling instructions for proper use of your lenses and lens care products, including the lens case. **EYE PROBLEMS, INCLUDING CORNEAL ULCERS, CAN DEVELOP RAPIDLY AND LEAD TO LOSS OF VISION.** Daily wear lenses are not indicated for overnight wear and should not be worn while sleeping. Clinical studies have shown the risk of serious adverse reactions is increased when these lenses are worn overnight.

Extended wear lenses should be regularly removed for cleaning and disinfection or for disposal and replacement on the schedule prescribed by your eye care practitioner. Clinical studies have shown that there is an increased incidence of serious adverse reactions in extended wear contact lens users as compared to daily wear contact lens users. Studies have also shown that the risk of serious adverse reactions increases the longer extended wear lenses are worn before removal for cleaning and disinfection or for disposal and replacement.

Studies have also shown that smokers had a higher incidence of adverse reactions. If you experience eye discomfort, excessive tearing, vision changes or redness of the eye, immediately remove your lenses and promptly contact your eye care practitioner.

It is recommended that contact lens wearers see their eye care practitioner twice each year or if directed, more frequently.

Precautions:

- Do not soak low water content (less than 55%) contact lenses longer than 12 hours. If you are unsure of the type of lens you wear, consult your eye care practitioner.
- Do not soak high water content (55% or more) contact lenses longer than 2 hours, otherwise ocular irritation may result. Should ocular irritation occur, immediately remove your contact lenses, clean and disinfect the lenses again and reapply. If irritation continues, remove your lenses and consult your eye care practitioner.
- KEEP OUT OF THE REACH OF CHILDREN.
- Do not take tablets internally.
- Do not use brown or otherwise discolored tablets.
- Avoid excessive heat.
- Always wash, rinse and dry hands before handling lenses.
- Lenses should **never** be placed on the eye directly from the enzymatic cleaning solution.
- **Use only sterile saline solution and the special vials provided to prepare the enzymatic cleaning solution. Do not use anything else to dissolve the tablets or any other containers.**
- Use only freshly prepared enzymatic cleaning solution and discard immediately after use.
- Use before expiration date on foil wrapper and unit carton.

Adverse Reactions (Possible Problems) and What to Do:

The following problems may occur:

- Eyes stinging, burning or itching (irritation)
- Excessive watering (tearing) of the eyes
- Unusual eye secretions
- Redness of the eyes
- Reduced sharpness of vision (visual acuity)
- Blurred vision
- Sensitivity to light (photophobia)
- Dry eyes

If you notice any of the above problems, a serious condition such as infection, corneal ulcer, neovascularization or iritis may be present. IMMEDIATELY remove and examine your lenses. If your lenses appear to be damaged, do not reapply; consult your eye care practitioner. If the problem stops and the lenses appear to be undamaged, thoroughly clean, rinse and disinfect the lenses and reapply them. If the problem continues, immediately remove the lenses and consult your eye care practitioner for identification of the problem and, if necessary, obtain treatment to avoid serious eye damage.

Directions: Your lenses must be cleaned using the special vials included in the cleaning kit. If you are using a refill package, transfer the vials from the previous kit you received to the receptacle in this package. Do not use any other containers.

Clean your lenses with ALLERGAN® ENZYMATIC Contact Lens Cleaner once a week, or more often if needed, as follows.

USE ONLY STERILE SALINE SOLUTION TO DISSOLVE THE TABLETS.

1. Vigorously rinse each vial with sterile saline solution. Then examine for cleanliness. Next, fill with sterile saline solution up to the fill line indicated on the vial. Drop one tablet into each vial. The tablet will effervesce (fizz) and quickly dissolve. Always use fresh solution for each enzymatic cleaning cycle.
2. Remove one lens at a time and clean with daily cleaner or sterile saline solution in the manner recommended by your eye care practitioner. Then rinse each lens thoroughly with sterile saline solution.
3. Place each lens in the appropriate vial (R for right. L for left lens).
4. Place the caps on the vials and shake to ensure thorough mixing.

   Low Water Content (less than 55%) Contact Lenses

   Soak lenses a minimum of 2 hours. Do not soak lenses in the enzymatic cleaning solution for more than 12 hours. (See Precautions)

   High Water Content (55% or more) Contact Lenses

   Soak lenses for 15 minutes to a maximum of 2 hours. (See Precautions)

   The enzymatic cleaning solution is not intended for the storage of lenses.
5. After the required soaking interval, remove the lenses from the enzymatic cleaning solution. **Rinse the lenses thoroughly with sterile saline solution and rub gently with your fingertips to remove debris and traces of the enzymatic cleaning solution. Disinfect lenses as directed by your eye care practitioner.**
6. Pour out the remaining solution, rinse the vials thoroughly with sterile saline solution and allow to air dry. **Do not use soap or detergent.**

Note: The enzymatic cleaning solution has a characteristic odor. This odor is normal. More than one enzymatic cleaning cycle may be required to adequately clean your lenses. Lenses must be disinfected in the usual way prior to reapplication.

How Supplied: In kits of 12 and 48 tablets including vials. (Promotional packages of tablets may not contain vials.) Also in refill packages of 24 and 36 tablets.

Avoid excessive heat.

Lenses: ALLERGAN® ENZYMATIC Contact Lens Cleaner is for use with soft (hydrophilic) contact lenses.

U.S. Patent 3,910,296

ALLERGAN®
SORBI•CARE®
SALINE SOLUTION

For rinsing, heat disinfection and storage of soft (hydrophilic) contact lenses. Regular use in your heat disinfection unit prevents calcium deposits from forming on soft contact lenses. May also be used as a rinsing solution in conjunction with chemical disinfection.

Description (ingredients): Allergan Sorbi-Care Saline Solution is a sterile, buffered, isotonic solution containing sodium chloride, sodium hexametaphosphate, boric acid and sodium borate, with sorbic acid (0.1%) as the preservative.

Allergan Sorbi-Care Saline Solution does *not* contain thimerosal, any other mercury-containing ingredients, or chlorhexidine. Therefore, the possibility of allergic hypersensitivity reaction to Allergan Sorbi-Care Saline Solution is reduced.

Actions: Rinsing lenses with Allergan Sorbi-Care Saline Solution after cleaning will remove loosened debris and traces of daily cleaning products. Disinfection of lenses is accomplished by immersing your lenses in Allergan Sorbi-Care Saline Solution in an appropriate carrying case and heating them in your heat disinfection (heating) unit.

When used with your heat disinfection unit, the special sequestering agent in Allergan Sorbi-Care Saline Solution prevents inorganic deposits such as calcium and rust from attaching to your soft contact lenses.

Indications (Uses): Allergan Sorbi-Care Saline Solution is for use with soft (hydrophilic)

Continued on next page

Allergan Optical—Cont.

contact lenses. It can be used for rinsing, heat disinfection, and storage. It may also serve as a rinsing solution in conjunction with chemical disinfection.

Regular use in your heat disinfection unit prevents calcium deposits from forming on soft contact lenses.

Contraindications (Reasons Not to Use): If you are allergic to any ingredient in Allergan Sorbi-Care Saline Solution do not use this product.

Warnings: PROBLEMS WITH CONTACT LENSES AND LENS CARE PRODUCTS COULD RESULT IN SERIOUS INJURY TO THE EYE. It is essential that you follow your eye care practitioner's directions and all labeling instructions for proper use of your lenses and lens care products. **EYE PROBLEMS, INCLUDING CORNEAL ULCERS, CAN DEVELOP RAPIDLY AND LEAD TO LOSS OF VISION; THEREFORE, IF YOU EXPERIENCE EYE DISCOMFORT, EXCESSIVE TEARING, VISION CHANGES, OR REDNESS OF THE EYE, IMMEDIATELY REMOVE YOUR LENSES AND PROMPTLY CONTACT YOUR EYE CARE PRACTITIONER.** All contact lens wearers must see their eye care practitioner as directed. If your lenses are for extended wear, your eye care practitioner may prescribe more frequent visits.

To avoid contamination, do not touch tip of container to any surface. Replace cap after using.

Precautions:

- Always wash, rinse and dry hands before handling lenses.
- Fresh Allergan Sorbi-Care Saline Solution should be used daily. Never reuse the solution.
- To prevent buildup of calcium deposits which can damage lenses, this solution should be used daily. Do not wait until buildup occurs, since removal of established calcium deposits may reveal that permanent damage to your lenses has already occurred.
- Keep out of the reach of children.
- After reapplying your lenses, always empty your lens storage case, rinse with sterile rinsing solution, and allow to air dry.
- Store at room temperature.
- Use before the expiration date marked on bottle and carton.

Adverse Reactions (Possible Problems) and What to Do: The following problems may occur:

- Eyes stinging, burning, or itching (irritation)
- Excessive watering (tearing) of the eye
- Unusual eye secretions
- Redness of the eyes
- Reduced sharpness of vision (visual acuity)
- Blurred vision
- Sensitivity to light (photophobia)
- Dry eyes

If you notice any of the above problems, immediately remove and examine your lenses. If a lens appears to be damaged, do not reapply; consult your eye care practitioner. If the problem stops and the lenses appear to be undamaged, thoroughly clean, rinse and disinfect the lenses and reapply them. If the problem continues, immediately remove your lenses and consult your eye care practitioner.

If any of the above symptoms occur, a serious condition such as infection, corneal ulcer, neovascularization, or iritis may be present. Immediately remove your lenses and seek immediate professional identification of the problem and, if necessary, obtain treatment to avoid serious eye damage. For more information, see your **Instructions for Wearers** booklet **for your specific contact lenses.**

Directions:

- Always wash, rinse and dry hands before you handle your lenses.
- Clean, rinse and disinfect your lenses each time you remove them.
- Clean and rinse the same lens first to avoid mix-ups and put that lens into the appropriate chamber (section) of the lens storage case. Then repeat the procedure for the other lens.
- After you clean your lens, rinse it thoroughly with Allergan® Sorbi-Care® Saline Solution by holding the lens between the forefinger and thumb of one hand and directing a steady stream onto the lens or placing the lens in the palm of one hand and directing a steady stream of Allergan Sorbi-Care Saline Solution onto the lens.

Heat (Thermal) Disinfection

- Prepare the empty lens storage case. Wet the chambers of the case with Allergan® Sorbi-Care® Saline Solution.
- Place each lens in its correct chamber of the storage case.
- Fill the chamber using enough Allergan Sorbi-Care Saline Solution to completely cover the lens.
- Tightly close the top on the chamber.
- Repeat the above procedure for the second lens.
- Put the lens storage case into the disinfection unit and follow the directions for operating your unit.

Emergency (Alternate) Method for Heat (Thermal) Disinfection

If your heat disinfection unit is not available, place the tightly closed storage case which contains the lenses into a pan of already boiling water. Leave the closed lens case in the pan of boiling water for at least 10 minutes. (Above an altitude of 7,000 feet, boil for at least 15 minutes.) Be careful not to allow the water to boil away. Remove the pan from the heat and allow it to cool for 30 minutes to complete the disinfection of the lenses.

NOTE: USE OF THE HEAT DISINFECTION UNIT SHOULD BE RESUMED AS SOON AS POSSIBLE.

- Leave the lenses in the unopened storage case until ready to put on your eyes. Rinsing is not necessary before reapplication of the lenses, unless your eye care practitioner recommends rinsing.
- Clean soft contact lenses weekly with ALLERGAN® ENZYMATIC Contact Lens Cleaner to remove tear-protein deposits which can damage your lenses, impair your vision and reduce comfort.

Chemical Disinfection (Not Heat)

- Disinfect and store your lenses as directed by your eye care practitioner.
- **Before reapplying** your lenses, **rinse** the lenses **thoroughly** with Allergan® Sorbi-Care® Saline Solution.
- After you remove your lenses from the lens case, empty and rinse your lens storage case and allow it to air dry. When you next use the case, refill it with **fresh** disinfecting solution.
- Clean soft contact lenses weekly with ALLERGAN® ENZYMATIC Contact Lens Cleaner to remove tear-protein deposits which can damage your lenses, impair vision and reduce comfort.

How Supplied: Allergan Sorbi-Care Saline Solution is supplied in 8 fl oz (237 mL) plastic bottles. Bottles and cartons are marked with lot number and expiration date.

Lenses: Allergan® Sorbi-Care® Saline Solution is for use with soft (hydrophilic) contact lenses.

U.S. Patent No. 4,395,346

BLINK-N-CLEAN®
Hard Contact Lens Solution

Description: Blink-N-Clean Hard Contact Lens Solution gives the lens wearer increased comfort by quickly cleaning and rewetting the lenses. . . while they are still in the eye.

Directions: 1–2 drops in eye(s) as needed, up to 6 times a day.

Contains: Polyoxyl 40 stearate and polyethylene glycol 300 in a sterile, buffered solution with chlorobutanol 0.5% (chloral deriv.) as a preservative.

Note: Not for use with soft contact lenses. Do not touch dropper tip to any surface, since this may contaminate the solution. Keep bottle tightly closed.

How Supplied: ¼ fl oz and ½ fl oz bottles.

CLEAN-N-SOAK®
Hard Contact Lens Cleaning and Soaking Solution

Description: Clean-N-Soak Hard Contact Lens Cleaning and Soaking Solution removes dirt and residue and provides an antiseptic soaking and conditioning solution for hard contact lenses.

Contains: Cleaning agent, phenylmercuric nitrate (0.004%) in a sterile, buffered solution.

Directions: Wash and rinse hands thoroughly before handling lenses. Fill storage case with enough solution to completely cover lenses. Soak lenses at least four hours. Rinse lenses with an appropriate rinsing solution as recommended by your eye care practitioner and wet with Liquifilm® Wetting Solution. Solution should be changed daily.

Use LC-65® Daily Contact Lens Cleaner as a super cleaner for stubborn deposits.

Warnings: To avoid contamination, do not touch tip of container to any surface. Replace cap after using. Not for use with soft (hydrophilic) contact lenses. Do not put this product in the eye. The red tip is to remind you not to put this product in your eye.

How Supplied: 4 fl oz bottle.

CLEAN-N-SOAKIT®
Hard Contact Lens Storage Case

Convenient to carry because it is leakproof and compact.

Ideal for overnight storage because it holds enough solution to completely immerse lenses for thorough cleaning and disinfecting.

Maintains good lens hygiene because it is boilable and its removable parts make it easy to clean.

Not for use with soft contact lenses.

CLEAN-N-STOW®
Hard Contact Lens Storage Case

Convenient to carry because it's leakproof and compact. Ideal for overnight storage because it holds enough solution to completely immerse contact lenses for thorough cleaning and disinfecting.

Maintains good lens hygiene because it is boilable and its removable parts make it easy to clean.

Not for use with soft contact lenses.

EASYCLEAN/GP®
Daily Cleaner
For use with rigid gas permeable contact lenses* and hard contact lenses.
Preservative Free.

Description: EasyClean/GP® Daily Cleaner is a sterile, surface-active buffered solution containing cocoamphocarboxyglycinate (and) sodium lauryl sulfate (and) hexylene glycol, sodium chloride, sodium phosphate and edetate disodium.

ctions: EasyClean/GP Daily Cleaner is pecially formulated for gentle but efficient leaning of rigid gas permeable contact lenses* nd hard contact lenses. It safely removes the ay's accumulation of undesirable film and eposits within seconds. Daily use of Easy-lean/GP Daily Cleaner leaves lenses opti-ally clear, more wettable and more comfort-ble.

asyClean/GP Daily Cleaner is useful for lens earers with a history of sensitivity to mer-ury (thimerosal) or other preservatives pres-nt in other daily cleaners.

ndications (Uses): Use EasyClean/GP Daily leaner every day to clean your rigid gas per-neable contact lenses* or hard contact lenses efore rinsing and disinfection.

ontraindications (Reasons Not to Use): If ou are allergic to any ingredient in Easy-lean/GP Daily Cleaner, do not use this prod-ct.

arnings: PROBLEMS WITH CONTACT ENSES AND LENS CARE PRODUCTS OULD RESULT IN SERIOUS INJURY TO HE EYE. It is essential that you follow your ye care practitioner's directions and all label-ng instructions for proper use of your lenses nd lens care products. **EYE PROBLEMS, IN-LUDING CORNEAL ULCERS, CAN DE-ELOP RAPIDLY AND LEAD TO LOSS OF ISION; THEREFORE, IF YOU EXPERIENCE YE DISCOMFORT, EXCESSIVE TEARING, ISION CHANGES, OR REDNESS OF THE YE, IMMEDIATELY REMOVE YOUR LENSES ND PROMPTLY CONTACT YOUR EYE ARE PRACTITIONER.**

ll contact lens wearers must see their eye are practitioner as directed. If your lenses are or extended wear, your eye care practitioner ay prescribe more frequent visits.

o avoid contamination, do not touch tip of ontainer to any surface. Replace cap after sing.

recautions

- Do not put this product in the eye.
- Always wash, rinse and dry hands before handling lenses.
- Do not allow EasyClean/GP Daily Cleaner to dry on your lenses.
- Keep out of the reach of children.
- Store at room temperature.
- Use before the expiration date stamped on the bottle.
- Never wet contact lenses with saliva or place lenses in your mouth.

dverse Reactions (Possible Problems) and hat to Do: The following problems may ccur:

- Eyes stinging, burning, or itching (irritation)
- Excessive watering (tearing) of the eye
- Unusual eye secretions
- Redness of the eyes
- Reduced sharpness of vision (visual acuity)
- Blurred vision
- Sensitivity to light (photophobia)
- Dry eyes

f you notice any of the above problems, imme-iately remove and examine your lenses. If a ens appears to be damaged, do not reapply; onsult your eye care practitioner. If the prob-em stops and the lenses appear to be unda-naged, thoroughly clean, rinse and disinfect he lenses and reapply them. If the problem ontinues, immediately remove your lenses nd consult your eye care practitioner.

f any of the above symptoms occur, a serious ondition such as infection, corneal ulcer, neo-ascularization, or iritis may be present. Im-nediately remove your lenses and seek imme-iate professional identification of the problem nd, if necessary, obtain treatment to avoid erious eye damage. For more information, see our *Instructions for Wearers* booklet for your pecific contact lenses.

Directions For Use:

- Clean, rinse and disinfect your lenses each time you remove them.
- Always wash, rinse and dry hands before handling contact lenses.
- Always remove and clean the same lens first to avoid any mix-ups.

Prepare The Storage Case For Lens Disinfection:

- Fill each chamber of your lens storage case with Wet-N-Soak™ Wetting and Soaking Solution or other appropriate soaking solution.

Clean and Rinse Your Lenses:

- After you remove one lens, place it in the palm of your hand. Place 3 drops of Easy-Clean/GP® Daily Cleaner on each lens surface and rub for 20 seconds in the palm with your forefinger or between your thumb and forefinger. Rinse lenses thoroughly with an appropriate rinsing solution as directed by your eye care practitioner. Place the lens in the appropriate chamber of your lens case. Repeat the cleaning and rinsing procedure with your other lens and place it in the proper chamber.

Disinfect And Store Your Lenses:

- Be sure the lenses are completely covered with soaking solution before firmly tightening the caps. Disinfect and store your lenses as recommended by your eye care practitioner.

Clean FluoroPerm® and silicone acrylate rigid gas permeable lenses weekly with Pro-Free/GP® Weekly Enzymatic Cleaner to reduce the buildup of tear-protein deposits which can impair vision and reduce comfort.

How Supplied: EasyClean/GP® Daily Cleaner is supplied in 1 fl oz (30 mL) plastic bottles. The bottles and cartons are marked with lot number and expiration date.

Lenses: EasyClean/GP® Daily Cleaner is for use with rigid gas permeable contact lenses* and hard contact lenses.

*The following rigid gas permeable contact lenses are recommended for use with Easy-Clean/GP: ALLERGAN ADVENT®, Fluoro-Perm® and silicone acrylate lenses (including Polycon®, Paraperm®, Ocusil™, Optacryl and Boston®). Consult your eye care practitioner to identify the lens you wear.

FluoroPerm, Polycon, Paraperm and Boston are trademarks of other companies.

EXTENZYME®

Protein Cleaner*

For use with extended wear soft (hydrophilic) contact lenses.

Description: EXTENZYME® Protein Cleaner is a round tablet containing the enzyme papain, sodium chloride, sodium carbonate, sodium borate, and edetate disodium.

Actions: EXTENZYME Protein Cleaner removes protein deposits from the surface of extended wear soft (hydrophilic) contact lenses. It safely and effectively removes protein and reduces its buildup on your lenses when used as directed.

Indications: Use EXTENZYME Protein Cleaner prepared with **sterile saline solution** once a week for 15 minutes when starting with new, clean lenses to reduce protein buildup for clear vision and comfortable soft contact lens wear. If lenses are worn for more than 7 days without removal or have heavy protein deposits, EXTENZYME Protein Cleaner prepared with sterile saline solution should be used for 2 hours.

Contraindications: Do not use this product if you are allergic to any of its ingredients. If you are allergic to any ingredient in one sterile saline solution, use another appropriate sterile saline solution for soft contact lenses to prepare the enzymatic cleaning solution.

Warnings: This product contains the enzyme papain. Do not use this product if you are allergic to papain.

Lenses must be rinsed and disinfected following each enzymatic cleaning cycle. **DO NOT INSTILL THE ENZYMATIC CLEANING SOLUTION DIRECTLY INTO THE EYE.**

NEVER USE DISTILLED WATER TO DISSOLVE THE TABLETS. DISTILLED WATER IS NOT STERILE. USE OF A NON-STERILE PRODUCT IN THE PREPARATION OF SOFT CONTACT LENS SOLUTIONS MAY LEAD TO MICROBIAL CONTAMINATION OF LENSES WHICH CAN CAUSE SERIOUS EYE INFECTIONS.

PROBLEMS WITH CONTACT LENSES AND LENS CARE PRODUCTS COULD RESULT IN SERIOUS INJURY TO THE EYE. It is essential that you follow your eye care practitioner's directions and all labeling instructions for proper use of your lenses and lens care products. **EYE PROBLEMS, INCLUDING CORNEAL ULCERS, CAN DEVELOP RAPIDLY AND LEAD TO LOSS OF VISION; THEREFORE, IF YOU EXPERIENCE EYE DISCOMFORT, EXCESSIVE TEARING, VISION CHANGES, OR REDNESS OF THE EYE, IMMEDIATELY REMOVE YOUR LENSES AND PROMPTLY CONTACT YOUR EYE CARE PRACTITIONER.**

All contact lens wearers must see their eye care practitioner as directed. If your lenses are for extended wear, your eye care practitioner may prescribe more frequent visits.

Do not soak lenses longer than 2 hours in sterile saline solution as directed. Soaking extended wear soft (hydrophilic) lenses for longer periods may result in ocular irritation. Should this occur, proceed to clean, rinse, and disinfect your lenses according to recommended procedures.

Precautions:

- KEEP OUT OF THE REACH OF CHILDREN.
- Do not take tablets internally.
- Do not use brown or otherwise discolored tablets.
- Avoid excessive heat.
- Always wash, rinse and dry hands before handling lenses.
- Lenses must be disinfected following each enzymatic cleaning cycle.
- Do not soak lenses longer than the required soaking times stated in the directions section of this insert. Soaking extended wear soft (hydrophilic) lenses for longer periods may result in ocular irritation.
- Lenses should never be placed on the eye directly from the enzymatic cleaning solution.
- THE ENZYMATIC CLEANING CYCLE IS NOT A SUBSTITUTE FOR DISINFECTION OF YOUR LENSES. After enzymatic cleaning, lenses must be gently rubbed, then rinsed with sterile saline solution, and disinfected in the usual way prior to reapplication.
- Use only sterile saline solution and the special vials provided to prepare the enzymatic cleaning solution. Do not use anything else to dissolve the tablets or any other containers.
- Use only freshly prepared enzymatic cleaning solution and discard immediately after use.
- Use before expiration date on foil wrapper and unit carton.

Adverse Reactions (Possible Problems) and What to Do:

The following problems may occur:

- Eyes stinging, burning or itching (irritation)
- Excessive watering (tearing) of the eyes
- Reduced sharpness of vision (visual acuity)
- Sensitivity to light (photophobia)
- Unusual eye secretions

Continued on next page

Allergan Optical—Cont.

- Redness of the eyes
- Blurred vision
- Dry eyes

If you notice any of the above problems, a serious condition such as infection, corneal ulcer, neovascularization or iritis may be present. IMMEDIATELY remove and examine your lenses. If a lens appears to be damaged, do not reapply; consult your eye care practitioner. If the problem stops and the lenses appear to be undamaged, thoroughly clean, rinse and disinfect the lenses and reapply them. If the problem continues, IMMEDIATELY remove the lenses and consult your eye care practitioner for identification of the problem and, if necessary, obtain treatment to avoid serious eye damage.

Directions: Your lenses must be cleaned using the special vials included in the cleaning kit. Do not use any other containers. If you are using a refill package, transfer the vials from the previous kit you received to the receptacle in this package.

USE ONLY STERILE SALINE SOLUTION TO DISSOLVE THE TABLETS.

1. Vigorously rinse each vial with sterile saline solution. Then examine for cleanliness. Next, fill with sterile saline solution‡ up to the fill line indicated on the vial. Drop one tablet into each vial. The tablet will effervesce (fizz) and quickly dissolve. Always prepare fresh solution for each enzymatic cleaning cycle.
2. Remove one lens at a time and clean with daily cleaner or sterile saline solution in the manner recommended by your eye care practitioner.† Then rinse each lens thoroughly with sterile saline solution.
3. Place each lens in the appropriate vial (R for right, L for left lens).
4. Place the caps on the vials and shake to ensure thorough mixing.
   If you remove your lenses at least once a week, and they are new or protein-free, soak lenses for 15 minutes.
   If you wear your lenses for more than 7 days in a row, or if your lenses have heavy protein deposits, soak lenses for 2 hours to ensure effective cleaning.
   The enzymatic cleaning solution is not intended for the storage of lenses.
5. After the required soaking interval, remove the lenses from the enzymatic cleaning solution. Rinse the lenses thoroughly with sterile saline solution and rub gently with your fingertips to remove debris and traces of the enzymatic cleaning solution. Disinfect lenses as directed by your eye care practitioner.
6. Pour out the remaining solution, rinse the vials thoroughly with sterile saline solution and allow to air dry. Do not use soap or detergent.
   Note: The enzymatic cleaning solution has a characteristic odor. This odor is normal. More than one complete enzymatic cleaning cycle may be required to adequately clean your lenses. Lenses must be disinfected in the usual way prior to reapplication.

How Supplied: In cartons of 24 EXTENZYME® Protein Cleaner tablets including vials.
Avoid excessive heat.

Lenses: EXTENZYME® Protein Cleaner is for use with extended wear soft (hydrophilic) contact lenses.

* U.S. Patent 3,910,296.

† LENS PLUS® Daily Cleaner, LC-65® Daily Contact Lens Cleaner, Lens Clear® Soft Contact Lens Cleaner or any other commercially available soft contact lens daily cleaner can be used in place of sterile saline solution to clean lenses. However, lenses should always be rinsed with sterile saline solution after cleaning.

‡ LENS PLUS® Sterile Saline Solution, Allergan® HYDROCARE® Preserved Saline Solution, Allergan® Sorbi-Care® Saline Solution or any other sterile saline solution for soft contact lenses may be used to prepare the enzymatic cleaning solution when indicated.

LC–65®

Daily Contact Lens Cleaner

For use with gas permeable*, hard and soft (hydrophilic) contact lenses.

Description: LC-65® Daily Contact Lens Cleaner is a sterile, surface active, stabilized, buffered solution containing a cleaning agent, thimerosal 0.001% as the preservative, and edetate disodium.

Actions: LC-65 is especially formulated for gentle but efficient cleaning of gas permeable, hard and soft (hydrophilic) contact lenses. It safely removes the day's accumulation of undesirable film and deposits within seconds. Daily use of LC-65 leaves lenses optically clear, more wettable and more comfortable.

Indications (Uses): Use LC-65 every day to clean your gas permeable*, hard and soft (hydrophilic) contact lenses before rinsing and disinfection.

Contraindications (Reasons Not to Use): If you are allergic to mercury (which is in thimerosal) or any other ingredient in LC-65, do not use this product.

Warnings: Problems with contact lenses and lens care products could result in serious injury to the eye. It is essential that you follow your eye care practitioner's directions and all labeling instructions for proper use of your lenses and lens care products, including the lens case. Eye problems, including corneal ulcers, can develop rapidly and lead to loss of vision. Daily wear lenses are not indicated for overnight wear and should not be worn while sleeping. Clinical studies have shown the risk of serious adverse reactions is increased when these lenses are worn overnight.

Extended wear lenses should be regularly removed for cleaning and disinfection or for disposal and replacement on the schedule prescribed by your eye care practitioner. Clinical studies have shown that there is an increased incidence of serious adverse reactions in extended wear contact lens users as compared to daily wear contact lens users. Studies have also shown that the risk of serious adverse reactions increases the longer extended wear lenses are worn before removal for cleaning and disinfection or for disposal and replacement.

Studies have also shown that smokers had a higher incidence of adverse reactions.

If you experience eye discomfort, excessive tearing, vision changes, or redness of the eye, immediately remove your lenses and promptly contact your eye care practitioner.

It is recommended that contact lens wearers see their eye care practitioner twice each year or if directed, more frequently.

To avoid contamination, do not touch tip of container to any surface. Replace cap after using.

Precautions:

- Do not put this product in the eye. The red tip is to remind you not to put this product in your eye.
- Always wash, rinse and dry hands before handling lenses.
- Do not allow LC-65 to dry on your lenses.
- Keep out of the reach of children.
- Store at room temperature.
- Use before the expiration date stamped on bottle.
- Never wet contact lenses with saliva or plac lenses in your mouth.
- Soft (hydrophilic) contact lenses shoul never be rinsed with water.

Adverse Reactions (Possible Problems) an What to Do: The following problems ma occur:

- Eyes stinging, burning, or itching (irritatior
- Excessive watering (tearing) of the eye
- Unusual eye secretions
- Redness of the eyes
- Reduced sharpness of vision (visual acuity
- Blurred vision
- Sensitivity to light (photophobia)
- Dry eyes

If you notice any of the above problems, immediately remove and examine your lenses. If lens appears to be damaged, do not reapply consult your eye care practitioner. If the problem stops and the lenses appear to be undamaged, thoroughly clean, rinse and disinfec the lenses and reapply them. If the problen continues, immediately remove your lense and consult your eye care practitioner.

If any of the above symptoms occur, a seriou condition such as infection, corneal ulcer, neovascularization, or iritis may be present. Immediately remove your lenses and seek immediate professional identification of the problen and, if necessary, obtain treatment to avoi serious eye damage. For more information, se your **Instructions for Wearers** booklet for you specific contact lenses.

Directions For Use:

- Clean, rinse and disinfect your lenses eac time you remove them.
- Always wash, rinse and dry hands befor handling contact lenses.
- Always remove and clean the same lens firs to avoid mix-ups.

Gas Permeable* And Hard Contact Lenses

Prepare The Storage Case For Lens Disinfection:

- Fill each chamber of your lens storage cas with Wet-N-Soak PLUS™ Wetting an Soaking Solution or other appropriate soaking solution.

Clean and Rinse Your Lenses:

- After you remove one lens, place it in th palm of your hand. Place three drops of LC 65® Daily Contact Lens Cleaner on eac lens surface and rub for 20 seconds in th palm with your forefinger or between you thumb and forefinger. Rinse hard and ga permeable lenses with Wet-N-Soak PLUS™ Wetting and Soaking Solution or other ap propriate rinsing solution. Place the lens i the appropriate chamber of your lens case Repeat the cleaning and rinsing procedur with your other lens and place it in th proper chamber.

Disinfect And Store Your Lenses:

- Be sure the lenses are completely coverec with soaking solution before firmly tightening the caps. Disinfect and store your lense as recommended by your eye care practitioner.

Clean gas permeable lenses** weekly with Pro Free/GP® Weekly Enzymatic Cleaner to re duce the buildup of tear-protein deposits whict can impair vision and reduce comfort.

Soft (Hydrophilic) Contact Lenses

Prepare The Storage Case For Lens Disinfection:

- For HEAT DISINFECTION, fill each chamber of your lens storage case with fresh LENS PLUS® Sterile Saline Solution o other appropriate saline solution. FOF CHEMICAL DISINFECTION, fill lens cas with Allergan® HYDROCARE® Cleaning and Disinfecting Solution or other appropri ate disinfecting solution.

Clean and Rinse Your Lenses:

- After you remove one lens, place it in th palm of your hand. Place 3 drops of LC-65® Daily Contact Lens Cleaner on each lens sur face and rub for 20 seconds in the palm with your forefinger or between your thumb and forefinger. Rinse thoroughly with LENS PLUS Sterile Saline Solution, other appropriate saline solution, or your disinfecting solution. Place the lens in the appropriate chamber of your lens storage case. Repeat the cleaning and rinsing procedure with your other lens and place it in the proper chamber.

Disinfect And Store Your Lenses:

- Be sure the lenses are completely covered with solution before firmly tightening the caps. Disinfect and store lenses as directed by your eye care practitioner.
- After lens application, always empty and rinse lens case with sterile rinsing solution and allow to air dry, to prevent contamination and to help avoid serious eye injury.

Clean soft (hydrophilic) lenses weekly with ALLERGAN® ENZYMATIC Contact Lens Cleaner to reduce the buildup of tear-protein deposits which can damage your lenses, impair vision and reduce comfort.

How Supplied: LC-65 Daily Contact Lens Cleaner is supplied in ½ fl oz (15 mL) and 2 fl oz (60 mL) plastic bottles. The bottles and cartons are marked with lot number and expiration date.

Lenses: LC-65® Daily Contact Lens Cleaner is for use with gas permeable*, hard and soft (hydrophilic) contact lenses.

*The following rigid gas permeable lenses are recommended for use with LC-65: ALLERGAN ADVENT®, FluoroPerm® and silicone acrylate lenses, such as Boston®, Paraperm® and Polycon®.

**See product labeling for list of lenses.

FluoroPerm, Boston, Paraperm and Polycon are trademarks of other companies.

LENS CLEAR®

Soft Contact Lens Cleaner

For use with daily wear and extended wear soft (hydrophilic) contact lenses.

Specially formulated* for eyes that are sensitive.

Description: **LENS CLEAR Soft Contact Lens Cleaner** is a sterile, isotonic solution containing cocoamphocarboxyglycinate (and) sodium lauryl sulfate (and) hexylene glycol, with sorbic acid (0.1%) and edetate disodium (0.2%) as the preservatives. **LENS CLEAR Soft Contact Lens Cleaner** does *not* contain thimerosal, any other mercury-containing ingredients or chlorhexidine. Therefore, the possibility of allergic reactions is reduced.

Actions: **LENS CLEAR Soft Contact Lens Cleaner** is specially formulated for gentle but efficient cleaning of daily wear and extended wear soft (hydrophilic) contact lenses. It safely removes accumulations of undesirable film and deposits within seconds. Use of **LENS CLEAR Soft Contact Lens Cleaner** leaves lenses optically clear, more wettable and more comfortable.

Indications (Uses): Use **LENS CLEAR Soft Contact Lens Cleaner** every day to clean your daily wear or extended wear soft (hydrophilic) contact lenses before rinsing and disinfection.

Contraindications (Reasons Not to Use): If you are allergic to any ingredient in **LENS CLEAR Soft Contact Lens Cleaner**, do not use this product.

Warnings: **PROBLEMS WITH CONTACT LENSES AND LENS CARE PRODUCTS COULD RESULT IN SERIOUS INJURY TO THE EYE.** It is essential that you follow your eye care practitioner's directions and all labeling instructions for proper use of your lenses and lens care products. **EYE PROBLEMS, INCLUDING CORNEAL ULCERS, CAN DEVELOP RAPIDLY AND LEAD TO LOSS OF VISION; THEREFORE, IF YOU EXPERIENCE EYE DISCOMFORT, EXCESSIVE TEARING, VISION CHANGES, OR REDNESS OF THE EYE, IMMEDIATELY REMOVE YOUR LENSES AND PROMPTLY CONTACT YOUR EYE CARE PRACTITIONER.**

All contact lens wearers must see their eye care practitioner as directed. If your lenses are for extended wear, your eye care practitioner may prescribe more frequent visits.

Use of this product with deltafilcon A contact lens materials may discolor your lenses when used in conjunction with a heat disinfection regimen. If you are uncertain of the material from which your lenses are made, consult your eye care practitioner.

To avoid contamination, do not touch tip of container to any surface. Replace cap after using.

Precautions:

- Do not put this product in the eye. The red tip is to remind you not to put this product in your eye.
- Always wash, rinse and dry hands before handling lenses.
- Do not allow **LENS CLEAR Soft Contact Lens Cleaner** to dry on your lenses.
- Keep out of the reach of children.
- Store at room temperature.
- Use before the expiration date stamped on the bottle and carton.
- Never wet contact lenses with saliva or place lenses in your mouth.
- Soft (hydrophilic) contact lenses should never be rinsed with tap water.

Adverse Reactions (Possible Problems) And What To Do:

The following problems may occur:

- Eyes stinging, burning, or itching (irritation)
- Excessive watering (tearing) of the eye
- Unusual eye secretions
- Redness of the eyes
- Reduced sharpness of vision (visual acuity)
- Blurred vision
- Sensitivity to light (photophobia)
- Dry eyes

If you notice any of the above problems, immediately remove and examine your lenses. If a lens appears to be damaged, do not reapply; consult your eye care practitioner. If the problem stops and the lenses appear to be undamaged, thoroughly clean, rinse and disinfect the lenses and reapply them. If the problem continues, immediately remove your lenses and consult your eye care practitioner.

If any of the above symptoms occur, a serious condition such as infection, corneal ulcer, neovascularization, or iritis may be present. Immediately remove your lenses and seek immediate professional identification of the problem and, if necessary, obtain treatment to avoid serious eye damage. For more information, see your Instructions for Wearers booklet for your specific contact lens.

Directions for Use:

- Clean, rinse and disinfect your lenses each time you remove them.
- Always wash, rinse and dry hands before handling contact lenses.
- Always remove and clean the same lens first to avoid any mix-ups.
- It is important to always clean, disinfect and store your lenses as directed by your eye care practitioner.

Prepare The Storage Case For Lens Disinfection:

- For HEAT (thermal) DISINFECTION, fill each chamber of your lens storage case with fresh **LENS PLUS® Sterile Saline Solution** or other appropriate saline solution. For CHEMICAL (not heat) DISINFECTION, fill lens case with your disinfecting solution.

Clean And Rinse Your Lenses:

- After you remove one lens, place it in the palm of your hand. Place three drops of **LENS CLEAR® Soft Contact Lens Cleaner** on each lens surface and rub for 20 seconds in the palm with your forefinger or between your thumb and forefinger. Rinse thoroughly with **LENS PLUS Sterile Saline Solution**, other appropriate saline solution or your disinfecting solution. Place the lens in the appropriate chamber of your lens storage case. Repeat the cleaning and rinsing procedure with your other lens and place it in the proper chamber.

Disinfect And Store Your Lenses:

- Be sure the lenses are completely covered with solution before firmly tightening the caps. Disinfect and store lenses as directed by your eye care practitioner.

Clean soft contact lenses weekly with **ALLERGAN® ENZYMATIC Contact Lens Cleaner** to reduce the buildup of tear-protein deposits which can damage your lenses, impair vision and reduce comfort.

How Supplied: **LENS CLEAR Soft Contact Lens Cleaner** is supplied in ½ fl oz (15 mL) plastic bottles. The bottles and cartons are marked with lot number and expiration date.

Lenses: **LENS CLEAR Soft Lens Contact Cleaner** is for use with daily wear and extended wear soft (hydrophilic) contact lenses.

*** thimerosal-free**

LENS FRESH® OTC

Lubricating and Rewetting Drops

For use with soft (hydrophilic) and hard contact lenses.

Description: Lens Fresh Lubricating and Rewetting Drops is a sterile, buffered, isotonic aqueous solution that contains hydroxyethyl cellulose, sodium chloride, boric acid and sodium borate, with sorbic acid (0.1%) and edetate disodium (0.2%) as the preservatives.

Lens Fresh does not contain thimerosal, any other mercury-containing ingredients, or chlorhexidine. Therefore, the possibility of allergic reactions to Lens Fresh is reduced.

Action: Lens Fresh cushions, lubricates and rewets your lenses and helps to remove particulate material that may cause irritation and/or discomfort. While wearing your lenses, use Lens Fresh to moisten them and reduce their friction against your cornea. Also, use Lens Fresh to relieve minor irritation, discomfort, and/or blurring which may occur while you wear your lenses. Use Lens Fresh to cushion hard contact lens application.

Indications: Use Lens Fresh Lubricating and Rewetting Drops to lubricate and rewet soft (hydrophilic) and hard contact lenses.

Contraindications (Reasons Not To Use): If you are allergic to any ingredient in Lens Fresh, do not use this product.

Warnings: **PROBLEMS WITH CONTACT LENSES AND LENS CARE PRODUCTS COULD RESULT IN SERIOUS INJURY TO THE EYE.** It is essential that you follow your eye care practitioner's directions and all labeling instructions for proper use of your lens care products. **EYE PROBLEMS, INCLUDING CORNEAL ULCERS, CAN DEVELOP RAPIDLY AND LEAD TO LOSS OF VISION; THEREFORE, IF YOU EXPERIENCE EYE DISCOMFORT, EXCESSIVE TEARING, VISION CHANGES, OR REDNESS OF THE EYE, IMMEDIATELY REMOVE YOUR LENSES AND PROMPTLY CONTACT YOUR EYE CARE PRACTITIONER.**

All contact lens wearers must see their eye care practitioner as directed. If your lenses are for extended wear, your eye care practitioner may prescribe more frequent visits.

If drops turn yellow, discard and use fresh (colorless) drops. To avoid contamination, do not touch tip of container to any surface. Replace cap after using.

Precautions: Always wash, rinse and dry hands before handling lenses. Store solution at room temperature. Use before the expiration

Continued on next page

Allergan Optical—Cont.

date marked on the bottle and carton. Keep out of the reach of children.

Adverse Reactions (Possible Problems) and What To Do:

The following problems may occur:

- Eyes stinging, burning, or itching (irritation)
- Excessive watering (tearing) of the eye
- Unusual eye secretions
- Redness of the eye
- Reduced sharpness of vision (visual acuity)
- Blurred vision
- Sensitivity to light (photophobia)
- Dry eyes

If you notice any of the above problems, immediately remove and examine your lenses. If the lenses appear to be damaged, do not reapply; consult your eye care practitioner. If the problem stops and the lenses appear to be undamaged, thoroughly clean, rinse, and disinfect the lenses as directed by the individual product package inserts and reapply them. If the problem continues, immediately remove the lenses and consult the eye care practitioner.

If any of the above symptoms occur, a serious condition such as infection, corneal ulcer, neovascularization or iritis may be present.Immediately remove your lenses and seek immediate professional identification of the problem and, if necessary, obtain treatment to avoid serious eye damage. For more information, see your **Instructions for Wearers** booklet for your specific contact lenses.

Directions: To rewet and lubricate your lenses and to relieve minor irritation, discomfort, and/or blurring, place one drop of Lens Fresh® in your eyes on each lens as needed.

To cushion hard contact lens application, rinse lenses with appropriate rinsing solution and place one drop of Lens Fresh on inner surface of each lens; apply lens.

Wipe any excess solution off eyelids.

Use ALLERGAN® ENZYMATIC Contact Lens Cleaner weekly to reduce the buildup of tear protein deposits on your soft (hydrophilic) lenses.

How Supplied: Lens Fresh is supplied in sterile ½ fl oz plastic dropper bottles. The bottles and cartons are marked with the lot number and expiration date.

Lenses: Lens Fresh is for use with soft (hydrophilic) and hard contact lenses.

LENS PLUS®
DAILY CLEANER

For use with soft (hydrophilic) contact lenses. Preservative Free.

Description: LENS PLUS Daily Cleaner is a sterile, surface-active buffered solution containing cocoamphocarboxyglycinate (and) sodium lauryl sulfate (and) hexylene glycol, sodium chloride and sodium phosphate.

Actions: LENS PLUS Daily Cleaner is specially formulated for gentle but efficient cleaning of soft (hydrophilic) contact lenses. It safely removes the day's accumulation of undesirable film and deposits within seconds. Daily use of LENS PLUS Daily Cleaner leaves lenses optically clear, more wettable and more comfortable.

Indications (Uses): Use LENS PLUS Daily Cleaner every day to clean your soft (hydrophilic) contact lenses, before rinsing and disinfection.

LENS PLUS Daily Cleaner is useful for lens wearers with a history of sensitivity to mercury (thimerosal) or other preservatives present in other daily cleaners.

Contraindications (Reasons Not To Use): If you are allergic to any ingredient in LENS PLUS Daily Cleaner, do not use this product.

Warnings: Problems with contact lenses and lens care products could result in serious injury to the eye. It is essential that you follow your eye care practitioner's directions and all labeling instructions for proper use of your lenses and lens care products, including the lens case. Eye problems, including corneal ulcers, can develop rapidly and lead to loss of vision.

Daily wear lenses are not indicated for overnight wear and should not be worn while sleeping. Clinical studies have shown the risk of serious adverse reactions is increased when these lenses are worn overnight.

Extended wear lenses should be regularly removed for cleaning and disinfection or for disposal and replacement on the schedule prescribed by your eye care practitioner. Clinical studies have shown that there is an increased incidence of serious adverse reactions in extended wear contact lens users as compared to daily wear contact lens users. Studies have also shown that the risk of serious adverse reactions increases the longer extended wear lenses are worn before removal for cleaning and disinfection or for disposal and replacement.

Studies have also shown that smokers had a higher incidence of adverse reactions.

If you experience eye discomfort, excessive tearing, vision changes, or redness of the eye, immediately remove your lenses and promptly contact your eye care practitioner.

It is recommended that contact lens wearers see their eye care practitioner twice each year or if directed, more frequently

To avoid contamination, do not touch tip of container to any surface. Replace cap after using.

Precautions:

- Do not put this product in the eye. The red tip is to remind you not to put this product in your eye.
- Always wash, rinse and dry hands before handling lenses.
- Do not allow LENS PLUS Daily Cleaner to dry on your lenses.
- Keep out of the reach of children.
- Store at room temperature.
- Use before the expiration date stamped on the bottle.
- Never wet contact lenses with saliva or place lenses in your mouth.
- Soft (hydrophilic) contact lenses should never be rinsed with water.

Adverse Reactions (Possible Problems) And What To Do:

The following problems may occur:

- Eyes stinging, burning, or itching (irritation)
- Excessive watering (tearing) of the eye
- Unusual eye secretions
- Redness of the eyes
- Reduced sharpness of vision (visual acuity)
- Blurred vision
- Sensitivity to light (photophobia)
- Dry eyes

If you notice any of the above problems, immediately remove and examine your lenses. If a lens appears to be damaged, do not reapply; consult your eye care practitioner. If the problem stops and the lenses appear to be undamaged, thoroughly clean, rinse and disinfect the lenses and reapply them. If the problem continues, immediately remove your lenses and consult your eye care practitioner.

If any of the above symptoms occur, a serious condition such as infection, corneal ulcer, neovascularization, or iritis may be present. Immediately remove your lenses and seek immediate professional identification of the problem and, if necessary, obtain treatment to avoid serious eye damage. For more information, see your Instructions for Wearers booklet for your specific contact lenses.

Directions For Use:

- Clean, rinse and disinfect your lenses each time you remove them.
- Always wash, rinse and dry hands before handling contact lenses.
- Always remove and clean the same lens first to avoid any mix-ups.

Prepare The Storage Case For Lens Disinfection:

- For HEAT DISINFECTION, fill each chamber of your lens storage case with fresh LENS PLUS® Sterile Saline Solution or other appropriate saline solution. For CHEMICAL DISINFECTION, fill lens case with your disinfecting solution.

Clean And Rinse Your Lenses:

- After you remove one lens, place it in the palm of your hand. Place 3 drops of LENS PLUS Daily Cleaner on each lens surface and rub for 20 seconds in the palm with your forefinger or between your thumb and forefinger. Rinse thoroughly with LENS PLUS Sterile Saline Solution, other appropriate saline solution or your disinfecting solution. Place the lens in the appropriate chamber of your lens storage case. Repeat the cleaning and rinsing procedure with your other lens and place it in the proper chamber.

Disinfect And Store Your Lenses:

- Be sure the lenses are completely covered with solution before firmly tightening the caps. Disinfect and store lenses as directed by your eye care practitioner.
- To prevent contamination and to help avoid serious eye injury, always empty and rinse lens case with sterile rinsing solution and allow to dry.

Clean soft (hydrophilic) lenses weekly with ALLERGAN® ENZYMATIC Contact Lens Cleaner to reduce the buildup of tear-protein deposits which can damage your lenses, impair vision and reduce comfort. For hydrogen peroxide disinfection systems, use Ultrazyme™ Enzymatic Cleaner.

How Supplied: LENS PLUS Daily Cleaner is supplied in ½ fl oz (15 mL) and 1 fl oz (30 mL) plastic bottles. The bottles and cartons are marked with lot number and expiration date.

Lenses: LENS PLUS® Daily Cleaner is for use with soft (hydrophilic) contact lenses.

LENS PLUS®
Oxysept®
DISINFECTION SYSTEM

A disinfecting, neutralizing and storage system for daily wear and extended wear soft (hydrophilic) contact lenses in a chemical (not heat) lens care system.

The LENS PLUS® Oxysept® DISINFECTION SYSTEM consists of:

- LENS PLUS® Oxysept® 1 Disinfecting Solution—a sterile 3% hydrogen peroxide solution for lens disinfection.
- LENS PLUS® Oxysept® 2 Neutralizing Tablets—a neutralizer in a tablet form designed specifically for use with LENS PLUS Oxysept 1 Disinfecting Solution.
- OxyTab™ Cup—a specially designed lens case that *must be used with this lens care system.*

Description (Ingredients):

- **LENS PLUS Oxysept 1 Disinfecting Solution** is a sterile solution that contains microfiltered hydrogen peroxide 3% (stabilized with sodium stannate and sodium nitrate, and buffered with phosphates) and purified water.
- **LENS PLUS Oxysept 2 Neutralizing Tablets** are smooth, round, off-white to bluish-gray, slightly mottled tablets that contain catalose, with buffering and tableting agents.
- **OxyTab Cup** is a specially designed lens case that must be used with this system. It consists of a single flared cup and a lens holder attached to the cap.

Actions:

- **LENS PLUS Oxysept 1 Disinfecting Solution** destroys and prevents the growth of harmful microorganisms on the surface of the lenses in a minimum of 10 minutes.

- **LENS PLUS Oxysept 2 Neutralizing Tablets** are used to neutralize the LENS PLUS Oxysept 1 Disinfecting Solution, in a minimum of 10 minutes, after disinfection.
- **OxyTab Cup** is a specially designed case that *must be used* with the LENS PLUS Oxysept DISINFECTION SYSTEM for proper disinfection, neutralization and storage of soft (hydrophilic) contact lenses.

Indications (Uses):
Use the **LENS PLUS Oxysept DISINFECTION SYSTEM** to disinfect, neutralize and store soft (hydrophilic) contact lenses.

- Use **LENS PLUS Oxysept 1 Disinfecting Solution** to destroy and prevent the growth of harmful microorganisms which may cause infections.
- Use **LENS PLUS Oxysept 2 Neutralizing Tablets** to neutralize the LENS PLUS Oxysept 1 Disinfecting Solution after disinfection.
- Use the OxyTab Cup to hold the lenses during disinfection, neutralization and storage.

Contraindications (Reasons Not To Use):
If you are allergic to any ingredient in the LENS PLUS Oxysept DISINFECTION SYSTEM, do not use this system.

Warnings:

- **KEEP LENS PLUS® Oxysept® 1 Disinfecting Solution (HYDROGEN PEROXIDE) OUT OF THE EYES.** If LENS PLUS Oxysept 1 Disinfecting Solution accidentally comes in contact with the eyes, it may cause burning, stinging or redness. Immediately remove the lenses and flush your eyes with water. If burning or irritation continues, seek professional assistance. **ALWAYS NEUTRALIZE LENSES WITH LENS PLUS® Oxysept® 2 Neutralizing Tablets BEFORE APPLYING LENSES TO YOUR EYES.**
- To avoid lens case cracking from excessive pressure, use only the OxyTab™ Cup. The OxyTab Cup is specially designed for use with LENS PLUS Oxysept 2 Neutralizing Tablets to allow venting of pressure during neutralization. Other lens cases may not have this venting feature.
- Do not use LENS PLUS Oxysept 2 Neutralizing Tablets that do not bubble (effervesce) when added to LENS PLUS Oxysept 1 Disinfecting Solution. Bubbling indicates that the solution is being neutralized. If the tablet does not bubble, refer to the "Directions For Use" for what to do.
- Keep LENS PLUS Oxysept 1 Disinfecting Solution out of the reach of children. If accidentally swallowed, an upset stomach and vomiting may result. Seek immediate professional medical assistance or contact a poison control center.

Problems with contact lenses and lens care products could result in serious injury to the eye. It is essential that you follow your eye care practitioner's directions and all labeling instructions for proper use of your lenses and lens care products, including the lens case. Eye problems, including corneal ulcers, can develop rapidly and lead to loss of vision.

Daily wear lenses are not indicated for overnight wear and should not be worn while sleeping. Clinical studies have shown the risk of serious adverse reactions is increased when these lenses are worn overnight.

Extended wear lenses should be regularly removed for cleaning and disinfection or for disposal and replacement on the schedule prescribed by your eye care practitioner. Clinical studies have shown that there is an increased incidence of serious adverse reactions in extended wear contact lens users as compared to daily wear contact lens users. Studies have also shown that the risk of serious adverse reactions increases the longer extended wear lenses are worn before removal for cleaning and disinfection or for disposal and replacement.

Studies have also shown that smokers had a higher incidence of adverse reactions.

If you experience eye discomfort, excessive tearing, vision changes, or redness of the eye, immediately remove your lenses and promptly contact your eye care practitioner.

It is recommended that contact lens wearers see their eye care practitioner twice each year or if directed, more frequently.

To avoid contamination, do not touch the LENS PLUS Oxysept 2 Neutralizing Tablets. Do not touch the tip of the LENS PLUS Oxysept 1 Disinfecting Solution bottle to any surface. Replace the LENS PLUS Oxysept 1 Disinfecting Solution cap after using.

Precautions:

- Always wash, rinse and dry hands before handling lenses.
- Always clean, disinfect, and neutralize your lenses each time they are removed.
- Use only LENS PLUS Oxysept 1 Disinfecting Solution for disinfection and LENS PLUS Oxysept 2 Neutralizing Tablets for neutralization.
- Use only the OxyTab Cup with this system and fill the OxyTab Cup exactly to the fill line. Do not overfill or overtighten the cap.
- Use only LENS PLUS® Oxysept® DISINFECTION SYSTEM components; do not substitute.
- Never reuse solutions.
- Do not use tablets that appear to be broken or chipped.
- Do not take tablets internally.
- After adding the LENS PLUS Oxysept 2 Neutralizing Tablet, do not allow lenses to soak in the solution for longer than 24 hours without disinfecting and neutralizing again before wearing.
- After reapplying your lenses, always empty the OxyTab Cup, rinse with sterile rinsing solution, and allow to air dry.
- Store solution and tablets at room temperature.
- Use before the expiration date marked on the bottle, foil pouch, blister card and cartons.
- Never use LENS PLUS Oxysept 1 Disinfecting Solution or LENS PLUS Oxysept 2 Neutralizing Tablets in a heat disinfection unit as these products are not designed for use with heat disinfection.

Adverse Reactions (Possible Problems) And What To Do:
The following problems may occur:

- Eyes stinging, burning, or itching (irritation)
- Excessive watering (tearing) of the eyes
- Unusual eye secretions
- Redness of the eyes
- Reduced sharpness of vision (visual acuity)
- Blurred vision
- Sensitivity to light (photophobia)
- Dry eyes

If you notice any of the above problems, **IMMEDIATELY** remove and examine your lenses. If a lens appears to be damaged, do not reapply; consult your eye care practitioner. If the problem stops and the lenses appear to be undamaged, follow the complete "**Directions For Use**," below, before reapplying them. If the problem continues, **IMMEDIATELY** remove the lenses, discontinue use of all lens care products that contact the eye, and consult your eye care practitioner.

If any of the above symptoms occur, a serious condition such as infection, corneal ulcer, neovascularization, or iritis may be present. Seek immediate professional identification of the problem, and obtain treatment, if necessary, to avoid serious eye damage. For more information, see your *Instructions for Wearers* booklet for your specific contact lens type.

Directions For Use:
Follow the instructions below each time you remove your contact lenses. Always wash and rinse your hands before handling contact lenses. Always remove the same lens first to avoid mix-ups.

1. **PREPARE THE OxyTab™ Cup FOR LENS DISINFECTION**
   Remove the cap of the OxyTab Cup. Fill the OxyTab Cup exactly to the fill line with LENS PLUS® Oxysept® 1 Disinfecting Solution. Do not overfill.
2. **RINSE, CLEAN AND RINSE YOUR LENSES**
   Remove and handle one lens at a time. Rinse with an appropriate sterile saline solution, such as LENS PLUS® Sterile Saline Solution, then gently rub with an appropriate daily cleaner, such as LENS PLUS® Daily Cleaner. Rinse thoroughly with more sterile saline solution. Place the lens in the appropriate basket of the lens holder attached to the cap and close the basket lid. Repeat with the remaining lens.
3. **DISINFECT YOUR LENSES**
   Place the lens holder into the OxyTab Cup filled with LENS PLUS Oxysept 1 Disinfecting Solution. Tighten the cap (do not overtighten). Allow the lenses to soak for a minimum of 10 minutes to overnight.
4. **NEUTRALIZE YOUR LENSES**
   After soaking the lenses in LENS PLUS Oxysept 1 Disinfecting Solution, open the OxyTab Cup and place the lens holder aside without allowing the lens basket to come in contact with any surface. DO NOT DISCARD the LENS PLUS Oxysept 1 Disinfecting Solution remaining in the case.

- Bend the blister card containing the tablets along the perforations and remove one section.
- Hold the section over the OxyTab Cup, with the tablet facing up.
- Grasp the foil backing underneath, at the corner where it is not sealed to the plastic.
- Then, carefully peel back the foil to allow the tablet to fall directly into the cup.
- To avoid contamination, DO NOT TOUCH THE TABLET. If you touch the tablet or the tablet misses the cup, discard the tablet and dispense a new tablet into the cup.
- Replace the lens holder in the cup, tighten the cap (do not overtighten) and allow the lenses to soak for a minimum of 10 minutes to overnight.
  Some foaming will occur. This means that the neutralizing tablet is working and is normal.

If the tablet does not vigorously bubble (effervesce) in the LENS PLUS Oxysept 1 Disinfecting Solution, or, if you are not sure whether you have neutralized your lenses, discard the solution and repeat steps 3 and 4.

5. **RINSE AND WEAR**
   When you are ready to wear your lenses, remove one lens at a time. Rinse briefly (2 to 3 seconds) with an appropriate sterile saline solution, such as LENS PLUS® Sterile Saline Solution, then apply lenses.

- To prevent contamination and to help avoid serious eye injury, always empty and rinse lens case with sterile rinsing solution and allow to air dry.

6. **STORE YOUR LENSES**
   Keep the OxyTab Cup closed until you are ready to wear your lenses. If you do not intend to wear your lenses immediately following disinfection and neutralization, you may store them in the *unopened* OxyTab Cup until ready to wear later in the day. However, lenses should not remain in the solution for longer than 24 hours.
   If the lenses have been stored in the unopened OxyTab Cup for more than 24 hours, disinfect and neutralize again before wear-

Continued on next page

Allergan Optical—Cont.

ing (repeat steps 3 and 4). If the lenses are left in the OxyTab Cup for longer periods of time, disinfect and neutralize once a week and again before wearing.

Note: Use an enzymatic cleaner such as Ultrazyme® Enzymatic Cleaner, weekly to reduce the buildup of protein on your soft contact lenses. For further information, see the Ultrazyme package insert, or ask your eye care practitioner.

How Supplied: LENS PLUS® Oxysept® 1 Disinfecting Solution is supplied in sterile 8 and 12 fl oz plastic bottles.

LENS PLUS® Oxysept® 2 Neutralizing Tablets are supplied in cartons of 12 and 36 tablets.

OxyTab® Cup is available in the 12-tablet size of LENS PLUS Oxysept 2 Neutralizing Tablets.

The bottles, foil pouches, blister cards and cartons are marked with lot number and expiration date.

Store LENS PLUS Oxysept 1 Disinfecting Solution and LENS PLUS Oxysept 2 Neutralizing Tablets at room temperature.

Lenses: The LENS PLUS® Oxysept® DISINFECTION SYSTEM is for use with daily wear and extended wear soft (hydrophilic) contact lenses.

LENS PLUS® Oxysept® 2 Neutralizing Tablets

For use in the LENS PLUS® Oxysept DISINFECTION SYSTEM—A disinfecting, neutralizing and storage system for daily wear and extended wear soft (hydrophilic) contact lenses in a chemical (not heat) lens care system.

The LENS PLUS® Oxysept® DISINFECTION SYSTEM consists of:

- LENS PLUS® Oxysept® 1 Disinfecting Solution—a sterile 3% hydrogen peroxide solution for lens disinfection.
- LENS PLUS® Oxysept® 2 Neutralizing Tablets—a neutralizer in a tablet form designed specifically for use with LENS PLUS Oxysept 1 Disinfecting Solution.
- OxyTab™ Cup—a specially designed lens case that *must be used with this lens care system.*

Description (Ingredients):

- **LENS PLUS Oxysept 1 Disinfecting Solution** is a sterile solution that contains microfiltered hydrogen peroxide 3% (stabilized with sodium stannate and sodium nitrate, and buffered with phosphates) and purified water.
- **LENS PLUS Oxysept 2 Neutralizing Tablets** are smooth, round, off-white to bluish-gray, slightly mottled tablets that contain catalase, with buffering and tableting agents.
- **OxyTab Cup** is a specially designed lens case that must be used with this system. It consists of a single flared cup and a lens holder attached to the cap.

Actions:

- **LENS PLUS Oxysept 1 Disinfecting Solution** destroys and prevents the growth of harmful microorganisms on the surface of the lenses in a minimum of 10 minutes.
- **LENS PLUS Oxysept 2 Neutralizing Tablets** are used to neutralize the LENS PLUS Oxysept 1 Disinfecting Solution, in a minimum of 10 minutes, after disinfection.
- **OxyTab Cup** is a specially designed case that *must be used* with the LENS PLUS Oxysept DISINFECTION SYSTEM for proper disinfection, neutralization and storage of soft (hydrophilic) contact lenses.

Indications (Uses):

Use the **LENS PLUS Oxysept DISINFECTION SYSTEM** to disinfect, neutralize and store soft (hydrophilic) contact lenses.

- Use **LENS PLUS Oxysept 1 Disinfecting Solution** to destroy and prevent the growth of harmful microorganisms which may cause infections.
- Use **LENS PLUS Oxysept 2 Neutralizing Tablets** to neutralize the LENS PLUS Oxysept 1 Disinfecting Solution after disinfection.
- Use the OxyTab Cup to hold the lenses during disinfection, neutralization and storage.

Contraindications (Reasons Not To Use):

If you are allergic to any ingredient in the LENS PLUS Oxysept DISINFECTION SYSTEM, do not use this system.

Warnings:

- **KEEP LENS PLUS® Oxysept® 1 Disinfecting Solution (HYDROGEN PEROXIDE) OUT OF THE EYES.** If LENS PLUS Oxysept 1 Disinfecting Solution accidentally comes in contact with the eyes, it may cause burning, stinging or redness. Immediately remove the lenses and flush your eyes with water. If burning or irritation continues, seek professional assistance. **ALWAYS NEUTRALIZE LENSES WITH LENS PLUS® Oxysept® 2 Neutralizing Tablets BEFORE APPLYING LENSES TO YOUR EYES.**
- To avoid lens case cracking from excessive pressure, use only the OxyTab™ Cup. The OxyTab Cup is specially designed for use with LENS PLUS Oxysept 2 Neutralizing Tablets to allow venting of pressure during neutralization. Other lens cases may not have this venting feature.
- Do not use LENS PLUS Oxysept 2 Neutralizing Tablets that do not bubble (effervesce) when added to LENS PLUS Oxysept 1 Disinfecting Solution. Bubbling indicates that the solution is being neutralized. If the tablet does not bubble, refer to the "Directions For Use" for what to do.
- Keep LENS PLUS Oxysept 1 Disinfecting Solution out of the reach of children. If accidentially swallowed, an upset stomach and vomiting may result. Seek immediate professional medical assistance or contact a poison control center.

Problems with contact lenses and lens care products could result in serious injury to the eye. It is essential that you follow your eye care practitioner's directions and all labeling instructions for proper use of your lenses and lens care products, including the lens case. Eye problems, including corneal ulcers, can develop rapidly and lead to loss of vision.

Daily wear lenses are not indicated for overnight wear and should not be worn while sleeping. Clinical studies have shown the risk of serious adverse reactions is increased when these lenses are worn overnight.

Extended wear lenses should be regularly removed for cleaning and disinfection or for disposal and replacement on the schedule prescribed by your eye care practitioner. Clinical studies have shown that there is an increased incidence of serious adverse reactions in extended wear contact lens users as compared to daily wear contact lens users. Studies have also shown that the risk of serious adverse reactions increases the longer extended wear lenses are worn before removal for cleaning and disinfection or for disposal and replacement.

Studies have also shown that smokers had a higher incidence of adverse reactions.

If you experience eye discomfort, excessive tearing, vision changes, or redness of the eye, immediately remove your lenses and promptly contact your eye care practitioner.

It is recommended that contact lens wearers see their eye care practitioner twice each year or if directed, more frequently.

To avoid contamination, do not touch the LENS PLUS Oxysept 2 Neutralizing Tablets. Do not touch the tip of the LENS PLUS Oxysept 1 Disinfecting Solution bottle to any surface. Replace the LENS PLUS Oxysept 1 Disinfecting Solution cap after using.

Precautions:

- Always wash, rinse and dry hands before handling lenses.
- Always clean, disinfect, and neutralize your lenses each time they are removed.
- Use only LENS PLUS Oxysept 1 Disinfecting Solution for disinfection and LENS PLUS Oxysept 2 Neutralizing Tablets for neutralization.
- Use only the OxyTab Cup with this system and fill the OxyTab Cup exactly to the fill line. Do not overfill or overtighten the cap.
- Use only LENS PLUS® Oxysept® DISINFECTION SYSTEM components; do not substitute.
- Never reuse solutions.
- Do not use tablets that appear to be broken or chipped.
- Do not take tablets internally.
- After adding the LENS PLUS Oxysept 2 Neutralizing Tablet, do not allow lenses to soak in the solution for longer than 24 hours without disinfecting and neutralizing again before wearing.
- After reapplying your lenses, always empty the OxyTab Cup, rinse with sterile rinsing solution, and allow to air dry.
- Store solution and tablets at room temperature.
- Use before the expiration date marked on the bottle, foil pouch, blister card and cartons.
- Never use LENS PLUS Oxysept 1 Disinfecting Solution or LENS PLUS Oxysept 2 Neutralizing Tablets in a heat disinfection unit as these products are not designed for use with heat disinfection.

Adverse Reactions (Possible Problems) And What To Do:

The following problems may occur:

- Eyes stinging, burning, or itching (irritation)
- Excessive watering (tearing) of the eyes
- Unusual eye secretions
- Redness of the eyes
- Reduced sharpness of vision (visual acuity)
- Blurred vision
- Sensitivity to light (photophobia)
- Dry eyes

If you notice any of the above problems, **IMMEDIATELY** remove and examine your lenses. If a lens appears to be damaged, do not reapply; consult your eye care practitioner. If the problem stops and the lenses appear to be undamaged, follow the complete "**Directions For Use**," below, before reapplying them. If the problem continues, **IMMEDIATELY** remove the lenses, discontinue use of all lens care products that contact the eye, and consult your eye care practitioner.

If any of the above symptoms occur, a serious condition such as infection, corneal ulcer, neovascularization, or iritis may be present. Seek immediate professional identification of the problem, and obtain treatment, if necessary, to avoid serious eye damage. For more information, see your *Instructions for Wearers* booklet for your specific contact lens type.

Directions For Use:

Follow the instructions below each time you remove your contact lenses. Always wash, rinse and dry hands before handling contact lenses. Always remove the same lens first to avoid mix-ups.

1. **PREPARE THE OxyTab™ Cup FOR LENS DISINFECTION**
   Remove the cap of the OxyTab Cup. Fill the OxyTab Cup exactly to the fill line with LENS PLUS® Oxysept® 1 Disinfecting Solution. Do not overfill.
2. **RINSE, CLEAN AND RINSE YOUR LENSES**
   Remove and handle one lens at a time. Rinse with an appropriate sterile saline solution, such as LENS PLUS® Sterile Saline Solution, then gently rub with an appropriate

daily cleaner, such as LENS PLUS® Daily Cleaner. Rinse thoroughly with more sterile saline solution. Place the lens in the appropriate basket of the lens holder attached to the cap and close the basket lid. Repeat with the remaining lens.

3. **DISINFECT YOUR LENSES**
Place the lens holder into the OxyTab Cup filled with LENS PLUS Oxysept 1 Disinfecting Solution. Tighten the cap (do not overtighten). Allow the lenses to soak for a minimum of 10 minutes to overnight.

4. **NEUTRALIZE YOUR LENSES**
After soaking the lenses in LENS PLUS Oxysept 1 Disinfecting Solution, open the OxyTab Cup and place the lens holder aside without allowing the lens basket to come in contact with any surface. DO NOT DISCARD the LENS PLUS Oxysept 1 Disinfecting Solution remaining in the case.

- Bend the blister card containing the tablets along the perforations and remove one section.
- Hold the section over the OxyTab Cup, with the tablet side facing up.
- Grasp the foil backing underneath, at the corner where it is not sealed to the plastic.
- Then, carefully peel back the foil to allow the tablet to fall directly into the cup.
- To avoid contamination, DO NOT TOUCH THE TABLET. If you touch the tablet or the tablet misses the cup, discard the tablet and dispense a new tablet into the cup.
- Replace the lens holder in the cup, tighten the cap (do not overtighten) and allow the lenses to soak for a minimum of 10 minutes to overnight.
Some foaming will occur. This means that the neutralizing tablet is working and is normal.

If the tablet does not vigorously bubble (effervesce) in the LENS PLUS Oxysept 1 Disinfecting Solution, or, if you are not sure whether you have neutralized your lenses, discard the solution and repeat steps 3 and 4.

5. **RINSE AND WEAR**
When you are ready to wear your lenses, remove one lens at a time. Rinse briefly (2 to 3 seconds) with an appropriate sterile saline solution, such as LENS PLUS® Sterile Saline Solution, then apply lenses.

- To prevent contamination and to help avoid serious eye injury, always empty and rinse lens case with sterile rinsing solution and allow to air dry.

6. **STORE YOUR LENSES**
Keep the OxyTab Cup closed until you are ready to wear your lenses. If you do not intend to wear your lenses immediately following disinfection and neutralization, you may store them in the *unopened* OxyTab Cup until ready to wear later in the day. However, lenses should not remain in the solution for longer than 24 hours.
If the lenses have been stored in the unopened OxyTab Cup for more than 24 hours, disinfect and neutralize again before wearing (repeat steps 3 and 4). If the lenses are left in the OxyTab Cup for longer periods of time, disinfect and neutralize once a week and again before wearing.

Note: Use an enzymatic cleaner such as Ultrazyme® Enzymatic Cleaner, weekly to reduce the buildup of protein on your soft contact lenses. For further information, see the Ultrazyme package insert, or ask your eye care practitioner.

How Supplied: LENS PLUS® Oxysept® 1 Disinfecting Solution is supplied in sterile 8 and 12 fl oz plastic bottles.
LENS PLUS® Oxysept® 2 Neutralizing Tablets are supplied in cartons of 12 and 36 tablets.
OxyTab® Cup is available in the 12-tablet size of LENS PLUS Oxysept 2 Neutralizing Tablets.
The bottles, foil pouches, blister cards and cartons are marked with lot number and expiration date.
Store LENS PLUS Oxysept 1 Disinfecting Solution and LENS PLUS Oxysept 2 Neutralizing Tablets at room temperature.
Lenses: The LENS PLUS® Oxysept® DISINFECTION SYSTEM is for use with daily wear and extended wear soft (hydrophilic) contact lenses.

LENS PLUS® Oxysept® 1 Disinfecting Solution — OTC

For use in the LENS PLUS® Oxysept® DISINFECTION SYSTEM, a disinfecting, neutralizing and storage system for daily wear and extended wear soft (hydrophilic) contact lenses in a chemical (not heat) lens care system.
The **LENS PLUS Oxysept DISINFECTION SYSTEM** consists of:

- **LENS PLUS® Oxysept® 1 Disinfecting Solution** for lens disinfection and a choice of either:
- **LENS PLUS® Oxysept® 2 Rinse and Neutralizer** for neutralization and rinsing and the OxyCup™ Lens Case.

OR

- **LENS PLUS® Oxysept® 2 Neutralizing Tablets**—a neutralizer in a tablet form designed specifically for use with LENS PLUS Oxysept 1 Disinfecting Solution and the OxyTab™ Cup, a specially designed lens case that **must be used when using the Oxysept Neutralizing Tablets to neutralize LENS PLUS Oxysept 1.**

Description (Ingredients):

- **LENS PLUS Oxysept 1 Disinfecting Solution** is a sterile solution that contains microfiltered hydrogen peroxide 3% (stabilized with sodium stannate, sodium nitrate, and buffered with phosphates) and purified water.

Actions:

- **LENS PLUS Oxysept 1 Disinfecting Solution** destroys and prevents the growth of harmful microorganisms on the surface of the lenses in a minimum of 10 minutes.

Indications (Uses):

- Use **LENS PLUS Oxysept 1 Disinfecting Solution** to destroy and prevent the growth of harmful microorganisms which may cause infections.

Contraindications (Reasons not to use): If you are allergic to any ingredient in LENS PLUS Oxysept 1 Disinfecting Solution, do not use this product.

Warnings:

- **KEEP LENS PLUS Oxysept 1 Disinfecting Solution (HYDROGEN PEROXIDE) OUT OF THE EYES.** The red tip is to remind you not to put this product in your eye. If LENS PLUS Oxysept 1 accidentally comes in contact with eyes, it may cause burning, stinging or redness. Immediately remove the lenses and flush out your eyes with water. If burning or irritation continues, seek professional assistance.
ALWAYS NEUTRALIZE LENSES WITH LENS PLUS Oxysept 2 Rinse and Neutralizer or LENS PLUS Oxysept 2 Neutralizing Tablets BEFORE APPLYING LENSES TO YOUR EYES.
- **KEEP OUT OF THE REACH OF CHILDREN. If LENS PLUS Oxysept 1 is accidentally swallowed, an upset stomach and vomiting may result. Seek immediate professional medical assistance or contact a poison control center.**
Problems with contact lenses and lens care products could result in serious injury to the eye. It is essential that you follow your eye care practitioner's directions and all labeling instructions for proper use and care of your lenses and lens care products, including the lens case. Eye problems, including corneal ulcers, can develop rapidly and lead to loss of vision.
Daily wear lenses are not indicated for overnight wear and should not be worn while sleeping. Clinical studies have shown the risk of serious adverse reactions is increased when these lenses are worn overnight.
Extended wear lenses should be regularly removed for cleaning and disinfection or for disposal and replacement on the schedule prescribed by your eye care practitioner. Clinical studies have shown that there is an increased incidence of serious adverse reactions in extended wear contact lens users as compared to daily wear contact lens users. Studies have also shown that the risk of serious adverse reactions increases the longer extended wear lenses are worn before removal for cleaning and disinfection or for disposal and replacement.
Studies have also shown that smokers had a higher incidence of adverse reactions.

If you experience eye discomfort, excessive tearing, vision changes, or redness of the eye, immediately remove your lenses and promptly contact your eye care practitioner.
It is recommended that contact lens wearers see their eye care practitioner twice each year or, if directed, more frequently.

- To avoid contamination, do not touch tip of container to any surface. Replace cap after using.

Precautions:

- Always wash, rinse and dry hands before handling lenses.
- Always clean, disinfect and neutralize your lenses each time they are removed.
- Fill the OxyCup™ Lens Case or OxyTab™ Cup exactly to the fill line. Do not overfill or overtighten the cap.
- Use only LENS PLUS Oxysept DISINFECTION SYSTEM components; do not substitute.
- Never reuse solution.
- After reapplying your lenses, always empty the OxyCup Lens Case or OxyTab Cup, rinse with sterile rinsing solution, and allow to air dry.
- Store solution at room temperature.
- Use before the expiration date marked on the bottle and carton.
- Never use LENS PLUS® Oxysept® 1 in a heat disinfection unit, as this product is not designed for use with heat disinfection.

Adverse Reactions (Possible Problems) and what to do: The following problems may occur:

- Eyes stinging, burning, or itching (irritation)
- Excessive watering (tearing) of the eyes
- Unusual eye secretions
- Redness of the eyes
- Reduced sharpness of vision (visual acuity)
- Blurred vision
- Sensitivity to light (photophobia)
- Dry eyes

If you notice any of the above problems, **IMMEDIATELY** remove and examine your lenses. If a lens appears to be damaged, do not reapply; consult your eye care practitioner. If the problem stops and the lenses appear to be undamaged, follow the complete **Directions for Use,** below, before reapplying them. If the problem continues, **IMMEDIATELY** remove the lenses, discontinue use of all lens care products that contact the eye, and consult your eye care practitioner.
If any of the above symptoms occur, a serious condition such as infection, corneal ulcer, neovascularization, or iritis may be present. Seek immediate professional identification of the problem, and obtain treatment, if necessary, to avoid serious eye damage. For more information, see your **Instructions for Wearers Booklet** for your specific contact lens type.

Continued on next page

Allergan Optical—Cont.

Directions For Use: Follow the instructions below each time you remove your lenses. Always wash, rinse and dry hands before handling contact lenses. Always remove the same lens first to avoid mix-ups.

1. **Prepare Your Lens Case for Lens Disinfection**
   If you will be using the **LENS PLUS® Oxysept® 2 Rinse and Neutralizer** to neutralize your lenses **after disinfection,** prepare your **OxyCup™ Lens Case** for lens disinfection. If you will be neutralizing your lenses with **LENS PLUS Oxysept 2 Neutralizing Tablets,** prepare your **OxyTab™ Cup** for lens disinfection.
   Fill the lens case cup exactly to the fill line with **LENS PLUS® Oxysept® 1 Disinfecting Solution. Do not overfill.**
2. **Rinse, Clean, and Rinse Your Lenses**
   Remove and handle one lens at a time. Rinse with a sterile solution such as LENS PLUS® Sterile Saline Solution, then gently rub with LENS PLUS® Daily Cleaner or other recommended daily cleaner. Rinse thoroughly with more saline solution. Place the lens in the appropriate basket and close the basket lid. Repeat with the remaining lens.
3. **Disinfect Your Lenses**
   Place the lens holder into the lens case filled with LENS PLUS Oxysept 1 Disinfecting Solution and tighten the cap. Do not overtighten. Allow the lenses to soak for a minimum of 10 minutes to overnight.
4. **Neutralize Your Lenses**
   After soaking the lenses in LENS PLUS Oxysept 1 Disinfecting Solution, hold the lens case over the sink, unscrew and remove the cap.
   ALWAYS USE LENS PLUS Oxysept 2 Rinse and Neutralizer OR LENS PLUS Oxysept 2 Neutralizing Tablets FOR A MINIMUM OF 10 MINUTES TO OVERNIGHT TO NEUTRALIZE LENSES AFTER DISINFECTION.
   Follow the Directions For Use contained in the package insert of **either** LENS PLUS Oxysept 2 Rinse and Neutralizer or LENS PLUS Oxysept 2 Neutralizing Tablets to neutralize your lenses.
5. **Store Your Lenses**
   Keep the lens case closed until you are ready to wear your lenses. If you do not intend to wear your lenses immediately following disinfection and neutralization, you may store them in the unopened lens case until ready to wear later in the day.
   See the Directions For Use in the package insert of **either** LENS PLUS Oxysept 2 Rinse and Neutralizer or LENS PLUS Oxysept 2 Neutralizing Tablets for additional storage directions.
   If lenses have been stored in the unopened lens case for more than the recommended time, disinfect and neutralize again before wearing. If lenses are left in the lens case for longer periods of time, disinfect and neutralize once a week and before wearing.
6. **Rinse and Wear**
   When you are ready to wear your lenses, remove one lens at a time. Rinse briefly (2 to 3 seconds) with LENS PLUS® Sterile Saline Solution, or other sterile saline solution, then apply lenses.
   To prevent contamination and to help avoid serious eye injury, always empty and rinse lens case with sterile rinsing solution and allow to air dry.

Note: Use an enzymatic cleaner, such as Ultrazyme® Enzymatic Cleaner, weekly to reduce the buildup of protein on your soft contact lenses. For further information, see the Ultrazyme package insert or ask your eye care practitioner.

How Supplied:
LENS PLUS Oxysept 1 Disinfecting Solution is supplied in sterile 8 fl oz and 12 fl oz plastic bottles.
The bottles and cartons are marked with lot number and expiration date. Store LENS PLUS Oxysept 1 Disinfecting Solution at room temperature.
Lenses:
LENS PLUS Oxysept 1 Disinfecting Solution and the LENS PLUS® Oxysept® DISINFECTION SYSTEM are for use with daily wear and extended wear soft (hydrophilic) contact lenses.

LENS PLUS® Rewetting Drops
Preservative free
For use with soft (hydrophilic) contact lenses while the lenses are on the eyes.

Description: LENS PLUS Rewetting Drops is a sterile, preservative-free, buffered, isotonic, aqueous solution containing sodium chloride and boric acid.
LENS PLUS Rewetting Drops contains no thimerosal, other mercury-containing ingredients, chlorhexidine or other preservatives.
Actions: LENS PLUS Rewetting Drops rehydrates and rewets soft (hydrophilic) contact lenses and helps to remove particulate material that may cause irritation and/or discomfort.
Indications (Uses): Use LENS PLUS Rewetting Drops while wearing your lenses to moisten and rehydrate them. Also, use LENS PLUS Drops to relieve minor irritation, discomfort and/or blurring which may occur while wearing your lenses.
Contraindications (Reasons Not To Use): Do not use this product if you are allergic to any ingredient.
Warnings: Use only if tab and single-use container are intact.
To avoid contamination, do not touch tip of container to any surface. **Discard container after each use.** Do not touch tip of container directly to the eye.
Problems with contact lenses and lens care products could result in serious injury to the eye. It is essential that you follow your eye care practitioner's directions and all labeling instructions for proper use of your lenses and lens care products, including the lens case. Eye problems, including corneal ulcers, can develop rapidly and lead to loss of vison.
Daily wear lenses are not indicated for overnight wear and should not be worn while sleeping. Clinical studies have shown the risk of serious adverse reactions is increased when these lenses are worn overnight.
Extended wear lenses should be regularly removed for cleaning and disinfection or for disposal and replacement on the schedule prescribed by your eye care practitioner. Clinical studies have shown that there is an increased incidence of serious adverse reactions in extended wear contact lens users as compared to daily wear contact lens users. Studies have also shown that the risk of serious adverse reactions increases the longer extended wear lenses are worn before removal for cleaning and disinfection or for disposal and replacement.
Studies have also shown that smokers had a higher incidence of adverse reactions.
If you experience eye discomfort, excessive tearing, vision changes, or redness of the eye, immediately remove your lenses and promptly contact your eye care practitioner.
It is recommended that contact lens wearers see their eye care practitioner twice each year or, if directed, more frequently.
Precautions: Use immediately after opening. Do not store opened container. Store solution at room temperature. Use before the expiration date marked on the container tab and carton.
Adverse Reactions (Possible Problems) And What To Do:
The following problems may occur:

- Eyes stinging, burning or itching (irritation)
- Excessive watering (tearing) of the eye
- Unusual eye secretions
- Redness of the eye
- Reduced sharpness of vision (visual acuity)
- Blurred vision
- Sensitivity to light (photophobia)
- Dry eyes

If you notice any of the above problems, immediately remove and examine your lenses. If a lens appears to be damaged, do not reapply; consult your eye care practitioner. If the problem stops and the lenses appear to be undamaged, thoroughly clean, rinse, and disinfect the lenses and reapply them. If the problem continues after replacing your lens, immediately remove the lens and consult your eye care practitioner.
If any of the above symptoms occur, a serious condition such as infection, corneal ulcer, neovascularization or iritis may be present. Immediately remove your lenses and seek immediate professional identification of the problem and, if necessary, obtain treatment to avoid serious eye damage. For more information, see your **Instructions for Wearers** booklet for your specific contact lenses.
Directions: To use LENS PLUS® Rewetting Drops while you wear your lenses, twist the tab off of the convenient single-use container.
To rewet and rehydrate your lenses and to relieve minor irritation, discomfort and/or blurring, apply one or two drops to each eye on each lens. **Discard container after each use.**
Additional units of LENS PLUS Rewetting Drops can be used as needed throughout the day.
How Supplied: LENS PLUS Rewetting Drops is supplied in sterile 0.01 fl oz (0.35 mL) disposable single-use plastic containers that are packaged in cartons of 30 units each.
The containers and cartons are marked with lot number and expiration date.
Lenses: LENS PLUS Rewetting Drops is for use with soft (hydrophilic) contact lenses.

LENS PLUS®
Sterile Saline Solution
PRESERVATIVE FREE: Gentle Buffered Formula

For rinsing, heat disinfection, and storage after heat disinfection of soft (hydrophilic) contact lenses. May also be used for rinsing in conjunction with chemical disinfection.

Description: LENS PLUS Sterile Saline Solution is a sterile, preservative-free, buffered, isotonic solution containing sodium chloride and boric acid in an aerosol container.
Indications (Uses): LENS PLUS Sterile Saline Solution is indicated for use with soft (hydrophilic) contact lenses. It can be used for rinsing, heat disinfection, and storage after heat disinfection. It may also serve as a rinsing solution in conjunction with chemical disinfection.
LENS PLUS Sterile Saline Solution is useful for patients with a history of sensitivity to mercury (thimerosal) or other substances present in preserved saline solutions.
Contraindications (Reasons Not to Use): Do not use this product if you are allergic to any ingredient.
Warnings: CONTENTS UNDER PRESSURE. DO NOT APPLY DIRECTLY TO EYE AS INJURY MAY RESULT.
PROBLEMS WITH CONTACT LENSES AND LENS CARE PRODUCTS COULD RESULT IN SERIOUS INJURY TO THE EYE. It is essential that you follow your eye care practitioner's directions and all labeling instructions for

proper use of your lenses and lens care products. **EYE PROBLEMS INCLUDING CORNEAL ULCERS, CAN DEVELOP RAPIDLY AND LEAD TO LOSS OF VISION; THEREFORE, IF YOU EXPERIENCE EYE DISCOMFORT, EXCESSIVE TEARING, VISION CHANGES, OR REDNESS OF THE EYE, IMMEDIATELY REMOVE YOUR LENSES AND PROMPTLY CONTACT YOUR EYE CARE PRACTITIONER.**

All contact lens wearers must see their eye care practitioner as directed. If your lenses are for extended wear, your eye care practitioner may prescribe more frequent visits.

To avoid contamination, do not touch tip of container to any surface or transfer the solution to any other storage bottle prior to use. Replace cap after using.

Precautions:

- Always wash, rinse and dry hands before handling lenses.
- Fresh LENS PLUS Sterile Saline Solution should be used daily. **Never reuse the solution.**
- DO NOT USE SOLUTION THAT HAS NOT BEEN HEAT DISINFECTED FOR STORAGE OF LENSES.
- Keep out of the reach of children.
- Do not puncture or incinerate. Do not store at temperatures above 120°F.
- LENS PLUS Sterile Saline Solution should be used before the expiration date stamped on the container.
- After reapplying your lenses, always empty your lens case, rinse with sterile rinsing solution, and allow to dry.

Adverse Reactions (Possible Problems) and What to Do: The following problems may occur:

- Eyes stinging, burning, or itching (irritation)
- Excessive watering (tearing) of the eye
- Unusual eye secretions
- Redness of the eye
- Reduced sharpness of vision (visual acuity)
- Blurred vision
- Sensitivity to light (photophobia)
- Dry eyes

If you notice any of the above problems, immediately remove and examine your lenses. If a lens appears to be damaged, do not reapply; consult your eye care practitioner. If the problem stops and the lenses appear to be undamaged, thoroughly clean, rinse and disinfect the lenses and reapply them. If the problem continues, immediately remove your lenses and consult your eye care practitioner.

If any of the above symptoms occur, a serious condition such as infection, corneal ulcer, neovascularization, or iritis may be present. Immediately remove your lenses and seek immediate professional identification of the problem and begin treatment, if necessary, to avoid serious eye damage. For more information, see your **Instructions for Wearers** booklet for your specific contact lenses.

Directions:

Heat (Thermal) Disinfection

- Always wash, rinse and dry hands before you handle your lenses.
- Clean, rinse, and disinfect your lenses each time you remove them.
- Use can with nozzle directed at dot on rim. DO NOT TILT CAN BEYOND HORIZONTAL.
- To dispense solution, aim nozzle and press. Before each use, always expel a short stream of LENS PLUS® Sterile Saline Solution from tube to clear nozzle.
- Prepare the empty lens case. Wet the chambers of the case with LENS PLUS saline.
- Clean and rinse one lens first (always the same lens first to avoid mix-ups).
- After you clean your lens, rinse it thoroughly with LENS PLUS saline by holding the lens between the forefinger and thumb of one hand and directing a steady stream onto the lens or placing the lens in the palm of one hand and directing a steady stream of LENS PLUS saline onto the lens.
- Put that lens into the correct chamber (section) of the lens case.
- Fill the chamber using enough LENS PLUS saline to completely cover the lens.
- Tightly close the top on the chamber.
- Repeat the above procedure for the second lens.
- Put the lens case into the disinfection unit and follow the directions for operating your heat disinfection unit.

Emergency (Alternate) Method for Heat (Thermal) Disinfection

If your heat disinfection unit is not available, place the tightly closed lens case which contains the lenses into a pan of already boiling water. Leave the closed lens case in the pan of boiling water for at least 10 minutes. (Above an altitude of 7,000 feet, boil for at least 15 minutes.) Be careful not to allow the water to boil away. Remove the pan from the heat and allow it to cool for 30 minutes to complete the disinfection of the lenses.

NOTE: USE OF THE HEAT DISINFECTION UNIT SHOULD BE RESUMED AS SOON AS POSSIBLE.

- Leave the lenses in the unopened lens case until ready to wear. Before lens reapplication rinsing is not necessary unless your eye care practitioner recommends rinsing.

Chemical Disinfection (not heat)

- Always wash, rinse and dry hands before you handle your lenses.
- Disinfect and store lenses as directed by your eye care practitioner.
- Before reapplying lenses that are chemically disinfected, expel a short stream of LENS PLUS saline from the tube to clear nozzle, then rinse the lenses thoroughly with LENS PLUS saline.

Use ALLERGAN® ENZYMATIC Contact Lens Cleaner weekly to reduce the buildup of tear protein deposits on your soft (hydrophilic) contact lenses.

How Supplied: LENS PLUS Sterile Saline Solution is supplied in sterile 3 fl oz, 8 fl oz, 12 fl oz and 15 fl oz aerosol containers. The containers are marked with lot number and expiration date.

Lenses: LENS PLUS Sterile Saline Solution is recommended for use with soft (hydrophilic) contact lenses.

LensKeeper®

Contact Lens Carrying Case

Directions For Use:

- Wash and rinse hands thoroughly before handling lenses.
- Rinse the lens case before each use and allow to air dry. Do not use soaps or detergents.
- Always follow the lens care procedures recommended by your eye care practitioner. For complete information on the use of a particular lens solution, consult the package insert accompanying the product, or ask your eye care practitioner.
- Use fresh solutions daily.

For easy identification, both the left cap and outer base of the left lens well are marked with a raised "L".

Warning: If you experience any unexplained eye discomfort, watering, vision change, or redness of the eye, immediately remove your lenses and consult your eye care practitioner to identify the cause.

For Heat Disinfection Of Soft (Hydrophilic) Contact Lenses: Clean lenses with LENS PLUS® Daily Cleaner. Fill the lens case wells with LENS PLUS® Sterile Saline Solution and place each lens in the appropriate well. Cover each lens with saline solution, then replace the caps tightly. Dry the outside of the lens case and place in your heat disinfection unit. Follow the directions for your particular unit.

For Chemical Disinfection of Soft (Hydrophilic) Contact Lenses: Clean lenses with LENS PLUS® Daily Cleaner. Fill the lens case wells with Allergan® HYDROCARE® Cleaning and Disinfecting Solution, and place each lens in the appropriate well. Cover each lens with solution, then replace caps tightly. Lenses must be stored in the case at least 4 hours. Before wearing lenses, rinse them with LENS PLUS® Sterile Saline Solution.

CAUTION: Never heat lenses in Allergan HYDROCARE Cleaning and Disinfecting Solution. Do not use hard contact lens solutions with soft (hydrophilic) contact lenses.

For Hard and Silicone Acrylate Rigid Gas Permeable Contact Lenses: Clean lenses with Resolve/GP® Daily Cleaner or LC-65® Daily Contact Lens Cleaner. Then fill the lens case wells with Wet-N-Soak PLUS™ Wetting and Soaking Solution. Place each lens in the appropriate well. Cover each lens with solution, then replace caps tightly. Store lenses for at least 4 hours.

LENSRINS®

PRESERVED SALINE SOLUTION

For rinsing, heat disinfection and storage of soft (hydrophilic) contact lenses and for rinsing in conjunction with chemical disinfection.

Description: Lensrins Preserved Saline Solution is a sterile, buffered, isotonic solution containing sodium chloride; sodium phosphate, monobasic, monohydrate; sodium phosphate, dibasic, anhydrous; with edetate disodium (0.1%) and thimerosal (0.001%) as preservatives; and purified water.

Actions: Rinsing lenses with Lensrins Preserved Saline Solution after cleaning will remove loosened debris and traces of daily cleaning products. Disinfection of lenses is accomplished by immersing your lenses in Lensrins Preserved Saline Solution in an appropriate carrying case and heating them in your heat disinfection (heating) unit or by the lens care procedure recommended by your eye care practitioner.

Indications (Uses): Lensrins Preserved Saline Solution is for use with soft (hydrophilic) contact lenses. It can be used for rinsing, heat disinfection, and storage. It may also serve as a rinsing solution in conjunction with chemical disinfection.

Contraindications (Reasons Not to Use): If you are allergic to mercury, which is in thimerosal, or to any other ingredient in Lensrins Preserved Saline Solution, do not use this product.

Warnings: This product contains thimerosal (0.001%) as a preservative. Do not use this product if you are sensitive to thimerosal or any other ingredient containing mercury.

Problems with contact lenses and lens care products could result in serious injury to the eye. It is essential that you follow your eye care practitioner's directions and all labeling instructions for proper use of your lenses and lens care products, including the lens case. Eye problems, including corneal ulcers, can develop rapidly and lead to loss of vision.

Daily wear lenses are not indicated for overnight wear and should not be worn while sleeping. Clinical studies have shown the risk of serious adverse reactions is increased when these lenses are worn overnight.

Extended wear lenses should be regularly removed for cleaning and disinfection or for disposal and replacement on the schedule prescribed by your eye care practitioner. Clinical studies have shown that there is an increased incidence of serious adverse reactions in extended wear contact lens users as compared to

Continued on next page

Allergan Optical—Cont.

daily wear contact lens users. Studies have also shown that the risk of serious adverse reactions increases the longer extended wear lenses are worn before removal for cleaning and disinfection or for disposal and replacement.
Studies have also shown that smokers had a higher incidence of adverse reactions.
If you experience eye discomfort, excessive tearing, vision changes or redness of the eye, immediately remove your lenses and promptly contact your eye care practitioner.
It is recommended that contact lens wearers see their eye care practitioner twice each year or if directed, more frequently.
To avoid contamination, do not touch tip of container to any surface. Replace cap after using.

Precautions:
- Never reuse this solution.
- Always wash, rinse and dry hands before handling your lenses.
- After reapplying your lenses, always empty your lens storage case, rinse with sterile rinsing solution, and allow to air dry.
- Store between 59°–86°F (15°–30°C).
- Use before the expiration date marked on bottle and carton.

Adverse Reactions (Possible Problems) and What to Do: The following problems may occur:
- Eyes stinging, burning, or itching (irritation)
- Excessive watering (tearing) of the eye
- Unusual eye secretions
- Redness of the eyes
- Reduced sharpness of vision (visual acuity)
- Blurred vision
- Sensitivity to light (photophobia)
- Dry eyes

If you notice any of the above problems, immediately remove and examine your lenses. If a lens appears to be damaged, do not reapply; consult your eye care practitioner. If the problem stops and the lenses appear to be undamaged, thoroughly clean, rinse and disinfect the lenses and reapply them. If the problem continues, immediately remove your lenses and consult your eye care practitioner.
If any of the above symptoms occur, a serious condition such as infection, corneal ulcer, neovascularization, or iritis may be present. Immediately remove your lenses and seek immediate professional identification of the problem and begin treatment, if necessary, to avoid serious eye damage. For more information, see your **Instructions for Wearers** booklet for your specific contact lenses.

Directions For Use:
- Always wash, rinse and dry hands before you handle your lenses.
- Clean, rinse, and disinfect your lenses each time you remove them.
- Clean and rinse one lens first (always the same lens first to avoid mix-ups) and put that lens into the correct chamber (section) of the lens storage case. Then repeat the procedure for the second lens.
- After you clean your lens, rinse it thoroughly with Lensrins® Preserved Saline Solution by holding the lens between the forefinger and thumb of one hand and directing a steady stream onto the lens or placing the lens in the palm of one hand and directing a steady stream of Lensrins Preserved Saline Solution onto the lens.

Heat (Thermal) Disinfection
- Prepare the empty lens storage case. Wet the chambers of the case with Lensrins Preserved Saline Solution.
- Place each lens in its correct chamber of the storage case.
- Fill the chamber using enough Lensrins® Preserved Saline Solution to completely cover the lens.
- Tightly close the top on the chamber.
- Repeat the above procedure for the second lens.
- Put the lens storage case into the disinfection unit and follow the operating directions for your unit.

Emergency (Alternate) Method for Heat (Thermal) Disinfection
If your heat disinfection unit is not available, place the tightly closed storage case which contains the lenses into a pan of already boiling water. Leave the closed lens case in the pan of boiling water for at least 10 minutes. (Above an altitude of 7,000 feet, boil for at least 15 minutes.) Be careful not to allow the water to boil away. Remove the pan from the heat and allow it to cool for 30 minutes to complete the disinfection of the lenses.
NOTE: USE OF THE HEAT DISINFECTION UNIT SHOULD BE RESUMED AS SOON AS POSSIBLE.
- Leave the lenses in the unopened storage case until ready to put on your eyes. Before reapplying the lenses, rinsing is not necessary unless your eye care practitioner recommends rinsing.

Chemical Disinfection (not heat)
- Disinfect and store your lenses as directed by your eye care practitioner.
- Before reapplying your lenses, rinse the lenses thoroughly with Lensrins Preserved Saline Solution.
- To prevent contamination and to help avoid serious eye injury, always empty and rinse lens case with sterile rinsing solution and allow to air dry.

How Supplied: Lensrins Preserved Saline Solution is supplied in sterile 8 fl oz plastic bottles. Bottles and cartons are marked with lot number and expiration date.
Lenses: Lensrins Preserved Saline Solution is for use with soft (hydrophilic) contact lenses.

LENS-WET®
Lubricating and Rewetting Solution

Description: Lens-Wet® Lubricating and Rewetting Solution is a sterile, buffered, isotonic, aqueous solution that contains polyvinyl alcohol, thimerosal (0.002%) and edetate disodium (0.01%) as the preservatives; sodium phosphate, dibasic, anhydrous; sodium phosphate, monobasic, monohydrate; sodium chloride; sodium hydroxide and/or hydrochloric acid to adjust the pH; and purified water. Lens-Wet is for use with hard and soft (hydrophilic) contact lenses in heat (thermal) and chemical (not heat) lens care systems.
Actions: Lens-Wet lubricates and rewets your lenses and helps to remove particulate material that may cause irritation and/or discomfort.
Indications (Uses): Use Lens-Wet while you wear your lenses to moisten them and reduce their friction against your cornea. Also use Lens-Wet to relieve minor irritation, discomfort, and/or blurring which may occur while you wear your lenses.
Contraindications (Reasons Not to Use): If you are allergic to mercury, which is in thimerosal, or to any other ingredient in Lens-Wet, do not use this product.
Warnings: This product contains thimerosal (0.002%) as a preservative. Do not use this product if you are sensitive to thimerosal or any other ingredient containing mercury.
PROBLEMS WITH CONTACT LENSES AND LENS CARE PRODUCTS COULD RESULT IN SERIOUS INJURY TO THE EYE. It is essential that you follow your eye care practitioner's directions and all labeling instructions for proper use of your lenses and lens care products. **EYE PROBLEMS, INCLUDING CORNEAL ULCERS, CAN DEVELOP RAPIDLY AND LEAD TO LOSS OF VISION; THEREFORE, IF YOU EXPERIENCE EYE DISCOMFORT, EXCESSIVE TEARING, VISION CHANGES, OR REDNESS OF THE EYE, IMMEDIATELY REMOVE YOUR LENSES AND PROMPTLY CONTACT YOUR EYE CARE PRACTITIONER.**
All contact lens wearers must see their eye care practitioner as directed. If your lenses are for extended wear, your eye care practitioner may prescribe more frequent visits.
To avoid contamination, do not touch tip of container to any surface. Replace cap after using.
Precautions: Always wash, rinse and dry hands before handling your lenses.
Store solution at room temperature.
Use before the expiration date marked on the bottle and carton.
Adverse Reactions (Possible Problems) and What to Do: The following problems may occur:
- Eyes stinging, burning, or itching (irritation)
- Excessive watering (tearing) of the eyes
- Unusual eye secretions
- Redness of the eyes
- Reduced sharpness of vision (visual acuity)
- Blurred vision
- Sensitivity to light (photophobia)
- Dry eyes

If you notice any of the above problems, immediately remove and examine your lenses. If a lens appears to be damaged, do not reapply; consult your eye care practitioner. If the problem stops and the lenses appear to be undamaged, thoroughly clean, rinse and disinfect the lenses and reapply them. If the problem continues, immediately remove the lenses and consult your eye care practitioner. If any of the above symptoms occur, a serious condition such as infection, corneal ulcer, neovascularization, or iritis may be present. Immediately remove your lenses and seek immediate professional identification of the problem and, if necessary, obtain treatment to avoid serious eye damage. For more information, see your **Instructions For Wearers** booklet for your specific contact lenses.
Directions: Use Lens-Wet® while you wear your lenses. To rewet and lubricate your lenses, place one drop in each eye on each lens as needed.
To relieve minor irritation, discomfort and/or blurring, place one drop on the eye, then blink several times.
Wipe any excess solution off eyelids.
Clean soft (hydrophilic) contact lenses weekly with ALLERGAN® ENZYMATIC Contact Lens Cleaner to reduce the buildup of tear-protein deposits which can damage your lenses, impair vision and reduce comfort.
How Supplied: Lens-Wet Lubricating and Rewetting Solution is supplied in sterile, ½ fl oz plastic dropper bottles. The bottles and cartons are marked with lot number and expiration date.
Lenses: Lens-Wet Lubricating and Rewetting Solution is for use with hard and soft (hydrophilic) contact lenses.

LIQUIFILM® Wetting Solution
for comfortable hard contact lens wear

LIQUIFILM Wetting Solution wets and lubricates hard contact lenses with a clear antiseptic film to increase wearing time and comfort.
Contains: Polyvinyl alcohol with hydroxypropyl methylcellulose, edetate disodium, sodium chloride, potassium chloride and benzalkonium chloride (0.004%).
Directions: Wash hands well. Apply to both surfaces of the lens. Rub gently between thumb and forefinger. Rinse with an appropriate rinsing solution as recommended by your eye care practitioner. Apply another drop to inner surface and apply lens.

Warnings: To avoid contamination, do not touch tip of container to any surface. Replace cap after using. Keep out of the reach of children.
Note: Not for use with soft (hydrophilic) contact lenses.
How Supplied: ⅔ fl oz and 2 fl oz plastic bottles.

OxyCup™

Lens Case
for use in the LENS PLUS® Oxysept® DISINFECTION SYSTEM
for use with daily wear and extended wear soft (hydrophilic) contact lenses

OxyCup™ Lens Case for use in the LENS PLUS® Oxysept® DISINFECTION SYSTEM
Directions: Always wash and rinse your hands before handling contact lenses. Use LENS PLUS® Oxysept® 1 Disinfecting Solution to disinfect lenses. Always use LENS PLUS® Oxysept® 2 Rinse and Neutralizer to neutralize lenses after disinfection. Use only the OxyCup Lens Case for proper disinfection, neutralization, and storage of your lenses. The OxyCup Lens Case should NOT be overfilled or cap overtightened.
SEE PACKAGE INSERT ACCOMPANYING THE LENS PLUS Oxysept DISINFECTION SYSTEM PRODUCTS FOR IMPORTANT SAFETY INFORMATION.
Note: Use Ultrazyme™ Enzymatic Cleaner weekly to remove protein and reduce its buildup on your soft (hydrophilic) contact lenses.

ProFree/GP®

Weekly Enzymatic Cleaner
For use with rigid gas permeable contact lenses.*

Description: **ProFree/GP®** Weekly Enzymatic Cleaner is a round tablet containing the enzyme papain, sodium chloride, sodium carbonate, sodium borate, and edetate disodium.
Action: **ProFree/GP** Weekly Enzymatic Cleaner removes protein deposits from the surface of rigid gas permeable contact lenses.* It safely and effectively removes protein and reduces its buildup on your lenses when used as directed.
Indications: Use **ProFree/GP** Weekly Enzymatic Cleaner once a week for as little as 2 hours to reduce protein buildup for clear vision and comfortable lens wear.
Contraindications: Do not use ProFree/-GP® Weekly Enzymatic Cleaner if you are allergic to any of the ingredients in the tablet. If you are allergic to any ingredient in one sterile saline solution, use another sterile saline solution as recommended by your eye care practitioner to prepare the enzymatic cleaning solution.
Warnings: This product contains the enzyme papain. Do not use this product if you are allergic to papain.
Lenses must be rinsed and disinfected following each enzymatic cleaning cycle. DO NOT INSTILL THE ENZYMATIC CLEANING SOLUTION DIRECTLY INTO THE EYE.
NEVER USE DISTILLED WATER TO DISSOLVE THE TABLETS. DISTILLED WATER IS NOT STERILE. USE OF A NON-STERILE PRODUCT IN THE PREPARATION OF CONTACT LENS SOLUTIONS MAY LEAD TO MICROBIAL CONTAMINATION OF LENSES WHICH CAN CAUSE SERIOUS EYE INFECTIONS.
PROBLEMS WITH CONTACT LENSES AND LENS CARE PRODUCTS COULD RESULT IN SERIOUS INJURY TO THE EYE. It is essential that you follow your eye care practitioner's directions and all labeling instructions for proper use of your lenses and lens care products. **EYE PROBLEMS, INCLUDING CORNEAL ULCERS, CAN DEVELOP RAPIDLY AND LEAD TO LOSS OF VISION; THEREFORE, IF YOU EXPERIENCE EYE DISCOMFORT, EXCESSIVE TEARING, VISION CHANGES, OR REDNESS OF THE EYE, IMMEDIATELY REMOVE YOUR LENSES AND PROMPTLY CONTACT YOUR EYE CARE PRACTITIONER.**
All contact lens wearers must see their eye care practitioner as directed. If your lenses are for extended wear, your eye care practitioner may prescribe more frequent visits.
Precautions:
- KEEP OUT OF THE REACH OF CHILDREN.
- Do not take tablets internally.
- Do not use brown or otherwise discolored tablets.
- Avoid excessive heat.
- Always wash, rinse and dry hands before handling your lenses.
- **Lenses must be disinfected following each enzymatic cleaning cycle. The enzymatic cleaning cycle is NOT a substitute for disinfection of your lenses.** After enzymatic cleaning, lenses must be gently rubbed, then rinsed with an appropriate solution and disinfected in the usual way prior to reapplication.
- Do not soak lenses longer than 12 hours.
- Lenses should **never** be placed on the eye directly from the enzymatic cleaning solution.
- Use only the special vials provided to prepare enzymatic cleaning solution. Do not use any other container.
- Use only freshly prepared enzymatic cleaning solution and discard immediately after use.
- Use before expiration date on foil wrapper and unit carton.

Adverse Reactions (Possible Problems) and What to Do: The following problems may occur:
- Eyes stinging, burning, or itching (irritation)
- Excessive watering (tearing) of the eyes
- Unusual eye secretions
- Redness of the eyes
- Reduced sharpness of vision (visual acuity)
- Blurred vision
- Sensitivity to light (photophobia)
- Dry eyes

If you notice any of the above problems, a serious condition such as infection, corneal ulcer, neovascularization or iritis may be present. Immediately remove and examine your lenses. If a lens appears to be damaged, do not reapply; consult your eye care practitioner. If the problem stops and the lenses appear to be undamaged, thoroughly clean, rinse and disinfect the lenses and reapply them. If the problem continues, immediately remove the lenses and consult your eye care practitioner for identification of the problem and, if necessary, obtain treatment to avoid serious eye damage.
Directions: Your lenses must be enzymatically cleaned using the special vials included in the cleaning kit. If you are using a refill package, transfer the vials from the previous kit you received to the receptacle in this package. Do not use any other containers.
Clean your lenses with **ProFree/GP®** Weekly Enzymatic Cleaner once a week, or more often if needed, as follows:

1. Rinse vials thoroughly with fresh rinsing solution. Then examine for cleanliness. Next, fill with sterile saline solution up to the fill line indicated on the vial. **Use only sterile saline solution to dissolve the tablets.** Drop one tablet into each vial. The tablet will effervesce (fizz) and quickly dissolve. Always prepare fresh solution for each enzymatic cleaning cycle.
2. After removing the lenses from your eyes, clean each lens with Resolve/GP® Daily Cleaner, LC-65® Daily Contact Lens Cleaner or other appropriate cleaner.** Rinse each lens thoroughly with Wet-N-Soak PLUS™ Wetting and Soaking Solution or other appropriate rinsing solution** as directed by your eye care practitioner.
3. Place each lens in the appropriate vial.
4. Place the caps on the vials and shake to ensure thorough mixing. Soak lenses a minimum of 2 hours. **The enzymatic cleaning solution is not intended for the storage of lenses.** Do not soak lenses in the enzymatic cleaning solution for more than twelve (12) hours.
5. After soaking your lenses, remove them from the vials. Thoroughly clean each lens and rinse as directed in Step 2. Then disinfect your lenses as directed by your eye care practitioner.
6. Pour out the remaining solution, rinse the vials thoroughly with fresh rinsing solution and allow to air dry. **Do not use soap or detergent.**

Note: The enzymatic cleaning solution has a characteristic odor. This odor is normal. In the case of unusually heavy protein deposits, more than one complete enzymatic cleaning cycle may be required to adequately clean your lenses. Lenses must be disinfected in the usual way prior to reapplication.
How Supplied: In cartons of 16 and 24 tablets including vials.
Avoid excessive heat.
Lenses: **ProFree/GP®** Weekly Enzymatic Cleaner is for use with rigid gas permeable contact lenses.*

*The following rigid gas permeable lenses are recommended for use with ProFree/GP® Weekly Enzymatic Cleaner: FluoroPerm® and silicone acrylate lenses (including Boston®, Paraperm®, Polycon®, Ocusil™ and Optacryl). Consult your eye care practitioner to identify the type of lens you wear. Fluoroperm, Boston, Paraperm, and Polycon are trademarks of other companies.

**See individual product packaging for list of lenses.

U.S. Patent 3,910,296.

RESOLVE/GP®

Daily Cleaner
For use with rigid gas permeable* and hard contact lenses.
PRESERVATIVE FREE**

Description: Resolve/GP Daily Cleaner is a sterile, buffered solution with a unique combination of cocoamphocarboxyglycinate, sodium lauryl sulfate, hexylene glycol, alkyl ether sulfate and fatty acid amide surfactant cleaning agents.
Actions: Resolve/GP Daily Cleaner effectively cleans by removing lipids, mucus and other undesirable film and surface deposits from rigid gas permeable and hard contact lenses. The unique combination of surfactant cleaning agents also provides antimicrobial activity to eliminate the need to add potentially sensitizing preservatives. For rigid gas permeable* lenses use Resolve/GP in conjunction with ProFree/GP® Weekly Enzymatic Cleaner to promote clean lenses, clear vision and comfortable lens wear.
Resolve/GP Daily Cleaner is useful for lens wearers who have experienced reactions to preservatives present in other daily cleaners.
Indications (Uses): Use Resolve/GP to clean your rigid gas permeable* and hard contact lenses before rinsing and disinfection.
Contraindications (Reasons Not To Use): Do not use this product if you are allergic to any ingredient.

Continued on next page

Allergan Optical—Cont.

Warnings: PROBLEMS WITH CONTACT LENSES AND LENS CARE PRODUCTS COULD RESULT IN SERIOUS INJURY TO THE EYE. It is essential that you follow your eye care practitioner's directions and all labeling instructions for proper use of your lenses and lens care products. **EYE PROBLEMS, INCLUDING CORNEAL ULCERS, CAN DEVELOP RAPIDLY AND LEAD TO LOSS OF VISION; THEREFORE, IF YOU EXPERIENCE EYE DISCOMFORT, EXCESSIVE TEARING, VISION CHANGES, OR REDNESS OF THE EYE, IMMEDIATELY REMOVE YOUR LENSES AND PROMPTLY CONTACT YOUR EYE CARE PRACTITIONER.**
All contact lens wearers must see their eye care practitioner as directed. If your lenses are for extended wear, your eye care practitioner may prescribe more frequent visits.
To avoid contamination, do not touch tip of container to any surface. Replace cap after using.
Precautions:
- DO NOT PUT THIS PRODUCT IN THE EYE. The red tip is to remind you not to put this product in your eye.
- NOT FOR USE WITH SOFT (hydrophilic) CONTACT LENSES.
- Always wash, rinse and dry hands before handling lenses.
- Keep out of the reach of children.
- Store at room temperature.
- Use before the expiration date stamped on the bottle.
- Never wet contact lenses with saliva or place lenses in your mouth.

Adverse Reactions (Possible Problems) And What To Do:
The following problems may occur:
- Eyes stinging, burning, or itching (irritation)
- Excessive watering (tearing) of the eye
- Unusual eye secretions
- Redness of the eyes
- Reduced sharpness of vision (visual acuity)
- Blurred vision
- Sensitivity to light (photophobia)
- Dry eyes

If you notice any of the above problems, IMMEDIATELY remove and examine your lenses. If a lens appears to be damaged, do not reapply; consult your eye care practitioner. If the problem stops and your lenses appear to be undamaged, thoroughly clean, rinse and disinfect the lenses, then reapply. If the problem continues, IMMEDIATELY remove your lenses, discontinue use of all lens care products that contact the eye, and consult your eye care practitioner.
If any of the above symptoms occur, a serious condition such as infection, corneal ulcer, neovascularization, or iritis may be present. Immediately remove your lenses and seek immediate professional identification of the problem. Obtain treatment, if necessary, to avoid serious eye damage. For more information, see your Instructions for Wearers booklet for your specific contact lens type.
Directions For Use:
- Clean, rinse and disinfect your lenses each time you remove them.
- Always wash, rinse and dry hands thoroughly before handling contact lenses.
- Always remove and clean the same lens first to avoid any mix-ups.

Prepare The Storage Case For Lens Disinfection:
- Fill each chamber of your lens storage case with Wet-N-Soak PLUS™ Wetting and Soaking Solution or other appropriate soaking solution.

Clean And Rinse Your Lenses:
- After you remove one lens, place it in the palm of your hand. Place 3 drops of Resolve/GP® on each lens surface and rub for 20 seconds in the palm with your forefinger or between your thumb and forefinger. Rinse thoroughly with an appropriate rinsing solution as recommended by your eye care practitioner. Place the lens in the appropriate chamber of your lens case. Repeat the cleaning and rinsing procedure with your other lens and place it in the proper chamber.

Disinfect And Store Your Lenses:
- Be sure the lenses are completely covered with soaking solution before tightening the caps. Disinfect and store your lenses as recommended by your eye care practitioner.

Clean rigid gas permeable contact lenses weekly with ProFree/GP® Weekly Enzymatic Cleaner to reduce the buildup of tear-protein deposits which can impair vision and reduce comfort.
How Supplied: Resolve/GP Daily Cleaner is supplied in sterile 1 fl oz (30 mL) plastic bottles. The bottles and cartons are marked with lot number and expiration date.
Lenses: Resolve/GP Daily Cleaner is for use with rigid gas permeable* and hard contact lenses.

* The following rigid gas permeable lenses are recommended for use with Resolve/GP: Boston®, Paraperm®, Polycon®, Ocusil™, Optacryl and other silicone acrylate lenses. Consult your eye care practitioner to identify the type of lenses you wear.

** The unique combination of surfactant cleaning agents provides antimicrobial activity which eliminates the need to add potentially sensitizing preservatives.
Boston, Paraperm and Polycon are trademarks of other companies.

SOAKARE®
Hard Contact Lens Soaking Solution

Description: Soakare is a disinfecting/soaking solution specially designed to provide maximum conditioning and protection for hard contact lenses.
Contains: Purified water, edetate disodium (0.25%), and benzalkonium chloride (0.01%).
Directions: Wash, rinse and dry hands before handling lenses. Fill storage case with enough Soakare Solution to completely cover lenses. Soak lenses four or more hours. Rinse lenses with an appropriate rinsing solution as recommended by your eye care practitioner and wet with Liquifilm® Wetting Solution. Change the solution daily. Use LC-65® Daily Contact Lens Cleaner as a super cleaner for stubborn deposits. **Note:** Not for use with soft contact lenses. Do not put this product in the eye. The red tip is to remind you not to put this product in your eye.
How Supplied: 4 fl oz bottle.

Style Keeper®
Contact Lens Carrying Case

Directions For Use:
- Always wash, rinse and dry hands before handling lenses.
- Rinse the lens case before each use and allow to air dry. Do not use soaps or detergents.
- Always follow the lens care procedures recommended by your eye care practitioner. For complete information on the use of a particular lens solution, consult the package insert accompanying the product, or ask your eye care practitioner.
- Use fresh solutions daily.
- For easy identification, both the left cap and outer base of left lens well are marked with a raised "L".

Warning: If you experience any unexplained eye discomfort, watering, vision change, or redness of the eye, immediately remove your lenses and consult your eye care practitioner to identify the cause.
FOR HEAT DISINFECTION OF SOFT (HYDROPHILIC) LENSES: Use LENS PLUS® Daily Cleaner and LENS PLUS® Sterile Saline Solution.
FOR CHEMICAL DISINFECTION OF SOFT (HYDROPHILIC) LENSES: Use Allergan® HYDROCARE® Cleaning and Disinfecting Solution.
FOR HARD AND RIGID GAS PERMEABLE LENSES: Use EasyClean/GP® Daily Cleaner and Wet-N-Soak™ Wetting and Soaking Solution.
CAUTION: Never heat lenses in Allergan HYDROCARE Cleaning and Disinfecting Solution. Do not use hard contact lens solutions with soft (hydrophilic) lenses. Do not use hydrogen peroxide disinfecting solutions with the Style Keeper Lens Case.

TOTAL®
The All-In-One Hard Contact Lens Solution

Total Solution is an all-purpose solution to wet, cushion, clean and soak hard contact lenses.
Contains: Polyvinyl alcohol, edetate disodium and benzalkonium chloride in a sterile, buffered, isotonic solution.
Directions: Always wash, rinse and dry hands.
To clean and wet lenses before wearing, cover lens surface with a few drops of Total Solution. Rub gently, then rinse with an appropriate rinsing solution as recommended by your eye care practitioner. Place a drop of Total Solution on inner lens surface and apply lens.
To store lenses, fill storage case with enough Total Solution to completely cover lenses. Soak overnight.
Keep case tightly closed while storing lenses. Change solution every day.
Warnings: To avoid contamination, do not touch dropper tip to any surface. Replace cap after using. Not for use with soft contact lenses.
For those stubborn, hard-to-remove deposits, use **LC-65® Daily Contact Lens Cleaner,** the super-cleaner.
How Supplied: 2 fl oz, 4 fl oz economy size.

ULTRAZYME® Enzymatic Cleaner
for use with soft (hydrophilic) contact lenses in combination with LENS PLUS® Oxysept® 1 Disinfecting Solution and other* (see instructions at the end of this insert) 3% hydrogen peroxide disinfecting solutions.

Description (Ingredients): ULTRAZYME Enzymatic Cleaner is an effervescent, smooth, oval, white tablet that contains the enzyme subtilisin A, with effervescing, buffering, and tableting agents.
Actions: ULTRAZYME Enzymatic Cleaner, dissolved in LENS PLUS® Oxysept® 1 Disinfecting Solution or other* 3% hydrogen peroxide disinfecting solutions, simultaneously removes protein deposits while lenses are being disinfected. When used as directed, one ULTRAZYME tablet safely and effectively removes protein and reduces its buildup on your lenses while enhancing the disinfection capability of your hydrogen peroxide disinfecting solution.
Indications (Uses): ULTRAZYME Enzymatic Cleaner is indicated for use in a recommended 3% hydrogen peroxide disinfecting solution such as LENS PLUS Oxysept 1 Disinfecting Solution, to remove protein and reduce its buildup on soft (hydrophilic) contact lenses.
Contraindications (Reasons Not To Use): Do not use ULTRAZYME tablets if you are allergic to the enzyme subtilisin A.

Warnings:

- After the enzymatic/disinfection and neutralization cycles, lenses must be gently rubbed and rinsed with an appropriate rinsing solution before applying to your eyes.
- KEEP THE ENZYMATIC/DISINFECTING SOLUTION OUT OF YOUR EYES. If the solution accidentally comes in contact with eyes, it may cause burning, stinging or redness. Immediately remove your lenses and flush your eyes with water. If burning or irritation continues, seek professional assistance.
- ALL ENZYMATIC/DISINFECTION, NEUTRALIZATION AND RINSING CYCLES MUST BE COMPLETED BEFORE REAPPLYING YOUR LENSES.

Problems with contact lenses and lens care products could result in serious injury to the eye. It is essential that you follow your eye care practitioner's directions and all labeling instructions for proper use of your lenses and lens care products, including the lens case. Eye problems, including corneal ulcers, can develop rapidly and lead to loss of vision.

Daily wear lenses are not indicated for overnight wear and should not be worn while sleeping. Clinical studies have shown the risk of serious adverse reactions is increased when these lenses are worn overnight.

Extended wear lenses should be regularly removed for cleaning and disinfection or for disposal and replacement on the schedule prescribed by your eye care practitioner. Clinical studies have shown that there is an increased incidence of serious adverse reactions in extended wear contact lens users as compared to daily wear contact lens users. Studies have also shown that the risk of serious adverse reactions increases the longer extended wear lenses are worn before removal for cleaning and disinfection or for disposal and replacement.

Studies have also shown that smokers had a higher incidence of adverse reactions.

If you experience eye discomfort, excessive tearing, vision changes, or redness of the eye, immediately remove your lenses and promptly contact your eye care practitioner.

It is recommended that contact lens wearers see their eye care practitioner twice each year or if directed, more frequently.

Precautions:

- KEEP OUT OF THE REACH OF CHILDREN.
- Always wash, rinse and dry hands before handling lenses.
- Use the lens case recommended for your disinfection system.
- Never interchange or reuse solutions.
- Do not use tablets that are soft and sticky or irregular in appearance.
- Do not take tablets internally.
- The weekly enzymatic/disinfection cycle is not a substitute for cleaning and disinfecting.
- After reapplying your lenses, always empty the lens case, rinse with sterile saline solution, and allow to air dry.
- Use before the expiration date on the foil, blister package and unit carton.
- Never use ULTRAZYME® Enzymatic Cleaner in a heat disinfection unit as this product is not designed for use with heat disinfection.
- Store at room temperature, 15°–30°C (59°–86°F), in a dry place.

Adverse Reactions (Possible Problems) And What To Do:

The following problems may occur:

- Eyes stinging, burning, or itching (irritation)
- Excessive watering (tearing) of the eyes
- Unusual eye secretions
- Redness of the eyes
- Reduced sharpness of vision (visual acuity)
- Blurred vision
- Sensitivity to light (photophobia)
- Dry eyes

If you notice any of the above problems, IMMEDIATELY remove and examine your lenses. If a lens appears to be damaged, do not reapply; consult your eye care practitioner. If the problem stops and your lenses appear to be undamaged, thoroughly clean, rinse, and disinfect the lenses; then reapply. If the problem continues, IMMEDIATELY remove your lenses, discontinue use of all lens care products that contact the eye, and consult your eye care practitioner.

If any of the above symptoms occur, a serious condition such as infection, corneal ulcer, neovascularization or iritis may be present. Immediately remove your lenses and seek immediate professional identification of the problem, and obtain treatment, if necessary, to avoid serious eye damage. For more information, see your **Instructions for Wearers** Booklet for your specific contact lens type.

Directions For Use With The LENS PLUS® Oxysept® DISINFECTION SYSTEM: Use ULTRAZYME Enzymatic Cleaner once a week or more often as recommended by your eye care practitioner.

Always wash, rinse and dry hands before handling contact lenses. Always remove the same lens first to avoid mix-ups.

Follow the instructions below each time you use the ULTRAZYME® Enzymatic Cleaner tablet with the LENS PLUS Oxysept DISINFECTION SYSTEM.

- If your disinfection system consists of LENS PLUS Oxysept 1 Disinfecting Solution and LENS PLUS Oxysept 2 Rinse and Neutralizer, use only the OxyCup Lens Case for weekly enzymatic cleaning/disinfection and neutralization. Do not substitute any other lens case.
- If your disinfection system consists of LENS PLUS Oxysept 1 Disinfecting Solution and LENS PLUS Oxysept 2 Neutralizing Tablets, use only the OxyTab Cup for weekly enzymatic cleaning/disinfection and neutralization. Do not substitute any other lens case.

1. PREPARE THE LENS CASE (OxyCup or OxyTab Cup) FOR WEEKLY ENZYMATIC CLEANING/DISINFECTION.
   Fill the cup of the lens case exactly to the fill line with LENS PLUS® Oxysept® 1 Disinfecting Solution. Do not overfill. Next, place one (1) ULTRAZYME tablet in the cup. The tablet will fizz and quickly dissolve.
2. CLEAN AND RINSE YOUR LENSES.
   Remove one lens at a time and clean with LENS PLUS® Daily Cleaner or other recommended daily cleaner. Rinse thoroughly with a sterile saline solution such as LENS PLUS® Sterile Saline Solution. Place the lenses in the proper lens baskets of the lens holder and close the basket lids.
3. ENZYMATICALLY CLEAN AND DISINFECT YOUR LENSES.
   Place the lens holder in the lens case (OxyCup or OxyTab Cup) and tighten the cap (do not overtighten). Allow the lenses to soak for at least 15 minutes to a maximum of overnight. Increasing the soak time up to a maximum of overnight will allow for increased protein removal. Consult your eye care practitioner to determine the best soak time for you, as individuals vary in the amount of protein they deposit.

FOLLOW THE NEUTRALIZATION STEPS FOR EITHER LENS PLUS® Oxysept® 2 Rinse and Neutralizer or LENS PLUS® Oxysept® 2 Neutralizing Tablets.

DIRECTIONS FOR NEUTRALIZING WITH LENS PLUS® Oxysept® 2 Rinse and Neutralizer:

4. RINSE AND NEUTRALIZE YOUR LENSES. After the required soaking time, open the OxyCup over a sink. DISCARD the enzymatic/disinfecting solution from the cup and fill exactly to the line with LENS PLUS® Oxysept® 2 Rinse and Neutralizer. Do not overfill. Do not remove the lenses from the lens holder. Hold the cap and shake the baskets downward to remove the excess enzymatic/disinfecting solution. Then rinse the lens baskets containing the lenses for 2 to 3 seconds with the remaining LENS PLUS® Oxysept 2 Rinse and Neutralizer. Replace the lens holder containing the lenses in the OxyCup, tighten the cap (do not overtighten) and shake gently for a few seconds. (Note: Bubbling is a signal that the remaining LENS PLUS Oxysept 1 is being neutralized.) Allow the lenses to soak in LENS PLUS Oxysept 2 Rinse and Neutralizer for a minimum of 10 minutes to a maximum of 12 hours.
   NOTE: If ever you are not sure whether you have neutralized your lenses, rinse and neutralize again with LENS PLUS Oxysept 2 Rinse and Neutralizer.

OR

DIRECTIONS FOR NEUTRALIZING WITH LENS PLUS® Oxysept® 2 Neutralizing Tablets:

4. NEUTRALIZE YOUR LENSES. After the required soaking time, open the OxyTab Cup and place the lens holder aside without allowing the baskets to come in contact with any surface. DO NOT DISCARD the LENS PLUS Oxysept 1 Disinfecting Solution remaining in the case.
   Detach one section of the blister card containing the LENS PLUS Oxysept 2 Neutralizing Tablets. Hold the section over the OxyTab Cup with the tablet side facing up. Grasp and peel back the foil to allow the tablet to fall directly into the cup. To avoid contamination, DO NOT TOUCH THE TABLET. If you touch the tablet or the tablet misses the cup, discard that tablet and dispense a new tablet into the cup.
   Replace the lens holder in the cup, tighten the cap (do not overtighten) and soak for a minimum of 10 minutes to overnight.
5. RUB, RINSE AND WEAR.
   When you are ready to wear your lenses, remove one lens at a time and gently rub and rinse thoroughly with LENS PLUS® Sterile Saline Solution, or other appropriate sterile rinsing solution; then apply lenses.
   To prevent contamination and to help avoid serious eye injury, always empty and rinse lens case with sterile rinsing solution and allow to air dry.

*DIRECTIONS FOR OTHER 3% HYDROGEN PEROXIDE SYSTEMS:
(AOSept®, Lensept®, MiraSept™, CONSEPT™, Quik-Sept™ and PureSept™)

Follow the directions for your particular disinfection system. Use the lens case designed for use with your 3% hydrogen peroxide disinfecting solution.

- Place one (1) ULTRAZYME® Enzymatic Cleaner tablet in your 3% hydrogen peroxide disinfecting solution.
- Allow lenses to soak as usual in your disinfecting solution. However, if your disinfecting solution calls for a disinfection soak time less than 15 minutes, **increase the soak time to a minimum of 15 minutes when using ULTRAZYME.** Increasing the soak time up to a maximum of overnight will allow for increased protein removal. Consult your eye care practitioner to determine the best soak time for you, as individuals vary in the amount of protein they deposit.

NOTE: FAILURE TO FOLLOW THE INSTRUCTIONS SPECIFIED FOR YOUR HYDROGEN PEROXIDE DISINFECTING SOLUTION MAY RESULT IN SERIOUS EYE INFECTION. THE MINIMUM SOAK TIME

Continued on next page

Allergan Optical—Cont.

WITH ULTRAZYME SHOULD NEVER BE LESS THAN THE MINIMUM RECOMMENDED DISINFECTION SOAK TIME FOR YOUR HYDROGEN PEROXIDE DISINFECTING SOLUTION.

- After your lenses have been enzymatically cleaned/disinfected and neutralized (following the directions for your particular disinfection system), they **must be gently rubbed and rinsed** with LENS PLUS® Sterile Saline Solution or other appropriate sterile rinsing solution before wearing.

How Supplied: ULTRAZYME Enzymatic Cleaner is supplied in packages of 5, 10 and 20 tablets. The foil packages and cartons are marked with lot number and expiration date.
Lenses: ULTRAZYME Enzymatic Cleaner is for use with soft (hydrophilic) contact lenses.
U.S. Patent 3,910,296, 4,585,488 and Re. 32,672.
AOSept, Lensept, MiraSept, CONSEPT, QuikSept and PureSept are trademarks of other companies.

WET-N-SOAK™

Wetting and Soaking Solution
For use with rigid gas permeable contact lenses* and hard contact lenses.

Description: Wet-N-Soak™ Wetting and Soaking Solution is a sterile, buffered, isotonic solution that contains polyvinyl alcohol, edetate disodium and benzalkonium chloride (0.004%) as the preservative.
Actions: Wet-N-Soak disinfects and wets rigid gas permeable contact lenses* and hard contact lenses. Also store your lenses in Wet-N-Soak following disinfection.
Indications (Uses): Wet-N-Soak is indicated for use in the chemical disinfection and storage of rigid gas permeable contact lenses* and hard contact lenses. Use Wet-N-Soak to wet and cushion your lenses before applying them to your eyes.
Contraindications (Reasons Not To Use): Do not use if you are allergic to any ingredient in this product.
Warnings: PROBLEMS WITH CONTACT LENSES AND LENS CARE PRODUCTS COULD RESULT IN SERIOUS INJURY TO THE EYE. It is essential that you follow your eye care practitioner's directions and all labeling instructions for proper use of your lenses and lens care products. EYE PROBLEMS, INCLUDING CORNEAL ULCERS, CAN DEVELOP RAPIDLY AND LEAD TO LOSS OF VISION; THEREFORE, IF YOU EXPERIENCE EYE DISCOMFORT, EXCESSIVE TEARING, VISION CHANGES, OR REDNESS OF THE EYE, IMMEDIATELY REMOVE YOUR LENSES AND PROMPTLY CONTACT YOUR EYE CARE PRACTITIONER.
All contact lens wearers must see their eye care practitioner as directed. If your lenses are for extended wear, your eye care practitioner may prescribe more frequent visits.
To avoid contamination, do not touch tip of container to any surface.
Replace cap after using.
Precautions:

- Always wash, rinse and dry hands before handling lenses
- Not for use with soft (hydrophilic) contact lenses.
- Never reuse solution.
- Keep out of the reach of children
- Store solution at room temperature.
- Use before the expiration date marked on the bottle and carton.

Adverse Reactions (Possible Problems) and What To Do: The following problems may occur:

- Eyes stinging, burning, or itching (irritation)
- Excessive watering (tearing) of the eye
- Unusual eye secretions
- Redness of the eye
- Reduced sharpness of vision (visual acuity)
- Blurred vision
- Sensitivity to light (photophobia)
- Dry eyes

If you notice any of the above problems, IMMEDIATELY remove and examine your lenses. If a lens appears to be damaged, do not reapply; consult your eye care practitioner. If the problem stops and the lenses appear to be undamaged, thoroughly clean, rinse, and disinfect the lenses and reapply them. If the problem continues, IMMEDIATELY remove your lenses and consult your eye care practitioner.
If any of the above symptoms occur, a serious condition such as infection, corneal ulcer, neovascularization or iritis may be present. Immediately remove your lenses and seek immediate practitioner identification of the problem and obtain treatment, if necessary, to avoid serious eye damage. For more information, see your <u>Instructions for Wearers</u> booklet for your specific contact lenses.
Directions:

- Clean, rinse, and disinfect your lenses each time you remove them.
- Always wash, rinse and dry hands before handling contact lenses.
- Always remove the same lens first to avoid any mix-ups.

Prepare The Storage Case For Lens Disinfection:

- Fill each chamber of your lens storage case with Wet-N-Soak™ Wetting and Soaking Solution.

Clean and Rinse Your Lenses:

- Remove one lens and clean it with an appropriate daily cleaner such as Resolve/GP® Daily Cleaner** as directed. Rinse thoroughly with an appropriate rinsing solution. Place the lens in the appropriate chamber of your lens storage case. Be sure the lens is completely covered with Wet-N-Soak before firmly tightening the cap. Repeat the entire procedure with your other lens.

Disinfect And Store Your Lenses:

- Allow lenses to soak overnight or a minimum of 4 hours in Wet-N-Soak.

Apply Your Lenses:

- After soaking, lenses may be removed from the case and placed directly on the eyes. For extra cushioning, place one drop of Wet-N-Soak on the inner surface of each lens before applying.
- After reapplying lenses, empty the lens case, rinse with fresh rinsing solution, and allow to air dry.

Use ProFree/GP® Weekly Enzymatic Cleaner to remove protein and reduce its buildup on your FluoroPerm® and silicone acrylate rigid gas permeable lenses. For further information, see the ProFree/GP package insert accompanying the product or ask your eye care practitioner.
If you do not intend to wear your lenses immediately following disinfection you may store them in the *unopened* lens case.
If the lenses have been stored in the *unopened* lens case for more than 1 week, put fresh solution in the lens case and disinfect before wearing. If left in the lens case for longer periods of time, disinfect once a week and before wearing.
How Supplied: Wet-N-Soak Wetting and Soaking Solution is supplied in sterile 6 fl oz plastic bottles. The bottles and cartons are marked with lot number and expiration date.
Lenses: Wet-N-Soak is for use with rigid gas permeable contact lenses* and hard contact lenses.

*The following rigid gas permeable lenses are recommended for use with Wet-N-Soak: ALLERGAN ADVENT®, FluoroPerm®, and silicone acrylate lenses (including Polycon®, Paraperm®, Boston®, Ocusil™ and Optacryl). Consult your eye care practitioner to identify the lens you wear.
**See product labeling for list of lenses.
FluoroPerm, Polycon, Paraperm and Boston are trademarks of other companies.

WET-N-SOAK PLUS™

Wetting and Soaking Solution
For use with gas permeable contact lenses* and hard contact lenses

Description: WET-N-SOAK PLUS™ Wetting and Soaking Solution is a sterile, buffered isotonic solution that contains polyvinyl alcohol, edetate disodium and benzalkonium chloride (0.003%) as the preservative.
Actions: Wet-N-Soak PLUS disinfects your lenses by destroying harmful microorganisms on the surface of the lens. Use Wet-N-Soak PLUS to store your lenses after disinfection. Wet-N-Soak PLUS also wets and provides cushioning of the lens when placed on the eye.
Indications (Uses): Wet-N-Soak PLUS is indicated for chemical disinfection and storage of gas permeable lenses* and hard contact lenses. Use Wet-N-Soak PLUS to wet and cushion your lenses before applying them to your eyes.
Contraindications (Reasons Not to Use): Do not use if you are allergic to any ingredient in this product.
Warnings: PROBLEMS WITH CONTACT LENSES AND LENS CARE PRODUCTS COULD RESULT IN SERIOUS INJURY TO THE EYE. It is essential that you follow your eye care practitioner's directions and all labeling instructions for proper use of your lenses and lens care products. **EYE PROBLEMS, INCLUDING CORNEAL ULCERS, CAN DEVELOP RAPIDLY AND LEAD TO LOSS OF VISION; THEREFORE, IF YOU EXPERIENCE EYE DISCOMFORT, EXCESSIVE TEARING, VISION CHANGES, OR REDNESS OF THE EYE, IMMEDIATELY REMOVE YOUR LENSES AND PROMPTLY CONTACT YOUR EYE CARE PRACTITIONER.**
All contact lens wearers must see their eye care practitioner as directed. If your lenses are for extended wear, your eye care practitioner may prescribe more frequent visits.
To avoid contamination, do not touch tip of container to any surface. Replace cap after using.
Precautions:

- Always wash, rinse and dry hands before handling your lenses.
- Always use fresh solution daily.
- Not for use with soft (hydrophilic) contact lenses.
- Keep out of the reach of children.
- Store solution at room temperature.
- Use before the expiration date marked on the bottle and carton.

Adverse Reactions (Possible Problems) and What to Do: The following problems may occur:

- Eyes stinging, burning, or itching (irritation)
- Excessive watering (tearing) of the eye
- Unusual eye secretions
- Redness of the eye
- Reduced sharpness of vision (visual acuity)
- Blurred vision
- Sensitivity to light (photophobia)
- Dry eyes

If you notice any of the above problems, IMMEDIATELY remove and examine your lenses. If a lens appear to be damaged, do not reapply; consult your eye care practitioner. If the problem stops and the lenses appear to be undamaged, thoroughly clean, rinse and disinfect the lenses and reapply them. If the problem continues, IMMEDIATELY remove your lenses and consult your eye care practitioner.
If any of the above symptoms occur, a serious condition such as infection, corneal ulcer, neo-

vascularization or iritis may be present. Immediately remove your lenses and seek immediate practitioner identification of the problem and obtain treatment, if necessary, to avoid serious eye damage. For more information, see your Instructions for Wearers booklet for your specific contact lenses.

Directions:
- Clean, rinse and disinfect your lenses each time you remove them.
- Always wash, rinse and dry hands before handling contact lenses.
- Always remove the same lens first to avoid any mix-ups.

Prepare The Storage Case For Lens Disinfection:
- Fill each chamber of your lens storage case with Wet-N-Soak PLUS™ Wetting and Soaking Solution.

Clean And Rinse Your Lenses:
- Remove one lens and clean it with an appropriate daily cleaner as directed by your eye care practitioner. Rinse thoroughly with an appropriate rinsing solution. Place the lens in the appropriate chamber of your lens storage case. Be sure the lens is completely covered with Wet-N-Soak PLUS™ before firmly tightening the cap. Repeat the entire procedure with your other lens.

Disinfect And Store Your Lenses:
Allow lenses to soak overnight or for a minimum of 4 hours in Wet-N-Soak PLUS.

Apply Your Lenses
- After soaking, lenses may be removed from the case and placed directly on the eyes. For cushioning, place one drop of Wet-N-Soak PLUS on the inner surface of each lens before applying.
  Note: Use ProFree/GP® Weekly Enzymatic Cleaner once a week to remove protein and reduce its buildup on your silicone acrylate or FluoroPerm® rigid gas permeable lenses. For further information, see the ProFree/GP package insert accompanying the product or ask your eye care practitioner.

If you do not intend to wear your lenses immediately following disinfection you may store them in the unopened lens case.

If the lenses have been stored in the unopened lens case for more than 1 week, put fresh solution in the lens case and disinfect before wearing. If left in the lens case for longer periods of time, disinfect once a week and before wearing.

After reapplying lenses, empty the lens case, rinse with fresh rinsing solution, and allow to air dry.

How Supplied: Wet-N-Soak PLUS Wetting and Soaking Solution is supplied in sterile 4 fl oz and 6 fl oz plastic bottles. The bottles and cartons are marked with lot number and expiration date.

Lenses: Wet-N-Soak PLUS is for use with gas permeable contact lenses* and hard contact lenses.

*The following gas permeable lenses are recommended for use with Wet-N-Soak PLUS: the ALLERGAN ADVENT® (flurofocon A) Contact Lens and silicone acrylate lenses (including Boston®, Paraperm®, Polycon®, Ocusil™ and Optacryl). Consult your eye care practitioner to identify the lens you wear.

Boston, FluoroPerm, Paraperm and Polycon are trademarks of other companies.

Refer to contents page for information on Pharmaceutical Products.

CIBA Vision Corporation

2910 AMWILER COURT
ATLANTA, GA 30360

AODISC®

INSTRUCTIONS FOR REPLACING THE AODISC®

The AODISC is **specially** designed for use only in the AOSEPT® Disinfection/Neutralization System with AOSEPT® Solution. For complete system instructions, refer to the Package Insert enclosed with the AOSEPT Solution. The AODISC should not be used with other lens care disinfection solutions or other cups or cases not specifically designed for use with the AODISC.

Important: Wash your hands thoroughly, and dry them with a clean, lint-free towel, before handling your AODISC.

AN AODISC MUST **ALWAYS** BE PRESENT TO NEUTRALIZE THE AOSEPT SOLUTION

1. Remove the used AODISC

A. If your cup has a lens holder **with** a stem, simply remove the AODISC by pulling it off the stem **(Figure A.1)**.

B. If your cup has a lens holder **without** a stem, invert the open cup and rap firmly on a table or smooth surface **(Figure B.1)**.

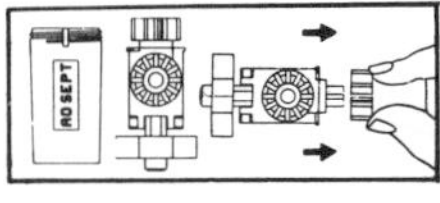

FIGURE A.1 (with a stem)

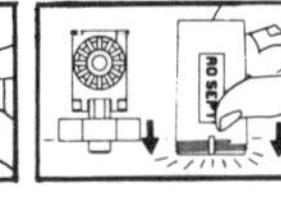

FIGURE B.1 (without a stem)

2. Replace with new AODISC®

A. If your cup has a lens holder **with** a stem, simply slide the new AODISC onto the stem **(Figure A.2)**. Your new AODISC is now ready for another 3 months of use.

B. If your cup has a lens holder **without** a stem, hold the open AOSEPT® cup horizontally and position the AODISC just inside the opening of the cup **(Figure B.2)** and push the AODISC with your index finger until it is firmly set in the base of the cup. Your new AODISC is now ready for another 3 months of use.

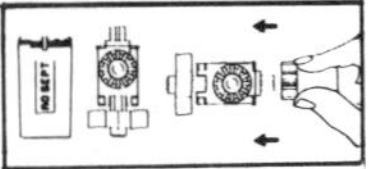

FIGURE A.2 (with a stem)

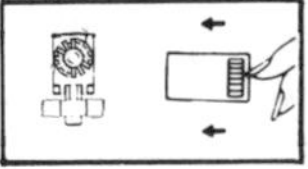

FIGURE B.2 (without a stem)

Remember:
- The AODISC must be replaced after 100 uses or three (3) months of daily use.
- Keep the AODISC at room temperature.
- There are no safe or acceptable substitutes for the AOSEPT® Solution, the AOSEPT® Lens Holder and Cup, or the AODISC, in the AOSEPT® Disinfection/Neutralization System.
- For further information regarding soft contact lens care, consult your eye practitioner or write to: Consumer Relations, CIBA Vision Corporation, P.O. Box 105069, Atlanta, GA 30348.

AOSEPT®

DISINFECTION/NEUTRALIZATION SOLUTION PACKAGE INSERT

AOSEPT® Disinfection/Neutralization Solution is for use in the AOSEPT® Disinfection/Neutralization System, an oxidation/chemical (not heat) system for the disinfection of soft (hydrophilic) contact lenses (including extended wear and tinted lenses). See **DESCRIPTION/INGREDIENTS** for contents.

The AOSEPT® System consists of the following:
- AOSEPT® Lens Holder and Cup
- AODISC®
- AOSEPT® Solution

Additional Products Available:
- CIBA Vision® Saline • CIBA Vision Cleaner • CIBA Vision Lens Drops • MiraFlow® Extra-Strength Daily Cleaner • Softwear® Saline.

Description/Ingredients: AOSEPT® Solution is a sterile ophthalmic solution containing microfiltered hydrogen peroxide 3%, sodium chloride 0.85%, stabilized with sodium stannate, sodium nitrate, buffered with phosphates.

Actions: Oxidation/chemical (not heat) disinfection/neutralization of soft (hydrophilic) contact lenses (including extended wear and tinted lenses) in the AOSEPT Solution kills microorganisms that could cause serious eye infections. THE AODISC MUST BE PRESENT FOR NEUTRALIZATION of the hydrogen peroxide to a sterile isotonic buffered saline solution before lenses are inserted on the eye.

NOTE: AOSEPT SOLUTION CONTAINS NO THIMEROSAL OR CHLORHEXIDINE, PRESERVATIVES TO WHICH SOME PEOPLE ARE SENSITIVE.

Indications/Uses: AOSEPT Solution is used in the AOSEPT System to disinfect soft (hydrophilic) contact lenses (including extended wear and tinted lenses) when used with the AODISC as directed.

Contraindications (Reasons not to use): None are known; however, if you are allergic to any ingredient in the AOSEPT Solution, do not use this product.

WARNINGS:

- **DO NOT PUT AOSEPT SOLUTION THAT HAS NOT BEEN NEUTRALIZED IN YOUR EYE.** Place lens on your eye only after neutralizing the AOSEPT Solution and rinsing your lens thoroughly with sterile saline solution. Neutralization of the AOSEPT Solution occurs by soaking the lenses for **SIX (6) hours with the AODISC.** Do not use the AODISC for more than 100 uses or three (3) months of daily use. Should AOSEPT Solution that has not been neutralized mistakenly get in your eye, REMOVE YOUR LENS IMMEDIATELY, FLUSH (WASH) YOUR EYE WITH A LARGE AMOUNT OF WATER OR STERILE SALINE for a few minutes. If burning and/or irritation persists, seek assistance from an eye care practitioner. Never touch the dropper tip of the bottle to any surface, since this may contaminate the solution.

- DO NOT TAKE AOSEPT SOLUTION INTERNALLY OR GASTRIC DISTRESS COULD RESULT. SEEK PROFESSIONAL ASSISTANCE OF A PHYSICIAN OR A POISON CONTROL CENTER IMMEDIATELY IF TAKEN INTERNALLY. KEEP OUT OF REACH OF CHILDREN.

PROBLEMS WITH CONTACT LENSES AND LENS CARE PRODUCTS COULD RESULT IN SERIOUS INJURY TO THE EYE. It is essential that you follow your eye care practitioner's directions and all labeling instructions for proper use of your lenses and lens care products including the lens case. **EYE PROBLEMS, INCLUDING CORNEAL ULCERS, CAN DEVELOP RAPIDLY AND LEAD TO LOSS OF VISION; THEREFORE, IF YOU EXPERIENCE EYE DISCOMFORT, EXCESSIVE TEAR-**

Continued on next page

CIBA Vision—Cont.

ING, VISION CHANGES, OR REDNESS OF THE EYE, IMMEDIATELY REMOVE YOUR LENSES AND PROMPTLY CONTACT YOUR EYE CARE PRACTITIONER. It is recommended that contact lens wearers see their eye care practitioner twice each year or, if directed, more frequently.

Precautions:

- **Never reuse AOSEPT Solution.**
- There is NO SAFE, ACCEPTABLE SUBSTITUTE IN THE AOSEPT SYSTEM FOR THE AOSEPT SOLUTION DUE TO ITS UNIQUE FORMULATION. DO NOT MIX OR SUBSTITUTE OTHER LENS CARE PRODUCTS CONTAINING HYDROGEN PEROXIDE. THESE PRODUCTS MAY NOT BE COMPATIBLE WITH THE AOSEPT SOLUTION. DO NOT USE OVER-THE-COUNTER GENERIC HYDROGEN PEROXIDE. Generic hydrogen peroxide solutions are not intended for use with contact lenses and may contain ingredients not tested for ocular safety and/or toxicity. Generic hydrogen peroxides are not intended for ophthalmic use and will cause DISCOLORATION and DAMAGE lenses.
- NEVER USE AOSEPT SOLUTION in a thermal (heat) disinfection unit.
- Store the AOSEPT Solution at room temperature: 59° to 86°F (15° to 30°C). Store upright.
- Use before the expiration date marked on the container and carton.
- To avoid the possibility of damage to your lenses, the following precautions should be taken when using the AOSEPT System:

1. **USE ONLY THE AOSEPT LENS HOLDER AND CUP WITH THE AOSEPT SYSTEM.**
2. Disinfection begins upon immediate contact between the AOSEPT Solution and the AODISC; lenses MUST be placed in the solution immediately.
3. DO NOT fill the AOSEPT Cup above the fill line. BE SURE TO FILL THE AOSEPT CUP ONLY TO THE FILL LINE WITH AOSEPT SOLUTION.

In addition:

1. DO NOT disinfect lens unless you have thoroughly rinsed the daily cleaner from the surface of the lens.
2. DO NOT use any solution in the AOSEPT Cup other than the AOSEPT Solution.
3. DO NOT overtighten the cup (only tighten finger-tight).
4. DO NOT use a damaged AOSEPT Cup.
5. Keep the bottle tightly closed when not in use.

Adverse Reactions: (Problems that may occur and what to do about them): With contact lens wear, the following problems may occur: eyes stinging, burning or itching (irritation), excessive watering (tearing) of the eyes, unusual eye secretions, redness of the eyes, reduced sharpness of vision (visual acuity), blurred vision, sensitivity to light (photophobia), or dry eyes. Studies have shown that smokers have a higher incidence of adverse reactions. If you notice any of the above problems, **immediately remove and examine your lenses for damage,** such as splits or tears. If the problem stops and the lenses appear to be undamaged, thoroughly clean/rinse and disinfect/neutralize the lenses and reinsert them. If the lens appears to be damaged, DO NOT USE THE LENS. If the lens does not seem to be damaged, but the problem continues, **STOP USE OF THE LENS IMMEDIATELY AND ALSO STOP USE OF ALL LENS CARE PRODUCTS. PROMPTLY consult your eye care practitioner.**

If any of the above symptoms persist, serious conditions such as infection, corneal ulcer, neovascularization, and iritis may be present. Seek immediate professional identification of the problem and treatment to avoid serious eye damage.

Directions For Use With Soft (HYDROPHILIC) Contact Lenses:

NOTE: If you are currently using a commercially available thermal (heat) disinfection system or chemical (not heat) disinfection system, the AOSEPT® System can be used interchangeably without damage to your lenses.

Clean, rinse, and disinfect/neutralize your contact lenses each time you remove them. Before handling your contact lenses, always wash your hands thoroughly and dry them with a clean, lint-free towel. To clean, rinse and disinfect/neutralize your lenses, the following two procedures must be followed:

PROCEDURE ONE—Clean your lenses after each removal.

1. Clean the surface of the right lens with Mira-Flow® Extra-Strength Daily Cleaner or other recommended cleaner. Follow the product instructions included with the cleaner.
2. Rinse the lens thoroughly with a steady stream of sterile saline solution, such as CIBA Vision Saline or Softwear® Saline and place the right lens on the dome in the unmarked side of the lens holder. (See note below.)
3. Repeat steps one and two with the left lens and place the lens on the other dome of the lens holder marked "L."

NOTE: To prevent damage to your lens, center the lens on the dome in the lens holder. Be sure the lens does not touch the basket rim, then close the basket lid.

PROCEDURE TWO—Disinfect/neutralize your lenses AFTER steps 1–3 above have been completed.

1. An AODISC® must always be present to neutralize the AOSEPT Solution. If your cup has a lens holder **with** a stem, place the AODISC onto the stem (Figure A). If your cup has a lens holder **without** a stem, place the AODISC in the bottom of the cup (Figure B).

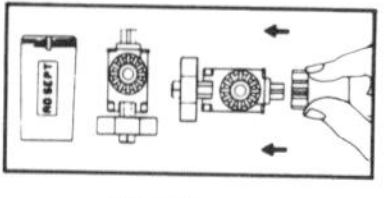
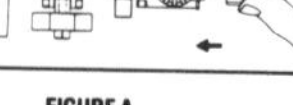

FIGURE A (with a stem)

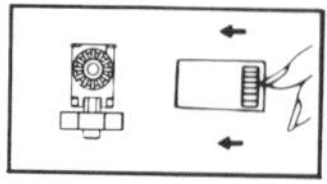

FIGURE B (without a stem)

2. After you've placed your lenses in the lens holder, fill the AOSEPT Cup with AOSEPT Solution to the fill line and **IMMEDIATELY** place the lens holder in the cup. Tighten (turn clockwise) the cap, and shake gently. DO NOT OVERFILL. Overfilling the cup will cause the AOSEPT Solution to overflow from the cup.
3. Allow the lenses to **soak for a minimum of six (6) hours or overnight.** After a minimum of six (6) hours, your lenses are ready to wear. If your lenses have been soaking in the AOSEPT Cup for more than 24 hours, you must repeat the disinfection/neutralization procedure again before wearing your lenses.
4. You must rinse your lens thoroughly with CIBA Vision Saline or Softwear® Saline prior to lens insertion on the eye.
5. After putting your lenses on, always discard the neutralized AOSEPT Solution from the AOSEPT Cup, rinse with AOSEPT Solution or CIBA Vision Saline, or Softwear® Saline, and **leave the cup open to air dry.** This rinsing and air drying will help to keep your cup free of microbial contaminants. The lens holder should be inverted (outside the cup) so it's not lying on its side, as shown below.

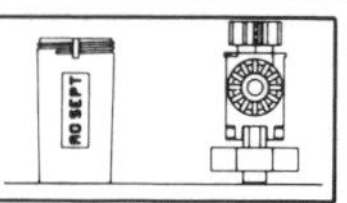

CORRECT WAY

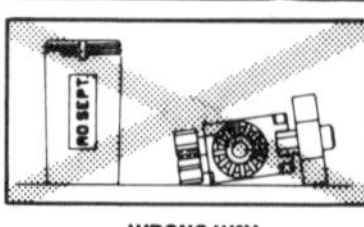

WRONG WAY

Direction Notes:

a. If bubbles flow from the hole on the top of the cap of the lens holder, this indicates that you have overfilled the cup or that you may not have thoroughly rinsed the cleaner off your lenses.
b. Never rinse your lenses in AOSEPT Solution and put directly on the eye.
c. **Lenses must always be disinfected/neutralized for a minimum of six (6) hours in the AOSEPT Cup with the AODISC and rinsed with saline before putting your lenses on.**
d. **The AODISC must be replaced with a new AODISC after 100 uses or three (3) months of daily use.**
e. If you use an enzymatic cleaner be sure to clean, disinfect/neutralize, and rinse your lenses before insertion on the eye.
f. Only an enzymatic cleaner that is recommended for use with hydrogen peroxide disinfecting solutions, such as Ultrazyme™, can be used with the AOSEPT Solution in the AOSEPT Cup. (NOTE: You must rinse your lenses with saline after enzyming.)
To prevent contamination and to help avoid serious eye injury, always empty and rinse lens case with fresh, sterile rinsing solution and allow to air dry.

How Supplied: AOSEPT Solution is supplied sterile in 4 oz. (120 mL), 8 oz. (237 mL), and 12 oz. (355 mL) plastic bottles. Bottles and cartons are marked with lot number and expiration date.

All system replacement products are sold separately.

For information regarding this product, consult your eye care practitioner or write to: Consumer Relations, CIBA Vision Corporation, P.O. Box 105069, Atlanta, GA 30348.

Ultrazyme™ is a trademark of Allergan, Inc.

CIBA VISION® SALINE

A sterile saline solution for use as a rinsing solution following chemical disinfection; or for rinsing, heat disinfection and storage after heat disinfection of soft (hydrophilic) contact lenses.

GENTLE ON YOUR EYES*
PRESERVATIVE-FREE

Description: CIBA Vision Saline is a sterile, preservative-free, buffered, isotonic solution containing sodium chloride and boric acid in an aerosol container.

Indications (Uses): CIBA Vision Saline is indicated for use with soft (hydrophilic) contact lenses. It can be used as a rinsing solution in conjunction with chemical disinfection. It may also be used for rinsing, heat disinfection, and storage after heat disinfection.

*CIBA Vision Saline is useful for patients sensitive to thimerosal or other substances present in preserved saline solutions.

Contraindications (Reasons not to use): If allergic to any ingredient in CIBA Vision® Saline, do not use.

Warnings: CONTENTS UNDER PRESSURE. DO NOT APPLY DIRECTLY TO EYE AS INJURY MAY RESULT.

PROBLEMS WITH CONTACT LENSES AND LENS CARE PRODUCTS COULD RESULT IN SERIOUS INJURY TO THE EYE. It is essential that you follow your eye care practitioner's directions and all labeling instructions for proper use of your lenses and lens care products. **EYE PROBLEMS, INCLUDING CORNEAL ULCERS, CAN DEVELOP RAPIDLY AND LEAD TO LOSS OF VISION; IF YOU EXPERIENCE**

EYE DISCOMFORT, EXCESSIVE TEARING, VISION CHANGES, OR REDNESS OF THE EYE, IMMEDIATELY REMOVE YOUR LENSES AND PROMPTLY CONTACT YOUR EYE CARE PRACTITIONER.

It is recommended that contact lens wearers see their eye care practitioner twice each year or, if directed, more frequently.

To avoid contamination, do not touch tip of container to any surface or transfer the solution to any other storage bottle prior to use. Replace cap after using.

Precautions:

- Always wash and rinse hands thoroughly before handling your lenses.
- Fresh CIBA Vision Saline should be used daily. **Never reuse the solution.**
- DO NOT STORE LENSES IN SOLUTION THAT HAS NOT BEEN THERMAL (HEAT) DISINFECTED.
- Keep out of the reach of children.
- Do not puncture or incinerate. Do not store at temperatures above 120° F.
- Use before the expiration date stamped on the container.
- After inserting your lenses, always empty and rinse your lens storage case with fresh rinsing solution and allow to air dry.

Adverse Reactions (Possible problems and what to do): The following problems may occur:

- Eyes stinging, burning, or itching (irritation)
- Excessive watering (tearing) of the eye
- Unusual eye secretions
- Redness of the eyes
- Reduced sharpness of vision (visual acuity)
- Blurred vision
- Sensitivity to light (photophobia)
- Dry eyes
- Studies have shown that smokers have a higher incidence of adverse reactions.

If you notice any of the above problems, immediately remove and examine your lenses. If a lens appears to be damaged, do not reinsert; consult your eye care practitioner. If the problem stops and the lenses appear to be undamaged, thoroughly clean, rinse and disinfect the lenses and reinsert them. If the problem continues, immediately remove your lenses and consult your eye care practitioner.

If any of the above problems occur, a serious condition such as infection, corneal ulcer, neovascularization, or iritis may be present. Immediately remove your lenses and seek immediate professional identification of the problem and begin treatment, if necessary, to avoid serious eye damage.

For more information, see your *Instructions for Wearers* booklet for your specific contact lenses.

To prevent contamination and to help avoid serious eye injury, always empty and rinse lens case with fresh rinsing solution and allow to air dry.

Directions

Chemical (Not heat) Disinfection:

- Always wash and rinse your hands before you handle your lenses.
- Disinfect and store lenses as directed by your eye care practitioner.
- Before reinserting lenses that are chemically disinfected, expel a short stream of CIBA Vision Saline to clear nozzle, then rinse the lenses thoroughly with CIBA Vision Saline.

Thermal (Heat) Disinfection:

- Always wash and rinse your hands before you handle your lenses.
- Clean, rinse, and disinfect your lenses each time you remove them.
- Use can with nozzle directed at dot on rim. DO NOT TILT CAN BEYOND HORIZONTAL.
- To dispense solution, aim nozzle and press. Before each use, always expel a short stream of CIBA Vision Saline from tube to clear nozzle.
- Prepare the empty lens case. Wet the chambers of the case with CIBA Vision Saline.
- Clean and rinse one lens first (always the same lens first to avoid mix-ups).
- After you clean your lens, rinse it thoroughly with CIBA Vision Saline by holding the lens between the forefinger and thumb of one hand and directing a steady stream onto the lens or placing the lens in the palm of one hand and directing a steady stream of CIBA Vision Saline onto the lens.
- Put that lens into the correct chamber (section) of the lens case.
- Fill the chamber using enough CIBA Vision Saline to completely cover the lens.
- Tightly close the top on the chamber.
- Repeat the above procedure for the second lens.
- Put the lens case into the disinfection unit and follow the directions for operating your heat disinfection unit.

Emergency (Alternate) Method for Thermal (Heat) Disinfection.

If your heat disinfection unit is not available, place the tightly closed lens case which contains the lenses into a pan of boiling water. Leave the closed lens case in the pan of boiling water for at least 10 minutes. (Above an altitude of 7,000 feet, boil for at least 15 minutes.) Be careful not to allow the water to boil away. Remove the pan from the heat and allow it to cool for 30 minutes to complete the disinfection of the lenses.

NOTE: USE OF THE HEAT DISINFECTION UNIT SHOULD BE RESUMED AS SOON AS POSSIBLE.

- Leave the lenses in the unopened lens case until ready to wear. Before reinsertion of the lenses, no rinsing is necessary unless your eye care practitioner recommends rinsing.

How Supplied: CIBA Vision Saline is supplied in sterile 3 fl.oz. (89 mL), 8 fl.oz. (237 mL), and 12 fl.oz. (355 mL) aerosol containers. The containers are marked with lot numbers and expiration date.

Lenses: CIBA Vision Saline is recommended for use with soft (hydrophilic) contact lenses.

For further information regarding this product, contact your eye care practitioner or write to: Consumer Relations, CIBA Vision Corporation, P.O. Box 105069, Atlanta, GA 30348.

LENSEPT® DISINFECTION SOLUTION and LENSEPT® NEUTRALIZER 5 MINUTE NEUTRALIZING AND RINSING/STORAGE SOLUTION

LENSEPT® Disinfection Solution is a microfiltered ophthalmic solution containing hydrogen peroxide for use in the LENSEPT Disinfection System, an oxidation/chemical (not heat) system for the disinfection of soft (hydrophilic) contact lenses.

LENSEPT® Neutralizer-5 Minute Neutralizing and Rinsing/Storage Solution is an ophthalmic solution containing bovine catalase as the neutralizer to neutralize the LENSEPT Disinfection Solution in the LENSEPT Disinfection System.

The LENSEPT Disinfection System consists of:

- LENSEPT Disinfection Solution
- LENSEPT Neutralizer-5 Minute Neutralizing and Rinsing/Storage Solution
- CIBA Vision® Lens Holder and Cup

Description/Ingredients: LENSEPT Disinfection Solution is a sterile ophthalmic solution containing microfiltered hydrogen peroxide 3%, stabilized with sodium stannate, sodium nitrate, buffered with phosphates.

LENSEPT Neutralizer is a sterile buffered, isotonic, aqueous ophthalmic solution containing sodium chloride, sodium borate decahydrate, boric acid and bovine catalase as the neutralizing agent, with sorbic acid and edetate disodium as preservatives.

The CIBA Vision® Lens Holder and Cup is a cup designed to hold soft lenses during disinfection, neutralization and storage.

Actions: LENSEPT Disinfection Solution is used after cleaning to provide oxidation/chemical (not heat) disinfection of soft (hydrophilic) contact lenses. Disinfection kills microorganisms that could cause serious eye infections. LENSEPT Disinfection Solution must be neutralized after the disinfection procedure with LENSEPT Neutralizer.

LENSEPT Neutralizer is for use after disinfection with LENSEPT Disinfection Solution to make the lenses safe for insertion into the eye.

The CIBA Vision Lens Holder and Cup is a cup designed to hold soft lenses during disinfection, neutralization and storage.

Note: THE LENSEPT DISINFECTION SYSTEM CONTAINS NO THIMEROSAL OR CHLORHEXIDINE, PRESERVATIVES TO WHICH SOME PEOPLE ARE SENSITIVE.

Indications/Uses: LENSEPT Disinfection Solution is used with the LENSEPT Disinfection System to disinfect soft (hydrophilic) contact lenses. The LENSEPT Disinfection Solution must be neutralized using LENSEPT Neutralizer 5 Minute Neutralizing and Rinsing/Storage Solution.

LENSEPT Neutralizer is used with the LENSEPT Disinfection System to neutralize soft (hydrophilic) contact lenses exposed to the LENSEPT Disinfection Solution, and for rinsing and storage of lenses.

Contraindications (Reasons not to use): None are known; however, if you are allergic to any ingredient in the LENSEPT Disinfection System, do not use these products.

Warnings:

DO NOT PUT LENSEPT DISINFECTION SOLUTION OR A LENS SOAKED WITH LENSEPT DISINFECTION SOLUTION IN YOUR EYE. Place lens on your eye ONLY after neutralization, by soaking a minimum of 5 minutes in LENSEPT Neutralizer. Should LENSEPT Disinfection Solution mistakenly get in your eye, burning and/or irritation will occur. REMOVE YOUR LENS IMMEDIATELY, FLUSH (WASH) YOUR EYE WITH A LARGE AMOUNT OF WATER OR STERILE SALINE FOR SEVERAL MINUTES. If burning and/or irritation persists, seek assistance from an eye care practitioner. Never touch the dropper tip of the bottle to any surface, since this may contaminate the solution. Replace cap after using.

DO NOT TAKE LENSEPT DISINFECTION SOLUTION INTERNALLY OR GASTRIC DISTRESS COULD RESULT. SEEK PROFESSIONAL ASSISTANCE OF A PHYSICIAN OR A POISON CONTROL CENTER IMMEDIATELY IF TAKEN INTERNALLY.

PROBLEMS WITH CONTACT LENSES AND LENS CARE PRODUCTS COULD RESULT IN SERIOUS INJURY TO THE EYE. It is essential that you follow your eye care practitioner's directions and all labeling instructions for proper use of your lenses and lens care products. EYE PROBLEMS, INCLUDING CORNEAL ULCERS, CAN DEVELOP RAPIDLY AND LEAD TO LOSS OF VISION; THEREFORE, IF YOU EXPERIENCE EYE DIS-

Continued on next page

CIBA Vision—Cont.

COMFORT, EXCESSIVE TEARING, VISION CHANGES, OR REDNESS OF THE EYE, IMMEDIATELY REMOVE YOUR LENSES AND PROMPTLY CONTACT YOUR EYE CARE PRACTITIONER.
All contact lens wearers must see their eye care practitioner as directed. If your lenses are for extended wear, your eye care practitioner may prescribe more frequent visits.

Keep out of the reach of children.
Precautions: Never reuse LENSEPT Disinfection Solution or LENSEPT Neutralizer.
There is NO SAFE, ACCEPTABLE, GENERIC SUBSTITUTE TO USE IN THE LENSEPT DISINFECTION SYSTEM FOR THE LENSEPT DISINFECTION SOLUTION OR THE LENSEPT NEUTRALIZER. DO NOT MIX OR SUBSTITUTE OTHER LENS CARE SYSTEMS CONTAINING HYDROGEN PEROXIDE OR CATALASE. THESE SYSTEMS MAY NOT BE COMPATIBLE WITH THE LENSEPT DISINFECTION SYSTEM. DO NOT USE OVER-THE-COUNTER GENERIC HYDROGEN PEROXIDE.
Generic hydrogen peroxide solutions are not intended for use with contact lenses and may contain ingredients not tested for ocular safety and/or toxicity. Generic hydrogen peroxides cause DISCOLORATION and DAMAGE lenses.
NEVER USE LENSEPT Disinfection Solution or LENSEPT Neutralizer in a thermal (heat) Disinfection Unit.
Keep the bottle tightly closed when not in use.
After reinserting your lenses always empty the lens cup and allow to air dry.
Store LENSEPT Neutralizer below 77°F (25°C). DO NOT FREEZE.
Store LENSEPT Disinfection Solution at room temperature: 59° to 86°F (15° to 30°C).
Adverse Reactions (Problems that may occur and what to do about them): With contact lens wear, the following problems may occur: eyes stinging, burning or itching (irritation), excessive watering (tearing) of the eyes, unusual eye secretions, redness of the eyes, reduced sharpness of vision (visual acuity), blurred vision, sensitivity to light (photophobia), or dry eyes. If you notice any of the above problems, *immediately remove and examine your lenses for damage,* such as splits or tears. If the problem stops and the lenses appear to be undamaged, thoroughly clean, disinfect, and neutralize the lenses and reinsert them. If the lens appears to be damaged, DO NOT USE THE LENS. If the lens does not appear to be damaged, but the problem continues, *IMMEDIATELY* STOP USE OF THE LENS AND ALL LENS CARE PRODUCTS. PROMPTLY consult your eye care practitioner.
If any of the above symptoms persist, serious conditions such as infection, corneal ulcer, neovascularization, and iritis may be present. Seek immediate professional identification of the problem and treatment to avoid serious eye damage.
Directions for Use: *Clean, disinfect, and neutralize your contact lenses each time you remove them.* Before handling your contact lenses, always clean and rinse your hands thoroughly and dry them with a clean towel. To clean, disinfect and neutralize your lenses, the following three procedures must be followed:
PROCEDURE ONE—Clean your lenses after each removal.
1. Clean surface of the left lens with a cleaner recommended by your eye care practitioner. Follow the product instructions.
2. Rinse the lens thoroughly with a steady stream of sterile saline solution and place lens in the basket of the CIBA Vision® Lens Holder marked "L."
NOTE: To prevent damage to your lens, place the lens on the center of the dome located in the lens basket; be sure the lens does not touch the basket rim, then close basket.
3. Repeat step one with the right lens, rinse as in step two and place the lens in the unmarked basket.

PROCEDURE TWO—Disinfect your lenses after lens cleaning steps 1–3 above have been completed for both lenses.
1. Fill the CIBA Vision Lens Cup to the fill line with LENSEPT Disinfection Solution and tighten (turn clockwise) the cap. Let stand for a minimum of fifty-five (55) minutes.

PROCEDURE THREE—Neutralize your lenses after lens disinfection has been completed.
1. After disinfection, empty the solution from the lens cup and gently shake excess solution from the baskets containing the lenses.
2. Fill the cup to the fill line with LENSEPT Neutralizer 5 Minute Neutralizing and Rinsing/Storage Solution. Place the lenses in the lens cup and close the lens cup. Gently shake the cup. Leave lenses in the lens cup for a minimum of 5 minutes.

DIRECTION NOTES:
a. Lenses must be soaked in the LENSEPT Disinfection Solution to disinfect the lenses.
b. Never rinse your lenses in the LENSEPT Disinfection Solution and insert on your eye. Lenses must always be neutralized with LENSEPT Neutralizer before being placed on the eye.
c. Should there be any confusion about where you are in the disinfection and neutralization procedure, start the entire procedure over from the beginning.
d. Lenses should be stored in an unopened lens cup until you are ready to wear them.
e. If you use an enzymatic cleaner, after enzyme treatment be sure to clean, disinfect, and neutralize before lens insertion.

STORE THE LENSEPT DISINFECTION SOLUTION AT ROOM TEMPERATURE BETWEEN 59° AND 86°F (15° AND 30°C). KEEP OUT OF THE REACH OF CHILDREN. STORE THE LENSEPT NEUTRALIZER 5 MINUTE NEUTRALIZING AND RINSING/STORAGE SOLUTION BELOW 77°F (25°C). DO NOT FREEZE.
How Supplied: LENSEPT Disinfection Solution is supplied sterile in 4 oz. (120 mL), 8 oz. (237 mL) and 12 oz. (355 mL) plastic bottles. Bottles and cartons are marked with lot number and expiration date.
LENSEPT Neutralizer 5 Minute Neutralizing and Rinsing/Storage Solution is supplied sterile in 4 oz. (120 mL) and 8 oz. (237 mL) plastic bottles. Bottles and cartons are marked with lot number and expiration date.
CIBA Vision Lens Holder and Cup is supplied in single-unit cartons.
All system components are available for replacement.
For information regarding this product, consult your eye care practitioner, or write to Consumer Relations, CIBA Vision Corporation, P.O. Box 105069, Atlanta, Georgia 30348.

MIRAFLOW®
Extra-Strength Daily Cleaner
For soft (hydrophilic) and hard contact lenses.
PRESERVATIVE-FREE

Description: MiraFlow® Extra-Strength Daily Cleaner is a sterile solution containing purified water, isopropyl alcohol 20% v/v, poloxamer 407, and amphoteric 10. MIRAFLOW CONTAINS NO CHLORHEXIDINE AND NO THIMEROSAL, PRESERVATIVES TO WHICH SOME PEOPLE ARE SENSITIVE.
Actions: MiraFlow Extra-Strength Daily Cleaner loosens and removes accumulations of film, deposits, and debris from your lenses.
Indications (Uses): MiraFlow Extra-Strength Daily Cleaner is indicated for use to clean soft (hydrophilic) and hard contact lenses each time they are removed for disinfecting. MiraFlow may be used with either thermal (heat) or chemical (not heat) lens disinfection systems, as recommended by your eye care practitioner.
Contraindications (Reasons not to use): None are known; however, if you are allergic to any ingredient in MiraFlow Extra-Strength Daily Cleaner do not use this product.
Note: MiraFlow Extra-Strength Daily Cleaner is not recommended for use with rigid gas permeable lenses.
Warnings:

DO NOT PUT MIRAFLOW EXTRA-STRENGTH DAILY CLEANER DIRECTLY IN THE EYE OR INSERT LENSES THAT HAVE NOT BEEN THOROUGHLY RINSED. If irritation or stinging occurs when the lens is inserted, immediately remove the lens and again rinse thoroughly prior to reinsertion.
Serious damage to the eye and loss of vision may result from wearing contaminated or damaged contact lenses. Immediately consult your eye care practitioner to identify the cause of any unexplained eye discomfort, watering, vision change, or redness, and to begin any necessary treatment.
Cleaning is not a substitute for disinfection.
Do not touch the tip of the container to any surface, since this may contaminate the solution. Replace cap after using.

KEEP OUT OF REACH OF CHILDREN.

PROBLEMS WITH CONTACT LENSES AND LENS CARE PRODUCTS COULD RESULT IN SERIOUS INJURY TO THE EYE. It is essential that you follow your eye care practitioner's directions and all labeling instructions for proper use of your lenses and lens care products including the lens case. EYE PROBLEMS, INCLUDING CORNEAL ULCERS, CAN DEVELOP RAPIDLY AND LEAD TO LOSS OF VISION; THEREFORE, IF YOU EXPERIENCE EYE DISCOMFORT, EXCESSIVE TEARING, VISION CHANGES, OR REDNESS OF THE EYE, IMMEDIATELY REMOVE YOUR LENSES AND PROMPLY CONTACT YOUR EYE CARE PRACTITIONER.
It is recommended that contact lens wearers see their eye care practitioner twice each year or if directed, more frequently.

Studies have shown that smoking increases the risk of ulcerative keratitis for contact lens users.
Precautions:
- Keep the bottle tightly closed when not in use.
- Before handling your contact lenses, always wash your hands thoroughly and dry them with a clean, lint-free towel.
- Store at room temperature: 59° to 86°F (15° to 30°C).
- Use before the expiration date marked on the bottle and carton.

Adverse Reactions (Possible problems and what to do about them): The following problems may occur:
- Eye pain, stinging, burning, or itching (irritation)

- Excessive watering (tearing) of the eyes
- Unusual eye secretions
- Redness of the eyes
- Reduced sharpness of vision (visual acuity)
- Blurred vision
- Sensitivity to light (photophobia)
- Dry eyes

If you notice any of the above problems, immediately remove and examine your lenses for damage, such as splits or tears. If the problem stops and the lenses appear to be undamaged, thoroughly clean, rinse, and disinfect/neutralize the lenses and reinsert them. If the problem continues or a lens appears to be damaged, IMMEDIATELY REMOVE THE LENS AND CONSULT YOUR EYE CARE PRACTITIONER.

If any of the above symptoms occur, serious conditions such as infection, corneal ulcers, neovascularization, or iritis may be present. Seek immediate professional identification of the problem and treatment to avoid serious eye damage.

Directions:

General: Wash and rinse your hands thoroughly before handling contact lenses. Clean and disinfect your lenses each time you remove them. Clean and rinse the right lens first to avoid mix-ups. To prevent contamination and to help avoid serious eye injury, always empty and rinse lens case with fresh rinsing solution and allow to air dry.

SOFT LENSES:

After removing your lens, place it in the palm of your hand. Apply 1 or 2 drops of MiraFlow Extra-Strength Daily Cleaner to each lens surface and gently rub the lens for 15–30 seconds in the palm using the forefinger of the other hand. Rinse the lens thoroughly by rubbing the lens in a stream of saline solution such as CIBA Vision ® Saline or SoftWear® Saline. (NEVER USE WATER to rinse soft lenses.) Place the lens in the appropriate chamber of the lens storage case. Repeat this procedure for the other lens. Disinfect according to the instructions of your eye care practitioner. Do not soak lenses in MiraFlow Extra-Strength Daily Cleaner.

Enzymatic tablets are compatible with MiraFlow Extra-Strength Daily Cleaner use and may be used for removal of protein deposits, if recommended by your eye care practitioner.

HARD LENSES:

Apply 1 or 2 drops to each lens surface and gently rub between fingers for at least 10 seconds or as directed by your eye care practitioner. Rinse lens thoroughly with water. Repeat this procedure for the other lens. (Note: Repeat procedure if accumulations are especially heavy.)

How Supplied: MiraFlow Extra-Strength Daily Cleaner is supplied in sterile 0.85 fl. oz. (25 mL) plastic bottles. The containers and cartons are marked with lot number and expiration date.

SOFTWEAR® SALINE

FORMULATED FOR SENSITIVE EYES*
pH AS NATURAL AS YOUR OWN TEARS
FOR HEAT USERS TOO!

A sterile saline solution for use with soft (hydrophilic) contact lenses (including daily wear, extended wear, and tinted lenses).

This saline can be used in soft lens care regimens using saline. For example:

- Rinsing following daily or weekly cleaning
- Rinsing following disinfection, prior to lens insertion
- Use with heat disinfection
- Dissolving enzyme tablets
- Storage of soft lenses after disinfection

Description: SoftWear® Saline is a buffered, sterile saline solution. A special buffer maintains SoftWear Saline's pH balance at the same natural level as your tears. Contains NO thimerosal or chlorhexidine. SoftWear Saline is useful for patients sensitive to thimerosal or other irritating preservatives used in sterile saline solutions.

Contents: SoftWear Saline is a sterile, isotonic saline solution containing an antimicrobial buffer system (A.B.S.®) consisting of sodium borate, boric acid, and sodium perborate (generating up to 0.006% hydrogen peroxide stabilized with phosphonic acid[1]). If you are allergic to any ingredient in SoftWear Saline do not use this product.

Actions: Rinsing with SoftWear Saline removes loosened deposits and traces of cleaning and disinfecting solutions remaining on your lenses. It keeps lenses wet (hydrated) during thermal (heat) disinfection and during storage. It may also be used to dissolve enzyme tablets when saline is required.

Indications (Uses): SoftWear Saline is indicated for use with soft (hydrophilic) contact lenses. It can be used as a rinsing solution following use of a daily or weekly cleaner or following disinfection, prior to lens insertion. SoftWear Saline can also be used for storage after disinfection and to dissolve enzyme tablets when sterile saline is required.

Contraindications (Reasons not to use): There are no known contraindications for use of this product.

Warnings:

PROBLEMS WITH CONTACT LENSES AND LENS CARE PRODUCTS COULD RESULT IN SERIOUS INJURY TO THE EYE. It is essential that you follow your eye care practitioner's directions and all labeling instructions for proper use of your lenses and lens care products including the lens case. EYE PROBLEMS, INCLUDING CORNEAL ULCERS, CAN DEVELOP RAPIDLY AND LEAD TO LOSS OF VISION. IF YOU EXPERIENCE EYE DISCOMFORT, EXCESSIVE TEARING, VISION CHANGES, OR REDNESS OF THE EYE, IMMEDIATELY REMOVE YOUR LENSES AND PROMPTLY CONTACT YOUR EYE CARE PRACTITIONER.

It is recommended that contact lens wearers see their eye care practitioner twice each year or, if directed, more frequently. To avoid contamination, never touch the tip of the bottle to any surface. Keep bottle tightly closed when not in use.

Precautions:

- ALWAYS wash and rinse hands thoroughly and dry with a clean, lint-free towel before handling your lenses.
- Fresh SoftWear Saline should be used daily. NEVER REUSE THE SOLUTION.
- Never rinse your lenses in water from the tap.
- Keep out of the reach of children.
- Store at room temperature.
- Use before the expiration date marked on the container.

Adverse Reactions (Possible problems and what to do):

The following problems may occur with contact lens wear:

- Eyes stinging, burning, or itching (irritation)
- Excessive watering (tearing) of the eye
- Unusual eye secretions
- Redness of the eyes
- Reduced sharpness of vision (visual acuity)
- Blurred vision or halos around objects
- Sensitivity to light (photophobia)
- Dry eyes

If you notice any of the above problems, remove and examine your lens. If a lens appears to be damaged, do not reinsert; **CONSULT YOUR EYE CARE PRACTITIONER.** If the problem stops and the lenses appear to be undamaged, thoroughly clean, rinse, and disinfect with the disinfection regimen recommended by your eye care practitioner prior to reinsertion. If the problem continues, immediately remove your lenses and **CONSULT YOUR EYE CARE PRACTITIONER.**

If any of the problems occur, a serious condition such as infection, corneal ulcer, neovascularization, or iritis may be present. Seek immediate professional identification of the problem and begin treatment, if necessary, to avoid serious eye damage.

Studies have shown that contact lens wearers who smoke have a higher incidence of adverse reactions.

General Directions:

- Always wash your hands and dry them with a clean, lint-free towel before handling your lenses.
- Each time you remove your lenses, clean and disinfect them with the disinfection regimen recommended by your eye care practitioner.
- Start with the same lens first each time to avoid mix-ups.
- To prevent contamination and to help avoid serious eye injury, always empty and rinse lens case with fresh SoftWear Saline and allow to air dry when wearing lenses.
- ALWAYS FOLLOW THE DIRECTIONS OF YOUR EYE CARE PRACTITIONER.
- If needed, use drops for soft contact lenses, such as CIBA Vision® Lens Drops, throughout the day for lubricating and rewetting your lenses.
- SoftWear Saline may be used to store lenses prior to and following disinfection as recommended by your eye care practitioner.

Chemical or Hydrogen Peroxide Disinfection Directions:

- Clean each lens with a daily cleaner, such as MiraFlow® Extra-Strength Daily Cleaner, or CIBA Vision® Cleaner and rinse each lens thoroughly with SoftWear Saline.
- Disinfect/neutralize your lenses with a product such as AOSEPT® or LENSEPT® Disinfection Solution.
- After disinfection/neutralization, lenses may be rinsed with SoftWear Saline before insertion.
- Before storing your lenses in SoftWear Saline after hydrogen peroxide disinfection, discard the solution rinse and fill the lens case with fresh SoftWear Saline, or discard the solution, remove the platinum disc from the lens case and fill with fresh SoftWear Saline.

Thermal (Heat) Disinfection Directions:

- Prepare the empty lens case by rinsing and filling with fresh SoftWear Saline.
- Clean each lens with a daily cleaner, such as MiraFlow Extra-Strength Daily Cleaner or CIBA Vision Cleaner and rinse each lens thoroughly with SoftWear Saline.
- Place the first lens into the correct chamber of the lens case. Be sure your lens is fully immersed in saline. Close the chamber securely. Repeat the above procedure for the second lens.
- Put the lens case into the disinfection unit and follow its directions for use.
- Leave the lenses in the unopened lens case until ready to wear.
- Lenses may be rinsed with SoftWear Saline before insertion.

Enzyme Cleaning Directions:

- SoftWear Saline may be used for dissolving enzyme tablets when saline is called for in the product directions.
- Follow the directions of your eye care practitioner.

How Supplied: SoftWear Saline is supplied in 4 fl. oz., 8 fl. oz., and 12 fl. oz. reclosable plastic containers. The containers are marked with lot number and expiration date.

Continued on next page

CIBA Vision—Cont.

Lenses: SoftWear Saline is recommended for use with soft (hydrophilic) contact lenses (including daily wear, extended wear, and tinted lenses).

*Does not contain thimerosal or chlorhexidine.
[1]U.S. Patent Pending

Polymer Technology Corporation

100 RESEARCH DRIVE
WILMINGTON, MA 01887

BOSTON Advance™ CLEANER

BOSTON Advance™ Cleaner for fluoro silicone acrylate and silicone acrylate rigid gas permeable contact lenses.

Description: BOSTON Advance Cleaner is a sterile, concentrated homogenous surfactant solution containing alkyl ether sulfate, ethoxylated alkyl phenol, tri-quarternary cocoa-based phospholipid and silica gel as cleaning agents.
Actions: BOSTON Advance Cleaner is a new formula that removes accumulated film, stubborn deposits (including proteins and lipids), and debris from fluoro silicone acrylate and silicone acrylate rigid gas permeable contact lenses.
Indications: BOSTON Advance Cleaner is indicated for use to clean fluoro silicone acrylate and silicone acrylate rigid gas permeable contact lenses before conditioning (wetting, soaking, disinfecting).
Contraindications: This solution is not for use with soft lenses. Do not use this solution if you are allergic to any component of this product.
Directions:

1. Wash hands thoroughly.
2. Rub lens carefully with several drops of BOSTON Advance Cleaner in the palm of your hand for twenty (20) seconds.
3. *REMOVE ALL TRACES OF BOSTON ADVANCE CLEANER BY THOROUGHLY RINSING WITH FRESH TAP WATER.*
4. Place lens in storage case and fill each compartment with a fresh supply of conditioning solution. Soak for at least 4 hours or overnight before wearing.
5. Always keep bottle tightly closed when not in use.
6. Carefully observe the precautions highlighted in the blue panels.

Warnings. BOSTON Advance Cleaner is not intended for use directly in the eye. This solution is potentially irritating if misused. Redness or other symptoms of irritation may occur if lens is inadvertantly inserted into the eye without thoroughly rinsing off BOSTON Advance Cleaner. If the BOSTON Advance Cleaner is accidentally instilled into the eye, remove your lenses (if being worn) and immediately rinse your eyes with cool fresh tap water until all the BOSTON Advance Cleaner is thoroughly removed from the eye. To avoid contamination, never touch the dropper tip of the container with your hands or to any surface. Keep this bottle tightly closed when not in use.
How Supplied: BOSTON Advance Cleaner is supplied in sterile 30 ml and 10 ml units. Bottles are either sealed with imprinted neckbands or packed in tamper-evident cartons. The bottles are marked with a lot number and expiration date.

Shown in Product Identification Section, page 104

BOSTON Advance™ CONDITIONING SOLUTION

BOSTON Advance Conditioning Solution for fluoro silicone acrylate and silicone acrylate rigid gas permeable contact lenses.

Description: BOSTON Advance Conditioning Solution has been specifically formulated for use with fluoro silicone acrylate and silicone acrylate rigid gas permeable contact lenses. It contains a patented hydrophilic polyelectrolyte and a cationic cellulose derivative polymer as a wetting agent. This binds to the surface of the lens enhancing wettability and neutralizing surface ionic charges. It is a sterile, buffered, slightly hypertonic solution with polyaminopropyl biguanide (0.0015%) and edetate disodium (0.05%) as preservatives.
Actions: BOSTON Advance Conditioning Solution is a new formula that enhances the wettability characteristics of rigid gas permeable contact lenses. It also reduces friction against the cornea and removes particulate matter that may cause irritation and discomfort. BOSTON Advance Conditioning Solution contains a new disinfecting agent which is effective in destroying harmful microorganisms on the surface of rigid gas permeable contact lenses and in contact lens cases.
Indications: BOSTON Advance Conditioning Solution is indicated for disinfecting and soaking after cleaning and rinsing of fluoro silicone acrylate and silicone acrylate rigid gas permeable contact lenses (as listed in the labeling).
Contraindications: This solution is not for use with soft lenses. Do not use this solution if you are allergic to any component of this product.
Directions:

1. Wash hands thoroughly.
2. Remove lens from storage case. Reapply fresh BOSTON Advance Conditioning Solution on both surfaces prior to reinsertion.
3. Thoroughly clean interior of storage case with hot water and air dry. Completely replace solutions every day. Soak for at least 4 hours (or overnight) before wearing.
4. To avoid contamination, always keep solution bottles tightly closed when not in use.
5. Discard bottle and solution ninety (90) days after opening. Record date opened in space provided on bottle label.
6. Carefully observe the precautions highlighted in the blue panels.

Warnings: To avoid contamination, never touch the dropper tip of the container with your hands or to any surface.
How Supplied: BOSTON Advance Conditioning Solution is supplied in sterile 4 fluid ounce (120ml) and 1 fluid ounce (30ml) bottles. Bottles are either sealed with imprinted neckbands or packed in tamper-evident cartons. The bottles are marked with a lot number and expiration date.

Shown in Product Identification Section, page 104

BOSTON Advance™ REWETTING DROPS

BOSTON Advance Rewetting Drops for fluoro silicone acrylate and silicone acrylate rigid gas permeable contact lenses.

Description: BOSTON Advance Rewetting Drops has been specifically formulated for use with fluoro silicone acrylate and silicone acrylate rigid gas permeable contact lenses. It contains a patented hydrophilic polyelectrolyte that binds to the surface of the lens enhancing wettability and neutralizing surface ionic charges. It is a sterile, buffered, slightly hypertonic solution with polyaminopropyl biguanide (0.0015%) and edetate disodium (0.05%) as preservaties.
Actions: BOSTON Advance Rewetting Drops is a new formula that enhances lens wettability to reduce friction against the cornea. It also removes particulate matter that may cause irritation, discomfort and blurring during lens wear.
Indications: BOSTON Advance Rewetting Drops is indicated for use directly in the eye to lubricate and rewet fluoro silicone acrylate and silicone acrylate rigid gas permeable contact lenses (as listed in the labeling), during lens wear.
Contraindications: This solution is not for use with soft lenses. Do not use this solution if you are allergic to any component of this product.
Directions:

1. Use while contact lenses are on the eyes. DO NOT TOUCH DROPPER TIP TO EYELIDS OR LASHES.
2. One to three drops should be instilled into each eye as needed or as directed by your eye care professional.
3. Always keep the bottle tightly closed when not in use.
4. Discard bottle and solution ninety (90) days after opening (record date opened in space provided on bottle label).
5. Carefully observe the precautions highlighted in the blue panels.

Warnings: To avoid contamination, never touch the dropper tip of the container with your hands or to any surface.
How Supplied: BOSTON Advance Rewetting Drops is supplied in sterile 10ml bottles. Bottles are either sealed with imprinted neckbands or packed in tamper-evidence cartons. The bottles are marked with a lot number and expiration date.

Shown in Product Identification Section, page 104

Part 4—Spectacle Lenses and Products

Rodenstock USA, Inc.
Lens Division
69 KENOSIA AVENUE
DANBURY, CT 06813

Address inquiries to:

National (800) 458-0620
Ct State (203) 748-4311
Fax (800) 422-1211

Rodenstock manufactures a complete line of ophthalmic products including Lenses, Frames and Diagnostic Equipment.
The Aspheric Advantage™ by Rodenstock includes Cosmolite, Cosmolit Bifo 28 and Progressives. They provide the highest visual acuity of any single vision, Bifocal and Progressive Lens.

COSMOLIT SINGLE VISION
COSMOLIT BIFO 28

The use of aspheric surfaces has become more and more popular over the past few years thanks to progressive methods in science and technology, and due to the increased use of sophisticated computers. Today's spectacle lenses are no longer "mere" corrective aids; a modern spectacle lens must also satisfy high cosmetic demands. Cosmolit, as an aspheric lens, meets all these demands and offers an optimum combination of all parameters in the lower to medium positive power ranges.
The aspheric surface is used to reduce the curvature and the center thickness of the lenses while, at the same time, keeping the good peripheral imaging qualities which we are accustomed to from spherical lenses with high front curvatures. With the flatter design and the reduction in weight we achieve that optimisation target so important for larger eye-shapes—a more appealing cosmetic effect and greater comfort in wear without any compromises in the image quality.

Advantages:

- Superior Cosmetics—Cosmolit allows for the use of flatter base curves. This decreases reflections, reduces unsightly bulging, and retains integrity of the eyewire and frame shapes.
- Superior Optics—Cosmolit's computer designed curves eliminate nearly all spherical abberations, and reduce magnification.
- Thinner—Cosmolit lenses provide plus prescriptions that appear dramatically thinner than hard resin.
- Lighter—Less overall lens mass for more comfortable lenses.
- Processing—Unlike high index resins and polycarbonates, Cosmolit requires no more special processing than regular hard resin. Material—Hard Resin with Index 1.500

PROGRESSIV S®

A Completely New Design Basis with a number of physiological, optical and technical innovations incorporating Cosmolt Technology, Progressiv S sets new standards in visual comfort and performance against which previous progressive lenses will have to be measured.

Clear View Over the Whole Viewing Field

A further increase in the size of the distance and near portion zones with unimpaired vision.
A widening of the progression corridor and the ensuring of optimum effectiveness irrespective of the fitting method or of the optical power.

Physiologically Free of Distortion

It has been possible to reduce the distortion of this progressive lens to a level equivalent to that of single-vision lenses.

Unimpaired Binocular Vision

Full consideration of binocular vision in the form of laterally disparate depth perception and of fusion, unimpaired spatial perception and full binocular vision.

More Elegance

Cosmetic improvements thanks to the use of a flatter and more closely stepped base curve system with a simultaneous improvement in image quality.
The use of a higher index material in the glass range to obtain thinner and lighter lenses.
The introduction of decentered lenses to improve visual comfort with the aid of thinner and lighter lenses.

Improved Processing

Restriction of the measuring and reference points to the essential and necessary indications. Predictable fitting thanks to the equal validity of distance and near fitting methods.
The lenses of the Progressiv S series are an impressive sum of meaningful advances in all fields. Creating a new direction in optical design, setting standards in appearance, exemplary in their price/performance ratio, and unsurpassed in quality, they take up a leading position in the field of progressive lenses.
Technically and scientifically exciting solutions in all individual areas which merge fully to create perfect total function:
Progressiv S—The progressive lens made to measure for the human eye.

PROGRESSIV R®

The Progressiv R lens offers a better view of the world because the design objective was Total Performance of all lens components.

- Large Distance Viewing Area—Progressiv R's unique design gives your patients a wide, spherical distance viewing area.
- Smooth Power Progression—The Progressiv R "channel" is so precisely designed, it is ideal for all multifocal wearers. Power progresses smoothly, closely matching the eye's changing needs at intermediate distances. The channel is wide, and virtually free of astigmatism.
- Total Prescription Integrity—Other progressive lenses provide prescribed power only at a precise point in the near vision area. Progressiv R provides stabilized power throughout the near vision area. And, Progressiv R's near vision area is wider where it is needed, not where it will be edged off.
- Improved Peripheral Zones—Progressiv R lenses were designed to significantly reduce astigmatism and "image swim" normally found in progressive lenses. This results in larger useable areas, increased patient comfort and easier adaptation.
- Left-to-right Integrity—Progressiv R's left and right lenses are identical. There are virtually no power variances common in other lenses.

COLORMATIC™ Hard Resin and PHOTOCOLOR™ Hard Resin

Rodenstock now provides its first plastic lenses with photo-reactive properties. With this successful combination of plastic lenses plus the photo-reactive effect Rodenstock has created a photochromic with a difference.

Advantages:

—Now photo-reactive properties are available for plastic spectacle lenses.
—Uniform color change over entire surface, independent of lens thickness or optical power.
—A darken and fade response rate that enhances physiological acceptance.
—Fashion, comfort, u.v. protecting, changeable lenses

Colormatic Hard Resin

Colormatic photo-reactive hard resin lenses change from light brown to medium grey. Furnished in finished Cosmolit, semi-finished Cosmolit and semi-finished Progressive R and conventional single vision for minus prescriptions.

Photocolor Hard Resin

Photocolor photo-reactive hard resin lenses change from a delicate hint of color to a jewel-like luminescence in Aquamarine, Emerald, and Amethyst. Furnished in finished Cosmolit, semi-finished Cosmolit and semi-finished Progressive R. Comes only with AR coating.
Colormatic and Photocolor lenses are not sunglass density.

Lenses and Lens Care Notes

SECTION 10

Instrumentation Equipment and Sutures

This section is divided into two parts:

Part I—Specialized Instruments and Equipment

Part II—Sutures

Participating companies have listed categories of their products and locations of their sales and service offices.

Part I—Specialized Instruments and Equipment

Alcon Surgical, Inc.

6201 SOUTH FREEWAY
FT. WORTH, TX 76134

Address Inquiries to:

Marketing Department (817) 293-0450
1-800-TO-ALCON
(1-800-862-5266)

BSS® AND BSS PLUS® IRRIGATION ADMINISTRATION SET

This is a sterile inside and out administration set for recommended use in ophthalmic surgical irrigation with BSS® and BSS PLUS® Sterile Irrigating Solutions. It may also be used in a variety of other surgical procedures where administration set tubing interfaces with a sterile field.

In addition to its sterility, the BSS® and BSS PLUS® Irrigation Solution Administration Set is 96″ in length and contains a terminal male luer connector and guard which adapts to most operative uses. Other features include a vented spike, drip chamber with 5 micron filter, and in-line ball check control. The set is packaged in a tyvek chevron pouch for optimum security and delivery onto the sterile field. Each box contains fifty product pouches.

SINGLE USE CRYOEXTRACTORS

CRYOPHAKE®, Sterile, Disposable Cryoextractor

Completely self-contained. The long-time dependable standard.

STERILE, SINGLE USE ITEMS FOR OPHTHALMIC SURGERY

ALCON OPHTHALMIC KNIFE

The Alcon Ophthalmic Knife System—It's A-OK™! Superior cutting edges and a unique design characterize the Alcon Ophthalmic Knife. A unique manufacturing process, with extreme standards for quality, features blades that are individually cold-forged and sharpened from surgical-grade steel, giving you the edge you need and unequaled sharpness.

The A-OK™ knife is available in a variety of shapes and configurations, all featuring the same exacting and unequaled sharpness. It is available in four popular blade angles with full handles or blades and tips that screw into a reusable handle.

The A-OK™ Phacoemulsification Slit Knife is designed because your precise needs require precision answers. The knife is available in precise width choices from 2.5mm to 3.5mm because precision entry into the anterior chamber is needed during phacoemulsification procedures.

The A-OK™ Corneal/Scleral V-LANCE® Knife is designed for optimum performance featuring smooth penetration and a fluid tight seal. The blade allows for penetration through the sclera with minimal tenting and is versatile enough for limbal and clear corneal incisions.

The A-OK™ Crescent Knife is rounded for control yet sharp for precision. This unique design provides for superior tactile sensation due to the microsmooth, polished bevel leading into the precision edge. The A-OK Crescent Knife is most often used for creating scleral flaps, bevel incisions, or clearing Tenon's capsule.

All of the Alcon Ophthalmic Knife products feature the unique BLADESAVER™closed-cell foam blade protector. The unique BLADESAVER device protects the delicate point and edge of each knife. This is the same closed-cell foam protection as found in the Alcon Closure System.

The Alcon Ophthalmic Knife System—unequaled sharpness and dependable quality—when you need it and where you need it.

EYE-PAK® Ophthalmic Drapes

Totally redesigned surgical drape line featuring fourteen new drapes, four of which are unique, custom designs. EYE-PAK drapes feature new thinner materials and innovative adhesives to give better conformity and drapeability.

EYE-PAK materials include a new thinner micro-embossed plastic and a new non-woven fabric. Most EYE-PAK drapes are offered with either a round incise or an oval aperture fenestration.

The micro-embossed plastic is offered in our micro-size drape (5″×10″), mini-size drape (16″×16″), midi-size drape (24″×16″), full-size drape (40″×48″), over-size drape (48″×55″), and the unique ½ and ½ full body-size drape (65″×100″).

The non-woven fabric is offered in our full-size drape, standard full body-size drape, and the ½ and ½ full body-size drape.

Our unique full body designs are large enough to cover the entire patient and feature fluid catch bags, as well as a ventilation bridge. These features eliminate the need for numerous procedure sheets and other extra cost items such as catch bags or drape supports.

The EYE-PAK ophthalmic drapes—redesigned with you in mind.

I-KNIFE® Microsurgical Knives

The redesigned I-KNIFE® and all new I-KNIFE® II comprise the I-KNIFE Family of disposable microsurgical knives which offer a less-expensive, quality alternative that does not compromise sharpness. The unique manufacturing process assures consistently easy tissue penetration and virtually no tissue drag.

The redesigned I-KNIFE is available in full handles with four popular blade angles at 5mm lengths. The all new I-KNIFE II is available with screw-in tip and blades in 15° angulation and 3mm and 5mm lengths.

The Alcon I-KNIFE Family features the unique BLADESAVER™ foam blade protector. This closed-cell foam protects the delicate point and edge of each blade.

IRRIGATION & ASPIRATION KITS

Single-use I&A kits in standard and single-use handpiece system configurations available. Dual tray sterility and optimal quality components minimize trauma and maximize effec-

Continued on next page

Alcon—Cont.

tiveness. All kits are designed to interface with CAVITRON® or KELMAN® equipment. Six kits per box.

MICROSPONGE®
Miniature Surgical Sponge

The Alcon MICROSPONGE® Teardrop is the most absorbent surgical sponge available today. Shaped like a teardrop, the MICROSPONGE is smooth with rounded corners so it won't snag on delicate sutures. It also features the regular flat shaped tip or the sharp tip to aid in precise application at the surgical site. The body has been trimmed to lessen the possibility of obstructing vision through the microscope. Finally, the MICROSPONGE is very convenient because it features a flexible handle, making it easily held and manipulated.

The MICROSPONGE Teardrop is delivered sterile in a Tyvek and plastic envelope which eliminates lint when opening packages. It is conveniently packed with ten sponges to the envelope.

OPTEMP®
Sterile Disposable Cautery

Lightweight, balanced design gives the feel of a fine surgical instrument. Fine gauge tip with temperature designed for ophthalmic surgery. Slim, serrated barrel allows precise, positive control and better visibility of surgical site. Supplied in boxes of twelve each.

PHACOEMULSIFICATION KITS

Single use Phacoemulsification Kits for use with all CAVITRON® or KELMAN® phacoemulsification equipment. All kits are packaged in sterile dual trays; six kits per box.

Allergan Humphrey

2992 ALVARADO STREET
SAN LEANDRO, CA 94577

Address inquiries to:

Toll Free	(800) 227-1508
In California	(800) 826-6566
Telex	470714
Fax	415-483-8025

HUMPHREY A/B SCAN SYSTEM

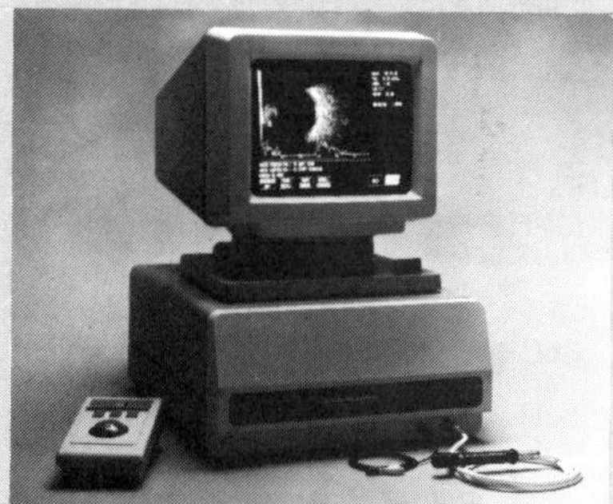

This micro-processor based digital instrument from Allergan Humphrey employs pulsed ultrasound to determine the axial length of the eye (A-mode), and to produce a two-dimensional plane view of the eye for diagnostic evaluation (B-mode). Modular in design, the A/B Scan System 835 features a CPU to drive the scanning transducers, an internal 40 Megabyte hard drive with a 3.5″ floppy disk drive for patient data and scan storage, and a large 12″, high-resolution CRT display. A simple trackball device/mouse and dual footpedal enable the sonographer to control scanning from the patient's chair or bedside. The display cues the operator on instrument set-up and scan performance by means of user-friendly, menu-driven software. The A/B Scan System 835 is loaded with features which benefit the general ophthalmic practice, cataract surgeon, and facilities specializing in detection of vitreo-retinal disease.

HUMPHREY AUTO KERATOMETER MODEL 420

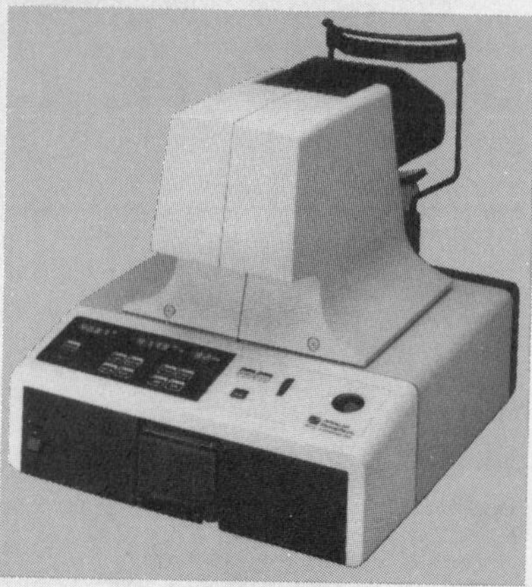

The Humphrey Auto Keratometer (AK) is an objective keratometer which automatically provides Central and peripheral K readings as well as an additional series of corneal analysis parameters. The AK is the only objective keratometer available that provides an interpretation of the corneal measurements. The AK enables any technician with minimal training to quickly provide accurate, repeatable K readings suitable for IOL power calculations. The Auto Keratometer interfaces electronically with the Humphrey Ultrasonic Biometer. The K measurements are automatically included in the desired IOL formula for increased speed and accuracy.

The peripheral K readings are processed by an internal microprocessor to give the corneal shape factor, the location of the apex and mire index. It also gives apical K readings and corneal astigmatism along the visual axis and at the apex. The unique Autofit function prints the recommended rigid contact lens base curve and optic zone diameter. Using Autofit, a technician can administer the routine, time consuming portions of the contact lens fitting procedure. This frees the doctor's time for patient consultation and evaluation of the lens fit on the eye.

A complete corneal analysis is provided and presented on a hard copy printout in seconds. Information of this type is valuable for in-depth corneal characterization and longitudinal patient records.

The AK provides a consistant objective method of monitoring pre and post operative corneal changes.

HUMPHREY AUTOMATIC REFRACTORS

Allergan Humphrey now has three new automatic refractors, the model 580, 585 and the model 590.

The Humphrey Automatic Refractor (HAR) model 570 is an objective refractor with complete subjective capabilities including glare testing and a low contrast acuity chart. Each model includes a preprogramed refracting sequence option as well as automatic P.D. calculation.

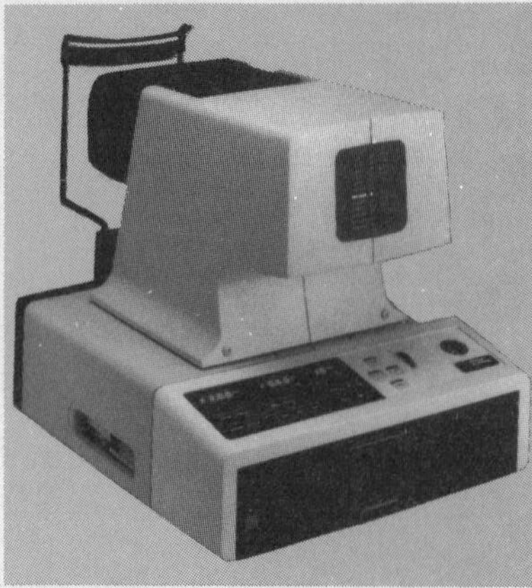

As an automatic refractor the HAR is unique. It allows both initial and final acuities to be taken at the instrument—without moving the patient to a phoropter. This is possible because the HAR contains an internal acuity chart and variable optics. A fast auto refraction is performed at the push of a button and the objective Rx immediately appears in front of the patient's eye and final acuity through the objective Rx can be taken.

The HAR contains several advanced design features which allow it to be operated by a technician with minimal training. Alignment is fully automatic and if the eye moves the instrument automatically follows it. In addition, if the patient accommodates during the objective refraction, the accommodation is "walked out" by an optional automatic plussing routine which occurs as the patient views the acuity chart. In determining final acuity, individual lines can be selected in order to eliminate confusion.

If additional refinement of the sphere and/or cylinder power and axis is desired, it can be made by manual adjustment as the patient views the acuity chart, duochrome, Jackson Cross Cylinder or PAM (Precision Astigmatic Measurement) targets. The instrument also has a unique recall capability which allows the operator to present the objective Rx and a subjective Rx to the patient for comparison. This feature, along with subjective verification, automatic alignment, spherical equivalence and optional automatic adjustment for accommodation places the Humphrey Automatic Refractor in a category which surpasses that of ordinary automatic refractors.

The model 585 is an objective refractor with the accuracy and ease of use of the 590. It includes spherical equivalence and modified line isolated Snellen and childrens targets. The sphere power can be changed subjectively and glare testing is included with a low contrast acuity chart.

The model 580 is an objective refractor with initial and final acuity measurement capabilities for the clinical practice that does not require subjective refracting features.

Clinical studies have shown that HAR refractions yield 20/20 acuity with comparable frequency and reliability to an experienced refractionist using a phoropter. The instrument can also be used for overrefraction of contact lenses and IOLs.

HUMPHREY FIELD ANALYZER

A computerized, projection perimeter which maps the entire visual field using Goldmann standard stimuli and Goldmann standard, self-adjusting, 31.5 asb background illumination.